MW00612010

Pharmacogenomics: An Introduction and Clinical Perspective

Notice

Medicine is an ever-changing science. As new research and clinical experience broaden our knowledge, changes in treatment and drug therapy are required. The authors and the publisher of this work have checked with sources believed to be reliable in their efforts to provide information that is complete and generally in accord with the standards accepted at the time of publication. However, in view of the possibility of human error or changes in medical sciences, neither the authors nor the publisher nor any other party who has been involved in the preparation or publication of this work warrants that the information contained herein is in every respect accurate or complete, and they disclaim all responsibility for any errors or omissions or for the results obtained from use of the information contained in this work. Readers are encouraged to confirm the information contained herein with other sources. For example and in particular, readers are advised to check the product information sheet included in the package of each drug they plan to administer to be certain that the information contained in this work is accurate and that changes have not been made in the recommended dose or in the contraindications for administration. This recommendation is of particular importance in connection with new or infrequently used drugs.

a LANGE medical book

Pharmacogenomics: An Introduction and Clinical Perspective

Edited by

Joseph S. Bertino Jr., PharmD, FCP, FCCP

Principal
Bertino Consulting
Schenectady, New York
and
Associate Professor of Pharmacology
College of Physicians and Surgeons
Columbia University
New York, New York

C. Lindsay DeVane, PharmD

Professor of Psychiatry and Behavioral Sciences
Medical University of South Carolina
Charleston, South Carolina

Uwe Fuhr, MD

Professor of Clinical Pharmacology
Department of Pharmacology
Faculty of Medicine at the University of Cologne
Cologne, Germany

Angela D. M. Kashuba, BScPhm, PharmD, DABCP

Professor of Pharmacy
Eshelman School of Pharmacy, Division of Pharmacotherapy and Experimental Therapeutics
Adjunct Professor of Medicine
School of Medicine, Division of Infectious Diseases
The University of North Carolina at Chapel Hill
Chapel Hill, North Carolina

Joseph D. Ma, PharmD

Assistant Professor of Clinical Pharmacy
University of California at San Diego
Skaggs School of Pharmacy & Pharmaceutical Sciences
San Diego, California

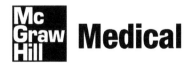

McGraw Hill **Medical**

New York   Chicago   San Francisco   Lisbon   London   Madrid   Mexico City
Milan   New Delhi   San Juan   Seoul   Singapore   Sydney   Toronto

The McGraw·Hill Companies

Pharmacogenomics: An Introduction and Clinical Perspective

Copyright © 2013 by The McGraw-Hill Companies, Inc. All rights reserved. Printed in the United States of America. Except as permitted under the United States Copyright Act of 1976, no part of this publication may be reproduced or distributed in any form or by any means, or stored in a data base or retrieval system, without the prior written permission of the publisher.

1 2 3 4 5 6 7 8 9 0   QDB/QDB   17 16 15 14 13 12

ISBN 978-0-07-174169-9
MHID 0-07-174169-0

This book was set in Adobe Garamond by Thomson Digital.
The editors were Michael Weitz and Brian Kearns.
The production supervisor was Catherine Saggese.
Project management was provided by Charu Bansal, Thomson Digital.
The cover designer was Barsoom Design.
Credit: © Mike Agliolo/Corbis
Quad/Graphics was the printer and binder.

This book is printed on acid-free paper.

Library of Congress Cataloging-in-Publication Data

Pharmacogenomics : an introduction and clinical perspective / edited by Joseph S. Bertino, Jr. ... [et al.].
   p. ; cm.
 Includes bibliographical references.
 ISBN-13: 978-0-07-174169-9 (soft cover : alk. paper)
 ISBN-10: 0-07-174169-0
 I. Bertino, Joseph S.
 [DNLM: 1. Pharmacogenetics. 2. Pharmaceutical Preparations—metabolism. 3. Pharmacological Phenomena—genetics. QV 38.5]
 LC classification not assigned
 615.1'9—dc23
                                                    2012024941

McGraw-Hill books are available at special quantity discounts to use as premiums and sales promotions, or for use in corporate training programs. To contact a representative please e-mail us at bulksales@mcgraw-hill.com.

Dedication

We dedicate this textbook to Dr. Werner Kalow, teacher, mentor, humanitarian, and one of the "fathers" of Pharmacogenomics.

Contents

Authors

Shashi Amur, PhD
Expert Regulatory Scientist
Genomics Group, Office of Clinical Pharmacology,
Office of Translational Sciences, Center for Drug
Evaluation and Research, Food Drug Administration,
Silver Spring, Maryland

Christina L. Aquilante, PharmD
Associate Professor, Department of Pharmaceutical
Sciences, School of Pharmacy, University of Colorado,
Denver, Aurora, Colorado

Dallas Bednarczyk, PhD
Investigator II
Department of Metabolism & Pharmacokinetics,
Novartis Institutes for BioMedical Research, Inc.,
Cambridge, Massachusetts

Joseph S. Bertino Jr., PharmD, FCP, FCCP
Principal
Bertino Consulting
Schenectady, New York
and
Associate Professor of Pharmacology
College of Physicians and Surgeons
Columbia University
New York, New York

Mark Bounthavong, PharmD
Pharmacoeconomics Clinical Specialist, Veterans Affairs
San Diego Healthcare System; Health Sciences Assistant
Clinical Professor, UCSD Skaggs School of Pharmacy
and Pharmaceutical Sciences, San Diego, California

Stefanie P. Ferreri, PharmD, BCACP, CDE
Clinical Associate Professor, Division of Pharmacy
Practice and Experiential Education, UNC Eshelman
School of Pharmacy, University of North Carolina at
Chapel Hill, Chapel Hill, North Carolina

Takahisa Furuta, MD, PhD
Center for Clinical Research,
Hamamatsu University School of Medicine,
Hamamatsu, Shizuoka Prefecture, Japan

Andrea Gaedigk, MS, PhD
Associate Professor, Division of Clinical Pharmacology
& Medical Toxicology, Children's Mercy Hospital &
Clinics, University of Missouri-Kansas City,
Kansas City, Missouri

Francis M. Gengo, PharmD, FCP
Associate Professor of Pharmacy and Neurology, Schools
of Pharmacy and Medicine, State University of New
York at Buffalo; Director of Clinical Research, Dent
Neurologic Institute, New Buffalo, New York

Christian Grimstein, PhD
Clinical Pharmacologist, Office of Clinical
Pharmacology, Office of Translational Sciences, CDER,
U.S. Food and Drug Administration, Silver Spring,
Maryland

Roy L. Hawke, PharmD, PhD
Clinical Assistant Professor, Division of
Pharmacotherapy & Experimental Therapeutics, UNC
Eshelman, School of Pharmacy, University of North
Carolina at Chapel Hill, Chapel Hill, North Carolina

Mary S. Hayney, PharmD, MPH, FCCP, BCPS
Professor of Pharmacy Practice, University of Wisconsin
School of Pharmacy, Madison, Wisconsin

Ogechi Ikediobi, PharmD, PhD
Assistant Professor, Department of Clinical Pharmacy,
School of Pharmacy, University of California, San
Francisco, San Francisco, California

Melanie S. Joy, PharmD, PhD
Associate Professor of Medicine, Associate Professor of
Pharmacy, University of North Carolina at Chapel Hill,
Chapel Hill, North Carolina

Lawrence Lee Soon-U, MD, PhD
Assistant Professor
National University of Singapore, National Healthcare
Group, Singapore

Sang-Seop Lee, PhD
Professor, Department of Pharmacology and Clinical
Pharmacology; Director, Pharmacogenomics Research
Center, Inje University College of Medicine; Director,
Clinical Trial Center, Inje University Busan Paik
Hospital, Busan, South Korea

Su-Jun Lee, PhD
Professor, Department of Pharmacology and Clinical
Pharmacology; Director, Pharmacogenomics Research
Center, Inje University College of Medicine; Director,
Clinical Trial Center, Inje University Busan Paik
Hospital, Busan, South Korea

Karen E. Lewis, MS, MM, CGC
Medical Policy and Technology Administrator, Priority Health, Adjunct Professor, Michigan State University College of Human Medicine, Grand Rapids, Michigan

Joseph D. Ma, PharmD
Assistant Professor of Clinical Pharmacy
University of California at San Diego
Skaggs School of Pharmacy & Pharmaceutical Sciences
San Diego, California

Marc Maliepaard, PhD
Medicines Evaluation Board, Radboud University Nijmegen Medical Centre, Nijmegen, The Netherlands
and
Medicines Evaluation Board, Utrecht, The Netherlands

Margaret Mendes, PharmD
Biologics and Pharmacogenomics Clinical Specialist, Pharmacoeconomics and Formulary Management, Veterans Affairs San Diego Healthcare System, San Diego, California

David A. Mrazek, MD, FRCPsych
Professor of Pediatrics and Psychiatry Consultant, Department of Psychiatry and Psychology, Mayo Clinic, Rochester, Minnesota

Michael Murray, PhD, DSc
Professor of Pharmacogenomics, Faculty of Pharmacy, University of Sydney, Sydney, Australia

Anne N. Nafziger, MD, PhD, MHS
Bertino Consulting, Schenectady, New York; Adjunct Research Professor, Department of Pharmacy Practice, School of Pharmacy & Pharmaceutical Sciences, State University of New York at Buffalo, Buffalo, New York

Julie Nangia, MD
Assistant Professor, Lester & Sue Smith Breast Cancer, Baylor College of Medicine, Houston, Texas

Christine M. Nguyen, PharmD, BCPS
Biologics and Pharmacogenomics Pharmacy Resident, Veterans Affairs San Diego Healthcare System, San Diego, California

Shanna K. O'Connor, PharmD, BCPS
Clinical Pharmacist, Kerr Drug, Clinical Instructor, UNC Eshelman School of Pharmacy, Chapel Hill, North Carolina

Hideaki Okochi, PhD
Associate Specialist, The Drug Studies Unit, School of Pharmacy and Medicine, University of California, San Francisco, San Francisco, California

Robert Lee Page II, PharmD, MSPH, FCCP, FAHA, BCPS
Associate Professor of Clinical Pharmacy & Physical Medicine, Clinical Specialist, Division of Cardiology, University of Colorado, School of Pharmacy, Denver, Colorado

Marisa Papaluca, MD
Section Head for Scientific Support and Projects
Human Medicines Development and Evaluation Unit
European Medicines Agency
London, United Kingdom

Markus Paulmichl, MD
Professor and Chairman, Institute of Pharmacology and Toxicology; Director of the Helga & Erich Kellerhals Research Laboratories for Novel Therapeutics, Paracelsus Medical University, Salzburg, Austria

Michelle M. Rainka, PharmD
Adjunct Instructor, University at Buffalo School of Pharmacy and Pharmaceutical Sciences, Amherst, New York

Mary W. Roederer, PharmD, BCPS
Assistant Professor, UNC Eshelman School of Pharmacy, UNC Department of Family Medicine, Institute for Pharmacogenomics and Individualized Therapy, Chapel Hill, North Carolina

Shirley K. Seo, PhD
Clinical Pharmacology Reviewer, Office of Clinical Pharmacology, Center for Drugs Evaluation and Research, U.S. Food and Drug Administration, Silver Spring, Maryland

Jae-Gook Shin, MD, PhD
Professor, Department of Pharmacology and Clinical Pharmacology; Director, Pharmacogenomics Research Center, Inje University College of Medicine; Director, Clinical Trial Center, Inje University Busan Paik Hospital, Busan, South Korea

Naohito Shirai, MD, PhD
Department of Gastroenterology
JA Shizuoka Kohseiren, Enshu Hospital
Hamamatsu, Shizuoka Prefecture, Japan

Mitsushige Sugimoto, MD, PhD
First Department of Medicine
Hamamtsu University, School of Medicine
Hamamatsu, Shizuoka Prefecture, Japan

Meghana V. Trivedi, PharmD, PhD
Assistant Professor, Department of Clinical Sciences and Administration, University of Houston College of Pharmacy; Adjunct Assistant Professor, Department of Medicine, Lester and Sue Smith Breast Center, Baylor College of Medicine, Houston, Texas

Shirley M. Tsunoda, PharmD
Assistant Professor, UCSD Skaggs School of Pharmacy and Pharmaceutical Sciences, University of California, San Diego, La Jolla, California

Xia Yang, PhD
Principal Scientist, Group Leader, Systems Biology, Sage Bionetworks, Seattle, Washington

Preface

In 2009 in San Antonio, Texas, I (JSB) was attending the annual meeting of American College of Clinical Pharmacology. My friend Bob Talbert (one of the authors of the *Pharmacotherapy: A Pathophysiologic Approach* textbook) and his wife took me and my wife out for dinner and, after sufficient Mexican food and drink, suggested that I edit a textbook on Pharmacogenomics. Bob made the point that the publisher of the textbook that he co-edits, McGraw-Hill, was very interested in this topic. The text would be meant for students, trainees, and others who were interested in the topic. This was a hard offer to turn down, a strong suggestion from an old colleague and friend, with a well-known and successful publisher!

However, I did know that this textbook had to have a broad editor and writer base. One of the jobs for the first editor is to beg (read "twist their arms") his friends and colleagues to help him as editors. Their job in turn is to convince their friends and colleagues to write chapters. So, I started making calls. My criteria for editors were individuals respected in the pharmacogenomic, clinical pharmacy, and clinical pharmacology communities, who had done sufficient research with original publications in the area of pharmacogenomics. These individuals also had to have the ability to beg their friends and colleagues (read this as "twist their arms") who also had done research and published in the area of pharmacogenomics, to write chapters. I was fortunate to be able to convince my four co-editors to contribute to this book. C. Lindsay DeVane, PharmD (Medical University of South Carolina School of Medicine), was a fellow when I was a student in Buffalo, NY, and had had an outstanding career in psychopharmacology. Lindsay is the ultimate southern gentleman. Uwe Fuhr, MD (University of Cologne, Faculty of Medicine), is a well-known and respected clinical pharmacologist from Cologne, Germany (a beautiful city), who is an editor for the European Journal of Clinical Pharmacology and has contributed greatly to the science of drug metabolism. I knew that Uwe could put forward a European perspective on this. Angela DM Kashuba, PharmD (University of North Carolina School of Pharmacy), is a pharmacist and clinical pharmacologist from Toronto, Canada (living in the USA for decades now), and has made substantial contributions to the pharmacogenomics literature. Additionally Angela works in the area of HIV eradication and prevention and has an international reputation. Joseph D Ma, PharmD (University of California at San Diego School of Pharmacy), is from Southern California. His contributions to pharmacogenomics have spanned both the medical and pharmacy literature and his passion for patient care, research, and teaching is contagious. Joe is always either devising or attempting to validate unique sampling methods to bring pharmacogenomics into the clinical setting. All of these outstanding individuals are teachers, scientists, and clinicians; thus, they discover, apply, and teach others pharmacogenomics. I could not have recruited a better group. We worked together well and complemented each other's knowledge.

The criteria that we as editors agreed upon for chapter authors was that the individuals must have contributed to original research in pharmacogenomics and that the book must have an appropriate international perspective. Chapter writers contribute to a textbook because of the pride of sharing knowledge; there is virtually no monetary gain. Again, we were fortunate to be able to recruit PharmD's, MDs, PhDs, and social scientists from 4 continents to contribute to this textbook. We are grateful to the individuals who, despite being "in demand" people, contributed to this textbook. The chapter authors are the experts in pharmacogenomics and we appreciate their contributions.

Along the way, when one puts a textbook together, things happen. We were fortunate in this regard and, in fact, lucky. We lost only one writer due to over-commitment (a gentleman who always apologizes profusely to this day but he did find a superb replacement). One of our writers suffered from breast cancer but successfully beat it (hooray!!), and another had a baby during the process (both her chapter and a baby picture showed up in my email box). Others changed jobs and moved on. But still, life goes on and they all came through on time with great work.

The science of pharmacogenomics has been described since the 10th century. It was then when the Pythagoreans (pupils of Pythagorus) were banned by him from eating fava beans (a staple at that time, still eaten today for its flavor and nutritional value) because of his observation of the development of hemolytic anemia in individuals with G6PD deficiency. These individuals endured endless societal criticism because they followed the life-saving directive of Pythagorus, as it was unheard of for such a basic food to be so deadly to a human being. This restriction, and its rationale, was discussed over the centuries, even by the philosopher Aristotle. But, most likely this restriction of the eating of fava beans saved the lives of many individuals with G6PD deficiency. This is the first known historical description of pharmacogenomics. Skip ahead to the 19th and 20th centuries with two very important developments in the field of genetics. The first was the description of inherited traits by Dr. Gregory Mendel and the second, a little recognized manuscript (at the time) published by Dr. Archbald Garrot on chemical individuality (sounds like one dose isn't right for everyone).

In the post-WWII world, an interesting discovery was made by a young physician-scientist from the University of Toronto. This physician-scientist, Dr. Werner Kalow, was a prisoner of war held in Arizona after he was "drafted" by the Nazi regime to be a German ship surgeon. The ship he was assigned to was captured in the Pacific by Allied Forces and prisoners were taken. In WWII America, Dr. Kalow served his time as the prisoner-of-war camp physician and would ride along with the prison ambulance until the end of the war. As Dr. Kalow stated "The Americans were smart, they knew that not all Germans in the military were supportive of the Nazi cause and it seemed that they easily picked out those of us that were not supportive, separated us and sent us to camps in the USA that allowed much more freedom." After WWII, Dr. Kalow returned to Berlin, and then moved to the University of Tornoto. In 1957, he, along with Dr. Natalie Staron, described prolonged skeletal muscle paralysis due to succinylcholine in a patient with cholinesterase deficiency. Kalow went on to describe the genetics of this finding by genotyping 135 patients and dividing them into extensive, intermediate, and poor metabolizers based on allele identification. Dr. Kalow went on to write the first textbook on "Pharmacogenetics," which was published in 1962. He worked until his passing at age 91 in 2008.

The science continued to evolve slowly until the 1980s with the availability of better analytical techniques to determine parent and metabolite drug concentrations more efficiently and cheaply. Additionally genetic advancements made finding genetic polymorphisms easier. These developments were followed by the Human Genome Project, which has provided some very valuable information that can be easily applied to pharmacogenomics. Many have contributed to the advancement of pharmacogenomics. Thus, the reader can get a sense of the volume of information that has been generated over 10 centuries.

This first edition of the book is meant to be a basic introduction to the topic of pharmacogenomics. The textbook has been written for students, trainees, scientists, and clinicians in pharmacy, medicine, nursing and other allied health professions. We did not intend this to be a comprehensive textbook covering all aspects of pharmacogenomics, but to give the user a general overview of the topic.

The textbook is divided into two sections. The first section covers more general aspects of pharmacogenomics. In these sections we attempted to cover areas such as ethics, regulatory science, and pharmacoeconomics among others. In particular, Chapters 2 and 3 provide a "mini" course in molecular genetics and testing. The second section reviews the role of pharmacogenomics in areas such as cardiovascular medicine and immunology. The book presents learning objectives for each chapter. The chapters in the second section also have cases for the reader to appreciate the clinical application of pharmacogenomics. We hope that the readers of this book understand that drug therapy must be individualized based on genetics and environmental factors. Rather than suggesting the same drug, biologic or vaccine dose for everyone, there are many instances where dosage individualization is essential.

The editors hope that you find this textbook informative. We always welcome suggestions to improve the textbook. Please email us if you have suggestions or comments.

Joseph S. Bertino Jr., PharmD, FCP, FCCP
C. Lindsay DeVane, PharmD
Uwe Fuhr, MD
Angela D. M. Kashuba, BScPhm, PharmD, DABCP
Joseph D. Ma, PharmD

Acknowledgments

A book like this could not have been completed without the support of others.

JSB would like to acknowledge the support of his wife, Anne Nafziger, and his (adult) children Jaimie and Christopher Bertino, who inspired and supported him. Also, the extensive assistance of Joe DiPiro is acknowledged. Joe's guidance and friendship were invaluable throughout the process.

ADMK acknowledges the support of her husband, Odin Naderer, and her wonderful children Skylar and Erik Naderer.

JDM acknowledges the support of his wife, Lois Sangmin Lee, and his daughter Chloe Ma.

And of course the editors acknowledge the participation of all chapter writers who are friends and colleagues to each of us.

Developing Perspectives on Pharmacogenomics

Roy L. Hawke, PharmD, PhD

LEARNING OBJECTIVES

- To present various perspectives on pharmacogenomics, from the professional student to the practitioner, as well as a historical perspective on this rapidly developing field. A case describing a potential scenario for a pharmacist not adequately prepared for the integration of pharmacogenomics into patient care is provided.

- To briefly describe the origins and evolution of pharmacogenomics.

- To discuss the reasons why, after a decade of research, pharmacogenetics and individualized therapy have not yet emerged as an important part of patient care.

- To offer a glimpse of the future where increasingly complex technologies and more rapid advances in pharmacogenetic research will simplify the use of a patient's genetic variation for the selection of drug therapy and prediction of outcomes.

PERSPECTIVES ON PHARMACOGENOMICS

At first glance, it may not be obvious that the title of the introductory chapter for this textbook is a play on words. Perspectives are needed to properly understand how and when to apply knowledge. In this regard, as you become familiar with the concepts developed in the various chapters of this textbook and acquire specific knowledge and skills for the assessment of pharmacogenomic information, you will develop your own perspective so that you can apply these to the care of your patients. However, pharmacogenomics is still a rapidly emerging field, and so the vast amount of current research effort will provide new knowledge and information, perhaps previously unimagined, that will continue to shape current perspectives on how pharmacogenomics is to be utilized and the extent in which it should be applied. In other words, the perspectives of the practitioner will need to continuously change as the field of pharmacogenomics changes. Therefore, use of this textbook is just a starting point, a necessary first step to becoming an enlightened, modern-day practitioner who uses pharmacogenomic information along with other traditional sources of data to make informed pharmacotherapy recommendations.

Student Perspectives

A common perspective shared by many professional pharmacy students is that application of pharmacogenomic information to patient care is complicated and requires an understanding of the various scientific methods used to discover and establish associations between genetic polymorphisms and an important human trait, drug response. This perspective, often encountered during the decade in which I have coordinated an elective course entitled *Introduction to Applied Pharmacogenomics*, is one of needless trepidation and erroneous assumptions and stems, in part, from confusion created when basic scientists jumped to offer new pharmacogenomics courses and textbooks to interested professional students. These initial efforts focused almost exclusively on the science of pharmacogenomics, principally because there were so few examples of application. Today, many courses are still taught by basic scientists who are more comfortable discussing the pros and cons of various genotyping methods than they are with discussing the strengths and weaknesses of the design of clinical trials that aim at validating the clinical utility of a genetic association. Another source for such perspective stems from the way pharmacogenomics has been introduced in most curriculums. Given the dearth of clinically oriented textbooks, pharmacogenomic topics are typically interspersed throughout the curriculum; therefore, clinical application and relevance are diluted. Unlike case discussions that take place in pharmacotherapy modules taught by practitioners, the professional student is left to form his or her own perspective on pharmacogenomics without structure or context. It is our intent that this textbook will provide the student and the practitioner with a common ground for integrating pharmacogenomic information and laboratory data, both of which are obtained with methodologies validated by basic scientists, for assessments and recommendations on patient care during case discussions.

Practitioner Perspectives

As has been previously suggested, pharmacists are uniquely positioned in the health care system to assume responsibility for advising providers and patients on the interpretation and application of results from pharmacogenomic tests because of their pivotal role as point-of-care providers and recognition as drug experts.[1] However, although pharmacogenomic topics are included in most professional curricula, there is some evidence to suggest that pharmacists may not feel prepared to assume such a responsibility. A recent assessment of the pharmacogenomics educational needs of pharmacists within a large, academic, multicampus health care system indicates pharmacists believe pharmacogenomics knowledge is important to the profession, but they lack the knowledge and self-confidence to act on the results of pharmacogenomics testing. Sixty-three percent felt they could not accurately apply the results of pharmacogenomics tests to drug-therapy selection, dosing, or monitoring.[2] The following case involving a community pharmacist illustrates the "pharmacogenomics shock" created when the pharmacogenomics educational needs of pharmacists are not met by a professional curriculum. This results in a perspective shared by many practitioners who feel unprepared to assume responsibility for interpreting and applying results from pharmacogenomic tests. This case illustrates many of the concepts, topics, and clinical issues addressed in this textbook that will prepare pharmacists for the new realities of practice in the age of pharmacogenomics.

Case: JT, A Community Pharmacist Given a Prescription for CYP2C19 Genotyping

JT is a recent graduate of a local School of Pharmacy and works at the only pharmacy in town. JT staffs the pharmacy alone on Tuesdays and receives a call from "Old Doc" Anderson who is worried about a patient whom he had prescribed Plavix last week following a recent MI. Doctor Anderson explains he has just learned that the US Food and Drug Administration (FDA) has added a black box warning to the Plavix label to advise physicians of the importance of genetics and the availability of testing. Doctor Anderson wants JT to take immediate steps to make sure Plavix is the right drug for this patient who is now on his way over to the pharmacy to have the appropriate genetic test done. Several thoughts run through JT's mind and he quickly identifies a number of questions he must find answers to before the patient arrives. Some of JT's immediate thoughts on this request for genotyping:

1. Is there any confidentiality or legal issue I should be aware of before I obtain a genetic test for this patient or share the results with anyone, including "Old Doc" Anderson?

2. Are there any liability issues if I do not do the genetic testing?

3. How accurate is this test (i.e., *positive predictive value*), and who are the CLIA-approved laboratories?

4. How clinically significant is this genetic effect (i.e., *penetrance*) anyway and what are the odds that this patient might actually have this genetic variation (i.e., *allelic and genotypic frequencies*)?

5. How do I interpret the genetic results when it comes back?

6. This patient is on a bunch of other drugs; how does a person's genetics influence his or her susceptibility for drug interactions?

JT is pretty sure that "Old Doc" Anderson knows something that he does not know, so JT begins to scramble for information he should have available before the patient arrives:

7. What types of samples are most commonly collected for genotyping?

8. Is it even possible to collect a sample for genotyping at a pharmacy, and what type and how much of a sample should I collect for Doctor Anderson's patient?

9. How quickly must the collected sample be sent out for genotyping before the DNA degrades?

10. How should the sample be stored and will it require freezing at ultracold temperatures?

11. Why do these unusual requests always seem to come up on my shift? I wonder where I can find a good case-based pharmacogenomics textbook?

Patient Perspectives

If practitioners feel unprepared to integrate pharmacogenomic tests into their practice, what perspectives might patients hold since they are even less informed and must rely on health care professionals for interpretation and application of genetic information? There are two factors to suggest that patient acceptance of pharmacogenomic testing may not represent a significant hurdle for pharmacists. A significantly greater percentage of Americans say pharmacists have "very high" or "high" honesty and ethical standards compared with the next-highest-rated professions, grade school teachers and medical doctors.[3] In addition, recent studies reveal use of pharmacogenomic-guided drug selection to facilitate personalized medicine has considerable support from patients who are even willing to pay out-of-pocket if the disease associated with a pharmacogenomic test for appropriate treatment represents a high risk for the patient's well-being.[4] Perhaps of greater concern to patients is that the drugs they are prescribed may actually harm them, and there is much discussion in the public sector about why so many patients fail to take their medications as prescribed. It has been suggested that as many as half of Americans do not adhere to their medication regimen because of out-of-pocket costs, concerns that a drug's ability to harm may outweigh its actual effectiveness, worries about drug side effects, and concerns for serious drug interactions since approximately 32 million Americans are prescribed three or more medications.[5] It has been estimated that poor patient compliance with prescribed medications costs the US health care system an estimated $290 billion in avoidable medical spending each year.[6] Therefore, it is apparent that pharmacy practitioners have the opportunity to greatly improve patient compliance and reduce health care costs by mastering the use of pharmacogenomics for individualizing selection of drug therapy to minimize potential harm to patients and to optimize clinical benefits for patients from whom pharmacists have their trust.

HISTORICAL PERSPECTIVE

So when should we pinpoint the origins of pharmacogenomics? Obviously, pharmacogenomics would never have evolved into a quantitative science without the seminal works of Charles Darwin[7] and Gregor Mendel,[8] or the discovery of the structure of DNA by Watson and Crick[9] almost 100 years later. Perhaps it is reasonable to suggest that the publication of the first completed sequence of the human genome by the Human Genome Project in 2003, a mere 50 years later, signaled the beginnings of the age of pharmacogenomics. During these 50 years, while the technological advancements needed to propel the field forward lagged behind, major theories and principles emerged following the discovery of genetic variation in drug response that led to the development of the field of pharmacogenomics. For example, in 1957, Motulsky[10] published his seminal study associating a number of human genetic conditions with toxic responses to drugs resulting from mutations in drug metabolism enzymes. His research led him to postulate that genetically determined adverse drug responses could serve as models for the interaction of heredity and environment in the pathogenesis of disease. Vogel[11] first coined the term "pharmacogenetics" in 1959 while describing current problems in human genetics, and the first pharmacogenetics textbook, *Pharmacogenetics: Heredity and the Response to Drugs*, was published by Kalow in 1962.[12] From the mid-1960s to the mid-1980s, several seminal twin and family study studies conducted by Vesell and Page[13] described the contribution of genetic and environmental factors for large interindividual variations in the metabolism and elimination of drugs with a latter focus on variation associated with the cytochrome P450 system.[14–17] During the last two decades preceding the "age of pharmacogenomics," much of the research to elucidate specific mechanisms for variation in drug response involved the isolation and characterization of polymorphic hepatic cytochrome P450 isozymes that has been described as "reverse genetics" since identification of the aberrant amino acid helped establish the specific mutations at the level of DNA and mRNA responsible for such pharmacogenetic differences.[18–22] Subsequent candidate gene association studies clearly established the clinical importance of genetic polymorphisms in proteins involved in the disposition of drugs as well as in the protein targets mediating pharmacodynamic response to drugs. All that was needed at this point were advances in technologies that would allow rapid and error-free sequencing of small amounts of DNA obtained from blood or tissue. Enter *Thermus aquaticus*, a species of bacterium discovered in the Lower Geyser Basin of Yellowstone National Park,[23] and the source of the heat-resistant enzyme Taq DNA Polymerase. Taq Polymerase was first isolated in 1976,[24] and named "Molecule of the Year" by *Science* in 1989 for its widespread application in the polymerase chain reaction DNA amplification reaction.

The Age of Pharmacogenomics

During the late 1990s, the publicly funded Human Genome Project led by Collins had been making slow progress until Craig Venter announced in May 1998 that Celera Genomics would sequence the genome within 2 years. Thus started a race to sequence the human genome that stimulated major advances in sequencing technologies.[25] Following the availability of powerful new technological platforms that enabled even more rapid and cheaper genome sequencing, government and industry began forming collaborative consortiums for obtaining and sharing genome sequence information.

One of the first significant research collaborations within the pharmaceutical industry was The SNP Consortium (TSC) that was established in 1999.[26] The program's overarching goal was to provide a high-quality, high-density single nucleotide polymorphism (SNP) map of the human genome. In 2002, the International HapMap Project, a collaboration involving academic centers, nonprofit biomedical research groups and private companies, was started with the goal of cataloging all of the common human genetic variation or SNPs (which are single base variations in the genetic code) as blocks of SNPs or haplotypes that tend to be inherited together.[27] In 2003, the US FDA began a concerted effort to raise the visibility of pharmacogenetics information in product labels as an effort to encourage the pharmaceutical industry to incorporate investigations of genetic influences on drug response during the early stages of drug development. Today, over 150 drugs have such information listed in their package inserts and that number is growing exponentially. More recently, the International Serious Adverse Events Consortium (SAEC) was established in 2007. This global, nonprofit partnership between leading pharmaceutical companies, the FDA, and academic institutions was established to identify and validate genetic markers to help predict individuals at risk for serious adverse drug events (SAEs). The goal of the consortium is to publish a set of predictive SNPs for all drug-related SAEs, which will reduce health care costs and improve the flow of safe and effective therapies by identifying safety issues for new drugs before they reach the market.[28] Collaborative projects such as HapMap and TSC provided a way for researchers to "tag" specific SNPs as representative of variation within blocks of DNA sequences (i.e., haplotype blocks) thereby reducing the number of SNPs that are needed to cover the entire human genome that contains millions of SNPs, as well as variations in the number of copies of large and small sections of the genome (i.e., copy number variation [CNV]).

This paved the way for genome-wide association studies (GWAS) and the development of the DNA gene chip that contains millions of "dots" of different DNA sequences that capture genetic variation across the genome to investigate associations between 500,000 or more SNPs and a specific disease or drug response. One of the most successful early examples of the power of GWAS was the discovery in 2005 of an association between age-related macular degeneration and an SNP in the complement factor H gene that was quite unexpected since it identified this disease as an inflammatory process.[29] By 2010, GWAS had become "state-of-the-art" for investigations on the mechanisms underlying complex diseases and drug response with over 1,200 human GWAS studies being conducted and more than 4,000 newly discovered SNP associations.[30,31]

The recent application of GWAS to investigations on liver disease illustrates how "discovery" GWAS studies can suddenly advance a field that had not made significant inroads in over a decade. Nonalcoholic fatty liver disease (NAFLD) is a complex disease, with obesity and diabetes being the most prevalent risk factors, that clusters in families and leads to cirrhosis and liver failure. There are no known effective therapies for NAFLD due to our poor understanding of the molecular basis for this disease. Unexpectedly, a single variant in the *PNPLA3* gene was found to be highly associated with the development of steatosis and NAFLD.[32] *PNPLA3* encodes a 481 amino acid protein of unknown function that belongs to the patatin-like phospholipase family and the cytosine to guanine substitution results in an amino acid substitution at codon 148. A follow-up study in 7,176 subjects confirmed the association between *PNPLA3* and susceptibility to NAFLD and identified variants in three additional loci that are associated with both increasing CT hepatic steatosis and histologic NAFLD.[33] These discoveries are likely to pave the way for the development of new and effective therapies for NAFLD due to the pharmacogenomic

elucidation of the molecular targets implicated in the development of the disease.

In another example, the development of the first effective therapies for chronic hepatitis C infection (HCV) was largely empirical and based on the known antiviral activity of human type I interferons that are produced by leukocytes and involve the innate immune response. Pegylated interferon-alpha plus ribavirin is now the first-line treatment for patients with HCV genotype 2 or 3 infections. However, sustained virologic response rates to peginterferon-based therapies, which are only 50% in patients with genotype 1 HCV infection, have not changed in over a decade until the recent development of HCV protease inhibitors that represent a new class of therapeutic agents for this disease. In spite of intense research efforts, little insight into the molecular mechanisms underlying large differences and resistance in patient response to peginterferon-based therapies was achieved until the successful application of GWAS that opened the door for individualizing therapy.[34] Unexpectedly, genetic polymorphisms near the human *IL28B* gene, which encodes for interferon lambda 3, were found to be associated with significant differences in response to the treatment[35] and with the natural clearance of the genotype 1 hepatitis C virus.[36]

Most recently, the discovery of "newer" types of non-SNP genetic variations such as indels, CNVs, and copy-neutral variations (inversions and translocations) has widened the scope of research to discover genetic markers of human diseases and drug response.[37] To enable such investigations, the 1000 Genomes Project, an international consortium which built on the data and technology generated by previous "big science" projects, was initiated to construct the most detailed map of genetic variations in the human genome by sequencing the genomes of at least 1,000 individuals from around the world.[38]

PHARMACOGENOMICS: WHERE ARE WE NOW AND WHAT DO WE KNOW?

The vast and concerted resources that have been invested in pharmacogenomics research over the past decade have resulted in a new understanding and appreciation of the complexity of the interacting influences controlling the expression of human phenotypes. As with all research, these efforts have produced some "surprises." Unexpectedly, results from the 1000 Genomes Project suggest that there are between 20 and 40 million SNPs scattered over the human genome instead of the earlier estimates of 1.5–2.0 million SNPs from the Human Genome Project. Clearly, the discoveries and progress being made in both the development of newer technologies and the elucidation of the molecular mechanism underlying disease susceptibility, progression, and response to drug therapies have entered an exponential growth phase. We now have chips containing 5 million SNPs instead of chips with 0.5–1 million SNPs. And while it took the Human Genome Project, with all its vast resources and international collaborations, 13 years to complete the first full sequence of the human genome, the 1000 Genomes Project was able to accomplish its goal at a rate of two human genomes sequenced per day!

Along with the rapid advances in pharmacogenomic tools and technologies, there has been an explosion of new information and new insights to our understanding of the complexities underlying human variation. For example, the numbers of genes identified in our genome and the mRNA transcripts identified in our transcriptome do not add up to the number of proteins in our proteome. Regulation of mRNA processing is more complex than previously thought (e.g., microRNAs) and some genes encode more than one protein, or a gene may encode only RNA that does not get translated into protein. Many of our earlier views or "perspectives" regarding where research efforts need to be focused have changed. For example, early on, the field of pharmacogenomics was "distracted" by extreme examples of interindividual differences in drug metabolism and drug outcomes that were thought to be more important because of their high penetrance than less penetrant genetic influences that were more prevalent. For example, drug-induced liver injury (DILI) is unpredictable and has serious consequences for those idiosyncratic drug reactions that result in death. However, the occurrence of DILI is estimated between 1 in 10,000 and 1 in 100,000;[39] therefore, the intense pharmacogenomic efforts in this area are not likely to have a large impact on human health and health care costs. Similarly, pharmacogenetic research was initially focused on the associations of CYP450 polymorphisms for many serious drug toxicities, and only through GWAS investigation have we recently gained an appreciation for the importance of the immune system for many serious drug reactions.[40] We have also developed a new understanding that genetics is not everything and perhaps even less than what we thought. Many human traits are essentially nonheritable due to overriding environmental influences and for some phenotypes the nongenetic component can be as much as 60% or greater, and as described below, we are only now attempting to quantify these effects. We have learned that GWAS will be much more helpful in elucidating causal factors for complex diseases than what we previously thought. For example, no one could have predicted that susceptibility to NAFLD, a complex disease involving insulin resistance, aberrant fatty acid metabolism, oxidative stress, and the features of metabolic syndrome, would be associated with just two to three genes as discussed above.

PHARMACOGENOMICS: WHAT LIES AHEAD AND WHEN WILL IT DELIVER ON ITS PROMISE OF INDIVIDUALIZED THERAPY?

Whole-genome sequencing is now being used to identify loss-of-function mutations in individuals with rare phenotypes that might provide new mechanistic insights and approaches for the treatment of common human diseases. For example, sequencing of the PCSK9 gene in 128 of the 2,877 subjects enrolled in the Dallas Heart Study who had the lowest plasma levels of LDL cholesterol led to the discovery of two nonsense mutations

that indicated the important role of this protein in coronary heart disease.[41] Similarly, sequencing of the human exome, the part of the genome comprising exons (i.e., the coding portions of genes that are expressed as proteins and other functional gene products), will be used to identify rare individuals with loss-of-function mutations in proteins that can be targeted for therapeutic intervention. Arrays to detect functional variants in the human exome are only now becoming available. Data are beginning to emerge from investigations on the genetic basis for human variation in gene expression. These investigations combine two pharmacogenomic "discovery" platforms (gene expression microarray analysis and GWAS) to identify regions of the genome that contribute to the expression of complex traits that are referred to as expression quantitative trait loci.[42] Given the accelerating pace of new technologies and discoveries in pharmacogenomics, there is no way to predict or "guess" that new breakthrough will provide the next quantum advance in our use of genetic information to obtain optimal drug outcomes in patients, or when it will likely occur. Clearly, a systems (biology) approach will be required for individualizing drug therapies for many complex diseases. In oncology, there will be methods that enable the integration of genetic variation in both somatic (i.e., tumor traits) and germ cells (i.e., human traits) for predicting how, together, they influence a patient's response to anticancer therapy. In addition to GWAS, other data-rich discovery strategies, from wide-scale quantification of epigenomic regulation of gene expression to comprehensive characterization of the human proteome and metabolome, will unveil common molecular pathways for diseases once considered distinct. In the future, therapeutics will target unique cellular networks and molecular pathways, rather than single protein targets, which in turn will require more sophisticated and higher level assessment of pharmacogenomic variation. For example, environmental exposures (e.g., an epigenetic factor) might increase/decrease the enzyme activity of the slowest step (or bottleneck) in a multiple-step pathway so that the genetic variation for a different gene, which now becomes the slowest step, unmasks a new genetic association for that multistep pathway and phenotype (i.e., disease progression or drug response). Therefore, eventual prediction of some phenotypic responses will require an understanding of how epigenetic controls on entire DNA expression programs can override genetic variation at a basal, homeostatic state. The influence on epigenetic factors can only be elucidated by large-scale, systematic epigenome-wide association studies (EWAS).[43] The epigenome is highly dynamic and regulated by a complex interplay between genetic and environmental factors, and epigenetic information is commonly expressed through DNA methylation, posttranslational modifications of histone proteins, and noncoding RNAs (e.g., short microRNAs). Although still in its infancy, technology is now available for DNA methylation EWAS investigations due to the discovery DNA methylation is correlated in blocks of up to 1 kb, which enabled the design of cost-effective EWASs,[44] leading to the first well-designed EWAS 5 years later (Breitling, LP et al, 2011).[45] Interactions between genetic and epigenetic variation have been recently described, and regions of the genome where genetic variants are known to influence methylation state have been termed methylation quantitative trait loci.[46]

For some drugs (e.g., clopidogrel and abacavir), pharmacogenomics has already delivered on its promise of individualizing drug therapy and ensuring optimal patient outcomes; however, it may never deliver for diseases where the phenotype is very complex and affected by either placebo (emotional) or temporary external influences. For example, posttraumatic epilepsy is an example where the severity of head trauma and the feedback mechanisms evoked may be so highly variable and patient-specific that perhaps no pharmacogenomic investigation, GWAS or otherwise, will be able to account for the vast heterogeneity of this patient population. The discovery that susceptibility to a number of sporadic epilepsy syndromes is associated with rare deletions in chromosome 16[47] may explain the failure of genetic association studies to identify highly penetrant SNP associations since the genetic variation is one of missing alleles instead of variant alleles. Depression is another example where placebo (e.g., patient's faith) or environmental influences (e.g., a highly emotional response to death of a parent) may be too difficult to adjust for in the design of a GWAS. The effect of genetic drift, which occurs in small populations or results from a population bottleneck, and can result in ethnic differences in how a common genetic variation, or the absence of one, can differently influence drug response in different areas of the world, has only been recently recognized. And the limited availability of some therapeutic options in these areas will require different algorithms and therefore the need for international cooperation and effort on a global scale.[48] Given the complexity and immensity of information that must be processed, new informatics approaches will certainly be needed before the dream of turning a genotype into a dose can be realized.

CLINICAL PERSPECTIVES AND LAG TIME

As we have tried to illustrate in the pages of this introductory chapter, we are in the exponential phase of the "age of pharmacogenomics" where advancements in technologies, and new insights of the complexities influencing human phenotype, are ever more rapidly altering our perspectives on how variation in the human genome can shape the clinical course of an individual's disease and his or her response to drug therapies. So how do we as clinicians cope with this flood of information, some if not most, which may become obsolete due to the rapidly shifting perspectives, so that we can begin to understand how to best integrate pharmacogenomic information into our practice? This is especially challenging since current paradigms for the discovery and development of new drug therapies are also rapidly changing so that newer, safer, and more effective "systems-based" therapies have the potential for outdating the advancements in pharmacogenomics.[49] Such a change in paradigm is needed given the immense difficulties and hurdles encountered in the scientific discovery and drug development processes, and the time and effort required for the successful translation of science into clinical practice even under the best of circumstances. It has been estimated that the median translation lag time between the

first reported discovery (e.g., a publication or awarded patent) of a therapeutic agent representing a new class with similar characteristics and mode of action and a highly impactful clinical intervention is 27 years, and lag time following a highly cited randomized trial for an agent, 16.5 years.[50] Unrealistic expectations and promises for the rapid translation of pharmacogenomics into patient care have the potential of creating negative public perspectives with respect to eventual acceptance or whether such a goal is possible. Therefore, practitioners must acquire the fundamental skills and knowledge that will enable them to critically evaluate evidence-based literature as it relates to the role of genetic variation on clinical outcomes. Through their acquired clinical and pharmacogenomic knowledge, clinicians will need to assess the impact of new developments in pharmacogenomics and pharmacotherapy on the current state of disease management and extrapolate future needs for ensuring optimal clinical outcomes. This "clinical perspective" will enable clinicians to form opinions on the future impact of new pharmacogenomic information on patient care in their chosen field.

For example, an immunologically mediated hypersensitivity reaction is the most serious adverse effect of abacavir, a nucleoside reverse transcriptase inhibitor developed as a treatment for human immunodeficiency virus (HIV). This reaction affects 5–8% of patients during the first 6 weeks of treatment, which limits its utility and requires careful monitoring whenever initiated. Immediate and permanent discontinuation of abacavir is mandated at the first sign of abacavir hypersensitivity that results in rapid reversal of symptoms. Subsequent rechallenge with abacavir is contraindicated since it can result in a more severe, rapid, and potentially life-threatening reaction. The discovery that screening of patients infected with HIV for an HLA-B*5701 variant allele[51] before initiating abacavir treatment could significantly reduce the incidence of hypersensitivity reaction to abacavir resulted in labeling changes by the FDA. Now, it is considered malpractice to not test for the HLA-B*5701 allele before prescribing abacavir. However, while this discovery was a significant validation of the use of pharmacogenomic information to ensure safe and effective drug outcomes, the clinical impact of this discovery was never fully realized as newer, more effective, and convenient HIV medications and newer classes of HIV therapeutic agents quickly offered better options for HIV therapy.

Similarly, the recent discovery that an SNP (i.e., rs12979860) upstream from the *interleukin 28B* gene,[52] which encodes for interferon lambda 3, strongly influences the rates of sustained virologic response in patients with chronic HCV treated with peginterferon and ribavirin was thought to bring new mechanistic insights that would provide new and more effective therapies. However, it is likely that the clinical impact of this discovery will also never be realized since new cases of HCV infection have fallen dramatically with the screening of blood products, and new classes of anti-HCV drugs, such as HCV protease inhibitors and polymerase inhibitors, are rapidly changing the pharmacotherapy landscape such that "experts" in the field suggest HCV may be the next human disease to be eradicated from the human population.

SUMMARY—DEVELOPING PERSPECTIVES ON PHARMACOGENOMICS

So where do we start? The most logical first step in acquiring the necessary pharmacogenomics knowledge, skills, and perspectives is to develop a fundamental understanding of basic genetic concepts underlying pharmacogenomics and its somewhat complex nomenclature. This includes knowledge of the analytical methods and the bioinformatics used for identifying associations with genetic variation, as well as an insight as to why such genetic associations do not always conform to "Mendelian law." An introduction to some of the complex ethical, legal, and social considerations surrounding the use of pharmacogenomic information, such as regulatory decisions on the use of genomics to inform decisions on the use of drugs in populations where drugs have not been studied, is needed before any perspective can be formed. Then, for a proper "historical perspective" the pharmacy practitioner should have a good understanding of the genetic variation underlying the absorption, disposition, metabolism, and elimination (aka ADME) of drugs with a focus on drug metabolism and transporter genes, including epigenetic influences due to inhibition, induction, and activation. To understand "patient or public" perspectives that shape public health policy, an understanding of the issues underlying public access to pharmacogenomic testing, patient counseling, as well as pharmacoeconomic implications is also needed. Finally, in order to develop appropriate "clinical perspectives," the pharmacy practitioner should have a good fundamental understanding of how pharmacogenomics is currently being applied in therapeutic areas such as cardiology, infectious diseases, oncology/hematology, psychiatry and addiction, vaccination, transplantation and immunology, pain management, and neurology, as well as insight on the major emerging areas of pharmacogenomic application such as in nephrology, pulmonary gastroenterology, and endocrinology. With the knowledge and skills obtained from the application of pharmacogenomics to the patient cases presented in the various chapters of this textbook, it is our hope pharmacy practitioners will be well equipped to assess and respond to rapidly shifting pharmacogenomic perspectives that will allow them to best integrate pharmacogenomic information in clinical practice.

REFERENCES

1. Lee KC, Ma JD, Kuo GM. Pharmacogenomics: bridging the gap between science and practice. *J Am Pharm Assoc.* 2010;50(1):e1–e14.

2. McCullough KB. Assessment of the pharmacogenomics educational needs of pharmacists. *Am J Pharm Educ.* 2011;75(3):51.

3. Jones JM. *Nurses Top Honesty and Ethics List for 11th Year.* Gallup Inc; December 3, 2010. Available at: http://www.gallup.com/poll/145043/nurses-top-honesty-ethics-list-11-year.aspx.

4. Issa AM, Tufaila W, Hutchinsond J, Tenorioc J, Poonam Baligaa M. Assessing patient readiness for the clinical adoption of personalized medicine. *Public Health Genomics.* 2009;12:163–169 [doi: 10.1159/000189629].

5. Landro L. Many pills, many not taken. *Wall Street Journal.* October 13, 2011. Available at: http://online.wsj.com/article/SB10001424052970203388804576616882856318782.html.

6. A NEHI Research Brief. *Thinking Outside the Pillbox: A System-wide Approach to Improving Patient Medication Adherence for Chronic Disease.* New England Healthcare Institute; August 2009. Available at: www.nehi.net/uploads/full_report/pa_issue_brief__final.pdf.

7. Darwin CR. *The Origin of Species. Vol. XI. The Harvard Classics.* New York: P.F. Collier & Son; 2001:1909–1914; Bartleby.com, www.bartleby.com/11/.

8. Mendel, J.G. (1866). Versuche über Pflanzenhybriden. Verhandlungen des naturforschenden Vereines in Brünn, Bd. IV für das Jahr, 1865, Abhandlungen, 3–47. For the English translation, see: Druery CT, Bateson W. Experiments in plant hybridization. *J R Hort Soc.* 1901;26:1–32. http://www.esp.org/foundations/genetics/classical/gm-65.pdf. Retrieved 2009-10-09.

9. Watson JD, Crick FHC. Molecular structure of nucleic acids: a structure for deoxyribose nucleic acid. *Nature.* 1953;171:737–738.

10. Motulsky AG. Drug reactions, enzymes, and biochemical genetics. *JAMA.* 1957;165:835–836.

11. Vogel F. Moderne probleme der humangenetik. *Ergeb Inn Med Kinderheilk.* 1959;12:52–125.

12. Kalow W. *Pharmacogenetics: Heredity and the Response to Drugs.* Philadelphia, PA: Saunders; 1962.

13. Vesell ES, Page JG. Genetic control of drug levels in man: phenylbutazone. *Science.* 1968;159:1479–1480.

14. Vesell ES. Advances in pharmacogenetics. *Prog Med Genet.* 1973;9:291–367.

15. Weinshilboum RM, Vesell ES. Pharmacogenetic symposia. *Fed Proc.* 1984;43:2295–2347.

16. Vesell ES, Penno MB. Assessment of methods to identify sources of interindividual pharmacokinetic variations. *Clin Pharmacokinet.* 1983;8:378–409.

17. Propping P. Pharmacogenetics. *Rev Physiol Biochem Pharmacol.* 1978;83:124–173.

18. Jaiswal AK, Gonzalez FJ, Neber DW. Human P1-450 gene sequence and correlation of mRNA with genetic difference in benzo(*a*)pyrene metabolism. *Nucleic Acids Res.* 1985;13:4503–4520.

19. Conney AH. Induction of microsomal cytochrome P-450 enzymes: the first Bernard B. Brodie lecture at Pennsylvania State University. *Life Sci.* 1986;39:2493–2518.

20. Song B-J, Gelboin HV, Park S-S. Complementary DNA and protein sequences of ethanol-inducible rat and human cytochrome P-450s: transcriptional and post-transcriptional regulation of the rat enzyme. *J Biol Chem.* 1986;261:16689–16697.

21. Beaune PH, Guengerich FP. Human drug metabolism *in vitro*. *Pharmacol Ther.* 1988;37:193–211.

22. Gonzalez FJ, Skoda RC, Kimura S, et al. Characterization of the common genetic defect in humans deficient in debrisoquine metabolism. *Nature.* 1988;331:442–446.

23. Brock TD, Freeze H. *Thermus aquaticus*, a nonsporulating extreme thermophile. *J Bacteriol.* 1969;98(1):289–297.

24. Chien A, Edgar DB, Trela JM. Deoxyribonucleic acid polymerase from the extreme thermophile. *Thermus aquaticus. J Bacteriol.* 1976;127(3):1550–1557.

25. Abbott A. The human race. *Nature.* 2010;464:668–669 [doi:10.1038/464668a].

26. Holden AL. The SNP Consortium: summary of a private consortium effort to develop an applied map of the human genome. *Biotechniques.* 2002;32:S22–S26.

27. McVean G, Spencer CCA, Chaix R. Perspectives on human genetic variation from the HapMap Project. *PLoS Genet.* 2005;1(4):e54 [doi:10.1371/journal.pgen.0010054].

28. http://www.saeconsortium.org.

29. Klein RJ, Zeiss C, Chew EY, et al. Complement factor H polymorphism in age-related macular degeneration. *Science.* 2005;308(5720):385–389 [doi:10.1126/science.1109557].

30. Manolio TA, Guttmacher AE, Manolio TA. Genomewide association studies and assessment of the risk of disease. *N Engl J Med.* 2010;363(2):166–176 [doi:10.1056/NEJMra0905980].

31. Hindorff LA, Junkins HA, Manolio TA. NHGRI catalog of published genome-wide association studies. 2010. http://www.genome.gov/gwastudies.

32. Romeo S, Kozlitina J, Xing C, et al. Genetic variation in PNPLA3 confers susceptibility to nonalcoholic fatty liver disease. *Nat Genet.* 2008;40(12): 1461–1465 [Epub September 25, 2008; doi: 10.1038/ng.257].

33. Speliotes EK, Yerges-Armstrong LM, Wu J, et al. Genome-wide association analysis identifies variants associated with nonalcoholic fatty liver disease that have distinct effects on metabolic traits. *PLoS Genet.* 2011;7(3):e1001324 [Epub March 10, 2011].

34. Ladonato SP, Katze MG. Genomics: hepatitis C virus gets personal. *Nature.* 2009;461(7262):357–358 [doi:10.1038/461357a].

35. Ge D, Fellay J, Thompson AJ, et al. Genetic variation in IL28B predicts hepatitis C treatment-induced viral clearance. *Nature.* 2009;461(7262): 399–401 [doi:10.1038/nature08309].

36. Thomas DL, Thio CL, Martin MP, et al. Genetic variation in IL28B and spontaneous clearance of hepatitis C virus. *Nature.* 2009;461(7265): 798–801 [doi:10.1038/nature08463].

37. Ku CS, Loy EY, Salim A, Pawitan Y, Chia KS. The discovery of human genetic variations and their use as disease markers: past, present and future. *J Hum Genet.* 2010;55:403–415 [doi:10.1038/jhg.2010.55].

38. Kuehn BM. 1000 Genomes Project promises closer look at variation in human genome. *JAMA.* 2008;300:2715.

39. Holt MP, Ju C. Mechanisms of drug-induced liver injury. *AAPS J.* 2006;8(1):E48–E54.

40. Daly AK. Using genome-wide association studies to identify genes important in serious adverse drug reactions. *Annu Rev Pharmacol Toxicol.* 2012;52: 21–35 [doi:10.1146/annurev-pharmtox-010611-134743].

41. Cohen J, Pertsemlidis A, Kotowski IK, Graham R, Garcia CK, Hobbs HH. Low LDL cholesterol in individuals of African descent resulting from frequent nonsense mutations in PCSK9. *Nat Genet.* 2005;37:161–165 [Erratum, *Nat Genet.* 2005;37:328].

42. Innocenti F, Cooper GM, Stanaway IB, et al. Identification, replication, and functional fine-mapping of expression quantitative trait loci in primary human liver tissue. *PLoS Genet.* 2011;7(5):e1002078 [Epub May 26, 2011].

43. Rakyan VK, Down TA, Balding DJ, Beck S. Epigenome-wide association studies for common human diseases. *Nat Rev Genet.* 2011;12:529–541.

44. Eckhardt F, Lewin J, Cortese R, et al. DNA methylation profiling of human chromosomes 6, 20 and 22. *Nat Genet.* 2006;38:1378–1385.

45. Breitling LP, Yang R, Korn B, Burwinkel B, Brenner H. Tobacco smoking related differential DNA methylation: 27k discovery and replication. *Am J Hum Genet.* 2011;88:450–457.

46. Zhang D, Cheng L, Badner JA, et al. Genetic control of individual differences in gene-specific methylation in human brain. *Am J Hum Genet.* 2010;86:411–419.

47. Heinzen EL, Radtke RA, Urban TJ, Cavalleri GL, Depondt C. Rare deletions at 16p13.11 predispose to a diverse spectrum of sporadic epilepsy syndromes. *Am J Hum Genet.* 2010;86(5):707–718 [Epub April 15, 2010].

48. Roederer MW, Sanchez-Giron F, Kalideen K, et al. Pharmacogenetics for Every Nation Initiative. Pharmacogenetics and rational drug use around the world. *Pharmacogenomics.* 2011;12(6):897–905.

49. Collins FS. Reengineering translational science: the time is right. *Sci Translational Med.* 2011;3(90):1–6.

50. Contopoulos-Ioannidis DG, Alexiou GA, Gouvias TC, Ioannidis JP. Life cycle of translational research for medical interventions. *Science.* 2008;321:1298–1299.

51. Mallal S, Phillips E, Carosi G, et al. HLA-B*5701 screening for hypersensitivity to abacavir. *N Engl J Med.* 2008;358:568–579.

52. Smith KR. Identification of improved IL28B SNPs and haplotypes for prediction of drug response in treatment of hepatitis C using massively parallel sequencing in a cross-sectional European cohort. *Genome Med.* 2011;3:57 [doi:10.1186/gm273].

2

Genetic Concepts of Pharmacogenomics: Basic Review of DNA, Genes, Polymorphisms, Haplotypes and Nomenclature

Andrea Gaedigk, MS, PhD

LEARNING OBJECTIVES

- Review concepts of DNA and genetics.
- Discuss genetic polymorphism and its implications.
- Outline nomenclature used in pharmacogenomics.

GENOMIC DNA

The double helix structure of deoxyribonucleic acid (DNA) was discovered in 1953 by Watson and Crick. The now famous structure is composed of two DNA molecules that run in opposite directions and are wound around each other in a clockwise direction. Each polynucleotide chain is composed of a phosphate backbone, sugars, and the four nucleotide bases adenine (A), cytosine (C), guanine (G), and thymine (T). One of the forces holding the two strands together are hydrogen bonds formed between the nucleotide bases of the opposite strands called base pairs (A and T form two and C and G form three hydrogen bonds). Within cells of higher organisms, genomic DNA (gDNA) is associated with many proteins, among them histones that help organize these macromolecules into chromosomes. Unless a eukaryotic cell is dividing, gDNA is highly condensed and almost exclusively located in the cell nucleus. In humans, there are approximately 3 billion base pairs (bp) that are organized in 46 chromosomes (two sets of 23, one set inherited from each parent). gDNA is also called the "blueprint" of life, because it encodes information

for proteins and RNA. Specifically, the sequence of the four base "letters" A, C, G, and T determines the sequence of amino acids in proteins and the sequence composition of RNAs in the cell. However, only a small portion of the gDNA serves this purpose. Other areas of the gDNA harbor binding sites for regulatory proteins such as transcription factors or encode noncoding RNAs such as microRNA that play a role in the regulation of gene and/ or protein expression.[1,2] More insight is also being gained about the role of epigenetics. The term epigenetics refers to changes in gene expression that are not explained by the DNA sequence itself, but by DNA modifications such as methylation and acetylation. Biological consequences may also arise from structural variations across the genome such as copy number variations (CNVs).

Sources of DNA Used for Genetic Analyses

gDNA can essentially be extracted from any part of the human body. The most widely utilized sources of gDNA are blood and saliva or cheek brushings (also known as mouth swabs or buccal brushes), because they are relatively easy to collect and bear only minimal risk. Whole blood is easy to handle and store and high-quality and sufficient amounts of gDNA are typically obtained from specimen as little as a few drops. Blood may also be collected in concert with clinical samples to minimize blood draws. Mouth swabs using cotton or bristle brushes collect saliva and/or mucosal epithelium cells by placing them into the mouth or brushing along the side of the cheek. The amount of DNA retrieved from such samples may vary considerably and may allow for only a limited number of genetic tests to be performed. Also, the integrity of gDNA may be compromised if swabs or brushes were not immediately processed or frozen for long-term storage. Therefore, saliva has become more popular as gDNA source as commercial collection devices have become available[3] that are not only convenient to use but also stabilize the specimen and allow for long-term storage under a variety of conditions making them an excellent choice for collection outside the clinical or laboratory setting including patient self-sampling. Other sources for pharmacogenetic studies may include tissues such as liver originating from organ donors, biopsies, tissue banks, and commercial sources. Especially when studying epigenetics, the gDNA must be derived from the tissue of interest because DNA modification patterns may be tissue-specific.

Purification of Genomic DNA, Quantity and Quality Assessment

DNA isolation or purification in simple terms refers to its removal from other cellular components. For many diagnostic analyses or research applications including DNA sequencing, genotyping, and cytogenetic testing, to name a few, DNA requires extraction and a minimum level of purity. Following are the essential steps included in a typical DNA isolation procedure: (1) lysis of the cells containing the DNA (by alkaline lysis, a detergent, or mechanical disruption), (2) degradation of proteins present in the sample including those associated with the DNA (using a protease), and (3) separation of the DNA from all other components (via ethanol precipitation or spin column). There are numerous commercially available kits accommodating wide ranges of sample types, volumes, and sizes. High gDNA quality and quantities can be obtained using both ethanol precipitation and silica membrane-based spin column procedures. Typical amounts of gDNA isolated from 0.2 mL of whole blood, 25 mg of tissue, and 0.2 mL of saliva are 1–12, 10–50, and 0.5–10 µg, respectively. Actual amounts may vary depending on tissue type, sample quality, and disease state of donor, to name a few (more detailed information can be obtained from kit manufacturers).

The overall quality of a gDNA sample is measured by its molecular integrity and the presence of impurities such as residual protein. Molecular integrity can be determined by agarose gel electrophoresis. A high-quality sample exhibits a well-defined band that migrates at approximately 50 kilobase (kb) while degraded DNA presents itself by a smear throughout the lane. The presence of protein can be assessed spectrophotometrically by the ratio of the absorbance of UV light at a wavelength of 260 and 280 nm ($A_{260/280}$). A ratio between 1.7 and 2 generally indicates a high-quality gDNA sample. Other impurities such as residual ethanol or salt are often only indirectly detected in otherwise high-quality samples, for example, if a sensitive downstream application performed only poorly or not at all.

The DNA yield can be estimated by agarose gel electrophoresis against calibrator samples or determined by measuring the absorbance at A_{260nm}. The concentration is calculated by the following equation: concentration (µg/mL) = (A_{260} reading − A_{320} reading) × dilution factor × 50 µg/mL. The total yield (µg) = DNA concentration (µg/mL) × total sample volume (mL). The drawbacks of spectrophotometry include the inability to distinguish between DNA, RNA, and other contaminants, single- and double-strand DNA, and its relative insensitivity. This can be overcome by utilizing fluorescent DNA-binding dyes such as the ultrasensitive nucleic acid stain PicoGreen that can detect and quantitate DNA concentrated as low as 10 ng/mL DNA (kits available from multiple sources).

An increasingly popular and widely used line of instruments is NanoDrop devices[4] that can measure absorbance and/or fluorescence in small sample volumes of 0.5–2 µL.

FROM GENE TO PROTEIN

Overview of the Basic Components of a Gene and Translation into Protein

The term "gene" was first used by the Danish geneticist Johannsen in a book he published in 1909 in which he described "elements of heritage."[5] Today, according to the HUGO Gene Nomenclature Committee (HGNC) guidelines, a gene is defined as "a DNA segment that contributes to phenotype/function. In the absence of demonstrated function a gene may be characterized by sequence, transcription or homology."[6] The number of human protein-coding genes is estimated to range between 20,000 and 25,000.[7] The exact number of genes remains elusive because defining a DNA segment as a gene can be challenging. For example, small genes or overlapping genes may elude annotation, some genes encode more than one protein, or a gene may encode only RNA that does not get translated into protein.[8]

The essential components of a protein-coding gene and a simplistic overview of the processes involved in gene expression, that is, gene transcription, splicing, translation, and posttranslational modifications, are provided in Figure 2–1. Regulatory elements constitute DNA sequences to which regulatory proteins bind. These include transcription factor binding sites and are mostly located in the upstream region of a gene, but can also occur within the gene. The promoter is typically in close proximity to the site from which RNA transcription initiates. It contains sequence that allows RNA polymerase and other factors crucial for transcription initiation to attach. DNA segments between the transcription start and stop sites are called exons

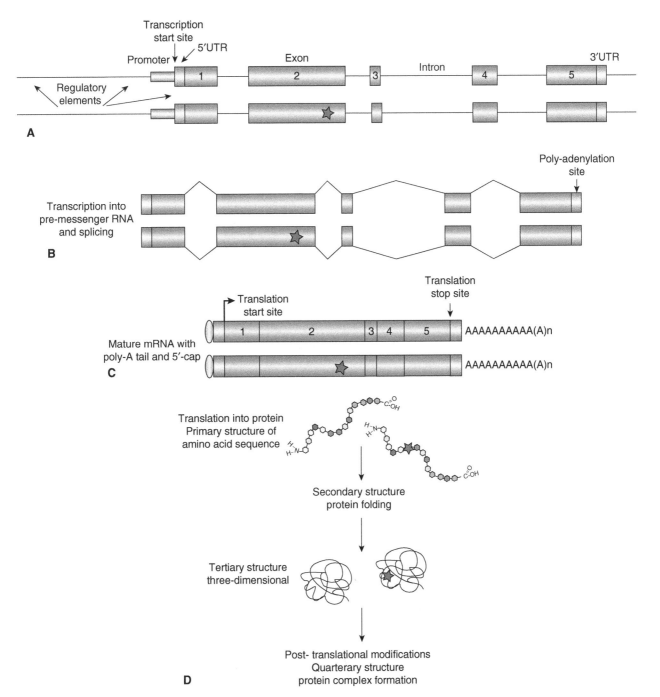

FIGURE 2-1 From gene to protein. (**A**) Depicts two allelic variants of a gene composed of five exons, four introns, a promoter, and regulatory regions. The red star indicates the presence of a SNP within an exon 2 that changes the code for an amino acid. 5′ and 3′ untranslated regions (UTRs) are as indicated. (**B** and **C**) The gene is transcribed into pre-messenger RNA, which is further processed by splicing (intron sequences are excised). This process produces mature mRNA, which is capped at the 5′ end and has a tail of multiple adenosine monophosphates at the 3′ end (poly-A tail). (**D**) Translation into a polypeptide is initiated at the ATG start codon and terminated at a stop codon. The peptide chain forms secondary structures (α-helices, β-sheets) that will assume a three-dimensional tertiary structure. The SNP present in exon 2 is causing an amino acid change in the protein that was translated from the mRNA that originated from the variant allele. Some proteins receive posttranslational modifications and/or may form a quaternary complex with other proteins.

and introns. A sequence is defined as exon if it is retained in mature messenger RNA (mRNA), while introns are intervening sequences that are removed in the mRNA splicing process. The number of exons and introns of a gene and their sizes vary considerably.[9] In the example shown in Figure 2–2, there are five exons and four introns. The 5′ and 3′ untranslated regions (UTRs) are exonic in nature, and are transcribed and retained in mRNA, but are not translated into protein. A gene also contains

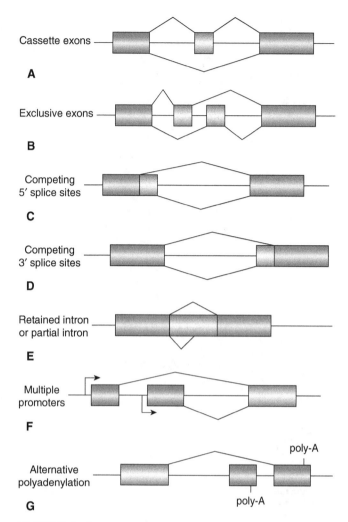

FIGURE 2–2 Alternative splicing. Elementary alternative splicing events represent binary choices. (**A**) Cassette exons are discrete exons that can be independently included or excluded from the mRNA. They can be further subdivided into "skipped" and "cryptic" exons according to whether the main observed variant includes or excludes the exon, respectively. (**B**) Mutually exclusive splicing involves the selection of only one from an array of two or more exon variants. (**C** and **D**) Competing 5′ and 3′ splice sites represent "exon modification" events. (**E**) Retention of entire or partial intronic sequences. (**F**) Alternative splicing in conjunction with the use of alternative promoters (or alternative first exons). (**G**) Alternative mRNA 3′ ends by using polyadenylation sites in different exons. Note that regulation of the last two categories need not be at the level of splicing. (Reprinted by permission from Macmillan Publishers Ltd. Adapted from Matlin AJ, Clark F, Smith CWJ. Understanding alternative splicing: towards a cellular code. *Nat Rev Mol Cell Biol.* 2005;6:386–398.)

a number of additional "signals" necessary to direct transcription and translation including transcription initiation and polyadenylation (poly-A) sites and translation start and stop sites.

In the process of transcription a complementary strand of so-called pre-mRNA is synthesized. The main steps of this process entail the unwinding of the DNA double helix and opening of the hydrogen bonds between base pairs, initiation and synthesis of complementary RNA strands using ribonucleotides

as building blocks (A, C, G, and uracil [U] that replaces T), and release from the DNA template. Before the pre-mRNA leaves the nucleus, the molecules receive a 3′ poly-A tail and a 5′ cap. These modifications protect mRNAs from degradation, and are important for mRNA export from the nucleus and mRNA translation into protein. In the next step, the intervening sequences (introns) are removed, and exons spliced together to generate a mature mRNA. Conserved sequences at the exon/intron junctions (exon 3′ splice acceptor and intron 5′ splice donor sites) are playing a vital part to direct spliceosomes, machineries of RNA, and proteins that carry out this task.

Finally, the mRNA is translated into protein by ribosomes, which takes place in the cytosol. Ribosomes are machineries composed of proteins and RNA. In the translation process, mRNA, ribosomes, transfer RNAs (tRNAs), and other proteins work together to translate the genetic code into a specific chain of amino acids, or polypeptide. Specifically, small RNA molecules that are covalently bound to an amino acid (tRNAs) recognize three-letter "words," or codons, on the mRNA via their anticodon. As the tRNAs line up along an mRNA molecule, the amino acids they carry are synthesized into a polypeptide chain by the ribosome. There are 64 codons of which 61 code for 1 of the 20 amino acids found in proteins. Three codons (UAA, UGA, and UAG) serve as stop codons and one codon, the AUG translation start codon, carries out dual function by signaling translation initiation and incorporating the amino acid methionine.[10] Additional and more detailed information about genes, how they are translated into protein, and the genetic code can be found at the HGNC and National Center for Biotechnology Information (NCBI) Web sites and links,[6,10] among many other online sources.

In Figure 2–1 the star indicates the presence of a nucleotide sequence variation in a region that is translated (exon). This variation changes an amino acid codon and hence directs the incorporation of an amino acid that differs from that encoded by the wild-type sequence. An amino acid change may have a dramatic effect on the protein structure and/or function or no impact at all depending on the position and nature of the change.

As the polypeptide chain is synthesized, secondary structures (β-sheets, helices) are formed, which are essential for a protein's folding into its three-dimensional, or tertiary structure. A protein may be further modified after translation by glycosylation, an enzymatic process that adds glycans, lipids, or other molecules to the protein. Other posttranslational modifications include the formation of disulfide bridges and covalent bonds between amino acid thiol groups. Some proteins also form complexes with another or multiple other protein molecules. Proteins may be more stable in complexes or exhibit different kinetics, while some enzymatic functions require complex protein complexes or structures.

Alternative Use of Exons Exemplified by the *UGT1* Gene

Alternative or differential splicing is a process by which more than one protein product can be generated from a single

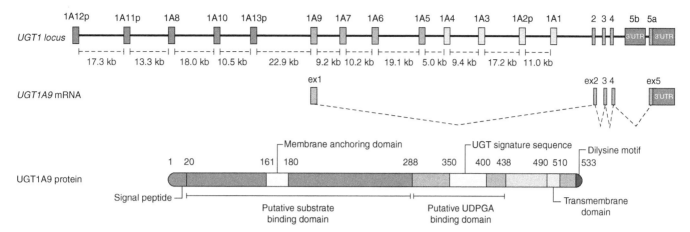

FIGURE 2-3   Alternative splicing of *UGT1A* and resulting protein structures. Numerous first exons are alternatively spliced to three mutual exons (exons 2–4). Exons that are not utilized are labeled as "pseudo-exons," for example, 1A1p. Additional variation is introduced by two alternative exons 5 (ex5a and ex5b). Each first exon has its own promoter allowing for tissue-specific expression. The first exon is believed to provide the substrate-binding and anchoring domains while exons 2–5 encode the cofactor and transmembrane binding domains. (Reproduced from Guillemette C, Levesque E, Harvey M, Bellemare J, Menard V. UGT genomic diversity: beyond gene duplication. *Drug Metab Rev.* 2010;42: 22–42. Reproduced with permission of Informa Healthcare.)

gene.[11,12] This process is relatively common in higher organisms and appears to play a role in not only the generation of complex proteomes but also the level of gene regulation and expression. Figure 2–2 shows basic alternative splicing events, which may result in functional protein, but could also generate nonfunctional polypeptides. As illustrated, exons and/or introns may be skipped or retained in their entirety or partially; exons may also be used alternatively and, finally, these events are not mutually exclusive. Whether a functional protein is encoded by a given mature mRNA molecule depends on which sequences are retained and excised during the splicing process.

The uridine diphospho (UDP)-glucuronosyltransferase (UGT) superfamily of enzymes is involved in the metabolism of not only numerous drugs and sex steroids but also endogenous compounds such as bilirubin and environmental toxins.[13] The genes within the *UGT1* and *UGT2* gene loci not only carry sequence variations leading to a wide range in enzymatic activity but also undergo extensive alternative splicing making them a good example for the context of this chapter.

The *UGT1A* gene utilizes 13 alternate promoters or first exons to produce 9 functional UGT1A enzymes named UGT1A1, 1A3, 1A4, 1A5, 1A6, 1A7, 1A8, 1A9, and 1A10. Each of these first exons encodes a substrate-binding domain that is spliced to four common exons (exons 2–5); these encode the highly conserved transmembrane domain and the binding domain of the cosubstrate (Figure 2–3). Exons *UGT1A2P*, *1A11P*, *1A12P*, and *1A13P* are pseudogenes and do not produce a functional protein. In addition to adding significant diversity to a single gene, the use of multiple promoters also allows to regulate the expression of the different UGT1 enzymes in a tissue-specific manner. The bilirubin-metabolizing UGT1A1, for instance, is ubiquitously expressed while other UGT1As are found in gastrointestinal tissues or are exclusively expressed in extrahepatic tissues. Only recently, it was discovered that

alternative splicing also involves exon 5 of the common gene region further explaining interindividual variability in UGT1-mediated glucuronidation.[13]

Single nucleotide polymorphisms (SNPs) that change amino acids can also be found in those first *UGT1A* exons providing yet another layer of variability in UGT1A function. Alternative splicing is also observed for UGT2 family members.[13] A comprehensive list for UGT allelic variation can be found at the UDP-glucuronosyltransferase alleles nomenclature page.[14]

GENETIC VARIATION

Sequence Variations Commonly Found in Genes that Impact Their Function

Sequence variations of various kinds are present in any given human genome. They include SNPs, insertions and deletions of one or few nucleotides (indels), larger deletions and insertions, CNVs, variable number tandem repeats (VNTRs), gene rearrangements, and de novo mutations. Whether a variation has a functional consequence depends on its location and nature.

Because one set of chromosomes is inherited from each parent, an individual can be homozygous for a given sequence (i.e., the sequence is the same on both chromosomes) or heterozygous (i.e., the sequence is different). The term allele is most often used to describe variable forms of the same gene or other defined regions of interest and the term genotype describes the combination of the two allelic variants of a gene in a given individual. In most instances, a common and functional gene version is referred to as the "wild-type" or "reference" allele and deviations thereof polymorphic or mutant variants. These and other genetic terms are described in more detail in genetic text books or online sources.[15–17]

Polymorphism versus Mutation

The term polymorphism is used when two or more different phenotypes are present in a population. Polymorphisms are frequently observed, because they contribute to the diversity and adaptability of a population to a changing environment. Examples are hair color or blood types. In the field of (pharmaco)genetics, this term describes sequence variations in a gene that occur at a frequency of at least 1%. If the variation occurs less frequently (<1%), it is referred to as mutation.[17] Examples include slow and fast acetylation of isoniazid, an antituberculosis medication that is metabolized by the polymorphically expressed *NAT2* gene[18] or glucose-6-phosphate dehydrogenase deficiency.[19]

Single Nucleotide Polymorphisms and Indels

A DNA sequence variation is called a SNP when a single nucleotide is changed to another at a particular position within a genome. SNPs are the most common sequence variations in the human genome with approximately 1 SNP per 1,000 base pairs, or >3 million per genome. For example, a particular sequence reads AGGTC**A**GT for one allele and AGGTC**G**GT for another (the SNP is A > G). In some cases one nucleotide can have not just one, but two or three allelic variants. One specific example is the SNP at position 2677 in the multidrug resistance gene 1 (*MDR1* or *ABCB1*) that is triallelic, meaning that T or A can be found instead of the wild-type G (G > T/A).

RefSNPs (rs) are reference SNPs that are catalogued by the NCBI in the Database for Short Genetic Variations (dbSNP database).[20] Each submitted SNP (ss) is mapped to the genome and a reference ID number (rs number) assigned to a short genetic variation. As implied by its name, the dbSNP database also catalogues short nucleotide insertions and deletions. As an example, the SNP in the *MDR1* gene mentioned above is catalogued as rs2032582.

Amino acid changes caused by nonsynonymous SNPs, or missense mutations can have a wide range of consequences on enzymatic function. A histamine to proline change encoded by the cytochrome P450 2D6 *(CYP2D6) *7* variant, for instance, obliterates function, while a proline to serine change on the *CYP2D6*10* variant impacts protein stability and leads to reduced *in vivo* function of the enzyme. Other amino acid changes may not exhibit an effect at all or only toward particular substrates (see Chapter 6). In contrast, synonymous or silent SNPs do not change an amino acid. Insertions and deletions of one or two nucleotides in coding regions will shift the three-letter code and, consequently, incorrect amino acids will be incorporated in the growing polypeptide. Often, such frameshifts also lead to premature termination due to the generation of stop codons. A SNP can also directly generate a stop codon (nonsense mutation). A deletion or insertion of three nucleotides leads to an amino acid loss or gain impacting enzymatic activity.

SNPs located in introns and exons can alter RNA splicing, which in turn impacts enzymatic activity. For example, the *CYP2D6*4* allele is characterized by a G > A SNP that causes aberrant splicing and loss of function (homozygous carriers are CYP2D6 poor metabolizers) while an intronic SNP in the *CYP2D6*41* reduced function allele is believed to interfere with a splice enhancer binding site that diminishes the amount of correctly spliced mRNA. SNPs in transcription factor binding sites or other regulatory gene regions can also have a profound consequence on enzyme activity by impacting RNA transcription levels. Gene expression and translation can also be affected by SNPs in the 5′ and 3′ untranslated gene region.

SNPs affecting gene expression are collectively also referred to as "expression" SNPs (eSNPs). These are typically located in noncoding gene regions and noncoding small RNAs that interact with a gene.

Haplotype and Tag SNPs

In genetics, haplotype describes the combination of alleles that are located on one chromosome and inherited together. The term is also used to describe all SNPs on a chromosome, which are statistically linked with each other. In pharmacogenetics, haplotype is used in the latter sense, but often applied to smaller regions of interest such as a part of a gene, an entire gene, or multiple genes within a locus as illustrated in Figure 2–4. In a given population, haplotypes can be inferred from individuals' genotype data by haplotype phasing methods such as the software package PHASE[21] or Haploview.[22]

Haplotype, tag SNPs, and utilization are exemplified on the vitamin K epoxide reductase complex 1 (*VKORC1*) gene that plays a crucial role in concert with *CYP2C9* in the response of the widely used anticoagulant warfarin.[23] The *VKORC1* gene has extensively been characterized. SNPs across the *VKORC1* gene can be found in different combinations, defining multiple haplotypes within two clades (or branches)[24] that associate with warfarin maintenance dose. A tag SNP is a SNP by which genetic variation across a particular region can be identified. Specifically, the SNPs at locations −1339 and 1173 of *VKORC1* are in complete linkage and equally informative.[25] Consequently, either one could be utilized to discriminate haplotypes that require lower warfarin dosage. The SNP most frequently used as a tag SNP for genotyping purposes is −1639G > A (rs9923231).

Copy Number Variation

New molecular techniques are driving the discovery and detection of CNVs along their characterization and contributions to human disease.[26] CNVs are abundant throughout the genome. Currently, the Database for Genomic Variants has catalogued 66,700 CNVs (>1 kb) and 34,000 indels (100 kb to 1 kb) at almost 16,000 loci.[27]

Many gene families were created through the mechanism of gene duplication allowing individuals to adapt to changing environments. Therefore, it is not surprising that many enzymes involved in the detoxification of xenobiotic substances and metabolism and disposition of many drugs are members of large gene families that comprise highly homologous genes. An

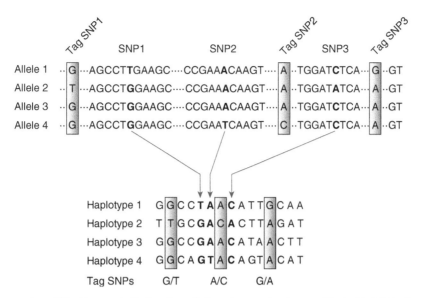

FIGURE 2–4 Haplotype and tag SNPs. The graph displays four allelic variants, or haplotypes. The bolded SNPs (SNPs 1, 2, and 3) may be located in a given gene region and of particular interest. Tag SNPs shown in boxes are sequence variations that allow discrimination of the different haplotypes, that is, genotype information of a tag SNP indirectly provides information regarding all other SNPs that are statistically linked to it.

example is the human cytochrome P450 (CYP) superfamily that contains 56 putatively functional and over 50 pseudogenes.[28–30] *CYP2D6*, a gene that harbors numerous SNPs and small indels, is also affected by extensive CNV along other gene rearrangements.[31–33] The *CYP2D6*5* allele lacks the entire *CYP2D6* gene and constitutes a nonfunctional variant. Duplications and multiplications of up to 13 functional gene copies have been observed. Respective alleles are denoted as, for example, *CYP2D6*2×2* and *CYP2D6*2×3*, if the copy number is known. An extension of ×*N* is utilized to indicate that the allele carries two or more copies. Duplications and multiplications of functional gene units contribute to increased activity and ultrarapid drug metabolism. However, duplications of reduced and nonfunctional genes and variants carrying duplications, or tandems of nonfunctional and functional genes, have also been described. The highest and lowest frequencies of gene duplications were observed in East Africans and East Asians, respectively, but overall *CYP2D6* CNV frequencies vary significantly across populations.[34] Other genes encoding drug-metabolizing enzymes with known CNVs include *CYP2A6*, the sulfotransferase *SULT1A1*, *UGT2B17*, and the glutathione *S*-transferases *GSTM1* and *GSTT1*.

The quantitative detection of specific CNVs such as those described above is more difficult compared with SNP genotyping owing to its quantitative nature. Methods including Southern blot analysis and long-range polymerase chain reaction (PCR) may only yield information regarding the presence or absence of the gene, but not how many copies are present. More sensitive methods such as real-time PCR in conjunction with fluorescent-labeled TaqMan probes, pyrosequencing, and multiplex PCR analysis successfully discriminated between zero, one, two, and three gene copies. The detection of three or more copies has been

reported on,[31] but is technically even more demanding, in part because of the lack of freely available, validated control samples. Genome-wide CNV analyses utilize array-based methods[35] that are typically detecting gene deletions and duplications, but not multiplications.

Repetitive DNA Sequences

Microsatellites (<5 bp in length), which may also be called short tandem repeats (STRs) or simple sequence repeats (SSRs), and minisatellites (>5 bp in length) constitute variable number tandem repeat (VNTR). These are found throughout the genome and can be highly variable in repeat number making them extremely informative targets especially for paternity[36] and forensic[37] testing.

Many VNTRs are located in intergenic regions without an apparent function; they can, however, also occur within a gene. One famous example is the dominant trinucleotide repeat disorder Huntington disease. Subjects with <29 CAG repeats encoding a polyglutamine tract are normal, while those with >35 repeats are affected by the disease. Another well-known example is the tandem TA dinucleotide repeat in the TATAA element of the gene promoter of *UGT1A1*. The presence of seven repeats $(TA)_7$ instead of the wild-type $(TA)_6$ causes significantly reduced protein expression that contributes to hyperbilirubinemia in Gilbert syndrome.[38] Finally, the drug-metabolizing enzyme *CYP2E1* gene carries a variable number of 42–60 bp long repeat elements in its promoter region that appear to play a role in the inducibility of gene expression[39] and thereby contribute to alcohol and nicotine dependence.[40]

Nomenclature

The HGNC is assigning unique gene symbols and names to genes and provides useful tables listing closely related genes of superfamilies.[41] However, this organization is not keeping track of the continually growing number of allelic variants and haplotypes that are still being discovered for many genes. In order to provide the science field with a unified nomenclature the so-called star (*) allele nomenclature have been devised to "encourage scientists worldwide to speak the same language" and to avoid "homemade" allelic designations that can confuse the nomenclature system and the scientific literature.[42] This quote is taken from the Human Cytochrome P450 (*CYP*) Allele Nomenclature Committee[42] that has taken on efforts to organize and share information for allelic variation of genes of the *CYP* superfamily. Web-based sites are also maintained for *UGT*,[14] *NAT*,[43] and *ALDH* gene nomenclature, while for other gene families including soluble *GSTs*,[44] *SULTs*,[45] and the multidrug transporter *MDR1* (*ABCB1*)[46,47] recommendations exist only in form of published manuscripts and may not be standardized and consistently applied throughout the literature. This is exemplified by *ABCB1* of which one frequent variant is typically cited as 3435C > T and not by its proposed star designation.

For naming a gene, the HUGO-assigned "root" gene symbol is followed by an Arabic number indicating the family, which is followed by a letter designating the enzyme subfamily and, finally, an Arabic number may differentiate an individual gene within a subfamily.[48,49] Examples are CYP2D6: CYP(root)2(family) D(subfamily)6(gene in subfamily) as shown in Figure 2–5, or NAT2: NAT(root)2(family). For P450s, members of different families exhibit ≤40% identity on the protein level and ≥59% if they are in the same subfamily. Notably, the genes of subfamily members are usually found in clusters on the same chromosome.[48]

Allelic variants of a gene are distinguished by asterisks and Arabic numbers as in *CYP2D6*1*, *CYP2D6*2*, etc., or *NAT2*4*, *NAT2*5*, etc. It has to be noted that the variant labeled *1*, in most cases, represents the reference gene sequence that encodes functional protein and is often also referred as "wild-type." One exception is the *NAT2*4* variant that constitutes the reference sequence for the functional enzyme. Furthermore, by convention, human gene and allele names are provided in upper case and in italics, for example "*CYP2D6*1* gene," while the corresponding protein is shown as "CYP2D6.1." Mouse counterparts are displayed as, for example, cyp2d9.[49]

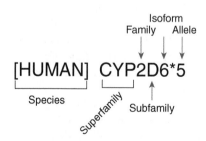

FIGURE 2–5 Gene nomenclature. The graph dissects gene nomenclature using an example of a human cytochrome P450 enzyme.

The nomenclature Web sites are useful recourses providing a range of information. The P450 nomenclature site, for instance, lists allele and protein names, the nucleotide changes on the corresponding cDNA and gene sequences, information regarding functional consequence if known, and relevant references for each variant. Hyperlinks allow quick access to reference sequences and rs numbers. The UGT Web site, on the other hand, offers two options for each *UGT* gene, one organized by haplotype and the other by SNPs.

Ethnic Differences of the Occurrence of Sequence Variations

Variability in drug metabolism among individuals of the same ethnic group or race can be substantial (10- to >40-fold) and is by far greater than the differences observed between ethnic groups or races (2- to 3-fold).[50] Examples including warfarin metabolism and response to β-blockers are provided by Urban[51] reviewing race, ethnicity, ancestry, and pharmacogenetics. More in-depth information can also be found in the book entitled *Pharmacogenomics in Admixed Populations*.[52]

CYP2D6 is a good example to illustrate interindividual and interethnic variability. The *CYP2D6* gene locus has been extensively studied in the past 20 years across populations and as of today over 100 allelic variants and sub-variants have been catalogued.[42] Mean activity toward CYP2D6 probe substrates varies among populations[53] and a large portion of the variability can be explained by the polymorphic expression of the enzyme.[54] The particular allelic variants causing this variability, however, are strikingly different between populations.[53,55] The nonfunctional *CYP2D6*4* allele, for instance, has not been detected in some Asian or sub-Saharan populations, but can reach over 20% in certain European populations and is also the most frequent variant causing poor metabolism in Europeans and Americans of European descent. On the other hand, *CYP2D6*10* is the most common variant in Asians ranging from approximately 25% to 60%[55] substantially contributing to lower mean activity compared with Caucasians.[53] Lower mean activity has also been observed for African Americans,[53,54,56] which is, however, mostly attributed to the reduced function alleles *CYP2D6*17* and *29* in addition to *CYP2D6*10* and other variants conveying reduced activity. Furthermore, certain allelic variants appear to be exclusive to certain populations and their descendents. Examples are *CYP2D6*17* and *29* that are routinely detected in black Africans and African Americans, but have also been found in Caucasian Americans, albeit at much lower frequencies (this is likely due to population admixture). There are also low-frequency nonfunctional variants that are population-specific such as *CYP2D6*40* and *42* (discovered in African Americans) and *CYP2D6*18*, *44*, and *49* that have only been reported in Asians.[42]

Based on the prevalence of alleles in a given population or geographic area, genotyping should be tailored toward the population tested to accurately predict phenotype. Most commercially available testing (tests or services) covers the most common and functionally important allelic variants, but not necessarily more rare and/or population-specific variants. Efforts have been made, however, to develop genotype panels that include *CYP2D6* variants predominantly or exclusively found in Asian populations.[57] By the same token, studies that include genotype analyses should always include test panels geared toward the populations investigated. This may be straightforward for Caucasians, which have often been extensively studied, but is certainly more challenging in genetically heterogeneous African populations and their descendents and populations with high degrees of admixture such as Brazilians.[58]

Hardy–Weinberg Equilibrium

The Hardy–Weinberg equilibrium (HWE) model was defined over 100 years ago by the work of an English mathematician, Godfrey Hardy, and a German physician, Wilhelm Weinberg. Based on probability modeling they concluded that gene frequencies are inherently stable while evolution is happening.[59] The work by Hardy, Weinberg, and other population geneticists let to the paradigm that evolution will not occur in a population when seven conditions are met: (1) mutations are absent, (2) natural selection is absent, (3) the population is infinitely large, (4) all members breed, (5) breeding occurs in a random fashion, (6) everyone has the same number of offspring, and (7) there is no migration in or out of the population. Since all these are impossible to meet at the same time, evolution is inevitable. From observations, Hardy and Weinberg developed an equation to describe the probable allele frequencies in a population and follow them from generation to generation. This equation is known as the HWE: $p^2 + 2pq + q^2 = 1$, where p represents the frequency of the major (or dominant) allele (A) and q the frequency of the minor or recessive allele encoding a trait (a). People having one of each are called heterozygous for the trait (Aa). Therefore, $p = AA + (1/2)Aa$ and $q = aa + (1/2)Aa$. Since there are only two alleles in this example, it follows that $p + q = 1$. If the frequency of p or q is known, the other can be calculated. Likewise, allele frequencies can be inferred from observations of phenotypes.

For example, in a Caucasian population, about 7% (7/100) of individuals are poor metabolizers for CYP2D6-mediated drugs. In this case $q^2 = 7/100 = 0.07$. The square root of 0.07 will provide the frequency of the alleles responsible for the trait, that is, $q = 0.27$. Consequently, the frequency of all alleles conferring metabolism is $1 - 0.27 = 0.73$. If we insert these values into the HW equation, we will get the following:

$$(0.73)^2 + 2(0.27 \times 0.73) + (0.27)^2 = 1$$

$$\text{or } 0.53 + 0.40 + 0.07 = 1$$

indicating that 0.53 (53%) of individuals are carriers of two alleles conferring function (trait AA), 0.4 (40%) carry 1 functional and 1 nonfunctional allele (trait Aa), and 0.07 (7%) have 2 nonfunctional alleles and are poor metabolizers (trait aa). In this example, all functional alleles, regardless of whether they are fully functional or have reduced function, are combined to represent p and all nonfunctional variants are represented by q. HWE can be modified to include additional variables to, for example, represent all alleles with reduced function or defined alleles of interest.

If the number of observed genotypes (p^2, $2pq$, and q^2) or phenotypes/traits (AA, Aa, and aa) deviates from that expected by HWE, the population sample may not be random (e.g., could include related subjects), or large enough or may be biased for a particular phenotype/trait. Frequencies that deviate from the HWE could also be caused when an assay fails to detect all alleles, for instance, when a SNP located on a subset of alleles interferes with allele detection.

Phenotype Prediction from Genotype Data

Within the context of pharmacogenetics, phenotype often refers to a person's activity of a drug-metabolizing enzyme, or metabolizer status. The terms poor/slow and extensive/fast metabolizers were coined when first studies described that portions of a population were distinct in their ability to metabolize certain drugs. The debrisoquine/sparteine polymorphism, for which the underlying cause is polymorphic expression for CYP2D6, is such an example.[60,61] Over the years different probe substrates were used for a given enzyme of interest to determine an individual's phenotype by measuring the compounds and/or their metabolites in body fluids such as urine, plasma, and saliva. Urinary ratios of drug/metabolite are popular measurements to classify individuals into different phenotype groups. Depending on the phenotyping procedure and probe drug used, two to four phenotype groups may be differentiated, that is, poor (PM), intermediate (IM), extensive (EM), and ultrarapid (UM); the latter three, however, often show substantial overlap and clear-cut antimodes may not be available. Phenotyping probe drugs and pharmacokinetic metrics for CYP2D6 phenotyping have been extensively assessed and reviewed by Frank et al. (2007);[62] the criteria described therein also apply for phenotyping procedures of other DMEs.

Polymorphisms in the gene of a DME may greatly impact a person's phenotype. It is therefore tempting to use genotype as a predictor for phenotype. One has to bear in mind, however, that additional environmental factors such as disease, infection, nutrition, concomitant mediation, and supplements may substantially contribute to the variability in drug metabolism, and a person's metabolizer status at a given time. In addition, a genotype test is only as good as the number of alleles tested and a person may carry additional sequence variations that are rare and were not tested or are unknown.

Subjects may be divided into subgroups based on genotype and their mean effect on phenotype. Individuals classified as genotypic PMs have two nonfunctional alleles and genotypic UMs have variants or additional gene copies that are anticipated to exceed activity conveyed by two fully functional allelic variants. Genotypic EMs typically include subjects carrying at least one fully functional allele, while genotypic IMs are characterized by the presence of a nonfunctional and/or reduced function allele. However, some genotypes may not consistently be classified and may be found in the EM or IM group. Classification based on genotype may also be hampered if insufficient data are available regarding the activity of an allele, and, lastly, one also has to consider substrate specificity, that is, one particular variant may have full activity toward one substrate, but altered pharmacokinetics toward another substrate.

To facilitate genotype grouping and prediction from genotype data, especially for highly polymorphic genes such as *CYP2D6*, alternative classification systems have been introduced, among them the "semiquantitative gene dose (GSD)"[63] and "activity score (AS)"[54] systems. Essentially, in these systems, a value is assigned to each allele reflecting no function (value = 0), reduced function (value = 0.5), and full function (value = 1). Gene duplications receive double the value of their single counterparts, for example, *CYP2D6*2×2*, value = 2. The sum of the values for both alleles represents the GSD or AS. For example, *CYP2D6*1/*2×2*, **1/*2*, **1/*4*, **5/*10*, and **3/*6* genotypes have scores of 3, 2, 1, 0.5, and 0, respectively. Advantages and clinical utility of these alternative classification systems have been discussed by Kirchheiner.[64] While these systems are being adopted by many experts in the field, further studies are necessary to better define the values assigned to an allele for a given drug to more accurately reflect its activity. As shown recently on data for drug clearance, the values currently assigned to *CYP2D6*2* and *41* may over-estimate actual activity.[65]

Regardless, however, of which system is used to classify individuals, it should always be clear whether "phenotype" is based on actual phenotype measurement or a genetically predicted phenotype and how subjects were grouped. Unfortunately, in many reports, it is not always clear which genotypes are in which group or whether the correct alleles were examined to determine the genotype in the population and the term phenotype is often employed to describe genetically predicted phenotype, which may not, as discussed above, reflect the actual phenotype of a person at a given time. Clearly, standardized systems for the prediction of phenotype from genotype data would be highly valuable especially for the individualization of drug therapy.

REFERENCES

1. Benes V, Castoldi M. Expression profiling of microRNA using real-time quantitative PCR, how to use it and what is available. *Methods.* 2010;50:244–249.
2. Bertino JR, Banerjee D, Mishra PJ. Pharmacogenomics of microRNA: a miRSNP towards individualized therapy. *Pharmacogenomics.* 2007;8:1625–1627.
3. DNA Genotek. Supplier of saliva collection kits. Available at: www.dnagenotek.com/.
4. NanoDrop Spectrophotometer. Available at: http://www.nanodrop.com/.
5. Johannsen W, ed. *Elemente der exakten Erblichkeitslehre.* Jena: Gustav Fischer; 1909. Available at: http://caliban.mpiz-koeln.mpg.de/johannsen/elemente/index.html.
6. HUGO Gene Nomenclature Committee. Available at: http://www.genenames.org/guidelines.html#genenames.
7. International Human Genome Sequencing Consortium. Finishing the euchromatic sequence of the human genome. *Nature.* 2004;431:931–945.
8. Pennisi E. Gene counters struggle to get the right answer. *Science.* 2003;301:1040–1041.
9. Scherer S. *Guide to the Human Genome.* Cold Spring Harbor, NY: Cold Spring Harbor Laboratory Press; 2008. Available at: http://www.cshlp.org/ghg5_all/section/gene.shtml.
10. National Center for Biotechnology Information (NCBI). Available at: http://www.ncbi.nlm.nih.gov/About/primer/genetics_genome.html.
11. Matlin AJ, Clark F, Smith CWJ. Understanding alternative splicing: towards a cellular code. *Nat Rev Mol Cell Biol.* 2005;6:386–398.
12. Hallegger M, Llorian M, Smith CWJ. Alternative splicing: global insights. *FEBS J.* 2010;277:856–866.
13. Guillemette C, Levesque E, Harvey M, Bellemare J, Menard V. UGT genomic diversity: beyond gene duplication. *Drug Metab Rev.* 2010;42:22–42.
14. UDP-glucuronosyltransferase alleles nomenclature page. Available at: http://www.pharmacogenomics.pha.ulaval.ca/sgc/ugt_alleles/.
15. Genetic Dictionary. Available at: www.biology-online.org/dictionary/Genetic.
16. Genetic Dictionary. Available at: www.merriam-webster.com/dictionary/genetic.
17. Speicher M, Antonarakis S, Motulsky AG, eds. *Vogel and Motulsky's Human Genetics.* 4th ed. Heidelberg: Springer; 2010.
18. Sim E, Lack N, Wang C-J, et al. Arylamine *N*-acetyltransferases: structural and functional implications of polymorphisms. *Toxicology.* 2008;254:170–183.
19. Glucose-6-phosphate. Glucose-6-phosphate dehydrogenase deficiency. Available at: http://g6pddeficiency.org/index.php.
20. NCBI Database for Short Genetic Variations. Available at: www.ncbi.nlm.nih.gov/projects/SNP/.
21. Stephens M, Donnelly P. A comparison of Bayesian methods for haplotype reconstruction from population genotype data. *Am J Hum Genet.* 2003;73:1162–1169.
22. Haploview. Program for haplotype analysis. Available at: http://www.broadinstitute.org/scientific-community/science/programs/medical-and-population-genetics/haploview/haploview.
23. International Warfarin Pharmacogenetics Consortium, Klein TE, Altman RB, et al. Estimation of the warfarin dose with clinical and pharmacogenetic data. *N Engl J Med.* 2009;360:753–764.
24. Rieder MJ, Reiner AP, Gage BF, et al. Effect of *VKORC1* haplotypes on transcriptional regulation and warfarin dose. *N Engl J Med.* 2005;352:2285–2293.
25. Limdi NA, Wadelius M, Cavallari L, et al. Warfarin pharmacogenetics: a single *VKORC1* polymorphism is predictive of dose across 3 racial groups. *Blood.* 2010;115:3827–3834.
26. Wain LV, Armour JAL, Tobin MD. Genomic copy number variation, human health, and disease. *Lancet.* 2009;374(9686):340–350.
27. Database for Genomic Variants. Available at: http://projects.tcag.ca/variation/.
28. Gonzalez FJ, Nebert DW. Evolution of the P450 gene superfamily: animal–plant 'warfare', molecular drive and human genetic differences in drug oxidation. *Trends Genet.* 1990;6:182–186.
29. Lewis DF, Watson E, Lake BG. Evolution of the cytochrome P450 superfamily: sequence alignments and pharmacogenetics. *Mutat Res.* 1998;410:245–270.
30. Nelson DR. The cytochrome P450 homepage. *Hum Genomics.* 2009;4:59–65.
31. Gaedigk A, Twist GP, Leeder JS. *CYP2D6, SULT1A1* and *UGT2B17* copy number variation (CNV): quantitative detection by multiplex PCR. *Pharmacogenomics.* 2012;13:91–111.
32. Zanger UM, Raimundo S, Eichelbaum M. Cytochrome P450 2D6: overview and update on pharmacology, genetics, biochemistry. *Naunyn Schmiedebergs Arch Pharmacol.* 2004;369:23–37.
33. Gaedigk A, Ndjountché L, Divakaran K, et al. Cytochrome P4502D6 (*CYP2D6*) gene locus heterogeneity: characterization of gene duplication events. *Clin Pharmacol Ther.* 2007;81:242–251.
34. Ingelman-Sundberg M, Sim SC, Gomez A, Rodriguez-Antona C. Influence of cytochrome P450 polymorphisms on drug therapies: pharmacogenetic, pharmacoepigenetic and clinical aspects. *Pharmacol Ther.* 2007;116:496–526.
35. Pinto D, Darvishi K, Shi X, et al. Comprehensive assessment of array-based platforms and calling algorithms for detection of copy number variants. *Nat Biotechnol.* 2011;29:512–520.

36. Orchid Cellmark paternity testing. Available at: http://www.orchid cellmark.com/.

37. Advancing criminal justice through DNA technology. Available at: http://www.dna.gov/basics/analysis/str.

38. Bosma PJ, Chowdhury JR, Bakker C, et al. The genetic basis of the reduced expression of bilirubin UDP-glucuronosyltransferase 1 in Gilbert's syndrome. *N Engl J Med.* 1995;333:1171–1175.

39. Uchimoto T, Itoga S, Nezu M, Sunaga M, Tomonaga T, Nomura F. Role of the genetic polymorphisms in the 5′-flanking region for transcriptional regulation of the human *CYP2E1* gene. *Alcohol Clin Exp Res.* 2007;31:36–42.

40. Howard LA, Sellers EM, Tyndale RF. The role of pharmacogenetically-variable cytochrome P450 enzymes in drug abuse and dependence. *Pharmacogenomics.* 2002;3:185–199.

41. HUGO Gene Nomenclature Committee. Available at: http://www.genenames.org/.

42. Home Page of the Human Cytochrome P450 (CYP) Allele Nomenclature Committee. Available at: http://www.cypalleles.ki.se/.

43. Consensus human arylamine *N*-acetyltransferase gene nomenclature. Available at: http://louisville.edu/medschool/pharmacology/consensus-human-arylamine-n-acetyltransferase-gene-nomenclature/.

44. Mannervik B, Board PG, Hayes JD, et al. Nomenclature for mammalian soluble glutathione transferases. *Methods Enzymol.* 2005;401:1–8.

45. Blanchard RL, Freimuth RR, Buck J, Weinshilboum RM, Coughtrie MW. A proposed nomenclature system for the cytosolic sulfotransferase (SULT) superfamily. *Pharmacogenetics.* 2004;14:199–211.

46. Kroetz DL, Pauli-Magnus C, Hodges LM, et al. Sequence diversity and haplotype structure in the human *ABCB1* (*MDR1*, multidrug resistance transporter) gene. *Pharmacogenetics.* 2003;13:481–494.

47. Kim RB, Leake BF, Choo EF, et al. Identification of functionally variant *MDR1* alleles among European Americans and African Americans. *Clin Pharmacol Ther.* 2001;70:189–199.

48. Nebert DW, Nelson DR, Adesnik M, et al. The P450 superfamily: updated listing of all genes and recommended nomenclature for the chromosomal loci. *DNA.* 1989;8:1–13.

49. Nelson DR, Kamataki T, Waxman DJ, et al. The P450 superfamily: update on new sequences, gene mapping, accession numbers, early trivial names of enzymes, and nomenclature. *DNA Cell Biol.* 1993;12:1–51.

50. Nebert DW, Menon AG. Pharmacogenomics, ethnicity, and susceptibility genes. *Pharmacogenomics.* 2001;1:19–22.

51. Urban TJ. Race, ethnicity, ancestry, and pharmacogenetics. *Mt Sinai J Med J Translational Personalized Med.* 2010;77:133–139.

52. Suarez-Kurtz G. *Pharmacogenomics in Admixed Populations.* Rio de Janeiro: Landes Bioscience; 2007.

53. Neafsey P, Ginsberg G, Hattis D, Sonawane B. Genetic polymorphism in cytochrome P450 2D6 (CYP2D6): population distribution of CYP2D6 activity. *J Toxicol Environ Health B Crit Rev.* 2009;12:334–361.

54. Gaedigk A, Simon SD, Pearce RE, Bradford LD, Kennedy MJ, Leeder JS. The CYP2D6 activity score: translating genotype information into a qualitative measure of phenotype. *Clin Pharmacol Ther.* 2008;83:234–242.

55. Sistonen J, Sajantila A, Lao O, Corander J, Barbujani G, Fuselli S. *CYP2D6* worldwide genetic variation shows high frequency of altered activity variants and no continental structure. *Pharmacogenet Genomics.* 2007;17:93–101.

56. Gaedigk A, Bradford LD, Marcucci KA, Leeder JS. Unique CYP2D6 activity distribution and genotype–phenotype discordance in African Americans. *Clin Pharmacol Ther.* 2002;72:76–89.

57. Kim EY, Lee SS, Jung HJ, et al. Robust *CYP2D6* genotype assay including copy number variation using multiplex single-base extension for Asian populations. *Clin Chim Acta.* 2010;411:2043–2048.

58. Suarez-Kurtz G. Pharmacogenetics in the Brazilian population. *Front Pharmacol.* 2010;1:118.

59. Weinberg W. Über den Nachweis der Vererbung beim Menschen. *Jahreshefte des Vereins für vaterländische Naturkunde in Württemberg.* 1908;64:368–382.

60. Mahgoub A, Idle JR, Dring LG, Lancaster R, Smith RL. Polymorphic hydroxylation of debrisoquine in man. *Lancet.* 1977;2:584–586.

61. Eichelbaum M, Spannbrucker N, Steincke B, Dengler HJ. Defective *N*-oxidation of sparteine in man: a new pharmacogenetic defect. *Eur J Clin Pharmacol.* 1979;16:183–187.

62. Frank D, Jaehde U, Fuhr U. Evaluation of probe drugs and pharmacokinetic metrics for CYP2D6 phenotyping. *Eur J Clin Pharmacol.* 2007;63:321–333.

63. Steimer W, Zopf K, von Amelunxen S, et al. Allele-specific change of concentration and functional gene dose for the prediction of steady-state serum concentrations of amitriptyline and nortriptyline in CYP2C19 and CYP2D6 extensive and intermediate metabolizers. *Clin Chem.* 2004;50:1623–1633.

64. Kirchheiner J. CYP2D6 phenotype prediction from genotype: which system is the best? *Clin Pharmacol Ther.* 2008;83:225–227.

65. Abduljalil K, Frank D, Gaedigk A, et al. Assessment of activity levels for *CYP2D6*1*, *CYP2D6*2*, and *CYP2D6*41* genes by population pharmacokinetics of dextromethorphan. *Clin Pharmacol Ther.* 2010;88:643–651.

Analytical Methods to Identify Genetic Variations and Bioinformatics

3

Andrea Gaedigk, MS, PhD, & Xia Yang, PhD

L E A R N I N G   O B J E C T I V E S

- Define terminology for pharmacogenomic testing.
- Outline methods used for genetic testing in pharmacogenomics.
- Provide information on informatics in pharmacogenomics.

METHODS TO DETECT SEQUENCE VARIATIONS

There are numerous methods or platforms to detect DNA sequence variations.[1] These can be divided into two categories, those designed to identify specific SNPs of interest, for example, to determine a person's genotype for a given drug-metabolizing enzyme or a panel of genes, and those supporting genome-wide analyses.

Following are brief descriptions of some popular methods that are frequently used to determine a person's genotype. All depend on the polymerase chain reaction (PCR), which is not described in further detail here; abundant information can be found online or in technical guides provided by manufacturers of PCR supplies.

Restriction-Fragment Length Polymorphisms (RFLPs)

This method exploits a sequence difference between the wild-type and variant that impacts the recognition site of a restriction enzyme. The region of interest is amplified by PCR and subsequently incubated with a restriction enzyme. Resulting fragments are then separated by agarose gel electrophoresis. Figure 3–1 provides an overview. This method was one of the earliest employed for genotyping detecting SNPs. It is simple to perform and requires only basic equipment. It is, however, time consuming due to the enzymatic digestion and electrophoresis step and cannot be automated. RFLP analysis can also be performed on restricted genomic DNA to identify fragment patterns associated with a disease or a phenotype. In that case, the procedure is often referred to as Southern blot analysis.[2]

Real-Time PCR

In real-time (RT) PCR, the formation of amplification product is detected at each cycle. This can be achieved by measuring fluorescent dyes that intercalate into DNA such as SYBR green,[3] fluorogenic-labeled probes such as TaqMan chemistry[3] (also known as "fluorogenic 5" nuclease chemistry), or molecular beacons,[4] to name a few. TaqMan® SNP Genotyping Assays are frequently utilized for ease of use and because over 4.5 million SNP assays are commercially available including 3.5 million HapMap SNPs, 70,000 cSNPs, and 160,000 validated assays.[5] Such assays can also be custom-designed and probes and primers obtained from a variety of sources.

Briefly, each TaqMan assay contains PCR primers and two probes containing different fluorescent dyes. The oligonucleotide probe has a fluorescent dye on the 5′ end that serves as reporter and a quencher dye on the 3′ end preventing it to emit any fluorescence while intact. One probe is designed to perfectly

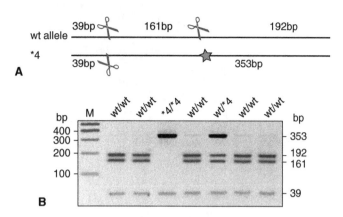

A

B

FIGURE 3–1 Genotyping by RFLP analysis. **(A)** To detect the *CYPD6*4* allelic variant, a 392 base pair (bp) long PCR product was amplified from genomic DNA. The wild-type allele carries two recognition sites for the *BstN*I restriction enzyme as indicated by scissors. The SNP characterizing the *CYP2D6*4* allele destroys one of those sites as indicated by the star. Consequently, the PCR products derived from the wild-type and variant alleles will be cut into three and two fragments, respectively. **(B)** The resulting digestion products were separated by size using agarose gel electrophoresis, visualized with ethidium bromide, a DNA-intercalating dye, and scanned for documentation. Subjects homozygous for the wild-type allele exhibit 192, 161, and 39 bp long fragments, subjects homozygous for *CYP2D6*4* have 363 and 39 bp long fragments, and heterozygous subjects exhibit a composite pattern. Genotypes of the subjects are as indicated. M denotes the 100 bp marker reference ladder.

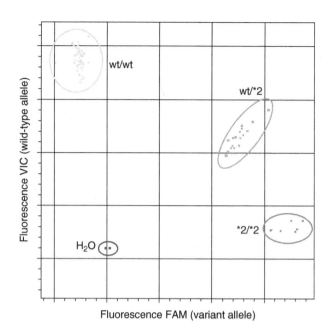

FIGURE 3–2 Genotyping by TaqMan® chemistry. The *CYP2C19*2* allele was genotyped using a commercially available TaqMan® assay from Applied Biosystems. The probes binding to the wild-type and *CYP2C19*2* alleles are labeled with VIC and FAM, respectively. Signal from VIC only indicates that a subject is homozygous for the wild-type allele while signal from FAM only indicates that a subject is homozygous for the *CYP2C19*2* allele. Heterozygous subjects exhibit signals from both dyes. Negative controls containing H_2O instead of DNA show little or no signal. A typical plot shows three distinct genotype clusters.

bind to the wild-type allele, the other to the variant allele. When a probe binds to its target sequence, it will be cleaved by the 5′ nuclease activity of Taq DNA polymerase as PCR takes place. In the process, the reporter dye is separated from the quencher dye generating a reporter dye signal. In each PCR cycle fluorescent dye is cleaved from one or both probes resulting in an increase in fluorescence intensity proportional to the amount of amplicon produced. Figure 3–2 shows the TaqMan assay for a *CYP2D6* SNP. There are three distinct clusters categorizing individuals as homozygous wild-type (FAM signal only) or variant (VIC signal only) or heterozygous (signal from both dyes).

RT-PCR using fluorescent dyes or the DNA-intercalating dye SYBR green is also a mainstay method for the quantitative measurement of RNA expression levels among other applications. RT-PCR-based applications require PCR instrumentation and software, which are available in many laboratories. Because it is set up in 96-well plates and can be automated to a certain extend, it allows for a significantly higher throughput compared with gel-based producers.

High-Resolution Melt (HRM) Curve Analysis

HRM is a powerful technique that allows the detection of sequence variations based on the melting properties of a PCR product. Sequence variations that may be difficult or impossible to detect by RFLP or by TaqMan® may be measured by this

procedure, which has significantly been improved by the development of second-generation dyes such as EvaGreen. Essentially, a PCR product is generated in the presence of the intercalating dye. After PCR, the fragments are melted over a precision gradient and fluoresce measured at tight intervals. Depending on the sequence variation present, heterozygous and homozygous variant PCR fragments exhibit melt characteristics that are slightly, but measurably different from those observed for the wild-type. Differences in the melt characteristics are often displayed as differential plots such as that shown in Figure 3–3.

HRM requires RT-PCR instrumentation capable of creating precise thermogradients and specialized software. This procedure is also performed in multiwell plates and allows for medium to higher throughput.

AmpliChip® CYP450 Test

The AmpliChip® CYP450 Test from Roche Molecular Diagnostics uses microarray technology to test for sequence variations in the *CYP2D6* and *CYP2C19* genes.[6] This test has been approved by the US Food and Drug Administration[7] and is often utilized for clinical testing. In this test, PCR amplicons are generated, fragmented, labeled, hybridized to the microarray, and the bound products stained. Finally, the array is scanned, data analyzed, and the genotype and predicted

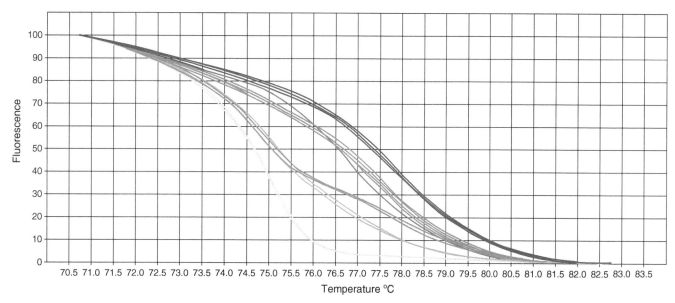

FIGURE 3-3 Genotyping by HRM. PCR fragments were generated from a gene that contains an SNP in a region that is deleted in some subjects. Combinations between the presence and absence of the SNP and the deletion give rise to six different allelic variants. Subjects (or genotypes) can be distinguished by their respective melt curve profiles. Each line in the graph represents a subject.

phenotype determined using the AmpliChip® CYP450 Test algorithm.[8] An advantage of this platform is that many allelic variants are tested side-by-side including some rarer variants. The *CYP2D6* gene deletion and presence of the most common gene duplications are also tested for, but it does not quantitate gene copy number. One downside is that the test requires specialized equipment. It should also be noted that the allele calling algorithm is based on haplotype information that was available at the time the product was developed. Since then, the definition has been updated for some *CYP2D6* allelic variants (haplotype information complemented, novel alleles described). An example is *CYP2D6*31*[9] that triggers a no-call due to a SNP that was not defined as being part of this allele's original haplotype.

Genome-Wide Association Studies (GWAS)

Microarray technology has made vast advances in the last decade and is now routinely utilized in the biomedical research landscape as demonstrated by an explosion of publications on GWAS alone. Early SNP arrays allowed testing for thousands of SNPs. Today, arrays can interrogate up to millions of genetic markers including SNPs and copy number variations (CNVs) throughout the genome. Two market leaders are Affymetrix[10] and Illumina[11] who utilize different technologies, GeneChip® and BeadChip®, respectively. Instead of going into technical details, we rather emphasize the importance of the design of any study that seeks to determine associations between genetic markers and a disease or quantitative trait (e.g., disease [obesity, diabetes], drug therapy [adverse drug reaction, response to a drug]). As reviewed by others,[12-18] success of GWAS studies is particularly based on using well-defined cohorts of subjects with and without the qualitative trait or disease. Furthermore, the

study also needs to be statistically robust and ideally is validated in a replication cohort. For a summary of examples of GWAS in pharmacogenomics, successes, and lessons, we refer to Daly[19] and Motsinger-Reif et al.[20]

Results of GWAS studies are often displayed in so-called Manhattan plots, which summarize the association of each tested genetic variation with the measured trait (Figure 3–4). One good example for a GWAS is a study in which the authors sought to identify gene variants that influence the response to clopidogrel, a drug that is often used to prevent ischemic events by inhibiting platelet aggregation. In the Manhattan plot of that particular study, the only SNPs with a significant association to the outcome measure, that is, inhibition of adenosine diphosphate (ADP)–dependent platelet activation, were within the *CYP2C* gene cluster containing the *CYP2C19* gene known to be involved in clopidogrel activation.[21]

Another example from the field of pharmacogenomics is a recent study that identified an association between drug-induced liver injury due to flucloxacillin and SNPs in the major histocompatibility complex (MHC) on chromosome 6.[22] This finding led to the discovery that the *HLA-B*5701* allele is a strong marker for this adverse event, which was replicated in a second cohort of subjects affected by the ADR. This study also demonstrated that GWAS not always requires large number of subjects, but can successfully be performed on subjects with well-defined phenotypes.

Detection of Copy Number Variation

On a genome-wide scale, CNVs, in particular deletions and duplications of larger chromosomal regions, can now be detected via microarray technology as described above. These arrays, however, may not detect CNVs of particular genes important

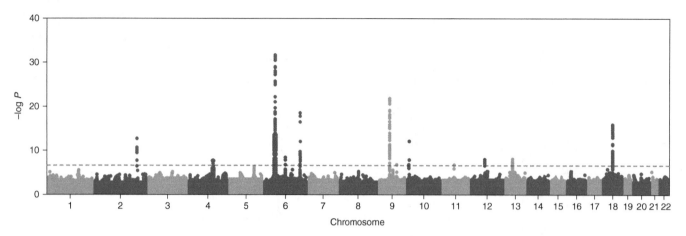

FIGURE 3–4 Representation of a Manhattan plot of a genome-wide association study (GWAS). In this example a number of sequence variations were associated with a trait of interest as indicated by peaks that reach *P*-values <10⁻⁷ (dotted line). (Reproduced with permission from Petukhova L, Duvic M, Hordinsky M, et. al. Genome-wide association study in *Alopecia areata* implicates both innate and adaptive immunity. *Nature.* 2010;466:113–117.)

for drug metabolism and disposition including members of the *CYP, UGT, GST,* and *SULT* gene families.

Subjects who are homozygous for a gene deletion can simply be identified by the absence of PCR product after gel electrophoresis or by generating long-range PCR products with primers binding to regions adjacent to the deletion or amplifying a duplication-specific product. However, these approaches do not allow discrimination between heterozygous carriers and those who are homozygous for the deletion or wild-type (depending on assay design). To determine gene copy number more accurately, quantitative PCR employing fluorescent probes (see Chapter 2) is probably the most commonly used method.[23–25] Other methods and platforms include pyrosequencing,[26] multiplex PCR analysis,[27,28] and LabChip microfluidic technology,[29,30] to name a few. Most of these methods are capable of discriminating between 0, 1, 2, and 3 copies; however, there is a paucity of information concerning how well platforms discriminate higher gene copy numbers, that is, 3, 4, 5, etc. Also, there are no gold standards for CNV detection for and the lack of validated samples, especially for higher copy numbers, makes the CNV assay validation process difficult. Furthermore, DNA quantity and quality is of utmost importance for these assays and may have crucial impact on assay accuracy as commented on by Shrestha et al.,[31] and references therein.

CYP2D6 is a gene that is not only highly polymorphic regarding SNPs and small indels but also affected by CNVs and gene rearrangements with *CYP2D7,* a highly homologous pseudogene. Taken together, this makes *CYP2D6* CNV determination rather difficult. In order to address challenges such as discrimination of higher copy number, variability in DNA quality, and presence of hybrid genes,[32–35] Gaedigk et al. have designed a multiplex PCR-based platform that determines *CYP2D6* copy number in four different gene regions[36] along CNVs of *UGT2B17* and *SULT1A1.* Figure 3–5 depicts gene copy number determined for the exon 1 region. The highlighted symbols

in the graph denote subjects who switch copy number clusters according to their genotype. For instance, the subject with the *CYP2D6*5/*66* genotype has one allele with the gene deletion (*5) and one hybrid allele composed of *CYP2D7* and *CYP2D6* (*66). Depending on which gene region is tested, the *CYP2D6* gene copy number for this individual is 0 or 1.

DNA Sequencing

DNA sequencing methods have first been described in the 1970s by Maxam and Gilbert[37] and Sanger et al.[38] The method described by Sanger et al, also referred to as "samger sequencing" or 'chain-terminator method', quickly became the method of choice. Essentially, a sequencing reaction contains DNA template (plasmid, PCR product, or other DNA template), a DNA primer (short oligonucleotide), DNA polymerase, and a mixture of deoxynucleotidephosphates (dNTPs) for DNA strand elongation and dideoxynucleotide triphosphates (ddNTP) for DNA strand termination. By strand extension and termination a ladder of products is generated from which the DNA nucleotide sequence can be inferred (Figure 3–6). Initially, one of the dNTPs or the sequencing primer was labeled radioactively and four separate reactions carried out, each of which contained one of the four ddNTPs (ddATP, ddCTP, ddGTP, or ddTTP). Resulting fragments were separated by acrylamide gel electrophoresis and fragments visualized by exposure to x-ray film. Read lengths per reaction averaged 200–500 base pairs (bp) depending on the length of the gel and run time. As fluorescent dye technology advanced, ddNTPs were synthesized with different fluorescent labels enabling single-tube reactions. Elongated fragments were detected by a laser as they migrated through a gel matrix. In the 1990s, slab gel electrophoresis was eventually replaced by more sophisticated instrumentation utilizing capillary electrophoresis (CE).[39] This technical evolution was significant to increase read length per reaction and throughput.

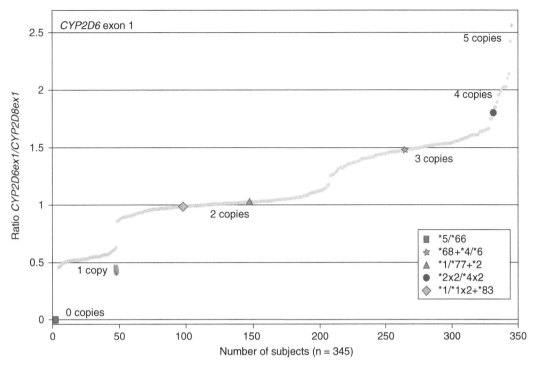

FIGURE 3–5 Quantitative PCR to determine gene copy number variation (CNV). To determine *CYP2D6* gene copy number, a region containing exon 1 was amplified simultaneously from *CYP2D6, 7,* and *8.* Because the size of the PCR product differs for each gene, they could be discriminated by capillary electrophoresis. The peak height of *CYP2D6* was normalized against that measured for *CYP2D8,* which is believed to always have two gene copies. A ratio of 0.5 indicates that there is one *CYP2D6* gene copy, a ratio of 1 indicates two gene copies, and so forth. For additional assay details including assay testing other *CYP2D6* gene regions, please see Ref.[36] Five subjects are highlighted by larger symbols because they switch clusters, that is, have different copy number results depending on the gene region tested. This observation is due to the presence of hybrid genes composed of *CYP2D6* and *CYP2D7.* The insert provides the *CYP2D6* genotypes for the highlighted subjects. (Adapted from Gaedigk et al. *Pharmacogenomics.* 2012;13:91–111.)

On average, read lengths exceed 500–700 bp per reaction, but can exceed 1,000 bp. Furthermore, in conjunction with a "shotgun" sequencing approach and the development of powerful and sophisticated software and DNA analysis tools (i.e., bioinformatics), CE revolutionized DNA sequence analysis as demonstrated by the generation of the first human consensus sequences of the Human Genome Project.[40,41] Today, capillary sequencing instruments are a mainstay in every molecular laboratory. In addition to DNA sequence analysis, CE is also frequently utilized to determine the size of PCR fragments, for example, in the analysis of repetitive DNA sequences (Chapter 2). CE was also utilized for the *CYP2D6* CNV assay described above and shown in Figure 3–5.

Next-generation sequencing (NGS), also known as massively parallel sequencing, constitutes yet another revolution in the genomic landscape. The first individual human genome sequence was obtained by NGS[42] in 2008 demonstrating the power of this technology that heavily relies on bioinformatics. For general overviews and technical details of major NGS platforms, please see Refs.[43–45] In addition to generating sequence data, NGS is also capable of reliably detecting SNPs, small deletions, and insertions ranging from 1 to ~1,000 bp in length as well as larger gene CNVs. Whole genome sequencing, however, is still relatively expensive and time consuming; therefore, many studies perform exome sequencing instead, that is, analyze the coding sequences only.[46] To use NGS even more cost-effectively, sequence analysis may comprise entire genes and adjacent sequences, but limit the number of genes interrogated.[47] NGS technology was also rapidly adapted to RNA sequencing to gain insights into the transcriptome (all RNAs expressed in a cell) on an unprecedented level.[48] Another area of research that profits immensely from NGS is epigenetics (the study of DNA modifications).[49]

There are a growing number of reports demonstrating the power of whole genome and exon sequencing using NGS. Recent cases include the discovery of sequence variations in patients with Charcot–Marie–Tooth neuropathy and intractable inflammatory bowel disease, respectively, explaining rare genetic conditions.[50–52] Whole genome sequencing, however, produces a wealth of information, which may not always be easy to interpret and immediately translate into clinical action. This is exemplified by a study entitled *Clinical Assessment Incorporating a Personal Genome.*[53,54] An integrated analysis of whole genome sequencing of "patient zero" within a clinical context revealed sequence variations that are consistent with family history, but issues related to translating population data to actionable information at the level of individual patients illustrate the future challenges for personalized medicine.

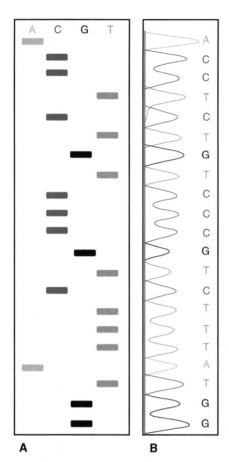

FIGURE 3–6 DNA sequence analysis. DNA sequence analysis using the chain-terminator method, also known as Sanger sequencing.[38] **(A)** Graphic display of a radioactive sequencing gel. Bands in respective lanes indicate the nucleotide sequence (starting at the bottom the first two bands are in the "G" lane followed by bands in the "T" and "A" lanes; the sequence is therefore "GGTA..."). Sequences were typically manually entered on file for data analysis. **(B)** Fluorescence is detected by a laser as fragments migrate through a capillary. Data are electronically captured and visualized as fluorescent peaks and can easily be imported into a variety of sequence analysis software packages.

Databases/Sources for Sequence Variation

Various databases have been developed to catalog sequence variations discovered to date, with some focusing on global collection of variations and some more specified for particular fields. The mostly used global databases include National Center for Biotechnology Information (NCBI) dbSNP,[55–57] Ensembl Variation database,[58] HapMap Project,[59,60] the 1000 Genomes Project,[61] Human Gene Mutation Database (HGMD),[62] and the Human Genome Variation Society (HGVS).[63] Databases focusing on structural variations include NCBI dbVAR,[64] Database of Genetic Variants (DGV),[65] and Human Genome Structural Variation Project.[66] Many disease-focused genetic variation databases such as the National Human Genome Research Institute (NHGRI) GWAS catalog[67,68] that systematically

compile suggestive and significant genetic variations associated with diseases or traits (including pharmacogenomic traits such as efficacy, adverse effects, dosage, and toxicity) from GWAS and Genetic Association Database[69] (GAD)[70] that catalogs all literature-based findings including those from candidate-gene-based genetic association studies are also available. There are also population-specific databases such as Pan SNPdb[71] that contains variations identified from 1,719 unrelated individuals from 71 populations from China (including Taiwan), India, Indonesia, Japan, Malaysia, the Philippines, Singapore, South Korea, and Thailand.[72] Examples of the databases emphasizing pharmacogenomic utilities include the Pharmacogenomics Knowledge Base (PharmGKB),[73] Cytochrome P450 (CYP) Allele Nomenclature Committee,[74] and Human Membrane Transporter Database (HMTD).[75] In this chapter, we focus on discussing selected global variation and pharmacogenomic-related databases.

Global Variation Databases

dbSNP

dbSNP[56,57] database was established by NCBI and NHGRI in 1998. It relies on submissions from various sources including individual laboratories, collaborative polymorphism discovery efforts, large-scale genome sequencing centers, and private industry. It archives genetic variations of 100 organisms as of August 1, 2011 and the list will continue to grow. The types of variations collected include SNPs, indels, microsatellites, short tandem repeats (STRs), multinucleotide polymorphisms (MNPs), and polymorphic insertion elements such as retrotransposons.[56] Although the name dbSNP does not reflect the fact that it covers many different types of sequence variations other than just SNPs, the majority of the variations are indeed SNPs. Of all species together, there are a total of 244 million submitted SNPs (ssSNPs with IDs starting with "ss"), ~88 million assigned reference SNPs (RefSNPs or rsSNPs with IDs starting with "rs"), and ~30 million validated SNPs. For the human genome, it currently holds over 143 million ssSNPs, >30 million rsSNPs, and ~20 million validated SNPs. The validated SNPs include those with supporting evidence from multiple independent submissions, frequency of genotype data, submitter confirmation, observation of all alleles in at least two chromosomes, and genotyped by HapMap and/or sequenced in the 1000 Genomes Project. For each rsSNP, the information available includes ss number ID, rs number ID, gene name, experimental method, population class, population detail, publication, marker, allele, chromosome, base position, heterozygosity range, build number, strain, heterozygosity, and genotype frequencies. Users can use various tools available at dbSNP to view the position of the variation in a gene, in the genome, in relation to introns, exons, other variants, codon changes, amino acid changes, predicted function of a gene such as synonymous or nonsynonymous, 3D structures of the encoded protein, etc. The dbSNP is also linked to other NCBI resources such as the nucleotide, protein, gene, taxonomy, and structure databases, PubMed, Online Mendelian Inheritance in Man (OMIM), and UniGene, allowing quick integration of information on a given variation. Likewise, dbSNP information can be easily accessed while surfing at other NCBI resources as well as non-NCBI bioinformatics sites such as UCSC Genome Browser[76–78] and Ensembl Variation database[58] that provides additional bioinformatic tools to access and analyze genetic variations.

As dbSNP entries originate from submissions of various resources, it is susceptible to false positives due to variable qualities of data from submitters. It has been estimated that the false-positive rate is between 15% and 17% for SNPs. Cautions are to be taken while using all submitted SNPs and restricting the attention to only validated SNPs may be necessary to reduce false discoveries.[79]

HapMap

The International HapMap Project[59,60] aims to identify the patterns of sequence variations in various populations. More specifically, it targets to identify haplotypes, that is, sets of associated SNP alleles in a chromosomal region that tend to be inherited together, as well as tag SNPs for each haplotype that most represent the pattern of genetic variations within each haplotype. Besides the importance of understanding the organization of human variations, the identified haplotypes and tag SNPs have substantial practical values in helping reduce genotyping cost and multiple testing issues (see detailed discussions in the section "Genetic Association of Pharmacogenomics Phenotypes"). For example, instead of genotyping or analyzing all 30 million validated SNPs in human genome, one can focus on testing a much smaller set of tag SNPs. HapMap was initiated in 2002 and to date has released three phases of data—HapMap1,[80] HapMap2,[81] and HapMap3[82]—into the public domain. HapMap1[80] was released in 2005 and identified more than 1 million SNPs with accurate and complete genotypes from 269 DNA samples from four populations—Yoruba people in Ibadan, Nigeria (YRI), Japanese in Tokyo (JPT), Chinese in Beijing (CHB), and the CEPH (residents with ancestry from Northern and Western Europe, collected in 1980 by the Centre d'Etude du Polymorphisme Humain) in the United States (CEU). HapMap1 demonstrated long segments of block-like structures of linkage disequilibrium (LD) and low haplotype diversity that leads to substantial correlations of SNPs with many of their neighboring SNPs, variations in haplotype frequency in different populations, and the feasibility of selecting and utilizing tag SNPs. HapMap2[81] was released in 2007 and reported 3.1 million SNPs from 270 samples of the same 4 populations as in HapMap1. It can capture ungenotyped common variations with an average maximum LD r^2 of between 0.9 and 0.96 depending on the population and can be used for imputation of ungenotyped SNPs to increase power of association studies, although up to 1% of all common variants are untaggable, primarily because they lie within recombination hotspots. HapMap3 was released in 2010 and presented both common and rare variants in 11 populations using a combination of genotyping and low-coverage DNA sequence data. The 11 populations include the 4 populations used in HapMap1 and HapMap2, African ancestry in the southwestern United States (ASW); Chinese in metropolitan Denver, Colorado, USA (CHD); Gujarati Indians in Houston, Texas, USA (GIH); Luhya in Webuye, Kenya (LWK); Maasai in Kinyawa, Kenya (MKK); Mexican ancestry in Los Angeles, California, USA (MXL); and Tuscans in Italy (Toscani in Italia, TSI). In total, 1.6 million common SNPs were genotyped in 1,184 reference individuals and ten 100-kilobase (kb) regions in 692 of these individuals were sequenced, with the later approach uncovering both novel SNPs and copy number polymorphisms (CNPs; CNVs with frequency of >1%). Imputation accuracy was found to be improved with this expanded reference panel and the feasibility of imputing novel CNPs and SNPs was also demonstrated. Compared with dbSNP, HapMap provides LD structure as well as tag SNPs. In addition, HapMap implements uniform and sophisticated quality control and therefore the false-positive rate is lower.

The 1000 Genomes Project

The 1000 Genomes Project[61] was initiated in 2008 on the maturation of NGS technologies with the aims to discover, genotype, and provide haplotype information on all types of sequence variations in about 2,500 unidentified people from over 20 populations using whole genome sequencing. The pilot study of HapMap samples representing five major population groups (populations in or with ancestry from Europe, East Asia, South Asia, West Africa, and the Americas) was completed in 2010[83] and the location, allele frequency, and local haplotype structure of approximately 15 million SNPs, 1 million indels, and 20,000 structural variants were reported.[83] It is estimated that each person on average carries 250–300 loss-of-function variants in annotated genes and 50–100 variants previously implicated in inherited disorders. The raw sequence files, alignment, variant calls, sample list, as well as sequencing progress can be obtained from the Web site. As sequencing can capture all types of variations, the completion of this project will symbolize a near-complete catalog of human variations.

Pharmacogenomics-Related Variation Databases

The Pharmacogenomics Knowledge Base

PharmGKB[73,84] is designed to curate human genetic variations that impact drug response as well as provide comprehensive relationships between genetic variations, genes, drugs, pathways, and diseases. Genomic, phenotype, and clinical information from ongoing pharmacogenetic and genomic studies is collected and is made accessible. SNPs are annotated by gene, drug, and disease and can be easily browsed and downloaded.

Cytochrome P450 (CYP) Allele Nomenclature Committee

This Web page is attributed to the allele nomenclatures of CYPs.[74] It collects known SNPs as well as their known functional consequences at amino acid and enzyme activity levels for each CYP isoform in each family. Although informative, the functionality of this site could be improved by implementing a database structure. This would not only facilitate batch downloading of all collections but also make cross-referencing of SNPs observed in the P450 genes with their official dbSNP

IDs more effective as well as enable direct mapping between databases.

Human Membrane Transporter Databases

The HMTD[85] is dedicated to membrane transporters and provides information on transporter family, chromosomal location, tissue distribution, genetic variants, disease association, 3D structure, and substrate/drug information. The UCSF–FDA TransPortal Database[86] is a recently established collaborative project between the University of California, San Francisco and the FDA. It serves as a repository of information on transporters that are important in the drug discovery process as a part of the US Food and Drug Administration–led Critical Path Initiative. This database contains information regarding the expression, localization, substrates, inhibitors, and drug–drug interactions of transporters.

BIOINFORMATIC TOOLS TO ANALYZE SEQUENCE VARIATIONS/PREDICT FUNCTIONAL CONSEQUENCE

Identification of genetic variations that affect a particular clinical phenotype such as drug metabolism or drug response does not directly infer the mechanisms through which the sequence changes manifest. Therefore, an understanding of the functional consequences of these variations on genes and/or proteins is necessary to explain why certain genetic polymorphisms influence specific phenotypes. Genetic variations can be either coding or noncoding. A coding sequence variation occurs in the coding region, that is, exons, of a gene and can be either synonymous or nonsynonymous. Nonsynonymous coding variations cause protein level changes such as single amino acid alterations resulting from single nucleotide changes, frameshift from insertions or deletions, or protein of abnormal length (even loss of protein product) via either gain or loss of stop codons. On the other hand, synonymous coding variations and noncoding variations may affect mRNA transcript levels by modulating the transcription factor binding sites (promoters, enhancers, and/or silencers) or sequences that are important for mRNA stability. Alternatively, they can cause variations in the mRNA transcript isoforms and hence protein isoforms by changing alternative splicing sites. Although in vivo or in vitro experiments provide reliable evidence for a particular functional mechanism, these wet-lab processes are laborious and costly and thus merit in silico methods that can help preselect candidate variations for experimental testing and guide experimental design.

Tools for Predicting Functional Consequences of Sequence Variation

Various bioinformatics tools have been developed to help predict the functional consequences of genetic variations.[87] A summary of available software packages including sequence variation categories, functional prediction categories, underlying algorithms and databases, and accessibility is provided in Table 3–1. As nonsynonymous coding variations impose changes in protein sequences and thus may have direct impact on the structures and functions of proteins, this type of variation has been the focus of a majority of the available tools such as SIFT,[88] SNAP,[89] PolyPhen,[90] SNPeffect,[91–93] LS-SNP,[94,95] and SNPs3D.[96] However, recent GWAS have revealed that nearly 40% of disease/trait-associated SNPs are located in intergenic regions and another 40% in intronic sequences. In contrast, only 12% are located in or close to protein-coding regions of genes and only <5% are nonsynonymous SNPs (nsSNPs).[107] Therefore, these nsSNP-focused tools are of very limited use for the majority of disease-associated variants.

In recent years, more integrative software packages that are capable of providing broader categorization of functional effects have been developed to not only help predict protein level changes but also assess many other aspects such as transcription factor binding sites, alternative splicing, and interactions with microRNAs (miRNAs) by leveraging multiple programs and databases. These include Variant Effect Predictor (formerly SNP Effect Predictor),[108] FastSNP,[109] SNPnexus,[110] ANNOVAR,[111] SNP function portal,[112] F-SNP,[113] Sequence Variant Analyzer (SVA),[114] and SeattleSeq Annotation[115] (Table 3–1). Among these, Variant Effect Predictor, FastSNP, SNPnexus, F-SNP, and SNP function portal mainly focus on known variants collected in public variant databases such as dbSNP[55] and the Ensembl Variation database,[58] and the others can also annotate novel variations from NGS data. Taking Variant Effect Predictor (link in Table 3–1) as an example, it utilizes the Ensembl Variation database to extract the relevant gene transcript(s) and corresponding gene of a variation, the relative location of the variation to the transcript(s), functional consequence types, and the predicted amino acid changes for a given list of sequence variations. The consequence types available through this tool include intergenic, regulatory region, upstream (within 5 kb), 5′ UTR, complex indel (spans intron/exon border), splice site (spans 1–3 bp into exon/3–8 bp into intron), synonymous coding, nonsynonymous coding, intronic, essential splice site (first/last 2 bp of intron), frameshift coding, stop gained, stop lost, 3′ UTR, downstream (within 5 kb), within noncoding gene, and within mature miRNA. Another tool, F-SNP (Table 3–1), borrows the strengths from 16 programs and databases and summarizes SNPs as functional or nonfunctional based on four functional categories, namely, protein coding, splicing regulation, transcriptional regulation, and posttranslation regulation.

With NGS technology becoming more mature and affordable, whole genome and exome sequencing studies have discovered millions of novel genetic variations[83] and additional novel rare variants associated with various diseases or traits will continue to be discovered, making the need for tools that can predict the function of novel variations as well as large numbers of variations (typically >3 million variants for a given human genome) more pressing. Tools such as ANNOVAR, SVA, and

TABLE 3–1 Bioinformatic tools to help predict functional consequences of genetic variations.

Variation Type	Software	Web Site	Function Prediction	Database	Algorithms/Programs	Special Notes
nsSNP	SIFT[88]	http://sift-dna.org	Whether an amino acid substitution affects protein function	SWISS-PROT, SWISS-PROT/TrEMBL, or NCBI's nonredundant protein databases	Based on sequence homology and conservation as well as the physical properties of amino acids	
nsSNP	SNAP[89]	http://www.rostlab.org/services/SNAP/	Classifies all nsSNPs in all proteins into non-neutral (effect on function) and neutral (no effect)	Protein Mutant Database, SWISS-PROT, UniProt, PROFacc, PROFsec, Pfam	Neural network (NN)–based method by incorporating sequence alignment, evolutionary information, predicted aspects of protein structure, family information	Includes predictions from SIFT and PolyPhen
nsSNP	PolyPhen[90]	http://genetics.bwh.harvard.edu/pph	Estimates the impact of an amino acid replacement on the three-dimensional structure and function of the protein	SWALL, Protein Data Bank (PDB), HSSP, SWISS-PROT	Uses a rule-based cutoff system on available data including 3D structures, SWISS-PROT annotations, and alignments	
nsSNP	SNPeffect[91-93]	http://snpeffect.vib.be	Structural, functional, and cellular effects on the amino acid change of a nonsynonymous coding SNP	UniProt knowledge base, PDB, Ensembl, dbSNP	Sequence- and structure-based position-specific scoring matrix	
nsSNP	LS-SNP[94,95]	http://www.salilab.org/LS-SNP	Predicts positions where nsSNPs destabilize proteins, interfere with the formation of domain–domain interfaces, have an effect on protein–ligand binding	SWISS-PROT, TrEMBL, MODBASE, PIBASE	Multiple sequence alignment (MSA) with an iterative database search	
nsSNP	SNPs3D[96]	http://www.SNPs3D.org	Identifies nsSNPs with deleterious effects on molecular function in vivo	HGMG, dbSNP, MutDB, protein databank	Requires coordinates of three-dimensional (3D) protein structures and utilizes support vector machines to recognize structural patterns	
nsSNP	PMUT[97]	http://mmb2.pcb.ub.es:8080/PMut/	Prediction (~80% success rate in humans) of the pathological character of single point amino acidic mutations based on the use of NNs	SWISS-PROT/TrEMBL, PDB, PMUT	Based on the use of NNs trained with a large database of neutral mutations (NEMUs) and pathological mutations	
nsSNP	PANTHER[98]	http://www.pantherdb.org/tools/csnpScoreForm.jsp	Estimates the likelihood of a particular nsSNP to cause a functional impact on the protein	PANTHER	Calculates the substitution position-specific evolutionary conservation (subPSEC) score based on an alignment of evolutionarily related proteins	
nsSNP	SNP@Domain[99]	http://snpnavigator.net	Annotates SNPs from dbSNP with protein structure-based as well as sequence-based domains	SCOP, Pfam, Ensembl, dbSNP, OMIM	Performs a structure-based domain assignment using the PDB-ISL method	

(Continued)

TABLE 3–1 Bioinformatic tools to help predict functional consequences of genetic variations. (*Continued*)

Variation Type	Software	Web Site	Function Prediction	Database	Algorithms/Programs	Special Notes
nsSNP	PolyDoms[100]	http://polydoms.cchmc.org/polydoms/	Predicts structural and functional impacts of all nsSNPs	NCBI CDD, PDB, NCBI Entrez Gene, OMIM, SwissChange, GAD, MGI	Uses SIFT, PolyPhen, and LS-SNP to predict impact of nsSNP on protein function	SIFT, PolyPhen, and LS-SNP combined
nsSNP	StSNP[101]	http://ilyinlab.org/StSNP/	Maps nsSNPs onto protein structures	dbSNP, PDB, NCBI protein, Entrez Gene, KEGG	Maps nsSNPs onto protein structures by comparative modeling of structure with nsSNPs by MODELLER (http://salilab.org) and visualizes their structural locations by using the multiple structure-sequence viewer Friend	
nsSNP	Snap[102]	http://snap.humgen.au.dk	Positions nsSNPs to sequences with protein features including protein sorting, posttranslational modifications, protein structure and function, amino acid modifications, change indicators, regions, secondary structures	Ensembl, UniProt/SWISS-PROT, Pfam, DAS-CBS, MINT, BIND, KEGG, CVDB, PigGIS, TreeFam	The protein features from SWISS-PROT and Pfam numbering 2 115 643 are mapped to the DNA sequence to assign further biological meaning	
nsSNP	MAPP	http://mendel.stanford.edu/SidowLab/downloads/MAPP/index.html	Predicts the impact of all nsSNPs on protein function		Prediction is based on the multisequence alignment and physiochemical properties of amino acid substitutions	
spSNP	AASsites[103]	http://genius.embnet.dkfz-heidelberg.de/menu/biounit/open-husar	Predicts SNPs that modify splicing	ssSNP target database, DBASS, Ensembl	GenScan, HMMgene, GeneID, GlimmerHMM, GrailEXP6, GeneWise, ESEfinder	Many programs combined
spSNP	Augustus[104]	http://augustus.gobics.de/	Predicts alternative splicing and alternative transcripts		Based on a Generalized Hidden Markov Model, a probabilistic model of a sequence and its gene structure	
Regulatory	PupaSuite[91,105]	http://pupasuite.bioinfo.cipf.es/.	Exonic splicing silencers (ESS), enhancers, transcription factor binding sites, new splice sites, miRNAs	ESS set from Wang et al,[106] JASPAR, TRANSFAC	Position weight matrices, MatScan, GeneID, miRanda, etc.	Interaccessibility with SNPeffect; human, mouse, and rat genomes
All	Variant Effect Predictor[108]	http://uswest.ensembl.org/tools.html	Predict both coding and noncoding effects of genetic variants	Ensembl Variation database, Ensembl Functional Genomics database	Ensembl API, Perl, MySQL	
All	FastSNP[109]	http://fastsnp.ibms.sinica.edu.tw	Predict both coding and noncoding effects of genetic variants and assess risk of SNPs	EnsemblMart, Ensembl Protein Report, SwissProg, dbSNP, UCSC GoldenPath, HapMap	Use TFSearch, PolyPhen, ESEfinder, RESCUE-ESE, FAS-ESS to predict functional category and use decision tree–based method to assess risk of SNPs	Many programs combined

Tool	Coverage	URL	Function	Databases	Implementation	Comments
SNPnexus[110]	All	http://www.snp-nexus.org/	Possible effects on the transcriptome and proteome levels are characterized and reported from five major annotation systems including gene/protein location and consequences, regulatory elements, structural variations, etc.	NCBI RefSeq, UCSC, Ensembl, the Vertebrate Genome Annotation (VEGA), AceView, EnsemblMart_48, GAD, miRBase, Database of Genomic Variants (DGV)	Perl annotation pipeline and MySQL database	
SNP function portal[112]	All	http://brainarray.mbni.med.umich.edu/Brainarray/Database/SearchSNP/snpfunc.aspx	Annotate SNPs using six major categories including genomic elements, transcription regulation, protein function, pathway, disease, and population genetics	dbSNP, UniSTS, NCBI ideogram, Entrez Gene, NCBI human genome assembly and HapMap2, TRANSFAC, InterPro, PubMed, Gene Ontology, KEGG, BioCarta, OMIM	Relational SNP database is built on Oracle 10g. Web function was implemented with Net, ASP, JSP, and Perl	
F-SNP[113]	All	http://compbio.cs.queensu.ca/F-SNP/	Integrate information from 16 bioinformatics tools and databases about the functional effects (splicing, transcriptional, translational, and posttranslational level) of SNPs	Ensembl, GoldenPath	PolyPhen, SIFT, SNPeffect, SNPs3D, and LS-SNP for nsSNPs; ESEfinder, RESCUE-ESE, ESRsearch, and PESX for SNPs in exonic splice regions; the Ensembl database for nonsense SNPs and SNPs in intronic splice sites; TFSearch and ConSite for transcriptional regulatory SNPs in promoter regions; the Ensembl and GoldenPath for other transcriptional regulatory regions, OGPET and Sulfinator for posttranslation modification sites. GoldenPath for conserved genomic regions	Integrate 16 tools and databases
ANNOVAR[111]	All	http://www.openbioinformatics.org/annovar/	Annotate functional effects of variants with respect to genes, conserved genomic regions, predicted transcription factor binding sites, microRNA target sites, and stable RNA secondary structures	UCSC Genome Browser, RefSeq genes, UCSC genes, Ensembl genes	Perl, SIFT, PolyPhen	Designed for sequencing data and can annotate novel variants
Sequence Variant Analyzer (SVA)[114]	All	http://www.svaproject.org/	Annotate SNPs, indels, and structural variants based on coding changes, splicing, regulatory regions, and noncoding RNA	NCBI RefSeq, Ensembl core and variation databases, UCSC Genome Browser, Go Ontology, KEGG, RefSNP, HapMap, 1000 Genomes Project, DGV	Java, NetBeans IDE, Java Swing	Annotate, visualize, and analyze the genetic variants identified through next-generation sequencing studies
SeattleSeq	All	http://gvs.gs.washington.edu/SeattleSeqAnnotation/	Annotate SNPs with protein positions, amino acid changes, conservation scores, distance to splice sites, PolyPhen predictions, microRNAs, and clinical association	Same as SVA		Include PolyPhen. Can annotate novel SNPs and are suitable for sequencing data

Note: nsSNP, nonsynonymous SNP; spSNP, SNP that may affect alternative splicing.

SeattleSeq have been developed to meet this need. ANNOVAR (Table 3–1) utilizes UCSC Genome Browser and Ensembl to identify variants within a gene and report closest genes, amino acid changes, mutations affecting the gain or loss of stop codons, changes in most conserved elements, and the predicted transcription factor binding sites. SVA uses NCBI reference sequences, the Ensembl core, and variation databases as the main source of annotation features for genes and variations. Other annotations such as transcription factor binding sites from the UCSC Genome Browser and known variants in HapMap, the 1000 Genomes Project, and the DGV databases are also included. One unique feature of SVA is that the annotation results can be linked with statistical tools to help further test the association between the predicted functional SNPs and a particular disease state. SeattleSeq Annotation (Table 3–1) annotates both known and novel SNPs with gene mapping, SNP functions, protein positions, and amino acid changes, conservation scores, allele frequencies, PolyPhen predictions, and clinical association. As the use of NGS continues to grow, we expect to see a growing list of such tools in the near future.

All the tools discussed above are freely available and each has its distinct features. The users need to choose the appropriate ones based on the types and number of variants under investigation, the functional category of focus, and the run time of the tools. As the underlying algorithms vary, the predictions may not be consistent between software packages. Therefore, it is necessary to test a few and summarize the results in order to obtain more reliable predictions. It is important to note that although these bioinformatics tools are useful for inferring how a genetic variation exerts its functional effect, the inferences they make can only be interpreted as speculative. Experimental testing is ultimately necessary to confirm the predictions.

BIOINFORMATICS APPROACHES TO ASSESSING ASSOCIATIONS BETWEEN GENOTYPE, INTERMEDIATE MOLECULAR TRAITS, AND PHENOTYPES

With advances in genotyping and sequencing technologies, genome-wide genotyping has become a reality and hence genetic association studies have largely deviated from the candidate gene approaches and entered the GWAS era. Based on the NHGRI GWAS catalog (accessed July 17, 2011),[67,116] a total of 48 pharmacogenomics GWAS studies had been conducted as of July 2011 to investigate the pharmacogenomics of various therapeutic agents in terms of dosage, therapeutic efficacy, adverse events, or hepatotoxicity. As most genotyping panels involve hundreds of thousands to a couple million SNPs, computationally and statistically intensive tools are needed to evaluate the association between SNPs and diseases/traits. An even more computationally intensive task is to study the genetics of intermediate molecular traits such as genetics of gene expression (GGE) as it requires the calculation of all pairwise relationships between millions of

SNPs and thousands of gene expression traits. Here we briefly discuss the computational and statistical considerations behind these analyses and introduce the PLINK toolset[117,118] for GWAS analysis.

Genetic Association of Pharmacogenomics Phenotypes

For pharmacogenomics GWAS, the traits of interest are therapeutic efficacy, dosage, adverse events, and toxicity. These traits can be categorical (such as responders and nonresponders) or quantitative (e.g., reduction in low-density lipoprotein [LDL] cholesterol levels). Different statistical tests are needed for such different types of traits. For categorical traits, chi-square test, Fisher's exact test, and Cochran–Armitage trend test can be used, whereas for quantitative traits, likelihood ratio test, Wald test, linear regression, and Kruskal–Wallis test can be used.[117,119] Besides consideration of statistical methods for single-SNP association tests to determine the significance of an association, a particular statistical issue that GWAS encounters is multiple comparison or multiple testing. Multiple testing refers to the situation where multiple statistical inferences are made simultaneously and by chance a certain proportion of the inferences is incorrect when all tests are considered together. For example, when 1 million SNPs are simultaneously tested for association with a trait, at a statistical level of $P < .05$, there could be 50,000 SNPs called significant simply by chance. Therefore, correction for multiple testing is critical to reduce false discoveries. In general, the genome-wide significance cutoff is set to $P < 5e-8$ and in most GWAS only a few or at most tens of SNPs can reach this level of significance. While keeping false discovery levels low, multiple testing correction also imposes high penalties to GWAS as it allows the detection of only signals of strong effect and may lose true causal SNPs conveying more subtle effects. Therefore, post-GWAS mining of smaller sets of SNPs driven by certain hypothesis such as pathways or functionally related gene sets is necessary to further differentiate true signals from noise. To this end, various SNP-set-based approaches have been developed (see Wang et al. for a comprehensive review).[120]

A powerful toolset, PLINK, has been developed to facilitate GWAS analysis.[88] PLINK is an open-source C/C++ toolset that supports data quality control, summary statistics, association analysis, and population stratification. Both command line–driven PLINK and a Java-based GUI version, gPLINK, are freely available for download with detailed instructions and tutorials. To date, PLINK has been the most widely used toolset for GWAS analysis.

Genetics of Intermediate Traits

As discussed earlier, the identification of association between genetic variations and clinical traits does not directly infer the mechanisms. Although a large number of bioinformatics tools have been developed to help predict the functional consequences of sequence variations as discussed in the previous section, empirical evidence is needed to support the predictions. Furthermore, functional variations that are not predicted by the bioinformatics tools may still exist. The study of the relationship between the genome and intermediate molecular traits such as gene expression, alternative splicing, and protein products can fill these gaps.

The most extensively studied intermediate molecular trait to date is the transcription levels of genes and the study of genetic variations that are associated with gene expression is termed GGE. Through such studies, one can simultaneously scan for associations between millions of SNPs and tens of thousands of genes of the human genome to determine which genetic loci are linked to the expression of which genes. Such genetic loci are termed expression quantitative loci (eQTLs) and individual SNPs under eQTLs are named expression SNPs (eSNPs). In a similar fashion, QTLs or SNPs that are associated with other molecular traits such as alternative splicing, allelic expression, and enzyme activity can also be identified. These QTLs or SNPs linking to intermediate molecular traits are useful in predicting the functions of the genetic variations.

GGE studies have been conducted primarily in lymphocytes or lymphoblastoid cell lines due to the ease of sample collection.[121–127] Recently, studies on additional tissues and cell types including monocytes,[128] fibroblast,[129] T cells,[129] liver,[119,130] and adipose tissues[130] have also been conducted. These studies support the presence of both shared eQTLs and tissue- or cell type-specific eQTLs. Moreover, only eQTLs from relevant tissues or cell types are more informative for a particular disease or trait.[130]

In addition to eQTLs through GGE studies, QTLs for other intermediate molecular traits such as alternative splicing (asQTLs),[124,131–133] allelic expression (aeQTLs),[134,135] DNA methylation (mQTLs),[136–141] and liver enzyme activity (aQTLs)[142] have also been pursued. As the technologies for genome-wide measurement of other intermediate traits such as miRNAs, proteomics, and metabolites mature, other types of QTLs can also be detected to further enrich the empirical annotation of functional variations.

As liver is the most relevant tissue for pharmacogenomic studies, functional variations identified in this particular tissue can of particular interest to these fields. In two recent studies, Schadt et al.[119] and Yang et al.[142] fully investigated the genetic architecture of liver gene expression as well as the enzyme activities of cytochrome P450s using ~500 human liver samples. More than 3,000 eQTLs for >6,000 distinct liver genes were reported, among which hundreds of genes encode drug-metabolizing enzymes and transporters. In addition to GGE analysis, genetics of activity measures of nine key drug-metabolizing P450 enzymes, namely, CYP1A2, CYP2A6, CYP2B6, CYP2C8, CYP2C9, CYP2C19, CYP2D6, CYP2E1, and CYP3A4, were also studied and ~60 aSNPs were found to be associated with the activities of all of these enzymes except for CYP2E1. These eSNPs and aSNPs discovered from the human liver studies are of importance for pharmacogenomic studies as they help to understand the impact of individual genetic variations on drug-metabolizing enzymes, transporters, and liver drug targets.

Integration of Genetics of Intermediate Molecular Traits and Phenotypes to Infer Causality and Mechanisms

Although correlation between an SNP and a molecular trait does not directly infer causal relationship, it is possible that a true functional SNP is in LD with the observed associated SNP. When the same genetic loci or SNPs are found to be associated with a human disease or trait, the genes that are linked to these QTLs or SNPs represent more plausible candidate causal genes. For instance, Schadt et al. identified three genes, namely, SORT1, CELSR2, and PSRC1, whose expression levels are associated with the 1p13 locus that was linked to coronary artery disease (CAD) and LDL, with SORT1 showing the strongest association.[119] While SORT1 is far more distant to the locus than three other reported candidate genes CELSR1, PSCR1, and MYBPHL, it was recently experimentally confirmed to be the causal gene underlying this locus for both LDL and CAD.[143,144]

Similarly, the genetic loci discovered from pharmacogenomic GWAS can be queried against the functional SNPs in relevant tissues such as liver to gain insights into the candidate causal genes and underlying mechanisms between the loci and drug response, adverse effect, or toxicity. Application of this approach has helped establish the mechanistic connections between sequence variations in the CYP2C9 and VKORC1 genes and warfarin dosage/response, HLA-DRB1 and lumiracoxib-related liver injury, SLCO1B1 and statin side effect, MICB/HLA-B/HLA-C and flucloxacillin-induced liver injury, SORT1/CELSR2/PSRC1 and statin response, and FAD1/FAD2/FAD3 and statin response[145] among others.

SUMMARY

The field of genetic testing and informatics is growing exponentially. Currently there are multiple resources available to researchers and clinicians. A basic understanding and referencing is provided here for the reader to use in an attempt to clarify this area.

REFERENCES

1. Morlighem JE, Harbers M, Traeger-Synodinos J, Lezhava A. DNA amplification techniques in pharmacogenomics. *Pharmacogenomics*. 2011;12(6): 845–860.
2. Restriction fragment length polymorphism (RFLP). Available at: http://www.ncbi.nlm.nih.gov/projects/genome/probe/doc/TechRFLP.shtml.
3. TaqMan. TaqMan and SYBR green chemistries. Available at: http://www.appliedbiosystems.com/absite/us/en/home/applications-technologies/real-time-pcr/taqman-and-sybr-green-chemistries.html?ICID=EDI-Lrn4.
4. Molecular beacons. Genotyping single nucleotide polymorphisms with molecular beacons. Available at: http://www.molecular-beacons.org/download/marras,m&p03%2821%29111.pdf.
5. Applied Biosystems. Available at: http://www.appliedbiosystems.com.
6. AmpliChip® CYP450 test. Available at: http://www.roche.com/products/product-details.htm?type=product&id=17.
7. Roche AmpliChip Cytochrome P450 Genotyping test and Affymetrix GeneChip Microarray Instrumentation System—K042259. FDA approval. Available at: http://www.fda.gov/MedicalDevices/ProductsandMedicalProcedures/DeviceApprovalsandClearances/Recently-ApprovedDevices/ucm078879.htm.

8. AmpliChip CYP450 test. CE-IVD [package insert]. Branchburg, NJ: Roche Molecular Systems Inc; January 2009.

9. Gaedigk A, Isidoro-Garcia M, Pearce RE, et al. Discovery of the non-functional *CYP2D6*31* allele in Spanish, Puerto Rican, and US Hispanic populations. *Eur J Clin Pharmacol.* 2010;66(9):859–864.

10. Affymetrix DNA microarray technology. Available at: http://www.affymetrix.com.

11. Illumina. DNA microarray technology. Available at: http://www.illumina.com.

12. DiStefano J, Taverna D. Technological issues and experimental design of gene association studies. *Methods Mol Biol.* 2011;700:3–16.

13. Iles M. Genome-wide association studies. *Methods Mol Biol.* 2011;713:89–103.

14. Pare G. Genome-wide association studies—data generation, storage, interpretation, and bioinformatics. *J Cardiovasc Transl Res.* 2010;3(3):183–188.

15. Roberts R, Wells GA, Stewart AF, Dandona S, Chen L. The genome-wide association study—a new era for common polygenic disorders. *J Cardiovasc Transl Res.* 2010;3(3):173–182.

16. Sale MM, Mychaleckyj JC, Chen WM. Planning and executing a genome wide association study (GWAS). *Methods Mol Biol.* 2009;590:403–418.

17. Smith J, Newton-Cheh C. Genome-wide association studies in humans. *Methods Mol Biol.* 2009;573:231–258.

18. Weale ME. Quality control for genome-wide association studies. *Methods Mol Biol.* 2010;628:341–372.

19. Daly AK. Genome-wide association studies in pharmacogenomics. *Nat Rev Genet.* 2010;11(4):241–246.

20. Motsinger-Reif AA, Jorgenson E, Relling MV, et al. Genome-wide association studies in pharmacogenomics: successes and lessons. *Pharmacogenet Genomics.* 2011, doi: 10.1097/FPC.0b013e32833d7b45.

21. Shuldiner AR, O'Connell JR, Bliden KP, et al. Association of cytochrome P450 2C19 genotype with the antiplatelet effect and clinical efficacy of clopidogrel therapy. *JAMA.* 2009;302(8):849–857.

22. Daly AK, Donaldson PT, Bhatnagar P, et al. HLA-B*5701 genotype is a major determinant of drug-induced liver injury due to flucloxacillin. *Nat Genet.* 2009;41(7):816–819.

23. Gallagher CJ, Kadlubar FF, Muscat JE, Ambrosone CB, Lang NP, Lazarus P. The *UGT2B17* gene deletion polymorphism and risk of prostate cancer. A case–control study in Caucasians. *Cancer Detect Prev.* 2007;31(4):310–315.

24. Hosono N, Kato M, Kiyotani K, et al. *CYP2D6* genotyping for functional-gene dosage analysis by allele copy number detection. *Clin Chem.* 2009;55(8):1546–1554.

25. Nguyen DL, Staeker J, Laika B, Steimer W. TaqMan real-time PCR quantification strategy of *CYP2D6* gene copy number for the LightCycler 2.0. *Clin Chim Acta.* 2009;403(1–2):207–211.

26. Söderbäck E, Zackrisson A-L, Lindblom B, Alderborn A. Determination of *CYP2D6* gene copy number by pyrosequencing. *Clin Chem.* 2005;51:522–531.

27. Hebbring SJ, Adjei AA, Baer JL, et al. Human *SULT1A1* gene: copy number differences and functional implications. *Hum Mol Genet.* 2006;16:463–470.

28. Leandro-Garcia LJ, Leskela S, Montero-Conde C, et al. Determination of *CYP2D6* gene copy number by multiplex polymerase chain reaction analysis. *Anal. Biochem.* 2009;389(1):74–76.

29. Gaedigk A, Gaedigk R, Leeder JS. *UGT2B17* and *SULT1A1* gene copy number variation (CNV) detection by LabChip microfluidic technology. *Clin Chem Lab Med.* 2010;48(5):627–633.

30. Nakamura N, Fukuda T, Nonen S, Hashimoto K, Azuma J, Gemma N. Simple and accurate determination of *CYP2D6* gene copy number by a loop-mediated isothermal amplification method and an electrochemical DNA chip. *Clin Chim Acta.* 2010;411(7–8):568–573.

31. Shrestha S, Tang J, Kaslow RA. Gene copy number: learning to count past two. *Nat Med.* 2009;15(10):1127–1129.

32. Gaedigk A, Fuhr U, Johnson C, Berard LA, Bradford D, Leeder JS. *CYP2D7-2D6* hybrid tandems: identification of novel *CYP2D6* duplication arrangements and implications for phenotype prediction. *Pharmacogenomics.* 2010;11(1):43–53.

33. Gaedigk A, Montane Jaime LK, Bertino JS, et al. Identification of novel *CYP2D7-2D6* hybrids: non-functional and functional variants. *Front Pharmacol.* 2010;1:121 [doi: 10.3389/fphar.2010.00121].

34. Ramamoorthy A, Flockhart DA, Hosono N, Kubo M, Nakamura Y, Skaar TC. Differential quantification of *CYP2D6* gene copy number by four different quantitative real-time PCR assays. *Pharmacogenet Genomics.* 2010 2010;20:451–454.

35. Ramamoorthy A, Skaar TC. Gene copy number variations: it is important to determine which allele is affected. *Pharmacogenomics.* 2011;12(3):299–301.

36. Gaedigk A, Twist GP, Leeder JS. *CYP2D6, SULT1A1* and *UGT2B17* copy number variation (CNV): quantitative detection by multiplex PCR. *Pharmacogenomics.* 2012;13(1):91–111.

37. Maxam AM, Gilbert W. A new method for sequencing DNA. *Proc Natl Acad Sci U S A.* 1977;74(2):560–564.

38. Sanger F, Nicklen S, Coulson AR. DNA sequencing with chain-terminating inhibitors. *Proc Natl Acad Sci U S A.* 1977;74(12):5463–5467.

39. Karger BL, Guttman A. DNA sequencing by CE. *Electrophoresis.* 2009;30(suppl 1):S196–S202.

40. Lander ES, Consortium IHGS. Initial sequencing and analysis of the human genome. *Nature.* 2001;409(6822):860–921.

41. Venter JC, Adams MD, Myers EW, et al. The sequence of the human genome. *Science.* 2001;291(5507):1304–1351.

42. Levy S, Sutton G, Ng PC, et al. The diploid genome sequence of an individual human. *PLoS Biol.* 2007;5(10):e254.

43. Zhang J, Chiodini R, Badr A, Zhang G. The impact of next-generation sequencing on genomics. *J Genet Genomics.* 2011;38(3):95–109.

44. Zhou X, Ren L, Meng Q, Li Y, Yu Y, Yu J. The next-generation sequencing technology and application. *Protein Cell.* 2010;1(6):520–536.

45. Metzker ML. Sequencing technologies—the next generation. *Nat Rev Genet.* 2010;11(1):31–46.

46. Teer JK, Mullikin JC. Exome sequencing: the sweet spot before whole genomes. *Hum Mol Genet.* 2010;19(R2):R145–R151.

47. Bell CJ, Dinwiddie DL, Miller NA, et al. Carrier testing for severe childhood recessive diseases by next-generation sequencing. *Sci Transl Med.* 2011;3(65):65ra64.

48. Costa V, Angelini C, De Feis I, Ciccodicola A. Uncovering the complexity of transcriptomes with RNA-Seq. *J Biomed Biotechnol.* 2010;2010:853916.

49. Bell JT, Spector TD. A twin approach to unraveling epigenetics. *Trends Genet.* 2011;27(3):116–125.

50. Lupski JR, Reid JG, Gonzaga-Jauregui C, et al. Whole-genome sequencing in a patient with Charcot–Marie–Tooth neuropathy. *N Engl J Med.* 2010;362(13):1181–1191.

51. Worthey EA, Mayer AN, Syverson GD, et al. Making a definitive diagnosis: successful clinical application of whole exome sequencing in a child with intractable inflammatory bowel disease. *Genet Med.* 2011;13(3):255–262. Also see http://www.jsonline.com/features/health/111224104.html.

52. Mayer AN, Dimmock DP, Arca MJ, et al. A timely arrival for genomic medicine. *Genet Med.* 2011;13(3):195–196.

53. Ashley EA, Butte AJ, Wheeler MT, et al. Clinical assessment incorporating a personal genome. *Lancet.* 2010;375(9725):1525–1535.

54. Ormond KE, Wheeler MT, Hudgins L, et al. Challenges in the clinical application of whole-genome sequencing. *Lancet.* 2010;375(9727):1749–1751.

55. Jaiswal AK. Human NAD(P)H:quinone oxidoreductase (NQO1) gene structure and induction by dioxin. *Biochemistry.* 1991;30:10647–10653.

56. Sherry ST, Ward M, Sirotkin K. dbSNP-database for single nucleotide polymorphisms and other classes of minor genetic variation. *Genome Res.* 1999;9(8):677–679.

57. Smigielski EM, Sirotkin K, Ward M, Sherry ST. dbSNP: a database of single nucleotide polymorphisms. *Nucleic Acids Res.* 2000;28(1):352–355.

58. Grant DM, Hughes NC, Janezic SA, et al. Human acetyltransferase polymorphisms. *Mutat Res.* 1997;376:61–70.

59. International HapMap Consortium. The International HapMap Project. *Nature.* 2003;426(6968):789–796.

60. de Morais SMF, Goldstein JA, Xie H-G, et al. Genetic analysis of the S-mephenytoin polymorphism in a Chinese population. *Clin Pharmacol Ther.* 1995;58:404–410.

61. Xie H-G, Xu Z-H, Luo X, Huang S-L, Zeng F-D, Zhou H-H. Genetic polymorphism of debrisoquine and S-mephenytoin oxidation metabolism in Chinese populations: a meta-analysis. *Pharmacogenetics.* 1996; 6:235–238.

62. Nowak MP, Tyndale RF, Sellers EM. CYP2D6 phenotype and genotype in a Canadian Native Indian population. *Pharmacogenetics.* 1997;7:145–148.

63. Vatsis KP, Weber WW, Bell DA, et al. Nomenclature for N-acetyltransferases. *Pharmacogenetics.* 1995;5:1–17.

64. Inoue K, Yamazaki H, Imiya K, Akasaka S, Guengerich FP, Shimada T. Relationship between CYP2C9 and 2C19 genotypes and tolbutamide methyl hydroxylation and S-mephenytoin 4′-hydroxylation activities in livers of Japanese and Caucasian populations. *Pharmacogenetics.* 1997;7:103–113.

65. Monaghan G, Foster B, Jurima-Romet M, Hume R, Burchell B. UGT1*1 genotyping in a Canadian Inuit population. *Pharmacogenetics.* 1997;7:153–156.

66. Jurima-Romet M, Foster BC, Rode A, et al. CYP2D6-related oxidation polymorphism in a Canadian Inuit population. *Can J Physiol Pharmacol.* 1997;75:165–172.

67. Hindorff LA, Sethupathy P, Junkins HA, et al. Potential etiologic and functional implications of genome-wide association loci for human diseases and traits. *Proc Natl Acad Sci U S A.* 2009;106(23):9362–9367.

68. Lind C, Hochstein P, Ernster L. DT-diaphorase as a quinone reductase: a cellular control device against semiquinone and superoxide radical formation. *Arch Biochem Biophys.* 1982;216:178–185.

69. Becker KG, Barnes KC, Bright TJ, Wang SA. The genetic association database. *Nat Genet.* 2004;36(5):431–432.

70. Siegel D, Gibson NW, Preusch PC, Ross D. Metabolism of mitomycin C by DT-diaphorase: role in mitomycin C-induced DNA damage and cytotoxicity in human colon carcinoma cells. *Cancer Res.* 1990;50: 7483–7489.

71. Ngamphiw C, Assawamakin A, Xu S, et al. PanSNPdb: the Pan-Asian SNP genotyping database. *PLoS One.* 2011;6(6):e21451.

72. Abdulla MA, Ahmed I, Assawamakin A, et al. Mapping human genetic diversity in Asia. *Science.* 2009;326(5959):1541–1545.

73. Siegel D, Gibson NW, Preusch PC, Ross D. Metabolism of diaziquone by NAD(P)H:(quinone acceptor)oxidoreductase (DT-diaphorase): role in diaziquone-induced DNA damage and cytotoxicity in human carcinoma cells. *Cancer Res.* 1990;50:7293–7300.

74. Walton MI, Smith PJ, Workman P. The role of NAD(P)H:quinone reductase (EC 1.6.99.2 DT-diaphorase) in the reductive bioactivation of the novel indoloquinone antitumor agent EO9. *Cancer Commun.* 1991;3:199–206.

75. Gibson NW, Hartley JA, Butler J, Siegel D, Ross D. Relationship between DT-diaphorase-mediated metabolism of a series of aziridinylbenzoquinones and DNA damage and cytotoxicity. *Mol. Pharmacol.* 1992;42:531–536.

76. Kent WJ, Sugnet CW, Furey TS, et al. The human genome browser at UCSC. *Genome Res.* 2002;12(6):996–1006.

77. Fujita PA, Rhead B, Zweig AS, et al. The UCSC Genome Browser database: update 2011. *Nucleic Acids Res.* 2011;39(database issue):D876–D882.

78. UCSC Genome Browser. Available at: http://genome.ucsc.edu/.

79. Mitchell AA, Zwick ME, Chakravarti A, Cutler DJ. Discrepancies in dbSNP confirmation rates and allele frequency distributions from varying genotyping error rates and patterns. *Bioinformatics.* 2004;20(7):1022–1032.

80. International HapMap Consortium. A haplotype map of the human genome. *Nature.* 2005;437(7063):1299–1320.

81. Frazer KA, Ballinger DG, Cox DR, et al. A second generation human haplotype map of over 3.1 million SNPs. *Nature.* 2007;449(7164):851–861.

82. Altshuler DM, Gibbs RA, Peltonen L, et al. Integrating common and rare genetic variation in diverse human populations. *Nature.* 2010; 467(7311):52–58.

83. 1000 Genomes Project Consortium. A map of human genome variation from population-scale sequencing. *Nature.* 2010;467(7319):1061–1073.

84. Hewett M, Oliver DE, Rubin DL, et al. PharmGKB: the Pharmacogenetics Knowledge Base. *Nucleic Acids Res.* 2002;30(1):163–165.

85. The Human Membrane Transporter Database. Available at: http://lab .digibench.net/transporter/.

86. Winner EJ, Prough RA, Brennan MD. Human NAD(P)H:quinone oxidoreductase induction in human hepatoma cells after exposure to industrial acylates, phenolics, and metals. *Drug Metab Dispos.* 1997;25: 175–181.

87. Karchin R. Next generation tools for the annotation of human SNPs. *Brief Bioinform.* 2009;10(1):35–52.

88. Ng PC, Henikoff S. SIFT: predicting amino acid changes that affect protein function. *Nucleic Acids Res.* 2003;31(13):3812–3814.

89. Bromberg Y, Rost B. SNAP: predict effect of non-synonymous polymorphisms on function. *Nucleic Acids Res.* 2007;35(11):3823–3835.

90. Sunyaev S, Ramensky V, Koch I, Lathe W 3rd, Kondrashov AS, Bork P. Prediction of deleterious human alleles. *Hum Mol Genet.* 2001;10(6): 591–597.

91. Reumers J, Conde L, Medina I, et al. Joint annotation of coding and non-coding single nucleotide polymorphisms and mutations in the SNPeffect and PupaSuite databases. *Nucleic Acids Res.* 2008;36(database issue):D825–D829.

92. Reumers J, Maurer-Stroh S, Schymkowitz J, Rousseau F. SNPeffect v2.0: a new step in investigating the molecular phenotypic effects of human non-synonymous SNPs. *Bioinformatics.* 2006;22(17):2183–2185.

93. Reumers J, Schymkowitz J, Ferkinghoff-Borg J, Stricher F, Serrano L, Rousseau F. SNPeffect: a database mapping molecular phenotypic effects of human non-synonymous coding SNPs. *Nucleic Acids Res.* 2005;33(database issue):D527–D532.

94. Ryan M, Diekhans M, Lien S, Liu Y, Karchin R. LS-SNP/PDB: annotated non-synonymous SNPs mapped to Protein Data Bank structures. *Bioinformatics.* 2009;25(11):1431–1432.

95. Karchin R, Diekhans M, Kelly L, et al. LS-SNP: large-scale annotation of coding non-synonymous SNPs based on multiple information sources. *Bioinformatics.* 2005;21(12):2814–2820.

96. Yue P, Melamud E, Moult J. SNPs3D: candidate gene and SNP selection for association studies. *BMC Bioinform.* 2006;7:166.

97. Ferrer-Costa C, Gelpi JL, Zamakola L, Parraga I, de la Cruz X, Orozco M. PMUT: a web-based tool for the annotation of pathological mutations on proteins. *Bioinformatics.* 2005;21(14):3176–3178.

98. Thomas PD, Campbell MJ, Kejariwal A, et al. PANTHER: a library of protein families and subfamilies indexed by function. *Genome Res.* 2003;13(9):2129–2141.

99. Han A, Kang HJ, Cho Y, Lee S, Kim YJ, Gong S. SNP@Domain: a web resource of single nucleotide polymorphisms (SNPs) within protein domain structures and sequences. *Nucleic Acids Res.* 2006;34(Web server issue):W642–W644.

100. Jegga AG, Gowrisankar S, Chen J, Aronow BJ. PolyDoms: a whole genome database for the identification of non-synonymous coding SNPs with the potential to impact disease. *Nucleic Acids Res.* 2007;35(database issue):D700–D706.

101. Uzun A, Leslin CM, Abyzov A, Ilyin V. Structure SNP (StSNP): a web server for mapping and modeling nsSNPs on protein structures with linkage to metabolic pathways. *Nucleic Acids Res.* 2007;35(Web server issue):W384–W392.

102. Li S, Ma L, Li H, et al. Snap: an integrated SNP annotation platform. *Nucleic Acids Res.* 2007;35(database issue):D707–D710.

103. Faber K, Glatting K, Mueller P, Risch A, Hotz-Wagenblatt A. Genome-wide prediction of splice-modifying SNPs in human genes using a new analysis pipeline called AASsites. *BMC Bioinform.* 2011;12(suppl 4):S2.

104. Stanke M, Keller O, Gunduz I, Hayes A, Waack S, Morgenstern B. AUGUSTUS: ab initio prediction of alternative transcripts. *Nucleic Acids Res.* 2006;34(Web server issue):W435–W439.

105. Conde L, Vaquerizas JM, Dopazo H, et al. PupaSuite: finding functional single nucleotide polymorphisms for large-scale genotyping purposes. *Nucleic Acids Res.* 2006;34(Web server issue):W621–W625.

106. Wang Z, Rolish ME, Yeo G, Tung V, Mawson M, Burge CB. Systematic identification and analysis of exonic splicing silencers. *Cell.* 2004;119(6):831–845.

107. Manolio TA. Genomewide association studies and assessment of the risk of disease. *N Engl J Med.* 2010;363(2):166–176.

108. McLaren W, Pritchard B, Rios D, Chen Y, Flicek P, Cunningham F. Deriving the consequences of genomic variants with the Ensembl API and SNP Effect Predictor. *Bioinformatics*. 2010;26(16):2069–2070.

109. Yuan HY, Chiou JJ, Tseng WH, et al. FASTSNP: an always up-to-date and extendable service for SNP function analysis and prioritization. *Nucleic Acids Res*. 2006;34(Web server issue):W635–W641.

110. Chelala C, Khan A, Lemoine NR. SNPnexus: a web database for functional annotation of newly discovered and public domain single nucleotide polymorphisms. *Bioinformatics*. 2009;25(5):655–661.

111. Wang K, Li M, Hakonarson H. ANNOVAR: functional annotation of genetic variants from high-throughput sequencing data. *Nucleic Acids Res*. 2010;38(16):e164.

112. Wang P, Dai M, Xuan W, et al. SNP Function Portal: a web database for exploring the function implication of SNP alleles. *Bioinformatics*. 2006;22(14):e523–e529.

113. Lee PH, Shatkay H. F-SNP: computationally predicted functional SNPs for disease association studies. *Nucleic Acids Res*. 2008;36(database issue):D820–D824.

114. Ge D, Ruzzo EK, Shianna KV, et al. SVA: software for annotating and visualizing sequenced human genomes. *Bioinformatics*. 2011;27(14):1998–2000.

115. Broly F, Gaedigk A, Heim U, Eichelbaum M, Mörike K, Meyer UA. Debrisoquine/sparteine hydroxylation genotype and phenotype: analysis of common mutations and alleles of CYP2D6 in European populations. *DNA Cell Biol*. 1991;10:545–557.

116. Hindorff L, Junkins H, Hall P, Mehta J, Manolio T. *A Catalog of Published Genome-Wide Association Studies*.

117. Purcell S, Neale B, Todd-Brown K, et al. PLINK: a tool set for whole-genome association and population-based linkage analyses. *Am J Hum Genet*. 2007;81(3):559–575.

118. Dahl ML, Yue Q-Y, Roh HK, et al. Genetic analysis of the CYP2D locus in relation to debrisoquine hydroxylation capacity in Korean, Japanese and Chinese subjects. *Pharmacogenetics*. 1995;5:159–164.

119. Schadt EE, Molony C, Chudin E, et al. Mapping the genetic architecture of gene expression in human liver. *PLoS Biol*. 2008;6(5):e107.

120. Wang K, Li M, Hakonarson H. Analysing biological pathways in genome-wide association studies. *Nat Rev Genet*. 2010;11(12):843–854.

121. Dixon AL, Liang L, Moffatt MF, et al. A genome-wide association study of global gene expression. *Nat Genet*. 2007;39(10):1202–1207.

122. Emilsson V, Thorleifsson G, Zhang B, et al. Genetics of gene expression and its effect on disease. *Nature*. 2008;452(7186):423–428.

123. Goring HH, Curran JE, Johnson MP, et al. Discovery of expression QTLs using large-scale transcriptional profiling in human lymphocytes. *Nat Genet*. 2007;39(10):1208–1216.

124. Montgomery SB, Sammeth M, Gutierrez-Arcelus M, et al. Transcriptome genetics using second generation sequencing in a Caucasian population. *Nature*. 2010;464(7289):773–777.

125. Pickrell JK, Marioni JC, Pai AA, et al. Understanding mechanisms underlying human gene expression variation with RNA sequencing. *Nature*. 2010;464(7289):768–772.

126. Stranger BE, Nica AC, Forrest MS, et al. Population genomics of human gene expression. *Nat Genet*. 2007;39(10):1217–1224.

127. Veyrieras JB, Kudaravalli S, Kim SY, et al. High-resolution mapping of expression-QTLs yields insight into human gene regulation. *PLoS Genet*. 2008;4(10):e1000214.

128. Zeller T, Wild P, Szymczak S, et al. Genetics and beyond—the transcriptome of human monocytes and disease susceptibility. *PLoS One*. 2010;5(5):e10693.

129. Dimas AS, Deutsch S, Stranger BE, et al. Common regulatory variation impacts gene expression in a cell type-dependent manner. *Science*. 2009;325(5945):1246–1250.

130. Zhong H, Beaulaurier J, Lum PY, et al. Liver and adipose expression associated SNPs are enriched for association to type 2 diabetes. *PLoS Genet*. 2010;6:e1000932.

131. Coulombe-Huntington J, Lam KC, Dias C, Majewski J. Fine-scale variation and genetic determinants of alternative splicing across individuals. *PLoS Genet*. 2009;5(12):e1000766.

132. Heinzen EL, Ge D, Cronin KD, et al. Tissue-specific genetic control of splicing: implications for the study of complex traits. *PLoS Biol*. 2008;6(12):e1.

133. Nembaware V, Lupindo B, Schouest K, Spillane C, Scheffler K, Seoighe C. Genome-wide survey of allele-specific splicing in humans. *BMC Genomics*. 2008;9:265.

134. Ge B, Pokholok DK, Kwan T, et al. Global patterns of cis variation in human cells revealed by high-density allelic expression analysis. *Nat Genet*. 2009;41(11):1216–1222.

135. Heap GA, Yang JH, Downes K, et al. Genome-wide analysis of allelic expression imbalance in human primary cells by high-throughput transcriptome resequencing. *Hum Mol Genet*. 2010;19(1):122–134.

136. Gibbs JR, van der Brug MP, Hernandez DG, et al. Abundant quantitative trait loci exist for DNA methylation and gene expression in human brain. *PLoS Genet*. 2010;6(5):e1000952.

137. Kerkel K, Spadola A, Yuan E, et al. Genomic surveys by methylation-sensitive SNP analysis identify sequence-dependent allele-specific DNA methylation. *Nat Genet*. 2008;40(7):904–908.

138. Ollikainen M, Smith KR, Joo EJ, et al. DNA methylation analysis of multiple tissues from newborn twins reveals both genetic and intrauterine components to variation in the human neonatal epigenome. *Hum Mol Genet*. 2010;19(21):4176–4188.

139. Schalkwyk LC, Meaburn EL, Smith R, et al. Allelic skewing of DNA methylation is widespread across the genome. *Am J Hum Genet*. 2010;86(2):196–212.

140. Shoemaker R, Deng J, Wang W, Zhang K. Allele-specific methylation is prevalent and is contributed by CpG-SNPs in the human genome. *Genome Res*. 2010;20(7):883–889.

141. Zhang D, Cheng L, Badner JA, et al. Genetic control of individual differences in gene-specific methylation in human brain. *Am J Hum Genet*. 2010;86(3):411–419.

142. Yang X, Zhang B, Molony C, et al. Systematic genetic and genomic analysis of cytochrome P450 enzyme activities in human liver. *Genome Res*. 2010;20(8):1020–1036.

143. Kjolby M, Andersen OM, Breiderhoff T, et al. Sort1, encoded by the cardiovascular risk locus 1p13.3, is a regulator of hepatic lipoprotein export. *Cell Metab*. 2010;12(3):213–223.

144. Musunuru K, Strong A, Frank-Kamenetsky M, et al. From noncoding variant to phenotype via SORT1 at the 1p13 cholesterol locus. *Nature*. 2010;466(7307):714–719.

145. Kasarskis A, Yang X, Schadt EE. Integrative genomics strategies to elucidate the complexity of drug response. *Pharmacogenomics*. 2011;12(12):1695–715.

Regulatory Considerations in Pharmacogenomics at EMA and US FDA

4

Markus Paulmichl, MD, Marc Maliepaard, PhD
Marisa Papaluca, MD, & Christian Grimstein, PhD

LEARNING OBJECTIVES

- Review and discuss the regulatory considerations for pharmacogenomics set forth by the European Medicines Agency (EMA).

- Review and discuss the regulatory considerations for pharmacogenomics set forth by the US Food and Drug Administration (FDA).

- Understand how these regulatory agencies have similarities and differences in their rules and application.

PHARMACOGENOMICS (PGx) AT THE EUROPEAN MEDICINES AGENCY (EMA)*

Introduction

It is inherent to any pharmacotherapy that there is no such thing like one drug or combination of drugs that can cure or alleviate symptoms of all patients suffering from the same defined disease. Drug action and safety is dependent on multiple factors inside and outside the human body; therefore, environment, lifestyle, age, organ function, xenobiotic intake, and our genetic makeup determine the efficacy, efficiency, and ultimately safety of a drug therapy in question. At the genetic level, both "global" and "local" variations must be considered; the former involving the karyotype (gender[1] and aneuploidy) and the latter involving polymorphisms in single or multiple genes.[2,3] Despite the

aforementioned genetic variations, additional conditions influencing the genetic contribution to drug action and safety are subsumed as "epigenetic factors."[4,5] In comparison to "global" and "local" genetic factors, the latter is much more difficult to "pinpoint" in terms of drug action and/or safety. One such example is the methylation pattern of CpG islands. In spite of a certain stability also propagated to next generations, the methylation pattern can change under different "internal" and/or "external" conditions relative to the human body, which are, up to now, only poorly understood.[6,7] Even more complex is the situation concerning the methylation of CpG sites adjacent to CpG islands (i.e. CpG shores). These regions seem to be able to change their methylation pattern within hours depending on different stimuli,[4] and perhaps drug therapies.[8,9] The methylation pattern of genomic DNA together with other epigenetic factors and/or noncoding (nc) RNAs (ncRNAs)[10] modulates the stability and amount of mRNA,[11] thereby altering the abundance of proteins crucial for drug efficacy, efficiency, and safety. Variations in the described genetic factors ultimately determine the interindividual variability and influence or predict the outcome of drug treatments and therefore provide an important

---

*The views expressed in this chapter are the personal views of the authors and may not be understood or quoted as being made on behalf of or reflecting the position of the European Medicines Agency, any of its committees or working parties, or the Medicines Evaluation Board.

framework for "personalized medicine,"[12] which is commonly acknowledged to form the foundation for a better matching between the available and future drugs with the individual situation of patients. Personalized medicine will optimally lead to more efficient and safer drug therapies that result in fewer adverse side effects, and allowing better selection of patients and more rational use of drugs. The new perspective of "personalized medicine" created the need for regulatory agencies to integrate the aspect of PGx into their regulatory framework. This section describes a brief history and gives insights into the "work in progress" regarding the implementation of PGx into the regulatory framework of the EMA.

History of PGx at the EMA

Following a workshop held in June 2000 with main stakeholder representatives, the EMA recognized the need of convening an expert group on PGx to address the priorities identified at the workshop, including terminology used in clinical trials for PGx-based medicinal product development. Therefore, in 2001, the Committee for Medical Products for Human Use (CHMP) established a multidisciplinary expert group, which was formalized in 2005 as the Pharmacogenetics Working Party (PGWP), the intention of which was to provide recommendations on all matters relating directly or indirectly to pharmacogenetics. Activities employed include (i) the hosting of workshops and briefing meetings, (ii) preparing, reviewing, and updating guidelines for the preparation and assessment of the PGx sections of regulatory submissions, (iii) supporting dossier evaluation, and (iv) providing advice to the CHMP on general and product-specific matters relating to PGx. Furthermore, at the request of the CHMP or of the Scientific Advice Working Party (SAWP), the PGWP may contribute to scientific advice on general and product-specific matters related to PGx. In 2001, the EMA also established a new informal regulatory forum called "The Innovation Task Force" (ITF), which hosts briefing meetings for encouraging scientific dialogue on emerging and innovative scientific issues with potential regulatory implications. These discussions enable the industry to discuss their PGx strategy and data prior to any formal decision making. In 2002–2003, based on preliminary experience the CHMP identified the need and adopted and published a technical document on terminology addressing the meaning and the implications of the most commonly used PGx-related terms, that is, pharmacogenetics and PGx, sample coding, followed by a version in layman's terms. In 2006, the EMA informal meeting platform for dialogue was expanded allowing the option for industry to have joint Food and Drug Administration (FDA)–EMA Voluntary Genomic Data Submission (VGDS) briefing meetings. Japanese authority Pharmaceuticals and Medical Devices Agency (PMDA) did participate as observers. In 2008 the terminology document published by the Agency in 2003 formed the basis for discussions within the International Conference on Harmonisation (ICH) of technical requirements for medicinal products and it is now incorporated in the ICH E15 guideline on the definition of genomic biomarkers: this guideline is aiming at facilitating the

integration of the PGx discipline into global drug development and approval processes. Following the adoption of the ICH E15 guideline in 2008, the name of the working party was modified to the Pharmacogenomics Working Party (PGWP; as opposed to *pharmacogenetics*; see above [http://www.ema.europa.eu/ema/index.jsp?curl=pages/contacts/CHMP/people_listing_000018.jsp&murl=menus/about_us/about_us.jsp&mid=WC0b01ac0580028d91]); the scientific remits and the mandate was extended accordingly in order to address the voluntary submissions of biomarkers.

PGx-Related CHMP Reflection Papers and Guidelines

As mentioned above, a number of technical documents have been adopted by the CHMP and released to the public. Those include reflection papers on (i) PGx sampling, testing, and data handling in the context of PGx studies, (ii) the impact of PGx in pharmacokinetic (PK) studies, their interpretation, and their potential labeling consequences, (iii) the EMA experience regarding Marketing Authorisation Applications in the oncology field, and (iv) the codevelopment of pharmacogenomic biomarkers and medicinal products. Beyond the ICH guidelines ICH E15 and ICH E16 focusing on PGx biomarkers terminology and on format of data submission, respectively, the first formal European guideline focused on PGx released by the CHMP is the one on the use of pharmacogenomic methodologies in the pharmacokinetic evaluation of medicinal products (EMA/CHMP/37646/2009; http://www.ema.europa.eu/docs/en_GB/document_library/Scientific_guideline/2012/02/WC500121954.pdf). Further documents designed to support the framework of PGx for drug development are currently under preparation at the EMA as per the PGWP Work Program. All technical documents adopted so far by the CHMP regarding PGx can be downloaded from the EMA Web site (www.ema.europa.eu) under Regulatory/Human medicines/Scientific guidelines/Multidisciplinary/Pharmacogenomics pathway. Currently, the PGWP is working on a PGx guideline for pharmacovigilance. Further guidelines will evolve with science in the field.

PGx in Drug Development

The "Guideline on the Use of Pharmacogenomic Methodologies in the Pharmacokinetic Evaluation of Medicinal Products" is coming into effect August 2012, and will contain substantial recommendations concerning PK for the development of new drugs. In the following section we would like to outline some sections that are extensively discussed jointly in the CHMP PGWP and in the Pharmacokinetics Working Party (PKWP). This guideline refers mainly to mutations of single genes coding for proteins involved in PK, a research field in which enough detailed insight has been obtained to translate the science from the workbench to the patient. Epigenetic factors, ncRNAs, karyotypes, and mutations in multiple genes involved in complex functional interplays within cells are, as mentioned, of undoubtful importance for drug action and safety; however, at the moment, the mechanisms underlying their impact in drug kinetics are poorly understood. Some considerations applicable to genetic biomarkers (gBMs) in PK may also be relevant to gBMs in pharmacodynamics (PD). At the moment, however, the EMA makes a clear distinction between PGx in PK, in PD, and in relation to clinical development and patient selection (see section "PGx Biomarkers and Patient Selection in Clinical Development"). The categories of proteins involved in PK include those involved in the absorption, distribution, metabolism, and elimination (ADME) of drugs. Within these ADME categories, PGx, at the moment, focuses most on drug metabolism (Phase I and Phase II enzymes), with less emphasis on the "transport" of drugs. This is to reflect requirements in an area where regulatory experience has been accumulated. However, it can be envisioned that PGx at the level of drug transport (absorption, distribution, and excretion, involving channels[13-17] and/or transporters[18,19]) may, in instances, play an even more important role than that of metabolizing enzymes.

PGx in Preclinical Studies

Human in vitro metabolism studies should optimally be conducted prior to Phase-I-studies (see also *Guideline on the investigation of drug–drug and food–drug interactions*, CPMP/EWP/560/95/Rev.1). Examples of such studies include, but are not limited to, (i) the identification of "important" enzymes responsible for catalyzing the bulk in vitro metabolism and (ii) the identification and characterization of metabolites created by the major candidate metabolic pathways. The difficulty is what "important" means in this context. Xenobiotic elimination from the body is essential for detoxification and guaranties species survival. Accordingly, xenobiotic metabolism is redundant (multiple enzymes are able to metabolize the same drug/xenobiotic). In an in vitro context, the metabolizing enzyme of an active parent drug could be considered "important" when ≥50% of the drug is predicted to be cleared by a single enzyme based on experimental data. In this case, it is reasonable to assume that polymorphic genes coding for such enzymes might have important implications on the safety of the respective drug. Percentages (cutoff values) below 50% will certainly apply to "flag" enzymes that lead to toxic metabolites. In vitro data (obtained prior to Phase-I-studies) regarding drug transporters may represent another target group for studying PGx. The impact of transporters may be implied in vivo through animal models, in vitro through cellular systems, or from information obtained on similar substances. The ability to make quantitative conjectures of the in vivo contribution of drug transporters remains underserved. Accordingly, no guidelines concerning transporters can be given at the moment.

PGx in the Pharmacokinetic Evaluation of Medicinal Products

The possibility of genetic influence on the drug PK should be considered early and throughout the Phase I program. If in vitro data indicate an important involvement of a known functionally polymorphic enzyme (see above), it seems to be reasonable to genotype the "first time in man" study population for the relevant genes to avoid safety issues related to genetically determined differences in active substance exposure. As extensively described in Chapter 2, single nucleotide polymorphisms (SNPs) and/or nucleotide insertion(s)/deletion(s) in respective genes may lead, compared with wild-type, to (i) increased or decreased clearance of the parent drug, (ii) increased or decreased production of active metabolites of the respective prodrug, or (iii) increased or decreased formation of toxic metabolites. Decreased metabolism seems only to be relevant for functions (i) and (ii), where in the former higher levels of the parent drug appear in the organism, and in the latter there is a loss of response. On the other hand, an increase in metabolism at each step (i–iii) always carries a potential clinical relevance, due to a loss of response in (i), higher levels of bioactive compound in (ii), or the production of toxic metabolites in (iii). Thirty to 50% of all clinically prescribed drugs are metabolized by enzymes having reported SNPs[20,21] that include both Phase I (cytochrome P450 enzymes such as CYP2C9, CYP2C19, and CYP2D6[22]) and Phase II (UDP-glucuronosyltransferases, *N*-acetyltransferase-2, and some methyltransferases) enzymes. Metabolizing enzymes account for 80% of those mentioned for pharmacogenetic purpose on current drug labels.[23] Recently, specific SNPs that impact drug efficacy and safety have been described within drug transporter. The impact of transporter polymorphisms on drug PKs has not yet been specified to the extent of those occurring in the Phase I and II metabolizing enzymes (one exception is the SLCO1B1 [OATP1B1] polymorphism which has been shown to significantly affect the PKs and adverse effects of some drugs, including some widely used statins[24-26]). The discrepancy is partly due to the difficulty in quantifying the role of specific transporters in vivo. More specific inhibitors and reliable methods for measuring drug transport are needed. Transporter polymorphisms have been shown to be more substrate-specific in their effects as compared with those observed with metabolizing enzymes. Therefore, the possibility of transporter polymorphism as a cause for altered drug PKs must always be considered throughout drug development. It is also important to mention that polymorphisms in drug transporters may affect systemic as well as local (target) exposure, the latter of which is even more complex to detect. It is anticipated that expansion within this area will occur in the near future, as knowledge on the role of drug transporters is rapidly developing. Investigations aimed at determining the effects of PGx on the PKs of a drug (proform and/or its active metabolite(s)) and their implications on efficacy and safety during development seem to be absolutely required when the magnitude of interindividual variation is likely to influence the efficacy and/or safety of the drug in genetically variable target populations. Factors identifying the *need* for such studies are: (i) in vitro and/or in vivo studies indicate that a known functionally polymorphic enzyme or transporter is likely to represent an important pathway in the metabolism or distribution of the drug, *or* (ii) in vitro and/or in vivo studies indicate that a known functionally polymorphic enzyme or transporter is likely to represent an important pathway in the formation, elimination, or distribution of a pharmacologically active or toxic metabolite, or (iii) in vivo studies indicate substantial interindividual differences in the PK of the drug that are *likely* to influence the efficacy or safety of the drug in the variable subpopulation, which cannot be explained by other intrinsic or extrinsic factors. Investigations aimed at determining the effects of PGx on the PKs of a drug should be generally *recommended* throughout drug development if: (i) available in vitro data indicate that a human polymorphic enzyme or transporter contributes to the PK of the active substances but the quantitative role may be low based on the in vitro data, *or* (ii) there is high interindividual PK variability, or there are PK outliers with higher or lower exposure to the active substances that cannot be attributed to other known intrinsic or extrinsic factors, but which *possibly* can give rise to clinical efficacy and safety concerns based on the existing knowledge, *or* (iii) major differences that cannot be attributed to other known intrinsic or extrinsic factors in PK are observed in different ethnic groups. An inherent difficulty is the formulation of stringent guidelines (cutoff values) for deciding when further investigations regarding PGx impact on drug behavior are justified. The PGWP at EMA is working toward the definition of principles guiding PGx-related research in drug development. What is in general consensus view is that the analysis of potentially responsible genes should be performed in situations where prominent (likely to have negative clinical or safety implications) PK variability cannot be justified by nongenetic intrinsic or extrinsic factors. Retrospective analyses may also play a key role in the identification of novel genetic variants that alter drug action and safety. Therefore, it would be optimal to acquire genetic samples (DNA, RNA, etc.) from patients participating in clinical trials so as to allow for both such types of analysis. Clinically relevant (in this setting defined as the situation that ≥25% of the drug is metabolized by a single polymorphic enzyme in an *in vivo situation*) influences of PGx on PK identified in Phase-I-studies should be considered in the design of Phase-II-studies. Where no genotype/phenotype-based dosing is applied to normalize for drug exposure, the exposure level obtained in the genotypically defined subpopulation should be investigated in the Phase-II-studies. If available data indicate that there is a significant difference in drug/metabolite exposure or distribution in the genetically/phenotypically defined subpopulation, genotyping for all of the relevant genes in all patients included in Phase-III-studies should be considered.

PGx Biomarkers and Patient Selection in Clinical Development

By sequencing the entire human genome and refining the techniques for doing so, our knowledge for gBMs relevant for increasing the efficacy, efficiency, and ultimately safety of pharmacotherapy has increased exponentially. In the former section we described the relevance of PGx-associated gBMs relative to PK; however, gBMs are important in the clinical context of (i) disease diagnosis and (ii) disease prognosis (prognostic gBMs): it is anticipated that on the basis of these two type of gBMs

even taxonomy of diseases and definition of phenotypes would change in the future. Prognostic gBMs (or markers) correlate with outcome of disease in either untreated or treated patients and frequently they are identified on the availability of biological samples collected for gBM studies. Prognostic BMs may or may not offer the basis for a clinical decision or influence the decision for treatment or intervention.

Genetic-BMs predicting response to treatment (predictive gBMs) play a crucial role in both drug development and therapy, as they identify individual pretreatment characteristics that allow the determination of whether or not a particular patient is a good candidate for treatment with a certain drug. Usually, predictive gBMs tend to be "binary" or depend on classifiers that translate the biomarker into a set of markers that predict clinical outcome.[27] They are, in their simplest definition, the abundance of a single gene product or point mutation(s) of an expressed single gene. Epigenetic factors, ncRNAs, karyotype, and mutations in multiple genes involved in complex functional interplays within cells are, as described in the former section, also important in this regard. However, at the moment, the underlining mechanisms are poorly understood and therefore less considered at the moment. Predictive gBMs allow for (i) patient selection and (ii) treatment algorithm allocation, thereby leading to a reduced heterogeneity of all phenotypic population.

Therefore, gBMs can be used in drug development program (i) *for the better definition of the disease and/or its prognosis* (e.g., HER2-overexpressing breast cancer [ErbB2], Philadelphia chromosome in chronic myeloid leukemia), (ii) *for excluding patients at increased risk* of experiencing serious adverse drug reactions (e.g., *HLA B* 5701* and abacavir use, or carbamazepine and *HLA-B*1502*), and (iii) *for drug response prediction*, via the identification of patients with a high likelihood of experiencing benefit with a particular medicinal product (see Tables 4–1 and 4–2). gBMs may also be used for selection of treatment dose and duration. For example, in treating HCV infections with PEG-IFN plus ribavirin, depending on the viral genome (viral genotype is considered a gBM) treatment duration would be of 48 weeks for genotypes 1 and 4, and 24 weeks for genotypes 2 and 3 (http://www.ema.europa.eu/docs/en_GB/document_library/Scientific_guideline/2011/07/WC500108672.pdf).

PGx biomarkers used to identify patients' population for centrally approved medicinal products (CAPs) and for some nationally approved products are shown in Tables 4–1 and 4–2.

The use of gBM in pharmaceuticals R&D opens the regulatory debate on key methodological aspects such as issues associated to the analytical platforms and assays used during drug development and after approval, regulatory acceptability of enrichment designs or of post hoc analyses in clinical studies, choice of suitable comparators, how to approach safety gBM validation in postapproval, impact on product information to patients and health care professionals, evidence required to qualify the gBMs and their clinical utility, and impact on the clinical setting of the larger patient population concerned.

Feasibility, timely availability, and affordability of the related test are of main importance along with some ethical aspects surrounding patient subgroups genomically defined.

TABLE 4–1 Examples of centrally approved products for which GBMs are included in the therapeutic indication of the product.

Product Name	Indication (As Described in EPAR)
Vectibix (Panitumumab)	Vectibix is indicated as monotherapy for the treatment of patients with epidermal growth factor receptor (EGFR) expressing metastatic colorectal carcinoma with nonmutated (wild-type) KRAS after failure of fluoropyrimidine-, oxaliplatin-, and irinotecan-containing chemotherapy regimens
Celsentri (maraviroc)	Celsentri is indicated for patients infected with only CCR5-tropic human immunodeficiency virus (HIV)-1 detectable. Before taking celsentri, it has to be confirmed that CCr5-tropic HIV-1 is detectable using an adequately validated and sensitive detection method on a newly drawn blood sample
Herceptin (trastuzumab)	Herceptin is indicated for the treatment of patients with HER2-positive early breast cancer, metastatic breast cancer, and metastatic gastric cancer
Erbitux (cetuximab)	Erbitux is indicated for the treatment of patients with EGFR-expressing, KRAS wild-type metastatic colorectal cancer: in combination with chemotherapy, or as a single agent in patients who have failed oxaliplatin- and irinotecan-based therapy and who are intolerant to irinotecan
Tyverb (lapatinib)	Tyverb is indicated for the treatment of patients with breast cancer, whose tumors overexpress HER2 (ErbB2)
Tarceva (erlotinib)	Tarceva is indicated for the treatment of patients with locally advanced or metastatic non-small cell lung cancer (NSCLC) after failure of at least one prior chemotherapy regimen. No survival benefit or other clinically relevant effects of the treatment have been demonstrated in patients with EGFR-negative tumors
Iressa (gefitinib)	Iressa is indicated for the treatment of adult patients with locally advanced or metastatic NSCLC with activating mutations of EGFR-TK
Sprycel (dasatinib)	Sprycel is indicated for the treatment of adults with chronic, accelerated, or blast phase chronic myeloid leukemia (CML) with resistance or intolerance to prior therapy including imatinib mesilate. It is also indicated for the treatment of adults with Philadelphia chromosome positive (Ph+) acute lymphoblastic leukemia (ALL) and lymphoid blast CML with resistance or intolerance to prior therapy
Tasigna (nilotinib)	Tasigna is indicated for the treatment of adults with chronic phase and accelerated phase Ph+ chronic myeloid leukemia (CML) with resistance or intolerance to prior therapy including imatinib. Efficacy data in patients with CML in blast crisis are not available
Trisenox (arsenic Trioxide)	Trisenox is indicated for induction of remission and consolidation in adult patients with relapsed/refractory acute promyelocytic leukemia (APL), characterized by the presence of the t(15;17) translocation and/or the presence of the promyelocytic leukemia/retinoic acid receptor α (PML/RAR-α) gene
Ziagen (abacavir)	Ziagen is indicated in antiretroviral combination therapy for the treatment of HIV infection. Before initiating treatment with abacavir, screening for carriage of the HLA-B*5701 allele should be performed in any HIV-infected patient, irrespective of racial origin. Screening is also recommended prior to reinitiation of abacavir in patients of unknown HLA-B*5701 status who have previously tolerated abacavir. Abacavir should not be used in patients known to carry the HLA-B*5701 allele, unless no other therapeutic option is available in these patients, based on the treatment history and resistance testing
Glivec (imatinib)	Glivec is indicated for: (a) Adult and pediatric patients with newly diagnosed Philadelphia chromosome (bcr-abl) positive (Ph+) CML for whom bone marrow transplantation is not considered as the first line of treatment (b) Adult and pediatric patients with Ph+ CML in chronic phase after failure of interferon-α therapy, or in accelerated phase or blast crisis (c) Adult patients with newly diagnosed Ph+ ALL integrated with chemotherapy (d) Adult patients with relapsed or refractory Ph+ ALL as monotherapy (e) Adult patients with myelodysplastic/myeloproliferative diseases (MDS/MPD) associated with platelet-derived growth factor receptor (PDGFR) gene rearrangements (f) Adult patients with advanced hypereosinophilic syndrome (HES) and/or chronic eosinophilic leukemia (CEL) with FIP1L1-PDGFR rearrangement (g) Adult patients with kit (CD 117) positive unresectable and/or metastatic malignant gastrointestinal stromal tumors (GIST)
Zelboraf (Vemurafenib)	Vemurafenib is indicated in monotherapy for the treatment of adult patients with BRAF V600 mutation-positive unresectable or metastatic melanoma.

Conclusions

It is becoming evident that the scientific knowledge of the human genome obtained only within one decade has influenced drug development in terms of both technology and applicability.

The potential applications of GBM and their impact on the development of medicinal products hold the promise of a more informed and more successful new drug development. At the same time they raise a range of methodological issues related to the generation of the clinical evidence supportive of a positive benefit/risk balance in clinical use. Those issues are discussed by the EMA Scientific Committees at various levels: in the early exploratory phase in the context of ITF informal briefing meetings (and joint voluntary genomic data submission with the US FDA); in a more advanced stage they are addressed formally on a case-by-case approach in scientific advice for specific drug

TABLE 4–2 Relevant GBMs and the scope of their inclusion in labeling.

Product	INN Name	Biomarker	Scope
Ziagen	Abacavir	HLA-B*5701	Safety
Herceptin	Trastuzumab	HER2 receptor	Efficacy
Glivec	Imatinib	Philadelphia chromosome (bcr-abl) positive	Efficacy
		PDGFR gene rearrangements	
		FIP1L1-PDGFR rearrangement	
		c-Kit	
Trisenox	Arsenic trioxide	PML/RAR-α	Efficacy
Erbitux	Cetuximab	EGFR/K-Ras	Efficacy
Tarceva	Erlotinib	EGFR	Efficacy
Sprycel	Dasatinib	Ph+ chromosome	Efficacy
Celsentri	Maraviroc	CCR5 coreceptor	Efficacy
Tasigna	Nilotinib	Ph+ chromosome	Efficacy
Vectibix	Panitumumab	K-Ras	Efficacy
Tyverb	Lapatinib	HER2	Efficacy
Iressa	Gefitinib	EGFR	Efficacy
Multiple trade names	Carbamazepine	HLA-B*1502	Safety
Multiple trade names	Phenytoin	HLA-B*1502	Safety
Multiple trade names	Tamoxifen	CYP2D6	Interactions
Multiple trade names	Clopidogrel	CYP2C19	Efficacy
Abilify	Aripiprazole	CYP2D6	Safety
Xeloda	Capecitabine	DPD	Safety
Onsenal[a]	Celecoxib	CYP2C9	Safety
Faslodex	Fulvestrant	Estrogen receptor	Efficacy
Viracept	Nelfinavir	CYP2C19	Safety
Fasturtec	Rasburicase	G6PD	Safety
Zelboraf	Vemurafenib	BRAF V600E	Efficacy

[a]Drug no longer registered

development plans or biomarker qualification. As regulatory experience matures, relevant guidelines in more advanced fields of PGx applications (e.g., PGx impact on a drug's PK) or reflection papers are prepared and published.

The EMA network developed and supported a series of activities in Europe, at international level (e.g., ICH), and within the context of bilateral arrangements with other competent authorities (e.g., US FDA and Japanese MHLW/PMDA), which allow the development of flexible and globally relevant regulatory approaches. New "personalized" medicinal products are currently approved and their use guided by genomic biomarkers. The prescribers are provided with more choices in selecting the most appropriate treatments and doses for subgroups or individual patients.

The significant and growing impact of GBM in drug development and use is documented by:

• The increasing number of products discovered and developed on the basis of genomic impact on cellular functional pathways (the "druggable" genome[28,29])

• The ability to identify patients:
  ○ At risks for serious ADRs in various populations (e.g., carbamazepine and serious cutaneous adverse reactions, serious hypersensitivity reaction to abacavir)
  ○ With special needs in terms of dose adjustments
  ○ Responding to treatment above the average clinical response observed in the general population
  ○ Responding to treatment when the general population would not respond

• The increasing inclusion of GBM in the indications for use of both newly authorized and established medicinal products

Further opportunities for optimizing benefit/risk balance of new and currently prescribed medicines are expected as scientific knowledge emerges on transporter genomics as well as in the area of epigenetics and ncRNAs.

PGx AT THE US FOOD AND DRUG ADMINISTRATION (US FDA)†

Overview of Drug Development and Regulatory Oversight

Drug approval in the United States is regulated by the US FDA. As part of its public health mission, the FDA is charged with protecting public health by ensuring the safety, efficacy, and security of human and veterinary drugs, biological products, and medical devices. FDA also promotes public health by helping to support innovations in drug development and providing the public with accurate, science-based information to ensure safe use of medicine and food.

When a drug developer (aka sponsor) intends to develop and promote a therapeutic product (e.g., drug or biologic), they must work with the FDA to reach general agreement on the types of studies, experiments, and data needed to support FDA approval. During drug development including Phase 1, 2, and 3 studies, sponsors submit protocols to receive feedback from FDA on their proposed studies. These protocol submissions are filed as Investigational New Drug (IND) New Drug Applications (NDAs). Initial IND submissions need to be submitted and reviewed prior to the start of a first in human study. Within 30 days following initial filing, the FDA determines based on the sponsor's provided data (usually from preclinical studies) whether the drug is safe to be administered to humans for the first time. For cases in which IND protocols are submitted during drug development (e.g., for Phase 2 or 3), sponsors intend to receive feedback from the agency regarding such aspects as the proposed trial design, dose, and patient or endpoint selection. When sufficient data are generated in order to seek final FDA approval for marketing, the sponsor will submit a New Drug Application (NDA) or Biologic License Application (BLA). Within 10 months (or 6 months for priority reviews), a multidisciplinary FDA review team determines (1) whether the drug is safe and effective for its proposed use and whether the proposed benefits outweigh the risks, (2) whether the drug's proposed labeling is appropriate, (3) whether the methods and controls used during manufacturing are adequate to preserve the drug's identity, strength, quality, and purity, and (4) whether additional postapproval studies are needed to address unresolved safety or efficacy concerns (e.g., in renal/hepatic impaired patients, pediatric patients) (The US Food and Drug Administration. *New Drug Application.* Silver Spring, MD: FDA; available at: http://www.fda.gov/Drugs/DevelopmentApprovalProcess/HowDrugsareDevelopedandApproved/ApprovalApplications/NewDrugApplicationNDA/default.htm; accessed July 26, 2011). The review is performed by a team of FDA reviewers in the Center of Drug Evaluation and Research (CDER) that consists of physicians, statisticians, chemists, pharmacologists, toxicologists, clinical pharmacologists (including pharmacogeneticists), and other scientists.

In order to provide guidelines to sponsors and FDA review staff, guidance documents that represent the agency's current thinking on processing, content, and evaluation/approval of applications as well as design, production, manufacturing, and testing of regulated products are available. Guidances are not regulations or laws and therefore not enforceable. However, they are a valuable tool to achieve consistency in the agency's regulatory approach and establish inspection and enforcement procedures.

Pharmacogenomics at the US Food and Drug Administration

The identification of the optimal combination of patient type (e.g., based on molecular determinants), drug choice, and dose optimization is a well-recognized challenge in drug development. Due to the impact of variable intrinsic (i.e., patient-specific) and extrinsic (i.e., environmental) factors on these parameters, differences in safety and/or efficacy outcomes among patients are often observed. The goal of personalized medicine is to identify the factors contributing to this variability and to predict safety and efficacy profiles for any given patient. Because relatively little is known for new drugs in development compared with already approved therapies, adequate and timely identification of variability in the above factors is necessary to inform a variety of drug development and regulatory decisions related to a therapeutic compound. These include choice of appropriate biomarkers for study, improved patient selection into clinical trials, informed dose selection for patient subgroups, and optimal trial design to demonstrate drug effects.

Incorporation of adequate trial designs and methodologies that help identify subpopulations that may have unique safety and efficacy profiles is increasingly recognized during drug development, especially in areas of oncology, antivirals, and cardiovascular diseases. For cases in which an association between a marker (e.g., genotype) and efficacy or safety is proposed (e.g., based on exploratory preclinical discovery studies or based on available scientific information), the hypothesis may be tested in early clinical studies (e.g., Phase-I and -II-studies). Generally, these studies are considered exploratory and may help to identify populations that should receive lower or higher doses, for example, due to excretory or metabolic differences. They may also help to identify responder populations that have a certain phenotypic, receptor, or genetic characteristic (e.g., in oncology). If differences in efficacy can be predicted early in development, enrichment strategies that are based on predictive markers may be employed in the more definitive safety and efficacy trials in later development. In addition, early studies can identify high-risk groups, for example, through identification of poor or rapid metabolizers whose blood levels of parent or relevant metabolites could be affected. During confirmatory studies, usually performed in later trials, the hypothesis that is based on data generated in early studies is tested. These trials may be conducted in the molecular marker-enriched patient population

---

†The views presented in this chapter are those of the author and do not necessarily reflect those of the US FDA. Official endorsement neither is intended nor should be inferred.

since a better response is assumed in this population. These trials can also further define the patient population, therapies, and other conditions under which the marker is predictive.

When pharmacogenetic strategies are employed, genes in the following three categories are usually assessed to investigate interpatient variability in PK, PD, response, or safety: (1) ADME genes relevant to PK of a drug (absorption, distribution, metabolism, excretion), (2) genes that affect the drug targets (including off-site targets) or related signaling pathways, and (3) genes that predict disease occurrence (prognostic markers). Furthermore, there is increased use of high-throughput methodologies (e.g., genome-wide association studies for hypothesis generation).

Adequate collection and retention of DNA samples from clinical trials is crucial to successfully use genetic information for drug development purposes. Because genomic hypotheses are usually explored under a separate voluntary informed consent, there is often incomplete DNA sample acquisition in clinical trials. Therefore, great care is needed to limit and understand the bias that could be potentially introduced from this voluntary DNA collection. Ideally, DNA samples should be collected at baseline (e.g., enrollment or randomization) and high sample acquisition rates should be achieved. Even for trials in which no genetic determinants are proposed a priori to influence response or safety, DNA should be collected prior to study initiation to facilitate pharmacogenomic analyses in the event that adverse events or meaningful (perhaps unexplained) differences in response are observed.

Besides the growing interest to identify and evaluate predictive and prognostic biomarkers in clinical studies, another rapidly evolving field with relevance to PGx at the FDA is the area of in vitro diagnostic regulation. For accurate identification of a biomarker to specify subpopulations, analytically validated assays need to be developed. The need for FDA-cleared or -approved diagnostics is particularly relevant for companion drug–diagnostic pairs. Regulatory review and subsequent marketing approval for these in vitro diagnostics is usually conducted by the Center of Devices and Radiological Health (CDRH).[30]

Contributing to the growing significance of PGx in clinical studies are several factors including (1) the rapidly advancing knowledge of molecular disease determinants, (2) the ability to economically evaluate genomic biomarkers in large patient cohorts, and (3) sponsor's increasing comfort with sharing genomic data with the FDA. This latter development is largely driven by early interaction with the FDA through the VGDS (later renamed the Voluntary Exploratory Data Submissions [VXDS] program). The FDA recognized in the early 2000s that the then emerging discipline of PGx had potential applications in drug development. Sponsors, however, hesitated to submit genomic data that they were generating to the FDA because of the concern that FDA scientists might compel companies to undertake additional research efforts based on review of highly exploratory data. In 2002, FDA introduced the concept of VGDS as a safe harbor for genomics data submissions and a draft guideline was released in November 2003 and finalized in March 2005.[31] In order to further advance PGx and to promote its uptake into

regulatory consideration, sponsors were encouraged to submit their exploratory genomic data that would be reviewed by FDA staff outside the formal regulatory framework; the goal was scientific exchange without specific binding advice on the part of FDA to any specific drug development issue. Partly as a consequence of the VXDS program, which is now in its 7th year, PGx is increasingly being considered in drug development and as part of regulatory review as evidenced by the rising numbers of IND, BLA, and NDA submissions with genomic data.[32] For example, in 2010 ($n = 210$), nearly four times the number of submissions were reviewed by Genomics Group review staff compared with that in 2008 ($n = 56$) and included all types of submissions (i.e., IND, NDA, BLA).

Regulatory Considerations: Review and Labeling Impact of Pharmacogenomic Studies

The increased importance of pharmacogenomic studies for drug development has been well recognized by FDA. For example, the Genomics Group, a review staff in the Office of Clinical Pharmacology at the FDA, developed an integrated, translational regulatory review scheme to provide an informed PGx-based assessment for IND as well as NDA/BLA submissions. As regulatory scientists, genomics reviewers have advanced knowledge of pharmacogenetics, clinical pharmacology, epidemiology, clinical trial design, and pharmacotherapy/clinical practice that is applied to develop regulatory policies and procedures to enhance incorporation of genomics and related disciplines in drug development, regulation, and clinical practice.

To enhance drug development through an efficient regulatory review process, genomics reviewers work with sponsors at the IND stage to increase likelihood that clinical studies generate unambiguous, uninterpretable data with respect to PGx and biomarkers. Regulatory advice is usually provided regarding sample collection, biomarker selection, and study design methodology. Furthermore, genomics reviewers analyze and interpret NDA and BLA submissions to support regulatory review as part of the CDER cross-disciplinary review team.[33]

Depending on several factors, pharmacogenomic information may be included in drug labels in order to make the prescriber aware of the impact of genetic information on drug response. The pharmacogenomic information in labeling may include (1) a description of polymorphic enzymes and their impact on PK and/or PD (e.g., reduced CYP P450 enzyme activity due to polymorphisms in CYP genes), (2) proper identification of subpopulations (e.g., through use of a diagnostic test) and information regarding allele frequencies, haplotypes, genotypes, or other genomic markers and their association with safety and/or efficacy, (3) description of PGx studies that provided evidence of genetically based differences in drug benefit or risk, and (4) dose changes based on genotype. Inclusion of genomic relevant information in drug labels is anticipated to increase in the future, given the enhanced inclusion of genomic studies in drug development.

Parallel Activities of European Medicines Agency (EMA) and FDA

Initiatives have been developed at both EMA and FDA for the need to share knowledge of emerging new genomic methodologies in drug development.[34] Besides supporting biomarker integration in research and development through providing scientific advice, these regulatory agencies also aim to establish a robust and predictable set of requirements for applications. Back in 2005, FDA (The Food and Drug Administration. Federal Register 69, 48876–48877; available at: http://www.fda.gov/OHRMS/DOCKETS/98fr/04-18360.htm; accessed July 26, 2011), EMA (EMEA/CHMP/PGxWP/20227/04 Guideline on Pharmacogenetics Briefing Meetings. London, UK: EMEA; available at: http://www.ema.europa.eu/pdfs/human/pharmacogenetics/2022704en.pdf; accessed July 26, 2011), and Japan's PMDA[35] published guidelines on how to adequately submit genomic information from drug development programs. Review of these submissions was performed under the VGDS program at the FDA and EMA that has been described elsewhere in this chapter. The VGDS initiative has led to an extensive progress in the development of exploratory biomarkers. However, most of the data generated during drug development were not submitted to the agencies or shared within the industry but remained within the companies. In response, the regulatory agencies were looking for a mechanism that encourages stakeholder to share biomarker data that would ultimately enhance the knowledge of biomarkers. They were also looking for a process on how to best apply biomarker information in preclinical and clinical drug development settings. The initiatives were ultimately realized with biomarker qualification programs (BQP) developed by EMA, FDA, and PMDA. Although these BQPs are administered independently by the respective agencies, the agencies often share information regarding biomarker qualification submissions in order to create efficiency in the review of the data.

In the past, biomarker qualification has been applied on a case-by-case basis. However, BQP offers the opportunity to qualify genomic and other biomarkers that are not tied to an individual product but have a wider relevance in the assessment of drug efficacy and safety. Today, consortia such as, but not limited to, the Predictive Safety Testing Consortium (PSTC) and EMA's Innovative Medicines Initiative create large amounts of data that complement and overlap and also have the potential to influence regulatory standards. A PSTC application for qualification of seven new renal biomarkers as predictors of drug-mediated nephrotoxicity was the first application of the new interagency review initiative (The EMA. *Final Report on the Pilot Joint EMEA/FDA VXDS Experience on Qualification of Nephrotoxicity Biomarkers*. London, UK: EMEA; available at: http://www.ema.europa.eu/pdfs/human/biomarkers/25088508en.pdf; accessed July 26, 2011). To guide stakeholders toward successful qualification of biomarkers and patient-reported outcome instruments, the FDA/CDER recently published a draft guidance on the qualification process for drug development tools (DDT). If a DDT is successfully qualified for a specific use, it can be used for the qualified purpose during drug development without the need to reconfirm the DDT's utility, resulting in expedited development of marketing applications.

In the future, the BQP needs to be tested with submissions from (1) a variety of platforms, (2) preclinical and clinical applications, (3) various disease areas, and (4) pharmaceutical companies, academic institutions, and diagnostic companies. A successful application in these settings would establish BQP as a valuable tool to identify new biomarkers able to accelerate drug development.

REFERENCES

1. Wang J, Huang Y. Pharmacogenomics of sex difference in chemotherapeutic toxicity. *Curr Drug Discov Technol.* 2007;4(1):59–68.
2. Bird A. Perceptions of epigenetics. *Nature.* 2007;447(7143):396–398.
3. Hattis D. Pharmacogenetics: ethnic differences in reactions to drugs and xenobiotics. *Science.* 1986;234(4773):222–223.
4. Riddihough G, Pennisi E. The evolution of epigenetics. *Science.* 2001;293(5532):1063.
5. Wolffe AP, Matzke MA. Epigenetics: regulation through repression. *Science.* 1999;286(5439):481–486.
6. Feinberg AP. Phenotypic plasticity and the epigenetics of human disease. *Nature.* 2007;447(7143):433–440.
7. Jones PA, Takai D. The role of DNA methylation in mammalian epigenetics. *Science.* 2001;293(5532):1068–1070.
8. Ingelman-Sundberg M, Gomez A. The past, present and future of pharmacoepigenomics. *Pharmacogenomics.* 2010;11(5):625–627.
9. Gomez A, Ingelman-Sundberg M. Pharmacoepigenetics: its role in interindividual differences in drug response. *Clin Pharmacol Ther.* 2009;85(4):426–430.
10. Zhou H, Hu H, Lai M. Non-coding RNAs and their epigenetic regulatory mechanisms. *Biol Cell.* 2010;102(12):645–655.
11. Eulalio A, Huntzinger E, Izaurralde E. Getting to the root of miRNA-mediated gene silencing. *Cell.* 2008;132(1):9–14.
12. Hamburg MA, Collins FS. The path to personalized medicine. *N Engl J Med.* 2010;363(4):301–304.
13. Catterall WA. Structure and function of voltage-sensitive ion channels. *Science.* 1988;242:50–61.
14. Clapham DE. SnapShot: mammalian TRP channels. *Cell.* 2007;129(1):220.
15. Jan L-Y, Jan Y-N. A superfamily of ion channels. *Nature.* 1990;345:672.
16. Jan LY, Jan YN. Tracing the roots of ion channels. *Cell.* 1992;69:715–718.
17. Paulmichl M, Li Y, Wickmann K, Ackerman M, Peralta E, Clapham D. New mammalian chloride channel identified by expression cloning. *Nature.* 1992;356:238–241.
18. Higgins CF. The ABC of channel regulation. *Cell.* 1995;82:693–696.
19. Pera A, Dossena S, Rodighiero S, et al. Functional assessment of allelic variants in the SLC26A4 gene involved in Pendred syndrome and nonsyndromic EVA. *Proc Natl Acad Sci U S A.* 2008;105(47):18608–18613.
20. Evans WE, Relling MV. Pharmacogenomics: translating functional genomics into rational therapeutics. *Science.* 1999;286(5439):487–491.
21. Eichelbaum M, Ingelman-Sundberg M, Evans WE. Pharmacogenomics and individualized drug therapy. *Annu Rev Med.* 2006;57:119–137.
22. Daly AK. Pharmacogenetics and human genetic polymorphisms. *Biochem J.* 2010;429(3):435–449.
23. Frueh FW, Amur S, Mummaneni P, et al. Pharmacogenomic biomarker information in drug labels approved by the United States Food and Drug Administration: prevalence of related drug use. *Pharmacotherapy.* 2008;28(8):992–998.
24. Pasanen MK, Neuvonen M, Neuvonen PJ, Niemi M. SLCO1B1 polymorphism markedly affects the pharmacokinetics of simvastatin acid. *Pharmacogenet Genomics.* 2006;16(12):873–879.

25. Ho RH, Tirona RG, Leake BF, et al. Drug and bile acid transporters in rosuvastatin hepatic uptake: function, expression, and pharmacogenetics. *Gastroenterology.* 2006;130(6):1793–1806.

26. Link E, Parish S, Armitage J, et al. SLCO1B1 variants and statin-induced myopathy—a genomewide study. *N Engl J Med.* 2008;359(8):789–799.

27. Simon R. Development and validation of biomarker classifiers for treatment selection. *J Stat Plan Inference.* 2008;138(2):308–320.

28. Russ AP, Lampel S. The druggable genome: an update. *Drug Discov Today.* 2005;10(23–24):1607–1610.

29. Hopkins AL, Groom CR. The druggable genome. *Nat Rev Drug Discov.* 2002;1(9):727–730.

30. Sapsford KE, Težak Ž, Kondratovich M, Pacanowski MA, Zineh I, Mansfield E. Biomarkers to improve the benefit/risk balance for approved therapeutics: a US FDA perspective on personalized medicine. *Ther Deliv.* 2010;1(5):631–641.

31. Lesko LJ, Zineh I. DNA, drugs and chariots: on a decade of pharmacogenomics at the US FDA. *Pharmacogenomics.* 2010;11(4):507–512.

32. Zineh I, Pacanowski MA. Pharmacogenomics in the assessment of therapeutic risks versus benefits: inside the United States Food and Drug Administration. *Pharmacotherapy.* 2011;31(8):729–735.

33. Zineh I, Woodcock J. The clinical pharmacogeneticist: an emerging regulatory scientist at the US Food and Drug Administration. *Hum Genomics.* 2010;4(4):221–225.

34. Goodsaid F, Papaluca M. Evolution of biomarker qualification at the health authorities. *Nature Biotechnol.* 2010;28(5):441–443.

35. Uyama Y. Tasks and expectations for drug design based on pharmacogenomics. *Nihon Yakurigaku Zasshi.* 2005;126(6):432–435.

5

Ethical, Legal, and Social Issues Associated with Pharmacogenomics

Joseph D. Ma, PharmD, Karen E. Lewis, MS, MM, CGC, & Joseph S. Bertino Jr., PharmD, FCP, FCCP

LEARNING OBJECTIVES

- To identify the current ethical, legal, and social issues associated with pharmacogenomics and pharmacogenomic testing.
- To understand how genetic discrimination, stigmatization, and privacy and confidentiality impact the implementation of pharmacogenomic testing into clinical practice.

- To understand the legal issues involving pharmacogenomic testing regarding the ownership of data and/or samples and intellectual property.
- To develop a knowledge base involving pharmacogenomic core competencies.

INTRODUCTION

On completion of the Human Genome Project in 2003, the field of pharmacogenetics and/or pharmacogenomics has rapidly developed with the intent of clinical application on individualizing therapy to maximize efficacy and/or minimize toxicity. There are numerous challenges and barriers that impact the implementation of pharmacogenomics into clinical practice. These include ethical, legal, and social issues that highlight risk, benefit, and public and professional acceptance.[1] Attempts to establish a framework of accelerating integration of appropriate pharmacogenomic and human genome discoveries into clinical practice have been reported.[2,3] Haddow and Palomaki[4] first reported the ACCE model for evaluating data on genetic tests. ACCE that takes its name from the four main criteria for evaluating a genetic test—analytic validity, clinical validity, clinical utility, and associated ethical, legal, and social implications—is a model process that includes collecting, evaluating, interpreting, and reporting

data about DNA (and related) testing for disorders with a genetic component in a format that allows policy makers to have access to up-to-date and reliable information for decision making. One of the major components for evaluation includes the associated ethical, legal, and social implications. The authors identified challenges and barriers to genetic testing including genetic discrimination, stigmatization, privacy/confidentiality, and personal/family social issues. Additional challenges highlighted legal issues regarding consent, ownership of data and/or samples, patents, licensing, disclosure obligations, and reporting requirements. Although the ethical, legal, and social issues revolve around establishing safeguards in the context of genetic testing, these components are applicable to pharmacogenomic testing.[5–7] Several examples in this chapter will highlight these issues in relation to genetic testing to aid in the understanding of specific concepts and application. The purpose of this chapter is to provide a framework of the ethical, legal, and social issues surrounding the rapidly evolving field of pharmacogenomics.

ETHICAL ISSUES

Genetic Discrimination

Individuals who obtain pharmacogenomic and/or genetic testing may be exposed to genetic discrimination. Genetic discrimination refers to when an individual, with a known genetic disorder or genetic polymorphism, is treated differently by his or her employer or insurance company.[8] Knowledge of genetic and/or pharmacogenomic information may be used to deny, limit, or cancel health insurance. There is suggestion that health insurers should have limited access to such information. Insurers would be able to use pharmacogenomic information for drug formulary management, but should be prohibited from using the same information in determining copayments or premiums, or negotiating contracts.[9] Additional concerns regarding genetic discrimination include employers using such information to only employ or retain individuals who do not have the genetic disorder or genetic polymorphism, limiting access to social services, and in the delivery of health care.[10] Consequently, genetic discrimination potentially generates social, health, and economic burdens for society due to decreasing opportunities of genetically predisposed individuals in a range of scenarios.

Several reports of genetic discrimination have been documented.[10–12] In 2001, the Equal Employment Opportunity Commission (EEOC) filed suit against the Burlington Northern State Santa Fe (BNSF) Railroad.[13] Without the knowledge and consent of its employees, BNSF tested 36 employees for a genetic condition associated with carpal tunnel syndrome as part of a comprehensive diagnostic exam. BNSF employees were examined by company-paid physicians and were not informed that genetic testing was being performed. Those employees who refused testing were also threatened with possible job termination.[14] BNSF defended such testing as a means of determining if repetitive stress injuries were work-related. Under the Americans with Disabilities Act, the EEOC argued that such testing as a basis for employment was unlawful and a cause for illegal discrimination.[13] The suit was eventually settled, with BNSF admitting that testing employees for a genetic condition was performed and that such testing was no longer being conducted.[13] In a case history study ($n = 41$), genetic discrimination involved insurance companies ($n = 32$) in areas of applications or coverage changes for health, life, disability, mortgage, and auto insurance. Seven cases involved employment in areas relating to hiring, termination, promotion, and transfer.[10] Due to the fear of discrimination, the authors also noted that respondents either withheld mentioning such information to health care providers, insurers, and employers or provided incomplete or dishonest information on insurance application forms.[10]

Stigmatization

Stigmatization is defined as "a social process that begins with distinguishing and labelling some feature of a person such as occupation, disease, or skin color."[15] An individual may experience stigmatization from family, friends, and coworkers on knowledge that a specific disease will not respond to therapy or if one is identified as a "poor metabolizer" of a specific medication. This may lead the individual to feeling lonely, isolated, hopeless, and depressed.[1] A classic example was during the 1980s, with human immunodeficiency virus/acquired immunodeficiency syndrome (HIV/AIDS) described as a sexually transmitted infection diagnosed in patients identified as homosexuals or intravenous drug users. Patients, as well as parents, children, and caregivers for HIV-positive patients, were susceptible to stigmatization. Negative connotations by the public included misperceptions that people associated with such behaviors were immoral, predatory, and dangerous.[15,16] Consequently, pharmacogenomic testing may also reveal similar negative connotations and public perceptions, as evidenced with traditional genetic testing.[17]

Privacy and Confidentiality

Patients, health care professionals, and policy makers are concerned about security and loss of privacy. The capacity for such information to be adequately stored and rapidly disseminated and the relative ease of accessibility all pose a risk for a loss of privacy.[18,19] Examples of methods to ensure privacy include use of de-identified subject data, use of password-protected and/or encrypted files, and limiting access. Additionally, federal legislation such as the Health Insurance Portability and Accountability Act (HIPAA) and private sector self-regulation exists. The HIPAA Privacy Rule provides federal protections for personal health information held by covered entities (e.g., health care providers, hospitals, pharmacies, insurance companies) and provides patients rights regarding personal health information. However, uncertainty remains in the capacity and ability of current systems to ensure privacy, security, and confidentiality. For example, health care practitioners who use telemedicine technologies to disseminate pharmacogenomic information may be faced with contrasting federal and state law privacy standards. In one scenario, if a provider orders a genetic test from one state and the results of the test are made available electronically to another out-of-state provider, clarification is warranted as to which state privacy laws are followed.[20,21] Additionally, HIPAA only applies to employer-based and commercially based issued health insurance and does not apply to individuals who seek private health insurance in the individual market.[14]

Balancing Harms and Benefits

Foreseeable harms should not outweigh anticipated benefits for participants in pharmacogenomic research. Minimizing harm implies a duty to ensure that research subjects are not subjected to unnecessary risks of harm and that their participation in research is essential to achieving the scientific outcomes necessary for future treatment for the subjects themselves, other individuals, or society as a whole.[22] Pharmacogenomic research includes the potential for physical risk and negative psychological impact. The physical risks are related to using a drug in which the drug itself has the potential to cause harms such as intolerable side effects. The psychological impact may include being excluded from enrolling in a clinical study if the individual does not have the genetic polymorphism or genotype, which may lead to despair if other treatments have failed or are not available. The implementation of a pharmacogenomic test to determine if an individual may respond appropriately to a given drug before beginning treatment may also result in a dilemma for health care providers and patients. For example, what is appropriate therapy for an individual who is not a candidate to receive a specific therapy based on a pharmacogenomic test result and for whom there are no other known treatments? Is it morally permissible to offer the treatment anyway with the knowledge of there being little chance for response or possibly even inducing harm? This is very unlikely to occur as most health care providers would find this option to be in conflict with their inherent duty to do no harm. However, this could theoretically create fear among consumers, which may result in patients unwilling to take the associated test for fear of being abandoned in their treatment.

LEGAL ISSUES

Informed Consent

With genetic testing, the DNA collected not just will include the known genetic polymorphisms obtained from participating in a research study but may also include information about the individual's entire genome. As a result, these DNA samples could provide invaluable information about not only the participant but also possibly his or her extended family, which could be entirely unrelated to the original study. Typically, such additional information would not be revealed to the original participants but rather be used in an anonymous fashion. However, this possibility should be discussed up front as part of obtaining informed consent. Although future use of such data may not be known at the time of consent, specific language should be described in the informed consent form. Consideration of using narrow (specific limited use) or broad (current and future use) terminology may be appropriate to help participants understand how their information may be used.[1,23]

In pharmacogenomic research one of the fundamental requirements to enter a study is to test individuals for a particular genotype of interest. Study participation in such research will reveal personal health information, which would not be known in other clinical studies. This particular knowledge does not necessarily compromise privacy and confidentiality but does require it be addressed in the consent process as well as dissemination of results that may or may not be revealed to the participants.[23]

Several issues related to the informed consent process for pharmacogenomic testing warrant discussion. First, there appears to be no standard at the national or international level concerning how to consent individuals for research that involves genetic testing. Although some have attempted to address these issues,[23] there currently exist two informed consent standards. The professional standard evaluates "what a reasonably prudent physician with the same background, training, and experience, practicing in the same community, would have disclosed to a patient in the same or similar situation."[1] In contrast, the patient standard attempts to address "what a reasonable patient in the same or similar situation would need or want to know to make an informed decision regarding a medical intervention or treatment."[1] Second, there is an inconsistency as to the placement of a consent form for genetic testing that was completed by the patient as part of a clinical study. Some advocate placement of the consent form in the patient's medical record, while others suggest that such information be kept separate from the patient's medical record. Our own experience has been that some institutional review boards (IRBs) do not recommend consent forms (for studies where genetic testing is to be done) to be placed in the medical record. Rather, such information should be kept in a file by both the investigator and the IRB. This attempts to ensure privacy by avoiding inadvertent disclosure of such information to anyone reviewing the patient's medical chart.

Ownership of Data and/or Samples

Pharmacogenomic testing requires collection of DNA. A biological specimen (e.g., blood, saliva, or tissue) is obtained from the patient. Due to genomic scale-up (e.g., genomic sequencing of patients), such specimens are stored in repositories known as biobanks. At times, biological specimens are aliquoted whereby material is used for pharmacogenomic testing and any remaining specimen is archived. The archiving of biological specimens in a biobank facilitates use of the same sample for future exploratory research with no defined time limit for use. These biological samples and their respective data are invaluable, not only to academic or medical geneticists but also to pharmaceutical companies and the biotechnology industry.

Claims of ownership of the biological specimen involve the subject-donor, the institution whereby research was conducted, and the individual investigator. Due to a lack of clearly defined regulations and multiple stakeholder involvement, the issue of ownership of biological specimens, such as those reserved for pharmacogenomic testing, remains contentious. From a subject-donor perspective, his or her biological specimen is considered a property right and denying such a right over biological material is unfair. The contrasting perspective "defends an absolute non-patrimonial view, denying the possibility of the existence of a property right."[24]

In the *Moore v Regents of the University of California* case,[25] the plaintiff sued the defendant claiming deprivation of property interest, lack of adequate informed consent, and breach of fiduciary duty. Mr Moore's biological specimens were collected by the defendant's physician for a research project. Unknown to the patient, the results of the research led to a patent application by the defendant. The state court ruled that Mr Moore did not retain the right of ownership of his biological specimen that was used to develop a new therapy/product. In addition, the court also noted that disclosure to the patient of additional research or economic interests was necessary.[25,26]

Research is underway to examine the issues related to the ownership of data and/or samples.[27,28] Legal writers have suggested theories related to trusteeship, benefit sharing, commodity, and "waste" models.[27] Current research is focused on understanding the different perspectives from the multiple stakeholders and to develop policies. Input should be acquired from all interested stakeholders including the general public, researchers, as well as the private sector. It also seems reasonable given the global nature of research and development that these regulations be formulated at an international level.[29]

Intellectual Property

Approximately 20% of all human genes are under US patents.[30] In 2005, this equated to 4,382 of the 23,688 genes described in the National Center for Biotechnology Information database.[30] US patent laws are intended to stimulate innovation and to protect the discoveries of inventors. For a period of 20 years, a patent provides the inventor the exclusive right to manufacture, use, and sell the discovery. To qualify for a patent, the invention needs to be useful, novel, and not obvious.[31,32] In the context of genomic medicine and pharmacogenomics, gene patents remain a contentious issue. The most common argument against gene patents is that since genes are naturally occurring biological processes, they exist to be discovered and not invented.[32] In contrast, such an argument is considered unpersuasive since isolating DNA does not occur naturally and that the "patent system has long recognized useful applications of discoveries as inventions."[32] In *Diamond v Chakrabarty*, the US Supreme Court ruled that genetically engineered bacteria were subject to patent protection as they did not occur in nature.[33] Although the genes themselves are not patentable, patent protection is allowable under the auspices of DNA that is modified, purified, or isolated resulting in a form that is nonexistent in nature.[31]

In 2009, a lawsuit was filed by the American Civil Liberties Union (ACLU) and others against Myriad Genetics for their US patent on the human genes BRCA1 and BRCA2. BRCA1 and BRCA2 mutations are associated with an increased risk of breast and ovarian cancers. Myriad Genetics currently owns at least seven patents directed at BRCA1 and BRCA2.[21,34] The plaintiffs argued that the BRCA genes were products of nature and were thus outside the realm of patent protection. Myriad Genetics cited the *Diamond v Chakrabarty* ruling and asked for dismissal. In a surprising ruling to many in the patent field, US District Court Judge Robert W. Sweet ruled in favor of the plaintiffs and invalidated seven BRCA patents by Myriad Genetics.[21] In June 2010, Myriad Genetics filed a notice of appeal in the US Court of Appeals for the Federal Circuit. In July 2011, the Federal Circuit ruled in favor of Myriad Genetics and declared that BRCA1 and BRCA2 genes were patent-eligible under Section 101 of the US Patent Act.[35]

Although it is not clear if the plaintiffs will appeal the Federal Circuit ruling, efforts are underway to consider regulatory and patent reform.[32,36,37] In 2011, the America Invents Act was signed into law and highlighted US patent reform. However, whether such law is applied to US patent cases involving pharmacogenomic and/or genetic testing remains to be seen. Others have suggested more stringent application of patent criteria for DNA sequences.[32] Expanding access to DNA sequences in publically available databases such as GenBank and the International HapMap Project will also provide researchers access and the ability to analyze genes associated with disease.[36]

Disclosure Obligations and Reporting Requirements

Ancillary information is defined as "additional information pertaining to the predisposition to diseases or conditions, prognostic information, or information relevant to other classes of drugs for which the individual is not currently seeking treatment or manifesting symptoms."[1] Pharmacogenomic testing potentially generates ancillary or incidental information unrelated to the original purpose for which the test was ordered. For research related to such testing, common practice has been to provide informed consent to individuals noting that genetic test results will not be disclosed, "incidental" or otherwise. However, some have expressed concerns that such a practice needs to be readdressed due to the advent of increasing technologies allowing for whole-genome sequencing, increasing accessibility of information, and increasing demand for the disclosure of such information.[38–40]

A recent study assessed the public perspectives regarding pharmacogenetics testing and managing ancillary information.[40] In a focused group session ($n = 45$), most participants agreed that physicians were obligated to disclose ancillary information.[40] Participants argued that the benefit of learning of ancillary risk information was an opportunity for preventive measures and a lack of knowledge of an individual's family history as reasons to warrant disclosure. However, participants also expressed concerns about insurance implications, the potential need for additional follow-up testing, and of the psychological harms, anxiety, and stress associated with the disclosure of ancillary information.[40] In another focus group study, perspectives regarding pharmacogenetics testing and managing ancillary information of primary care professionals and geneticists ($n = 21$) were also examined.[41] Among physicians, agreement was noted regarding the obligation to disclose ancillary information. Interestingly, geneticists believed that disclosure was not always necessary due to the complexities of genetic risk results.[41]

There is currently no consensus or system in place for communicating information to research participants that could have either a direct or indirect influence on care, especially when these findings are discovered years after the original study.[38] Should ancillary findings be returned to parents when children have been the subject in research? Do parents have an ethical duty to disclose the results to their child? Do researchers have an ethical duty to communicate research results? Communicating pharmacogenomic or genomic test results to children raises some questions such as who should receive the results (e.g., the child, his or her legal representative, his or her doctor) and in what capacity. These questions are particularly important because the information could have an impact on a child's clinical care and the parents may not be equipped to understand the impact on the overall health of their child. Because of the potential psychological effect on the participants' siblings and other family members, it is essential that the information and its implications be properly explained to the research participants and their parents. This raises similar issues in the consent process: how can complex information be simplified without distorting their meaning, or how can it be presented without sounding too optimistic.

SOCIAL ISSUES

Race and Ethnicity

Numerous examples exist regarding the prevalence of genetic polymorphisms varying between ethnic groups. *CYP2C19* is responsible for the metabolism of numerous drugs, including proton pump inhibitors (PPIs), tricyclic antidepressants, diazepam, and antiplatelet therapies (e.g., clopidogrel). At least 27 *CYP2C19* variant alleles have been identified,[42] with a higher prevalence of the *CYP2C19*2* and *CYP2C19*3* variants observed in Asians versus Caucasians and African Americans.[43,44] These variant alleles result in a functional loss of *CYP2C19* enzyme activity.[45,46] This may be of clinical significance regarding PPI efficacy as pharmacokinetic variability and *Helicobactor pylori* eradication rates are attributed, in part, to *CYP2C19* genetic polymorphisms. In several studies, *H. pylori* eradication rates were reported to be higher in Asians.[47–51]

Carbamazepine is an anticonvulsant and has been linked to life-threatening hypersensitivity reactions such as Stevens–Johnson syndrome (SJS) and toxic epidermal necrolysis (TEN).[52] The risk of a carbamazepine-induced SJS/TEN has been associated with individuals who possess the human leukocyte antigen *(HLA)-B*1502* allele. Interestingly, Caucasians who test positive for the *HLA-B*1502* allele may not be at risk for carbamazepine-induced hypersensitivity.[53] This is in contrast to Asian populations (e.g., Han Chinese, Indonesia, Malaysia, Taiwan, Thailand, the Philippines, and Vietnam), whereby the prevalence of the *HLA-B*1502* allele is approximately 10–15%.[54,55] In Han Chinese patients, there was 100% association with the *HLA-B*1502* allele and carbamazepine-induced SJS/TEN.[56] In a follow-up study, 59 of 60 patients who reported a carbamazepine-induced SJS/TEN were positive for *HLA-B*1502*.[57] In individuals of Thai ancestry, the odds ratio for developing carbamazepine-induced SJS/TEN was 54.76 (95% CI: 14.62–205.13, $P = 2.89 \times 10^{-12}$) for those who were positive for *HLA-B*1502*.[58] Based on the strength of these data and others, the US Food and Drug Administration and prescribing information recommend that individuals of Asian ancestry be tested for the *HLA-B*1502* allele prior to initiating carbamazepine.[58]

The association of pharmacogenomic testing with race and ethnicity is a contentious issue. Pharmacogenomic testing and/or research may stratify patients according to racial or ethnic groups resulting in genetic discrimination and stigmatization.[7,59]

With known health disparities regarding access to medical care among ethnic groups, there is concern that there will also be limited accessibility to pharmacogenomic testing. Regarding drug development and research, the population prevalence for certain genetic polymorphisms may result in the use of race as a primary criterion for participation in pharmacogenomic research.[1,7] Although the passage of the National Revitalization Act of 1993 mandated inclusion of racially identified groups into research,[60] theoretically, drug development may compromise the availability and access to pharmacogenomic testing and/or research in ethnic groups among industrialized and nonindustrialized countries. However, new guidelines, procedures, and practices are in development for engaging with the scientific community that offer opportunities to bridge the gap between genomic science and indigenous and/or developing communities.[61]

Testing in Vulnerable Populations

Pharmacogenomic research that is being performed needs to adhere to the principle that all individuals involved in any type of medical research are presumed to have the capacity and right to make free and informed decisions. Certain populations, such as children, may not have the capacity to make free and informed decisions. The majority of drugs used by children are done so without actually being tested specifically for their use. Assuming a drug that is safe and effective in adults will also be safe and effective in children is problematic due to known differences in developmental factors between children and adults. The Better Pharmaceuticals for Children Act of 1997 (renewed in 2002 as the Best Pharmaceuticals for Children Act [BPCA]) and the Pediatric Research Equity Act (PREA) have supported more direct research on existing and new drugs for use in children and have led to significant improvements in safety and efficacy.[62]

One method to protect children against the possible negative effects of participation in research is to use both consent and assent. Research protocols recognize that children should participate and want to participate in important decisions about their lives when developmentally appropriate, and that if they are too young to consent, their assent should be obtained.[63] In a pediatric research setting, the decision-making process regarding subject participation is more complex than when working with an adult population. It is generally accepted that children do not have the maturity or experience necessary to make an informed decision regarding their participation and therefore should include the input of a parent or adult guardian, the child (when appropriate), and the researcher.[64,65] The input of the researcher may be particularly useful when determining the medical benefits and risks of the child's research participation.[66] This is helpful because parents may find it difficult to weigh the possible advantages and disadvantages of their child's participation in pharmacogenomics research.

Vulnerable persons also include those with diminished competence and/or decision-making capacity due to medical conditions. This may include individuals diagnosed with schizophrenia, bipolar disorders, depressive disorders, and some dementias. At times, these medical conditions result in the affected individual having variable patterns of coherence for which decision making is known to follow a general pattern of decline. Most individuals with limited capacity are in some way still able to object or assent to research. However, individuals who have permanently lost the ability to self-reflect may be decisionally incapable. These individuals will need to involve assistance from family members and caregivers in order to participate in research. The participation of persons from such groups will be vital to ensure that drug development is specific to the predisposing genetic factors for a disease.[67–69]

Availability of Testing

A major barrier to implementing pharmacogenomics into clinical practice is the availability of pharmacogenomic testing.[6,70–72] In one study, questionnaires were sent to 629 individuals representing hospitals, laboratories, and universities throughout New Zealand and Australia. The objective of the study was to determine utilization rates of pharmacogenomic testing for drug metabolizing enzymes.[70] The results reported that 2% of respondents had genotyping tests available. In another study, poor availability of 20% was reported in North America medical practices for warfarin pharmacogenomic testing.[73]

Numerous factors that influence the availability of pharmacogenomic testing include assay equipment, training of staff, and cost. Conducting pharmacogenomic testing requires specialized genotyping equipment and training of personnel on site.[74] Practice settings may not have access to testing kits and laboratories in order to conduct testing. Although centralized laboratories (e.g., LabCorp) where testing can be performed are available, feasibility information such as the turnaround time for test results or test sensitivity and specificity varies or is lacking from laboratory sources. For example, anywhere from 5 to 10 days may be needed from obtaining the blood sample to determining and disseminating $CYP2C9$ and $CYP2D6$ genotyping test results.[75]

Knowledge and Education of Health Care Professionals

Knowledge deficiencies in genetics and pharmacogenomics exist among health care professionals in all disciplines.[76] In a survey on warfarin pharmacogenomic testing, five knowledge-based questions were developed and surveyed among health care professionals who provide anticoagulation services.[73] The survey response rate was low (22%), with participants including mostly pharmacists (64%) and nurses/nurse practitioners (23%). Knowledge was poor in areas of $CYP2C9$ and $VKORC1$ allele frequencies, the length of time required to perform a test, and interpreting test results. Approximately one third of respondents correctly answered the knowledge-based questions.[73] In an Internet-based survey of genetics education in psychiatry residency programs, more than 50% of respondents felt that their training in pharmacogenomics was minimal.[77] A recent systematic review also concluded similar findings that health care professionals generally

felt limited in their knowledge of pharmacogenomics.[76] The lack of knowledge in pharmacogenomics is also consistent among pharmacy, medical, and nursing students.[78–81]

Various initiatives are underway in order to train and educate health care professionals on pharmacogenomics. The National Coalition for Health Professional Education in Genetics (NCHPEG) is a working group of specialists with experience in genetics and health professions. NCHPEG identified 18 core competencies, with the purpose of encouraging health care professionals to "integrate genetics knowledge, skills, and attitudes into routine health care."[82] Examples in knowledge competencies include understanding basic genetics terminology, identifying genetic variations that facilitates prevention, diagnosis, and treatment options, and identifying available resources to assist those seeking genetic information or services.[82] Such competencies have been adapted in part by professional organizations. In 2002, the American Association of Colleges of Pharmacy (AACP) Academic Affairs Committee reported pharmacist-specific competencies in pharmacogenetics and pharmacogenomics, which were derived from 2001 NCHPEG competencies. Examples include a pharmacist being able to identify patients in whom pharmacogenetic testing is indicated, identify an appropriate pharmacogenomic test for a patient, and provide recommendations based on pharmacogenomic testing results.[83] Other professional organizations have also developed recommendations or position statements for pharmacogenomics education. These include the American Academy of Family Physicians *Core Educational Guidelines* and the Association of American Medical Colleges *Contemporary Issues in Medicine: Genetics Education Report.*[84,85]

CONCLUSIONS

While the science of pharmacogenomics has moved along rapidly, particularly since the completion of the Human Genome Project, a thorough plan to address the ethical, legal, and social issues remains to be developed and implemented. Currently there is no international standard for genetic testing. Input is required from the multiple stakeholders such as the subject-donor, the institution whereby research was conducted, regulatory agencies, professional organizations, health care professionals, and those involved in pharmacogenomic research. Guidelines need to be considered and harmonized internationally to protect individuals and reduce the chance of discrimination based on genetic testing, and be synchronized with the advancing field of pharmacogenomics.

REFERENCES

1. Haga SB. Ethical, legal, and social challenges to applied pharmacogenetics. In: McLeod HL, DeVane CL, Haga SB, et al., eds. *Pharmacogenomics. Applications to Patient Care.* Lenexa: American College of Clinical Pharmacy; 2009:273–297.
2. Berg JS, Khoury MJ, Evans JP. Deploying whole genome sequencing in clinical practice and public health: meeting the challenge one bin at a time. *Genet Med.* 2011;13(6):499–504.

3. Khoury MJ, Gwinn M, Yoon PW, Dowling N, Moore CA, Bradley L. The continuum of translation research in genomic medicine: how can we accelerate the appropriate integration of human genome discoveries into health care and disease prevention? *Genet Med.* 2007;9(10):665–674.

4. Haddow JE, Palomaki GE. ACCE: a model process for evaluating data on emerging genetic tests. In: Khoury MJ, Little J, Burke W, eds. *Human Genome Epidemiology: A Scientific Foundation for Using Genetic Information to Improve Health and Prevent Disease.* New York: Oxford University Press; 2004:217–233.

5. Goldman BR. Pharmacogenomics: privacy in the era of personalized medicine. *Northwest J Technol Intellect Property.* 2005;4:83–89. Available at: http://www.law.northwestern.edu/journals/njtip/v4/n1/4/Goldman.pdf.

6. Ikediobi ON, Shin J, Nussbaum RL, et al. Addressing the challenges of the clinical application of pharmacogenetic testing. *Clin Pharmacol Ther.* 2009;86(1):28–31.

7. Lipton P. Pharmacogenetics: the ethical issues. *Pharmacogenomics J.* 2003;3(1):14–16.

8. U.S. National Library of Medicine. Genetics Home Reference. What is genetic discrimination? 2011. Available at: http://ghr.nlm.nih.gov/handbook/testing/discrimination. Accessed November 22, 2011.

9. Zachry WM, Armstrong EP. Health care professionals' perceptions of the role of pharmacogenomic data. *J Manag Care Pharm.* 2002;8(4):278–284.

10. Billings PR, Kohn MA, de Cuevas M, Beckwith J, Alper JS, Natowicz MR. Discrimination as a consequence of genetic testing. *Am J Hum Genet.* 1992;50(3):476–482.

11. Otlowski MF, Taylor SD, Barlow-Stewart KK. Genetic discrimination: too few data. *Eur J Hum Genet.* 2003;11(1):1–2.

12. Low L, King S, Wilkie T. Genetic discrimination in life insurance: empirical evidence from a cross sectional survey of genetic support groups in the United Kingdom. *BMJ.* 1998;317(7173):1632–1635.

13. U.S. Equal Employment Opportunity Commission. EEOC settles ADA suit against BNSF for genetic bias. 2001. Available at: http://www.eeoc.gov/eeoc/newsroom/release/4-18-01.cfm. Accessed November 22, 2011.

14. Human Genome Project Information. Genetics privacy and legislation. 2008. Available at: http://www.ornl.gov/sci/techresources/Human_Genome/elsi/legislat.shtml. Accessed November 25, 2011.

15. Sankar P, Cho MK, Wolpe PR, Schairer C. What is in a cause? Exploring the relationship between genetic cause and felt stigma. *Genet Med.* 2006;8(1):33–42.

16. Bunting SM. Sources of stigma associated with women with HIV. *ANS Adv Nurs Sci.* 1996;19(2):64–73.

17. Wertz DC. Ethical, social and legal issues in pharmacogenomics. *Pharmacogenomics J.* 2003;3(4):194–196.

18. Bashshur RL, Reardon TG, Shannon GW. Telemedicine: a new health care delivery system. *Annu Rev Public Health.* 2000;21:613–637.

19. Liaw ST, Schattner P. eConsulting. *Methods Mol Med.* 2008;141:353–373.

20. Kuo GM, Ma JD, Lee KC, Bourne PE. Telemedicine, genomics and personalized medicine: synergies and challenges. *Curr Pharmacogenomics Personalized Med.* 2010;9:6–13.

21. Schwartz J, Pollack A. Judge invalidates human gene patent. *The New York Times.* 2010. Available at: http://www.nytimes.com/2010/03/30/business/30gene.html. Accessed December 2, 2011.

22. Freund CL, Clayton EW. Pharmacogenomics and children: meeting the ethical challenges. *Am J Pharmacogenomics.* 2003;3(6):399–404.

23. Robertson JA. Consent and privacy in pharmacogenetic testing. *Nat Genet.* 2001;28(3):207–209.

24. Lobato de Faria P. Ownership rights in research biobanks: do we need a new kind of 'biological property'? In: Solbakk JH, Holm S, Hofmann B, eds. *The Ethics of Research Biobanking.* New York: Springer Science; 2009:263–276.

25. *Moore v Regents of the University of California*, 51 Cal3d 120, 793 P2d 479, 271 Cal Rptr 146 (1990).

26. Hakimian R, Korn D. Ownership and use of tissue specimens for research. *JAMA.* 2004;292(20):2500–2505.

27. Center for Genomics and Society at UNC-Chapel Hill. Legal frameworks for the storage and use of genetic samples and information. Available at: http://genomics.unc.edu/genomicsandsociety/html/legal_frameworks_for_storage_a.html. Accessed December 20, 2011.

28. Center for Genomics and Society at UNC-Chapel Hill. Perceptions of ownership of biological samples. Available at: http://genomics.unc.edu/genomicsandsociety/html/perceptions_of_ownership_of_bi.html. Accessed December 20, 2011.

29. O'Doherty KC, Hawkins A. Structuring public engagement for effective input in policy development on human tissue biobanking. *Public Health Genomics.* 2010;13(4):197–206.

30. Jensen K, Murray F. Intellectual property. Enhanced: intellectual property landscape of the human genome. *Science.* 2005;310(5746):239–240.

31. Solomon LM, Sieczkiewicz GJ. Impact of the US Patent System on the promise of personalized medicine. *Gend Med.* 2007;4(3):187–192.

32. Williams N. New thinking on gene patents. *Curr Biol.* 2002;12(17):R577–R578.

33. *Diamond v Chakrabarty*, 447 U.S. 303 (1980).

34. Kepler TB, Crossman C, Cook-Deegan R. Metastasizing patent claims on BRCA1. *Genomics.* 2010;95(5):312–314.

35. Myriad applauds the court of appeals' decision to uphold gene patenting. 2011. Available at: http://investor.myriad.com/releasedetail.cfm?ReleaseID=595288. Accessed December 2, 2011.

36. Davis AF, Long RM. Pharmacogenetics research network and knowledge base second scientific meeting. *Pharmacogenomics J.* 2002;2(5):293–296.

37. Herder M. Patents & the progress of personalized medicine: biomarkers research as lens. *Ann Health Law.* 2009;18(2):187–229 [8 p preceding i].

38. Cho MK. Understanding incidental findings in the context of genetics and genomics. *J Law Med Ethics.* 2008;36(2):280–285, 212.

39. Haga SB, O'Daniel JM, Tindall GM, Lipkus IR, Agans R. Public attitudes toward ancillary information revealed by pharmacogenetic testing under limited information conditions. *Genet Med.* 2011;13(8):723–728.

40. Haga SB, Tindall G, O'Daniel JM. Public perspectives about pharmacogenetic testing and managing ancillary findings. *Genet Test Mol Biomarkers.* 2012;16(3):193–197.

41. Haga SB, Tindall G, O'Daniel JM. Professional perspectives about pharmacogenetic testing and managing ancillary findings. *Genet Test Mol Biomarkers.* 2012;16(1):21–24.

42. Home page of human cytochrome P450 (CYP) Allele Nomenclature Committee. Available at: http://www.cypalleles.ki.se/. Accessed November 30, 2011.

43. Desta Z, Zhao X, Shin JG, Flockhart DA. Clinical significance of the cytochrome P450 2C19 genetic polymorphism. *Clin Pharmacokinet.* 2002;41(12):913–958.

44. Mizutani T. PM frequencies of major CYPs in Asians and Caucasians. *Drug Metab Rev.* 2003;35(2–3):99–106.

45. de Morais SM, Wilkinson GR, Blaisdell J, Meyer UA, Nakamura K, Goldstein JA. Identification of a new genetic defect responsible for the polymorphism of (S)-mephenytoin metabolism in Japanese. *Mol Pharmacol.* 1994;46(4):594–598.

46. de Morais SM, Wilkinson GR, Blaisdell J, Nakamura K, Meyer UA, Goldstein JA. The major genetic defect responsible for the polymorphism of S-mephenytoin metabolism in humans. *J Biol Chem.* 1994;269(22):15419–15422.

47. Furuta T, Ohashi K, Kamata T, et al. Effect of genetic differences in omeprazole metabolism on cure rates for *Helicobacter pylori* infection and peptic ulcer. *Ann Intern Med.* 1998;129(12):1027–1030.

48. Furuta T, Ohashi K, Kobayashi K, et al. Effects of clarithromycin on the metabolism of omeprazole in relation to CYP2C19 genotype status in humans. *Clin Pharmacol Ther.* 1999;66(3):265–274.

49. Furuta T, Ohashi K, Kosuge K, et al. CYP2C19 genotype status and effect of omeprazole on intragastric pH in humans. *Clin Pharmacol Ther.* 1999;65(5):552–561.

50. Furuta T, Shirai N, Takashima M, et al. Effects of genotypic differences in CYP2C19 status on cure rates for *Helicobacter pylori* infection by dual therapy with rabeprazole plus amoxicillin. *Pharmacogenetics.* 2001;11(4):341–348.

51. Furuta T, Shirai N, Takashima M, et al. Effect of genotypic differences in CYP2C19 on cure rates for *Helicobacter pylori* infection by triple therapy with a proton pump inhibitor, amoxicillin, and clarithromycin. *Clin Pharmacol Ther.* 2001;69(3):158–168.

52. Kaniwa N, Saito Y, Aihara M, et al. HLA-B*1511 is a risk factor for carbamazepine-induced Stevens–Johnson syndrome and toxic epidermal necrolysis in Japanese patients. *Epilepsia.* 2010;51(12):2461–2465.

53. Alfirevic A, Jorgensen AL, Williamson PR, Chadwick DW, Park BK, Pirmohamed M. HLA-B locus in Caucasian patients with carbamazepine hypersensitivity. *Pharmacogenomics*. 2006;7(6):813–818.

54. Lee MT, Hung SI, Wei CY, Chen YT. Pharmacogenetics of toxic epidermal necrolysis. *Expert Opin Pharmacother*. 2010;11(13):2153–2162.

55. Lonjou C, Thomas L, Borot N, et al. A marker for Stevens–Johnson syndrome…: ethnicity matters. *Pharmacogenomics J*. 2006;6(4):265–268.

56. Chung WH, Hung SI, Hong HS, et al. Medical genetics: a marker for Stevens–Johnson syndrome. *Nature*. 2004;428(6982):486.

57. Hung SI, Chung WH, Jee SH, et al. Genetic susceptibility to carbamazepine-induced cutaneous adverse drug reactions. *Pharmacogenet Genomics*. 2006;16(4):297–306.

58. Food and Drug Administration. Information on carbamazepine (marketed as Carbatrol, Equetro, Tegretol, and generics) with FDA alerts. Available at: http://www.fda.gov/Drugs/DrugSafety/PostmarketDrugSafety InformationforPatientsandProviders/ucm107834.htm. Accessed November 30, 2011.

59. Lipton P. Nuffield Council on Bioethics consultation. *Pharmacogenomics*. 2003;4(1):91–95.

60. Lee SS. Racializing drug design: implications of pharmacogenomics for health disparities. *Am J Public Health*. 2005;95(12):2133–2138.

61. Jacobs B, Roffenbender J, Collmann J, et al. Bridging the divide between genomic science and indigenous peoples. *J Law Med Ethics*. 2010;38(3):684–696.

62. American Academy of Pediatrics. Best Pharmaceuticals for Children Act. Pediatric Research Equity Act. 2007 REAUTHORIZATION Improvements to Existing Law. 110th Congress: H.R. 3580, Public Law 110-85. Available at: http://www.aap.org/advocacy/washing/therapeutics/. Accessed November 21, 2011.

63. Avard D, Silverstein T, Sillon G, Joly Y. Researchers' perceptions of the ethical implications of pharmacogenomics research with children. *Public Health Genomics*. 2009;12(3):191–201.

64. Ross LF. Genetic testing of adolescents: is it in their best interest? *Arch Pediatr Adolesc Med*. 2000;154(8):850–852.

65. Ross LF, Moon MR. Ethical issues in genetic testing of children. *Arch Pediatr Adolesc Med*. 2000;154(9):873–879.

66. Wilfond BS, Carpenter KJ. Incidental findings in pediatric research. *J Law Med Ethics*. 2008;36(2):332–340, 213.

67. The National Commission for the Protection of Human Subjects of Biomedical and Behavioral Research. *The Belmont Report: Ethical Principles and Guidelines for the Protection of Human Subjects of Research*. Available at: http://www.hhs.gov/ohrp/humansubjects/guidance/belmont.html. Accessed November 21, 2011.

68. Chen DT, Miller FG, Rosenstein DL. Enrolling decisionally impaired adults in clinical research. *Med Care*. 2002;40(9 suppl):V20–V29.

69. Moser DJ, Schultz SK, Arndt S, et al. Capacity to provide informed consent for participation in schizophrenia and HIV research. *Am J Psychiatry*. 2002;159(7):1201–1207.

70. Gardiner SJ, Begg EJ. Pharmacogenetic testing for drug metabolizing enzymes: is it happening in practice? *Pharmacogenet Genomics*. 2005;15(5):365–369.

71. McKinnon RA, Ward MB, Sorich MJ. A critical analysis of barriers to the clinical implementation of pharmacogenomics. *Ther Clin Risk Manag*. 2007;3(5):751–759.

72. Newman W, Payne K. Removing barriers to a clinical pharmacogenetics service. *Personalized Med*. 2008;5(5):471–480.

73. Kadafour M, Haugh R, Posin M, Kayser SR, Shin J. Survey on warfarin pharmacogenetic testing among anticoagulation providers. *Pharmacogenomics*. 2009;10(11):1853–1860.

74. Marsh S, van Rooij T. Challenges of incorporating pharmacogenomics into clinical practice. *Gastrointest Cancer Res*. 2009;3(5):206–207.

75. Lee KC, Ma JD, Kuo GM. Pharmacogenomics: bridging the gap between science and practice. *J Am Pharm Assoc (2003)*. 2010;50(1):e1–e14 [quiz e15–e17].

76. Dodson C. Knowledge and attitudes concerning pharmacogenomics among healthcare professionals. *Personalized Med*. 2011;8(4):421–428.

77. Hoop JG, Savla G, Roberts LW, Zisook S, Dunn LB. The current state of genetics training in psychiatric residency: views of 235 U.S. educators and trainees. *Acad Psychiatry*. 2010;34(2):109–114.

78. Dodson CH, Lewallen LP. Nursing students' perceived knowledge and attitude towards genetics. *Nurse Educ Today*. 2011;31(4):333–339.

79. Green JS, O'Brien TJ, Chiappinelli VA, Harralson AF. Pharmacogenomics instruction in US and Canadian medical schools: implications for personalized medicine. *Pharmacogenomics*. 2010;11(9):1331–1340.

80. Latif DA. Pharmacogenetics and pharmacogenomics instruction in schools of pharmacy in the USA: is it adequate? *Pharmacogenomics*. 2005;6(4):317–319.

81. Murphy JE, Green JS, Adams LA, Squire RB, Kuo GM, McKay A. Pharmacogenomics in the curricula of colleges and schools of pharmacy in the United States. *Am J Pharm Educ*. 2010;74(1):7.

82. NCHPEG. Core competencies for all health care professionals. 2007. Available at: http://www.nchpeg.org/index.php?option=com_content& view=article&id=94&Itemid=84. Accessed September 30, 2011.

83. Johnson JA, Bootman JL, Evans WE, et al. Pharmacogenomics: a scientific revolution in pharmaceutical sciences and pharmacy practice. Report of the 2001–2002 Academic Affairs Committee. *Am J Pharm Educ*. 2002;66:12S–15S.

84. American Academy of Family Physicians (AAFP). Core educational guidelines. Medical genetics: recommended core educational guidelines for family practice residents. 1999. Available at: http://www.aafp.org/afp/1999/0701/p305.html. Accessed November 27, 2011.

85. Association of American Medical Colleges (AAMC). Contemporary issues in medicine: genetic education. 2004. Available at: https://members.aamc.org/eweb/DynamicPage.aspx?webcode=PubHome. Accessed November 27, 2011.

Pharmacogenetics of Cytochrome P450

Su-Jun Lee, PhD, Sang-Seop Lee, PhD, & Jae-Gook Shin, MD, PhD

LEARNING OBJECTIVES

- Discuss relevant genetic polymorphisms of important CYPs.
- Outline potential ethnic and racial differences in CYP genetics.

- Discuss potential clinical implications of genetic polymorphism.

Cytochrome P450s (CYPs) are a heme-containing superfamily of enzymes responsible for the metabolism of a wide range of structurally diverse substrates. In addition to the metabolism of human drugs, they also have biologically important roles, such as metabolism of several hormones, synthesis and elimination of cholesterol, regulation of blood homeostasis, metabolism of arachidonic acid, and detoxification of foreign pollutants. Genetic polymorphisms in genes encoding drug-metabolizing enzymes can result in variability in drug metabolism and drug elimination, which often affect treatment outcome at various degrees, depending on the severity of mutation and the extent of penetrance of that gene. There are large environmental factors, drug–drug interactions, and clinical factors that influence clinical outcomes, providing further complexity in understanding individual differences in drug responses. Because CYPs play a critical role in the metabolism of human drugs, accounting for approximately 80% of all phase I drug metabolism, CYP genes have been important targets for pharmacogenetics and pharmacogenomics research. Tremendous efforts on pharmacogenetics and pharmacogenomics during the last several decades have led to the discovery of many clinically relevant genetic polymorphisms in CYPs. This chapter presents an overview of functional CYP polymorphisms with regard to biochemical aspects as well as clinical consequences.

PHARMACOGENOMICS OF CYP2C9

Introduction

Among the four *CYP2C* genes in humans, *CYP2C9* is the most abundantly expressed enzyme in the human liver,[1,2] accounting for the metabolism of approximately 15–20% of prescribed and over-the-counter drugs.[3] CYP2C9 metabolizes a number of clinically important drugs, including the antidiabetic drugs tolbutamide and glipizide,[4,5] the anticonvulsant phenytoin,[6] the anticoagulant warfarin,[7] the antihypertensive drug losartan,[8] the diuretic torasemide,[9] and nonsteroidal anti-inflammatory drugs (NSAIDs) such as ibuprofen, diclofenac, piroxicam, tenoxicam, and mefenamic acid.[10] CYP2C9 also metabolizes endogenous substrates, such as arachidonic acid and linoleic acid.[11] Since CYP2C9 is polymorphic, it is involved in interindividual variation in the metabolism and disposition of the drugs described above. In particular, drugs with a narrow therapeutic index, such as *S*-warfarin and phenytoin, can present serious problems in dose adjustments while achieving appropriate drug concentrations without causing high dose–induced drug toxicity.

Functional Polymorphism of CYP2C9

A number of polymorphisms of CYP2C9 have been shown to contribute to altered CYP2C9 activity. The two most prevalent

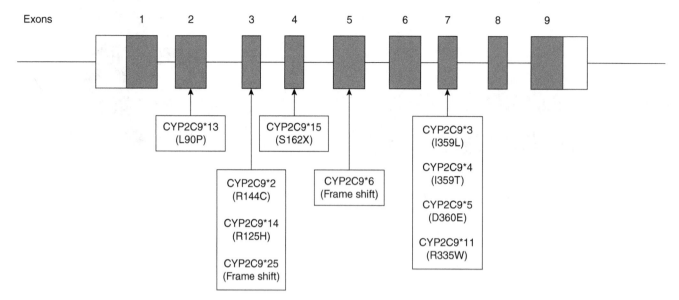

FIGURE 6A–1 Functional CYP2C9 alleles that were identified and evidenced in phenotyped human subjects. White boxes are 5'- and 3'-untranslated regions. Black boxes are exons in open reading frame. Arrow heads indicate mutated locations that result in amino acid change, stop codon (X), or frameshift.

and clinically relevant defective variants in white populations are CYP2C9*2 and *3.[12–15] Null variant alleles include CYP2C9*6, *15, and *25.[16–18] CYP2C9 variants identified from phenotyped individuals include CYP2C9*2, *3, *4, *5, *6, *11, *13, and *14[19–22] (Figure 6A–1). The frequency of CYP2C9*2 is 11% in whites and about 1% in blacks.[23,24] However, the frequency of

CYP2C9*2 in Asians is very rare or not detected in certain populations, such as Korean, Japanese, Taiwanese, and Chinese.[25–28] The frequency of CYP2C9*3 is 7% in whites, 1% in blacks, and 3% in Asians.[29] Ethnic differences in the frequency of these CYP2C9 genotypes are summarized in Table 6A–1. CYP2C9*2 carries an Arg144Cys mutation and CYP2C9*3 encodes an

TABLE 6A–1 Distribution of major CYP2C9 genotypes in different ethnic populations.

Ethnic Group	N	*1/*1	*1/*2	*1/*3	*2/*2	*2/*3	*3/*3	Reference
Whites								
American	140	94 (67.2%)	31 (22.1%)	12 (8.6%)	3 (2.1%)	0 (0%)	0 (0%)	Dickmann et al.[30]
British	561	392 (69.9%)	107 (19.1%)	53 (9.4%)	3 (0.5%)	6 (1.1%)	0 (0%)	Taube et al.[23]
Spanish	157	78 (49.7%)	25 (15.9%)	37 (23.5%)	3 (1.9%)	14 (8.9%)	0 (0%)	Garcia-Martin et al.[31]
Turkish	499	308 (61.7%)	90 (18.0%)	86 (17.2%)	5 (1.0%)	6 (1.1%)	4 (0.8%)	Aynacioglu et al.[32]
Italian	157	102 (65%)	24 (15.3%)	22 (14.0%)	4 (2.5%)	3 (1.9%)	2 (1.3%)	Scordo et al.[14]
Black								
African American	100	97 (97%)	2 (2%)	1 (1%)	0 (0%)	0 (0%)	0 (0%)	Sullivan-Klose et al.[26]
Ethiopian	150	130 (86.7%)	13 (8.7%)	7 (4.6%)	0 (0%)	0 (0%)	0 (0%)	Scordo et al.[14]
Asian								
Korean	574	561 (97.7%)	0 (0%)	13 (2.3%)	0 (0%)	0 (0%)	0 (0%)	Yoon et al.[28]
Korean	50	45 (90%)	0 (0%)	4 (8%)	0 (0%)	0 (0%)	1 (2%)	Lee et al.[33]
Chinese	115	111 (96.5%)	0 (0%)	4 (3.5%)	0 (0%)	0 (0%)	0 (0%)	Wang et al.[27]
Japanese	218	209 (95.9%)	0 (0%)	9 (4.1%)	0 (0%)	0 (0%)	0 (0%)	Nasu et al.[25]
Taiwanese	98	93 (91.8%)	0 (0%)	5 (8.2%)	0 (0%)	0 (0%)	0 (0%)	Sullivan-Klose et al.[26]
Indian	481	375 (78%)	24 (5%)	72 (15%)	5 (1%)	5 (1%)	0 (0%)	Jose et al.[34]
Malay	209	191 (91.4%)	8 (3.8%)	10 (4.8%)	0 (0%)	0 (0%)	0 (0%)	Ngow et al.[35]
Vietnamese	157	150 (95.5%)	0 (0%)	7 (4.5%)	0 (0%)	0 (0%)	0 (0%)	Lee et al.[36]
Iranian	200	164 (82%)	21 (10.5%)	0 (0%)	15 (7.5%)	0 (0%)	0 (0%)	Zand et al.[37]

Ile359Leu change. The investigation of CYP2C9*2 and *3 alleles showed that these variants are associated with significantly reduced S-warfarin 7'-hydroxylation in the various recombinant enzyme assay systems as well as the genotyped human liver microsomes.[13,15,30,38] However, no single in vitro system has been adopted as the standard method for exact evaluation of the functional change of the CYP2C9 polymorphisms compared with the wild-type CYP2C9*1. Therefore, quantitative comparisons of CYP2C9 variants with the wild-type CYP2C9 should be interpreted with great caution. Many functional studies evaluating the activity of CYP2C9*2 and *3 have consistently demonstrated a significantly reduced CYP2C9 activity compared with CYP2C9*1.[13,38–41] In general, the CYP2C9*3 variant has consistently exhibited a greater reduction, a 10–30% activity of the wild-type CLint, in the metabolism of all CYP2C9 substrate drugs than the CYP2C9*2 allele that exhibits a 70–90% activity of the wild-type CLint in various in vitro studies.[21] In most CYP2C9 substrates, individuals with the CYP2C9*3 heterozygous mutation exhibited approximately 50% of the wild-type total oral clearance and individuals carrying the CYP2C9*3 homozygous mutation showed a 5- to 10-fold reduction.[42–44] Therefore, it is believed that the CYP2C9*3 allele is a more defective allele affecting drug pharmacokinetics and pharmacodynamics. Substrate-specific differences in the metabolic activity of CYP2C9 alleles were reported,[42] suggesting that the particular CYP2C9 alleles can affect drug metabolism differently depending on the substrate. Although in vitro systems provide characterization of CYP2C9 alleles in regard to many substrates, the corresponding response of the drug by these alleles in vivo is still a difficult issue. However, for detecting changes in the metabolic activity of the CYP2C9 allele for certain drugs such as warfarin and phenytoin, in vitro systems are a useful predictor of the drug response in vivo.

Clinical Relevance of CYP2C9 Genetic Polymorphism

The clinical relevance of CYP2C9 polymorphisms was initiated and identified by two main coding variants, CYP2C9*2 and *3. A number of individual case reports with CYP2C9 substrate drugs have described the clinical significance of CYP2C9 polymorphisms with the new discovery of CYP2C9 defective alleles (official CYP2C9 allele nomenclature: http://www.cypalleles.ki.se/cyp2c9.htm). Among these case reports, most clinical problems with toxicity and dose adjustment have resulted from warfarin and phenytoin administration in CYP2C9 "poor metabolizer" (PM) genotypes.[45,46] Warfarin consists of equal amount of R- and S-warfarin. S-Warfarin is more potent and metabolized principally by CYP2C9, whereas R-warfarin is metabolized by CYP1A1, CYP2C19, and CYP3A4.[47] Patients having a CYP2C9*2 or *3 allele are significantly prone to experience a bleeding event and prolonged hospitalization due to unstable anticoagulation when compared with the wild-type. Therefore, it is suggested that lower warfarin doses need to be employed in patients having defective alleles. For example, in a similar demographic condition, stable warfarin daily dose requirements were differently observed as an average value of 7.9 mg per day for CYP2C9*1/*1 patients

(n = 49) and 2.2 mg per day for CYP2C9*1/*3 patients (n = 10).[48] Genotyping for CYP2C9 is a significant factor during the unstable period of warfarin dose initiation.[23,49,50] However, it appears that once antithrombotic stability is attained, experienced clinicians are likely to maintain a patient's INR and minimize his or her bleeding risk with less dependence on CYP2C9 genotype.[23] Studies from meta-analysis indicated that the CYP2C9 genotype accounted for 12% of the variability of warfarin dosing and VKORC1 polymorphisms accounted for 25%.[51] CYP2C9 genotyping prior to warfarin initiation improves the safety profile. The FDA has approved warfarin pharmacogenetic tests, which can be used for initial dose determination. Although cost-effectiveness with the CYP2C9 genotype testing remains to be determined, warfarin dosing models incorporating clinical factors and genetic profiles are under strong investigation.

Although both CYP2C9 and CYP2C19 metabolize phenytoin, CYP2C9 is responsible for the major pathway of phenytoin metabolism, accounting for approximately 80–90% of its elimination.[52,53] Since phenytoin exhibits a narrow therapeutic range with a concentration-related toxicity, small changes of CYP2C9 activity can lead to nervous system intoxication.[4,45] Multiple case reports and clinical observations suggested that the CYP2C9 genotype is an important determinant for the prediction of phenytoin disposition in humans.[16,32,54] For example, patients carrying at least one variant of defective CYP2C9 allele required a 30% lower phenytoin maintenance dose than the patients carrying CYP2C9*1/*1 genotype.[55] Similarly, individuals having CYP2C9*3/*3 exhibited a 3-fold increase in half-life and a 4-fold increase in AUC (area under the plasma concentration vs. time curves) compared with individuals having CYP2C9*1/*1.[4] The importance of CYP2C9 in the metabolism of phenytoin was evidenced by a case report of an individual who had a homozygous mutation for CYP2C9*6 null allele, indicating that this individual has no active CYP2C9 protein.[16] This individual was taken to the emergency department with severe phenytoin toxicity. Clearance of phenytoin in this individual was estimated to be 17% of the general population with 13 days of elimination half-life.[16] Clinical implications of CYP2C9 genotype are evident in phenytoin therapy. However, since there are many different CYP2C9 variant alleles, the impact of each variant on the clinical outcome of phenytoin remains to be determined.

Tolbutamide has been used as a phenotypic probe for CYP2C9 activity in vivo and as a prototypic substrate for the assessment of hepatic CYP2C9 activity in vitro.[5,56] Therefore, tolbutamide "PM" phenotype could be attributed to the homozygous mutation for CYP2C9 defective alleles. Investigations using CYP2C9 variants demonstrate that functional CYP2C9 polymorphisms are associated with significant changes in tolbutamide pharmacokinetics.[26] Similarly, pharmacokinetics of the antidiabetic drug glibenclamide and glimepiride has been significantly affected by CYP2C9 genotypes, indicating that individuals having CYP2C9*3 exhibited higher AUC and reduced oral clearance.[57,58] However, clinical consequences, such as blood glucose response, of CYP2C9 polymorphisms in the treatment of type 2 diabetic patients using oral hypoglycemic agents remain unclear.[57,58] Further prospective studies for the relationship between pharmacokinetics and pharmacodynamics would be necessary to approach the dose adjustment strategy on the basis of CYP2C9 genotype in diabetic patients.

Perspective of Clinical Application

A number of investigations have evaluated the clinical significance of CYP2C9*2 and *3 on the various CYP2C9 substrate drugs. In particular, individuals homozygous for CYP2C9*2 or *3 were associated with significant alterations in pharmacokinetics and pharmacodynamics of the drugs such as warfarin and phenytoin. Contribution of CYP2C9 genotype to drug metabolism is dependent on the substrate specificity, because most CYP2C9 substrates are also metabolized to certain degrees by other enzymes. For example, phenytoin is predominantly metabolized by CYP2C9, but minor metabolic pathway includes CYP2C19.[52] The metabolism of tolbutamide includes CYP2C19 as a minor metabolic pathway and the same is true of losartan with CYP3A4.[8,59] Since CYP2C9 metabolizes a wide range of clinically used drugs with different degrees of specificity,[42] comprehensive pharmacogenomics information together with the extent of CYP2C9's contribution to the total drug metabolism would be necessary to understand interindividual variations when taking CYP2C9-dependent drugs.

PHARMACOGENOMICS OF CYP2C19

Introduction

The cytochrome P450 CYP2C19 is a clinically important enzyme that metabolizes a number of drugs such as the antiulcer drug omeprazole,[60] the anticonvulsant mephenytoin,[60,61] the antimalarial proguanil,[62,63] the anxiolytic drug diazepam,[61,64,65] and certain antidepressants such as citalopram,[66] imipramine,[67] amitriptyline,[68] and clomipramine.[69] The metabolism of these drugs has been reported as polymorphic in humans.[12] The metabolic

ratio (MR) between the plasma concentration of omeprazole and that of its 5-hydroxy metabolite is used as a measure of CYP2C19 activity in vivo.[70] Because mephenytoin, a racemic mixture of R- and S-enantiomers, is metabolized differently and S-mephenytoin is much more rapidly hydroxylated by the CYP2C19, the S-/R-ratio has been used as a measure of CYP2C19 activity in humans.[1,70,71] Individuals can be categorized as "extensive metabolizers" (EMs) or "PMs" of drugs metabolized by CYP2C19 in population studies. Genetic polymorphisms of CYP2C19 have been shown to cause clinical consequences resulting in undesirable side effects, such as prolonged sedation and unconsciousness after administration of diazepam in CYP2C19 PMs.[61,64,65] In contrast, the proton pump inhibitor (PPI) drugs such as omeprazole and lansoprazole exhibit a greater cure rate for gastric ulcers with *Helicobacter pylori* infections in PMs than in EMs due to higher plasma concentration of the parent drugs in PMs.[72,73]

Functional Polymorphism of CYP2C19

The CYP2C subfamily in humans consists of four CYP2C genes that include CYP2C8, CYP2C9, CYP2C18, and CYP2C19. Among the four CYP2C genes, CYP2C19 is a major polymorphic P450.[74] A number of polymorphisms of CYP2C19 have been shown to contribute to the altered CYP2C19 activity. The most common defective variants are CYP2C19*2 and *3.[74,75] CYP2C19*2 is a splice mutation in exon 5 that produces a truncated nonfunctional protein and CYP2C19*3 produces a stop codon in exon 4.[76,77] Other null variant alleles include CYP2C19*4 (a mutation in the initiation codon) and CYP2C19*7 (a splice mutation in intron 5).[78,79] PMs can be defined as individuals carrying two defective CYP2C19 alleles. Several CYP2C19 variants were discovered by DNA sequencing of CYP2C19 gene in individuals who had been characterized by clinicians as PMs by phenotyping with mephenytoin or omeprazole.[70,71] These functional variants identified from phenotype studies include CYP2C19*5, *6, *8, *16, and *26[79–84] (Figure 6A–2). Among the

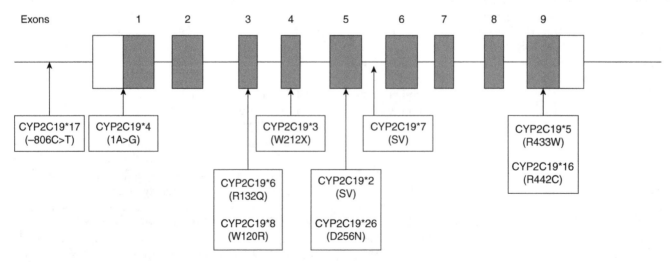

FIGURE 6A–2 Summary of CYP2C19 alleles that exhibited altered functions compared with the wild-type in phenotyped human subjects. White boxes are 5'- and 3'-untranslated regions. Black boxes are exons in open reading frame. Arrow heads indicate mutated locations that result in amino acid change, stop codon (X), or splicing variant (SV).

TABLE 6A–2 Frequencies of CYP2C19 *2, *3, and *17 alleles in different ethnic populations.

Ethnic Group	Allele No.	*1	*2	*3	*17	Reference
Whites						
Faroese	622	410 (65.9%)	116 (18.7%)	N.D	96 (15.4%)	Pedersen et al.[87]
Danish	552	358 (64.9%)	83 (15.0%)	N.D	111 (20.1%)	Pedersen et al.[87]
French	48	28 (58.3%)	10 (20.8%)	N.D	10 (20.8%)	Berge et al.[88]
Italian	720	646 (89.7%)	68 (9.4%)	6 (0.8%)	N.D	Scordo et al.[89]
Polish	250	153 (61.2%)	29 (11.6%)	N.D	68 (27.2%)	Kurzawski et al.[90]
Norwegian	664	394 (59.3%)	120 (18.1%)	4 (0.6%)	146 (22%)	Rudberg et al.[91]
Black						
African American	216	162 (75%)	54 (25%)	0 (0%)	N.D	Bravo-Villalta et al.[92]
Ethiopian	380	312 (82.1)	N.D	N.D	68 (17.9%)	Sim et al.[93]
Nigerian	86	73 (84.9%)	13 (15.1%)	0 (0%)	N.D	Babalola et al.[94]
Asian						
Korean	542	325 (60%)	154 (28.4%)	55 (10.1%)	8 (1.5%)	Kim et al.[95]
Korean	100	64 (64%)	29 (29%)	5 (5%)	2 (2%)	Lee et al.[82]
Chinese	136	130 (95.6%)	N.D	N.D	6 (4.4%)	Sim et al.[93]
Japanese	530	307 (57.9%)	148 (27.9%)	68 (12.8%)	7 (1.3%)	Sugimoto et al.[96]
Indian	40	25 (62.5%)	15 (37.5%)	0 (0%)	N.D	Lamba et al.[97]
Vietnamese	330	227 (68.8%)	87 (26.4%)	16 (4.8%)	N.D	Lee et al.[98]

defective CYP2C19 alleles, CYP2C19*2 and *3 are responsible for the majority of PM genotypes in the metabolism of CYP2C19 substrate drugs.[75,85] The PM trait is inherited as an autosomal recessive mutation and these polymorphisms are apparently different among ethnic groups. PMs represent 3–6% of whites and blacks, 13–23% of Asians, and 38–79% of Polynesians and Micronesians.[75,86] Ethnic differences in the frequency of functional CYP2C19 alleles are summarized in Table 6A–2. High interindividual variations in subjects homozygous for CYP2C19*1 are also observed and part of these variations can be explained by the genotyping for CYP2C19*17.[93] CYP2C19*17 confers an increased CYP2C19 activity due to an increase in CYP2C19 transcription and therefore individuals with homozygous carriers of CYP2C19*17 exhibit the rapid clearance of CYP2C19 substrate drugs.[91,93,99] Individuals having CYP2C19*17 are likely to exhibit a lack of response to certain PPIs and antidepressants when compared with the EMs (CYP2C19*1/*1).

Clinical Relevance of CYP2C19 Genetic Polymorphism

Lack or low activity of CYP2C19 enzyme can result in the prolonged accumulation of the CYP2C19 substrate drugs and this would lead to the drug toxicities or therapeutic failures. The altered CYP2C19 activity can be, at least in part, predicted by CYP2C19 genotype. The most extensively studied polymorphic variants of CYP2C19 are CYP2C19*2, *3, and *17 in clinical settings.[12,75,85] For example, the low extent of biotransformation

from the antimalarial drug proguanil to its active metabolite cycloguanil can lead to the insufficient efficacy of proguanil response.[100,101] However, clinical implications of CYP2C19 genotype on the efficacy of proguanil are uncertain.[12,102,103] This stems from the fact that other P450s such as CYP3A4 and CYP1A2 contribute to the formation of the active metabolite.[104,105]

Diazepam is demethylated by CYP2C19.[106] The plasma half-life of diazepam is about 4-fold longer in individuals for PM genotypes than in individuals homozygous for the wild-type CYP2C19*1.[64,65] Many Hong Kong physicians routinely prescribe a lower dose of diazepam for Chinese patients than for Caucasisans,[107] which is now attributed to the high frequency of CYP2C19*2 and *3 in Asians.[61] Toxic doses of diazepam may occur in PMs and therefore more care would be required for the decision of diazepam dose, particularly in Asians.

Individual variations in plasma concentrations of various PPIs can be accounted for the degree of CYP2C19 activity determined by *S*-mephenytoin 4′-hydroxylation assay.[108] After oral administration of omeprazole, the AUC of *S*-mephenytoin is much higher in PMs than in the EMs.[109] The extent of the contribution of CYP2C19 to the metabolism of various PPIs is different. For example, the ratios of the AUC values in PMs versus EMs are different in the decreasing order of omeprazole, pantoprazole, lansoprazole, and rabeprazole.[101,110] Although all of these PPIs are affected by CYP2C19 genotypes, rabeprazole is less dependent on the CYP2C19 genotype compared with the other PPIs, since rabeprazole can be nonenzymatically converted to its metabolite. CYP2C19 genotype affects cure rates for *H. pylori* infection in peptic ulcer patients. For example, the cure rate of peptic or duodenal ulcers for Japanese patients who received dual therapy with omeprazole (20 mg per day for 2 weeks) and amoxicillin (2,000 mg per day for 2 weeks) was 100% in CYP2C19 PMs, 60% in individuals heterozygous for one mutant allele, and 29% in individuals homozygous for CYP2C19*1 allele.[72] All of the past and current studies suggest that CYP2C19 PM genotype is beneficial in the treatment of gastric ulcer and gastroesophageal reflux disease due to the impaired metabolism of PPIs and therefore higher plasma concentrations of the PPIs in individuals having the CYP2C19 PM genotype.[110]

Increased enzyme activity of CYP2C19 can cause drug toxicity or increased drug efficacy. For instance, enhanced response to clopidogrel with the increased risk of bleeding was reported from CYP2C19*17 carriers due to the higher rate of biotransformation into the active metabolite.[111] However, another study reported an improved protective effect of clopidogrel after myocardial infarction in patients carrying the CYP2C19*17 allele.[112] The major contributors of clopidogrel activation have been identified by not only CYP2C19 but also CYP3A4 and paraoxonase-1.[68,113] Furthermore, clopidogrel itself is a potent inhibitor of CYP2C19 and CYP3A4.[114] Clinical relevance of CYP2C19 genotype on the efficacy of clopidogrel is under strong investigation for the genotype-guided therapy.[115] In general, patients who carry one or two CYP2C19 loss-of-function alleles exhibit a higher adverse event rate and diminished platelet inhibition than those with the EM genotype in the use of clopidogrel.[115–118] CYP2C19 PMs may not benefit from clopidogrel and therefore it is recommended to consider alternative treatments. However, no definitive recommendations have been established regarding dose adjustment of clopidogrel with CYP2C19 genotype testing. Further investigation on a large scale using genotype-guided clopidogrel therapy compared with other therapy options would reveal the cost-effectiveness of CYP2C19 genotype testing for clopidogrel therapy.

Perspective of Clinical Application

Translation of genetic information into the clinical practice requires two important issues, clinical significance and cost-effectiveness. CYP2C19 polymorphisms have been reported to affect the pharmacokinetics of the CYP2C19 substrate drugs such as diazepam, various PPIs, clopidogrel, and certain antidepressants (moclobemide, amitriptyline, clomipramine, sertraline, and citalopram). However, a significant relationship between CYP2C19 genotype and the clinical outcome has been limited to certain cases. CYP2C19 PMs have a markedly longer half-life of the common anxiolytic drug diazepam and the anti-ulcer drug omeprazole. Individuals with CYP2C19 PMs would require a much lower dose of diazepam for clinical relevance. Patients with CYP2C19 PMs exhibited an increased efficacy of omeprazole. However, CYP2C19 PMs have less benefit from the use of clopidogrel. The varied frequencies of CYP2C19 polymorphisms in different ethnic groups are evident, which results in variations in risk and efficacy of CYP2C19 substrate drugs in different ethnic populations. Many rare defective alleles have

been reported in the CYP2C19 gene. Although there is a lack of statistically significant data, such as in vivo pharmacokinetics and pharmacodynamics, due to their low incidences in populations, these rare polymorphisms are important since CYP2C19 metabolizes many important clinical drugs with great penetrance. Functional studies of CYP2C19 polymorphisms and their genotype/phenotype relationships need to be established with respect to their contributions to the toxicity or efficacy of the CYP2C19 drugs, which would be useful in the development of a dose prediction model for personalized medicine in the future.

PHARMACOGENOMICS OF CYP2D6

Introduction

CYP2D6 is one of the most polymorphic P450s and metabolizes approximately 20% of currently prescribed drugs.[99,119,120] However, hepatic content of CYP2D6 compared with major metabolic P450s is relatively small, about 2–4% of all P450 content.[121–123] CYP2D6 is located in a highly polymorphic gene cluster together with two inactive pseudogenes, CYP2D7P and CYP2D8P.[124–126] Although an active form of CYP2D7, a 138delT in exon 1 of CYP2D7P, was reported,[127] it is generally accepted that humans carry only one active CYP2D6 gene.[123,128] Representative substrates of CYP2D6 include antipsychotic drugs (haloperidol, clozapine, and risperidone), antiarrhythmic agents (flecainide and perphenazine), tricyclic antidepressants (imipramine, clomipramine, nortriptyline, and amitriptyline), β-adrenoreceptor antagonists (metoprolol, propranolol, bupranolol, and carvedilol), opioids (codeine and tramadol), and the estrogen receptor antagonist tamoxifen.[122,123,129] Since CYP2D6 is not inducible, genetic polymorphisms greatly contribute to the interindividual variations in enzyme activity. Five of the prototypic substrates for CYP2D6 activity assessment are sparteine,[129] debrisoquine,[130–132] dextromethorphan,[133–135] bufuralol,[129,136,137] and tramadol.[138–140] Among the five probe substrates, bufuralol and dextromethorphan are commonly used substrates in in vitro studies. The phenotype of CYP2D6 metabolism can be categorized based on genotypes such as UM (more than two functional alleles), EM (at least one or two normal functional alleles), IM (two reduced functional alleles or one null allele and the other allele with reduced function), and PM (two nonfunctional alleles). The phenotype of CYP2D6 metabolism shows ethnic differences; while UMs are mainly found in North Africa and Oceania, IMs are mainly from Asia, and high incidences of PMs are found in whites.[75,122,123,129,141]

Functional Polymorphism of CYP2D6

Currently, 81 CYP2D6 variant alleles were assigned to the Human Cytochrome P450 Allele Nomenclature Committee. Among them, the null alleles of CYP2D6 include *3, *4, *5, *6, *7, *8, *11, *12, *13, *14, *15, *16, *18, *19, *20, *21, *38, *40, *42, *44, *56, *60, and *62.[126,142–170] Since the null allele has no activity, its clinical impact is greater than any of the other functional alleles and therefore most of the null alleles are related to the PM phenotype. Among these null alleles, the most frequently studied alleles that are responsible for most of the CYP2D6 PM phenotype are CYP2D6*3 (frameshift), CYP2D6*4 (splice variant), CYP2D6*5 (gene deletion), and CYP2D6*6 (frameshift). The most common CYP2D6 variants having reduced function include CYP2D6*10, *17, and *41. Some of these CYP2D6 variants exhibit a clear ethnic disposition. For example, CYP2D6*4 is found at a frequency of about 15% in whites[171]; however, this variant occurs at a frequency of about <5% in blacks[172,173] and <1% in Asians.[174] This varying frequency of CYP2D6*4 is the major reason for the ethnically different PM distributions, accounting for 5–10% PMs in whites,[61,75,175] 0–19% PM in blacks,[75,176,177] and <1% PMs in Asians.[75,141,178] The CYP2D6*10 allele is a reduced functional allele, most commonly found in Asians at up to the frequency of 63%.[156,174,179–183] This allele contributes to a great extent of IM phenotype in Asians compared with the other ethnic populations. The highest prevalence of UM phenotype is found in Northeast Africa and the Oceania regions where individuals carrying duplication of CYP2D6*1 or *2 are high. For example, the frequency of CYP2D6*2xN is about 28% in the Mozabite population in Algeria and about 22% of CYP2D6*1xN has been found in Oceania,[122,184,185] whereas the frequency of CYP2D6*5 is similar in different ethnic populations ranging from 4% to 7%.[122,123,141] Ethnic differences in the frequency of functional CYP2D6 alleles are summarized in Table 6A–3. Genetic mutations of CYP2D6 can cause altered enzyme activity through various ways, which include changes in substrate recognition,

enzyme affinity for substrates, protein stability, and regulation of expression. CYP2D6 alleles with reduced activity include CYP2D6*10, *14, *17, *18, *36, *41, *47, *49, *50, *51, *54, *55, *57, *59, *62, and *72 (http://www.cypalleles.ki.se/cyp2d6.htm). Alleles with similar activity to the wild-type include *27, *39, and *48.[195] Most of these variant alleles are characterized in different labs with different protocols. Therefore, absolute determination of expressed activity through a quantitative manner is currently difficult. CYP2D6 gene exhibits copy number variations. For example, carriers of CYP2D6*2xN or CYP2D6*1xN show extremely high activity compared with the wild-type. Individuals having duplication or multiplication of the CYP2D6 active gene are expected to express significantly increased CYP2D6 substrate drug clearance, resulting in a lack of therapeutic effect or adverse drug reaction in some cases due to the significantly increased metabolism of the precursor into the active form of drug.

Clinical Relevance of CYP2D6 Genetic Polymorphism

Various systems have been developed to categorize CYP2D6 activity based on its genotype, such as UM, EM, IM, PM, and activity scores.[99,141,196] Many clinical drugs are greatly influenced by CYP2D6 genetic polymorphisms. First, antidepressants and antipsychotics exhibit significant differences in plasma concentrations, depending on CYP2D6 polymorphisms.[197–199] Several studies have shown that CYP2D6 PMs exhibit a higher incidence of undesirable side effects when taking CYP2D6-dependent

TABLE 6A–3 Frequencies of major CYP2D6 alleles in different ethnic populations.

Ethnic Group	Allele No.	*3	*4	*5	*6	*10	*17	*41	*1xN	*2xN	Reference
White											
American	416	4 (1)	73 (17.5)	16 (3.8)	4 (1)	79 (19)	1 (0.2)	N.D	1 (0.2)	3 (0.7)	Gaedigk et al.[186]
Spanish	210	2 (1)	29 (13.8)	7 (3.3)	2 (1)	4 (1.9)	N.D	N.D	4 (1.9)	4 (1.9)	Menoyo et al.[187]
Turkish	808	N.D	89 (11)	8 (1)	N.D	48 (5.9)	8 (1)	N.D	N.D	5 (0.6)	Aynacioglu et al.[188]
Italian	720	5 (0.7)	110 (15.3)	25 (3.5)	101 (14)	N.D	N.D	N.D	N.D	30 (4.2)	Scordo et al.[89]
Black											
African American	262	1 (0.4)	20 (7.6)	13 (5.0)	1 (0.4)	7 (2.7)	41 (15.6)	39 (14.9)	0 (0)	6 (2.3)	Cai et al.[189]
Ethiopian	244	0 (0)	3 (1.2)	8 (3.3)	N.D	21 (8.6)	22 (9)	53 (21.7)	N.D	33 (13.5)	Aklillu et al.[190]
Mozabite	60	N.D	7 (11.7)	2 (3.3)	N.D	N.D	5 (8.3)	5 (8.3)	N.D	17 (28.3)	Sistonen et al.[185]
Asian											
Korean	1516	N.D	N.D	85 (5.6)	N.D	691 (45.6)	N.D	34 (2.2)	2 (0.1)	15 (1)	Lee et al.[156]
Chinese	200	0 (0)	2 (1)	14 (7)	1 (0.5)	98 (49)	0 (0)	8 (4)	N.D	1 (0.5)	Zhou et al.[191]
Japanese	196	N.D	4 (2)	12 (6.1)	N.D	80 (40.8)	0 (0)	5 (2.6)	1 (0.5)	1 (0.5)	Tateishi et al.[183]
Taiwanese	360	N.D	N.D	19 (5.3)	N.D	227 (63.1)	N.D	N.D	N.D	N.D	Liou et al.[192]
Indian	894	0 (0)	65 (7.3)	17 (1.9)	N.D	91 (10.2)	0 (0)	N.D	N.D	N.D	Naveen et al.[193]
Malay	214	0 (0)	6 (2.8)	11 (5.1)	N.D	106 (49.5)	1 (0.5)	N.D	N.D	2 (0.9)	Teh et al.[194]

Numbers in parentheses indicate allele frequency (%). N.D, not determined.

TABLE 6A–4 List of the top 10 antidepressants and antipsychotic drugs that are greatly influenced by CYP2D6 genotypes.

Antidepressants	Antipsychotics
Imipramine	Perphenazine
Trimipramine	Thioridazine
Doxepin	Olanzapine
Maprotiline	Zuclopenthixol
Desipramine	Flupentixol
Nortriptyline	Aripiprazole
Clomipramine	Haloperidol
Paroxetine	Risperidone
Amitriptyline	Perazine
Fluoxetine	Pimozide

antidepressants,[200–208] antipsychotic drugs,[209–216] and selective serotonin reuptake inhibitors (SSRIs).[217–220] Similarly, multiple studies have found that CYP2D6 UMs experience diminished response to these drugs.[198,202,221,222] A list of the top 10 antidepressants and antipsychotic drugs whose plasma concentrations are greatly influenced by CYP2D6 polymorphisms is presented in Table 6A–4. Several articles suggest that physicians might consider reducing the dose of tricyclic antidepressants by about 50% of the normally prescribed dose for PMs and 140–180% for UMs.[141,198,223] However, routine testing for CYP2D6 genotype has not been approved by the FDA or endorsed by an expert panel, since the clinical significance and cost-effectiveness of genotyping have not been demonstrated.

Tamoxifen metabolism by CYP2D6 into its active agent is critical for its antitumor activity in breast cancer patients.[224–226] Data from numerous studies support that the relationship between CYP2D6 genotype and tamoxifen response is clinically relevant.[227–230] The CYP2D6 "PM" genotype has been associated with poor clinical outcome with tamoxifen.[225,231–236] Tamoxifen-treated patients homozygous for CYP2D6*4 exhibited a shorter disease- and relapse-free survival rate.[233,234,237,238] Similarly, patients carrying the CYP2D6 "poor" and "intermediate metabolizer" genotypes showed a significantly increased incidence of recurrence, shorter relapse-free survival, and shorter event-free survival rates.[229,239,240] In addition, patients having CYP2D6 UM genotype were associated with significantly longer relapse-free time, less breast cancer recurrences, and higher event-free survival compared with CYP2D6 EM carriers.[229,237,239,241]

Increased codeine metabolism by CYP2D6 to morphine has been shown to cause serious morphine toxicity.[242,243] CYP2D6 UM genotype exhibited about a 50% higher concentration of morphine compared with the EM genotype. However, individuals having defective alleles of CYP2D6 exhibited very low or undetectable morphine concentrations with a lack of analgesia.[244–246] A case report that a breastfed infant died from toxic levels of morphine strongly suggested an association between CYP2D6 genotype and morphine toxicity.[243] Both the mother and infant were CYP2D6 UM genotypes, resulting in high concentrations of morphine in the breast milk and blood due to the rapid and extensive conversion of codeine to morphine.

Tramadol is metabolized by CYP2D6 to generate a pharmacologically active O-desmethyltramadol and CYP2D6 genotype is shown to be linked to the concentration of O-desmethyltramadol, resulting in the different efficacy of tramadol treatment.[247–249] Individuals with the CYP2D6 PM genotypes exhibited lesser analgesic effect than the EM genotypes.[250–252] Patients carrying CYP2D6 UM genotype have higher concentrations of O-desmethyltramadol and better pain control than those carrying the EM genotype, but higher incidences of the side effects (i.e., nausea, respiratory depression) have been reported.[253,254] Therefore, CYP2D6 UMs might be at greater risk from regular tramadol doses and might benefit from a lower dose of tramadol.

Pharmacokinetic parameters for beta-adrenergic receptor antagonists, such as carvedilol, metoprolol, propranolol, and timolol, have been reported to be linked to CYP2D6 genetic polymorphisms.[123,255] Metoprolol consists of a racemic mixture of S- and R-metoprolol with the S-metoprolol exhibiting about a 500-fold greater affinity for beta1-adrenergic receptors than the R-form.[256] Alpha-hydroxylation of metoprolol is converted by CYP2D6 and O-demethylation is metabolized by CYP2D6 and CYP3A4.[257,258] Among the several metabolic pathways of carvedilol, 4'- and 5'-hydroxylations of carvedilol are mainly catalyzed by CYP2D6 with a minor contribution of these reactions catalyzed by CYP2E1 and CYP2C9.[259] Propranolol undergoes several metabolic pathways involving glucuronidation, ring hydroxylation, and side chain oxidation. Ring hydroxylation of propranolol is mainly catalyzed by CYP2D6.[260,261] Multiple studies indicated that patients carrying CYP2D6 PMs exhibited a decreased amount of the active metabolite 4-hydroxypropranolol.[262–264] Timolol is primarily metabolized by CYP2D6 (>90%) with minor metabolism by CYP2C19.[265] Individuals having CYP2D6 PM phenotype showed a higher plasma AUC of timolol than those having the EM and UM phenotypes in multiple studies.[266,267] In general, beta-adrenergic receptor antagonists are found at higher plasma concentrations in PMs than in the EMs. Although consistent association results between CYP2D6 genotypes and AUC values of the beta-adrenergic receptor antagonists have been reported in several studies, there is a lack of significant associations between CYP2D6 genotypes and the clinical incidence of adverse effects.[123,268–270] Further information would enable clinicians to incorporate the CYP2D6 genomic data into clinical practice with increased confidence.

Perspective of Clinical Application

CYP2D6 polymorphisms create differences in the clinical outcomes of the CYP2D6 substrate drugs. Significant advances in understanding the relationship between CYP2D6 genotypes and adverse drug reactions have been achieved in certain drugs, such as debrisoquine, tamoxifen, codeine, and tramadol. The CYP2D6 "PM" genotype has been associated with poor clinical

TABLE 6A-5 Genetic polymorphisms in CYP2C9, 2C19, and 2D6 with clinical consequences of drugs.

P450s	Drug	Consequences
CYP2C9	Warfarin	Increased risk of breeding episodes in PMs caused by reduced metabolism of S-warfarin and therefore increased S-warfarin concentration at normal dose
	Phenytoin	Increased risk of ataxia, unconsciousness, and mental confusion in PMs caused by increased phenytoin level
	Glimepiride, tolbutamide, glyburide	Increased risk potential of hypoglycemia in PMs due to increased drug level and low blood sugar level
CYP2C19	Diazepam	Increased risk of sedation time and unconsciousness in PMs caused by prolonged half-life of diazepam
	Omeprazole, pantoprazole, lansoprazole	Increased cure rates due to increased half-life of the parent drugs in PMs Decreased cure rates in EMs and UMs
	Clopidogrel	Decreased response to clopidogrel in PMs due to low transformation into active metabolite
CYP2D6	Imipramine, trimipramine, doxepin	Diminished response to the drugs in UMs and increased risk of adverse effects in the CNS and others in PMs
	Perphenazine, thioridazine, olanzapine	Diminished response to the drugs in UMs and increased risk of extrapyramidal side effect and others in PMs
	Tamoxifen	Poor drug efficacy in PMs due to low transformation into the active metabolite
	Codeine	Increased risk of adverse effects in UMs due to unacceptable concentration of active metabolite morphine
	Tramadol	Increased risk of respiratory depression or severe nausea in UMs due to unacceptable concentration of the active metabolite; lesser analgesic effect in PMs
	Carvedilol, metoprolol, propranolol, timolol	Increased risk potential of various side effects in PMs due to reduced metabolism and increased drug concentrations

outcomes with tamoxifen. CYP2D6 UM genotypes exhibited a higher concentration of morphine compared with the EM genotype, which is responsible for morphine toxicity in some case studies. Patients carrying CYP2D6 UM genotypes exhibited better pain control than those carrying the EM genotypes after tramadol administration, but higher incidences of nausea were observed. Clinical outcomes of drug studies, such as beta-adrenergic receptor antagonists and psychotropic medications, have been suggested to be associated with CYP2D6 polymorphisms. However, the extent of clinical impact by each allele on the drug responses is not clear and the statistical significance of CTP2D6 genotypes on clinical outcomes is different depending on researchers, clinical situations, and populations. This discrepancy might be from unequivocal definitions of phenotypes among different researchers. In order for clinicians to make a decision to incorporate CYP2D6 genetics into clinical practice, more clinical studies with clearly defined and consistent phenotype data are required. Many factors influence drug action, and this is the case with CYP2D6. Various upstream and downstream genes, as well as interactions with target enzymes, receptors, and the CYP2D6 genetics, will influence the ultimate clinical outcome. Particularly, clinical outcomes for CYP2D6-metabolized drugs such as beta-adrenergic receptor antagonists and psychotropic medications are greatly influenced by many other genes with numerous modulation factors. Integration of the genetics unique to each individual with clinical factors into a single model system would be a future direction for understanding the

relative contribution of CYP2D6 to the final clinical outcome. Effects of genetic polymorphisms in CYP2C9, CYP2C19, and CYP2D6 on clinical consequences of drugs are summarized in Table 6A–5.

PHARMACOGENOMICS OF OTHER P450s

CYP1A2 is involved in the metabolism of coffee, estrogen, clozapine, theophylline, olanzapine, and certain procarcinogens such as 2-aminoacetylfluorene (2-AAF), 2-amino-3,8-dimethylimidazo[4,5-f]quinoline (MeIQ), and 2-amino-1-methyl-6-phenylimidazo-[4,5-b]pyridine (PhIP).[271–273] It is predominantly expressed in the liver, accounting for about 10% of total hepatic P450 content.[274,275] CYP1A2*1F has been shown to increase the inducibility of CYP1A2 expression by caffeine, smoking, and omeprazole treatment than that of CYP1A2*1A.[276–280] This enhanced induction affects the increased metabolism of CYP1A2 substrate drugs with altered therapeutic outcomes[276,277] or increased risk of certain cancers.[281–283]

CYP2A6 metabolizes nicotine, cotinine, coumarin, methyl-n-amylnitrosamine (MNAN), and nicotine-derived nitrosamine ketone (NNK).[271–273,284] Therefore, high expresser individuals have been suggested to experience increased susceptibility to nicotine addiction, which has been proposed to be linked to the increased risk of smoking-related cancers.[99,285,286] Apparent ethnic variations in the CYP2A6 polymorphisms were found with about 1% of PMs in whites, but approximately 20% of PMs in Asians.[287-289] The majority of PMs in Asians are explained by the high frequency of CYP2A6*4 allele.[99,289] CYP2A6 alleles having no activity include CYP2A6*4, *5, and *20 (http://www.cypalleles.ki.se/cyp2a6.htm). Functionally altered CYP2A6 alleles in vivo are *2, *6, *10, *11, *12, *17, *18, *19, *23, *26, *27, *35A, and *35B (http://www.cypalleles.ki.se/cyp2a6.htm).

CYP2B6 is involved in the metabolism of bupropion, efavirenz, nevirapine, cyclophosphamide, and ifosfamide.[290,291] It is a highly polymorphic gene with different ethnic frequencies. The most common CYP2B6 variant is the CYP2B6*6 allele that varies 15–60% across different ethnic populations.[292,293] CYP2B6*6 is a coding variant with two amino acid changes, resulting in ~75% decrease in hepatic expression[292,293] and different enzyme activity depending on the substrates.[294-296] Among the CYP2B6 polymorphisms, CYP2B6*6, *16, and *18 consistently exhibit lower activity for efavirenz in vitro and in vivo.[297-299] A number of HIV patients receiving efavirenz experience central nervous system side effects, which are suggested to be from the varying concentration of efavirenz in plasma.[275,299] Individuals, particularly in Africa where CYP2B6*6 and *18 are common, may get help from genotyping for these alleles to minimize the possibility of adverse drug effects from efavirenz.

CYP3A4 and CYP3A5 are major CYP3A enzymes in humans and are responsible for the metabolism of more than 50% of currently used drugs.[300-302] Their similar activities and overlapping expressions have hampered the assessment of each gene's contribution to the total CYP3A metabolism.[300,301,303] Most of the in vivo phenotyping substrates for CYP3A enzymes used are midazolam and erythromycin (which is not a useful probe due to the influence of P-glycoprotein on its pharmacokinetics).[304,305] Although there are large interindividual variations in the expression and oral clearances of CYP3A substrate drugs, the genetic polymorphisms responsible for these large variations are not yet reported, even after combining the polymorphisms of CYP3A4 and CYP3A5. The null allele of the CYP3A4 variant is CYP3A4*20 and only occurs as a rare allele.[306] CYP3A4 alleles with significantly decreased activity in vitro include *8, *11, *13, *16, and *17.[303,307] Particularly, CYP3A4*17 exhibited a 95% decreased activity in the metabolism of nifedipine in vitro.[308] CYP3A5 is a more polymorphic enzyme when compared with the CYP3A4 gene.[309,310] Among the null alleles of CYP3A5 (*3, *5, *6, and *7), CYP3A5*3 is the most common defective allele with ethnically different frequencies.[309] The CYP3A5*3 allele generates an incorrectly spliced mRNA, which produces a truncated, nonfunctional protein. Individuals carrying CYP3A5*3 have been associated with a greatly reduced expression of CYP3A5 protein.[309] CYP3A5*3 has been found at a frequency of 90% in whites, 75% in Asians, and 20–50% in blacks.[303,310] CYP3A5*6 and *7 are prevalently found in blacks at a frequency of 17% and 6%, respectively, whereas they are not found in whites or Asians.[310,311] Immunosuppressive agents, such as tacrolimus and cyclosporine A, exhibit a wide range of interpatient variations in pharmacokinetics, with multiple adverse reactions in renal transplant recipients.[312,313] They are primarily metabolized by CYP3As and effluxed by P-glycoprotein (ABCB1).[313,314]

Multiple association studies have been conducted to investigate the relationship between CYP3A5 genotype and the dose requirements of these drugs to achieve appropriate target concentrations. Tacrolimus appears to have more clinical relevance with CYP3A5 genotype than cyclosporine A.[314-316] Several studies consistently indicate that oral clearance of tacrolimus in renal transplant recipients is lower in patients with CYP3A5*3/*3 genotype than in the CYP3A5*1 heterozygotes or homozygotes, suggesting that lower doses of tacrolimus in patients having CYP3A5*3/*3 genotype would be beneficial in initial dosing strategies.[315,317-319] However, it is not determined to what extent of pharmacokinetic variability can affect a clinical outcome with or without side effects.[314] Further studies with the advanced knowledge of CYP3A and other genotyping would improve clinical outcome without the side effects.

REFERENCES

1. Goldstein JA, de Morais SM. Biochemistry and molecular biology of the human CYP2C subfamily. *Pharmacogenetics.* 1994;4:285–299.
2. Wrighton SA, Stevens JC. The human hepatic cytochromes P450 involved in drug metabolism. *Crit Rev Toxicol.* 1992;22:1–21.
3. Rendic S, Di Carlo FJ. Human cytochrome P450 enzymes: a status report summarizing their reactions, substrates, inducers, and inhibitors. *Drug Metab Rev.* 1997;29:413–580.
4. Kidd RS, Straughn AB, Meyer MC, Blaisdell J, Goldstein JA, Dalton JT. Pharmacokinetics of chlorpheniramine, phenytoin, glipizide and nifedipine in an individual homozygous for the CYP2C9*3 allele. *Pharmacogenetics.* 1999;9:71–80.
5. Miners JO, Birkett DJ. Use of tolbutamide as a substrate probe for human hepatic cytochrome P450 2C9. *Methods Enzymol.* 1996;272:139–145.
6. Bajpai M, Roskos LK, Shen DD, Levy RH. Roles of cytochrome P4502C9 and cytochrome P4502C19 in the stereoselective metabolism of phenytoin to its major metabolite. *Drug Metab Dispos.* 1996;24:1401–1403.
7. Rettie AE, Korzekwa KR, Kunze KL, et al. Hydroxylation of warfarin by human cDNA-expressed cytochrome P-450: a role for P-4502C9 in the etiology of (S)-warfarin–drug interactions. *Chem Res Toxicol.* 1992;5:54–59.
8. Stearns RA, Chakravarty PK, Chen R, Chiu SH. Biotransformation of losartan to its active carboxylic acid metabolite in human liver microsomes. Role of cytochrome P4502C and 3A subfamily members. *Drug Metab Dispos.* 1995;23:207–215.
9. Miners JO, Rees DL, Valente L, Veronese ME, Birkett DJ. Human hepatic cytochrome P450 2C9 catalyzes the rate-limiting pathway of torsemide metabolism. *J Pharmacol Exp Ther.* 1995;272:1076–1081.
10. Rendic S. Summary of information on human CYP enzymes: human P450 metabolism data. *Drug Metab Rev.* 2002;34:83–448.
11. Bylund J, Ericsson J, Oliw EH. Analysis of cytochrome P450 metabolites of arachidonic and linoleic acids by liquid chromatography–mass spectrometry with ion trap MS. *Anal Biochem.* 1998;265:55–68.
12. Goldstein JA. Clinical relevance of genetic polymorphisms in the human CYP2C subfamily. *Br J Clin Pharmacol.* 2001;52:349–355.
13. Rettie AE, Haining RL, Bajpai M, Levy RH. A common genetic basis for idiosyncratic toxicity of warfarin and phenytoin. *Epilepsy Res.* 1999;35:253–255.
14. Scordo MG, Aklillu E, Yasar U, Dahl ML, Spina E, Ingelman-Sundberg M. Genetic polymorphism of cytochrome P450 2C9 in a Caucasian and a black African population. *Br J Clin Pharmacol.* 2001;52:447–450.
15. Takanashi K, Tainaka H, Kobayashi K, Yasumori T, Hosakawa M, Chiba K. CYP2C9 Ile359 and Leu359 variants: enzyme kinetic study with seven substrates. *Pharmacogenetics.* 2000;10:95–104.
16. Kidd RS, Curry TB, Gallagher S, Edeki T, Blaisdell J, Goldstein JA. Identification of a null allele of CYP2C9 in an African-American exhibiting toxicity to phenytoin. *Pharmacogenetics.* 2001;11:803–808.

17. Maekawa K, Fukushima-Uesaka H, Tohkin M, et al. Four novel defective alleles and comprehensive haplotype analysis of CYP2C9 in Japanese. *Pharmacogenet Genomics.* 2006;16:497–514.

18. Zhao F, Loke C, Rankin SC, et al. Novel CYP2C9 genetic variants in Asian subjects and their influence on maintenance warfarin dose. *Clin Pharmacol Ther.* 2004;76:210–219.

19. Allabi AC, Gala JL, Horsmans Y, et al. Functional impact of CYP2C95, CYP2C96, CYP2C98, and CYP2C911 in vivo among black Africans. *Clin Pharmacol Ther.* 2004;76:113–118.

20. King BP, Khan TI, Aithal GP, Kamali F, Daly AK. Upstream and coding region CYP2C9 polymorphisms: correlation with warfarin dose and metabolism. *Pharmacogenetics.* 2004;14:813–822.

21. Lee CR, Goldstein JA, Pieper JA. Cytochrome P450 2C9 polymorphisms: a comprehensive review of the in-vitro and human data. *Pharmacogenetics.* 2002;12:251–263.

22. Si D, Guo Y, Zhang Y, Yang L, Zhou H, Zhong D. Identification of a novel variant CYP2C9 allele in Chinese. *Pharmacogenetics.* 2004;14:465–469.

23. Taube J, Halsall D, Baglin T. Influence of cytochrome P-450 CYP2C9 polymorphisms on warfarin sensitivity and risk of over-anticoagulation in patients on long-term treatment. *Blood.* 2000;96:1816–1819.

24. Yasar U, Eliasson E, Dahl ML, Johansson I, Ingelman-Sundberg M, Sjoqvist F. Validation of methods for CYP2C9 genotyping: frequencies of mutant alleles in a Swedish population. *Biochem Biophys Res Commun.* 1999;254:628–631.

25. Nasu K, Kubota T, Ishizaki T. Genetic analysis of CYP2C9 polymorphism in a Japanese population. *Pharmacogenetics.* 1997;7:405–409.

26. Sullivan-Klose TH, Ghanayem BI, Bell DA, et al. The role of the CYP2C9-Leu359 allelic variant in the tolbutamide polymorphism. *Pharmacogenetics.* 1996;6:341–349.

27. Wang SL, Huang J, Lai MD, Tsai JJ. Detection of CYP2C9 polymorphism based on the polymerase chain reaction in Chinese. *Pharmacogenetics.* 1995;5:37–42.

28. Yoon YR, Shon JH, Kim MK, et al. Frequency of cytochrome P450 2C9 mutant alleles in a Korean population. *Br J Clin Pharmacol.* 2001;51:277–280.

29. Schwarz UI. Clinical relevance of genetic polymorphisms in the human CYP2C9 gene. *Eur J Clin Invest.* 2003;33(suppl 2):23–30.

30. Dickmann LJ, Rettie AE, Kneller MB, et al. Identification and functional characterization of a new CYP2C9 variant (CYP2C9*5) expressed among African Americans. *Mol Pharmacol.* 2001;60:382–387.

31. Garcia-Martin E, Martinez C, Ladero JM, Gamito FJ, Agundez JA. High frequency of mutations related to impaired CYP2C9 metabolism in a Caucasian population. *Eur J Clin Pharmacol.* 2001;57:47–49.

32. Aynacioglu AS, Brockmoller J, Bauer S, et al. Frequency of cytochrome P450 CYP2C9 variants in a Turkish population and functional relevance for phenytoin. *Br J Clin Pharmacol.* 1999;48:409–415.

33. Lee SJ, Jang YJ, Cha EY, Kim HS, Lee SS, Shin JG. A haplotype of CYP2C9 associated with warfarin sensitivity in mechanical heart valve replacement patients. *Br J Clin Pharmacol.* 2010;70:213–221.

34. Jose R, Chandrasekaran A, Sam SS, et al. CYP2C9 and CYP2C19 genetic polymorphisms: frequencies in the south Indian population. *Fundam Clin Pharmacol.* 2005;19:101–105.

35. Ngow HA, Wan Khairina WM, Teh LK, et al. CYP2C9 polymorphism: prevalence in healthy and warfarin-treated Malay and Chinese in Malaysia. *Singapore Med J.* 2009;50:490–493.

36. Lee SS, Kim KM, Thi-Le H, Yea SS, Cha IJ, Shin JG. Genetic polymorphism of CYP2C9 in a Vietnamese Kinh population. *Ther Drug Monit.* 2005;27:208–210.

37. Zand N, Tajik N, Moghaddam AS, Milanian I. Genetic polymorphisms of cytochrome P450 enzymes 2C9 and 2C19 in a healthy Iranian population. *Clin Exp Pharmacol Physiol.* 2007;34:102–105.

38. Yamazaki H, Inoue K, Chiba K, et al. Comparative studies on the catalytic roles of cytochrome P450 2C9 and its Cys- and Leu-variants in the oxidation of warfarin, flurbiprofen, and diclofenac by human liver microsomes. *Biochem Pharmacol.* 1998;56:243–251.

39. Gill HJ, Tjia JF, Kitteringham NR, Pirmohamed M, Back DJ, Park BK. The effect of genetic polymorphisms in CYP2C9 on sulphamethoxazole N-hydroxylation. *Pharmacogenetics.* 1999;9:43–53.

40. Miners JO, Coulter S, Birkett DJ, Goldstein JA. Torsemide metabolism by CYP2C9 variants and other human CYP2C subfamily enzymes. *Pharmacogenetics.* 2000;10:267–270.

41. Takahashi H, Echizen H. Pharmacogenetics of warfarin elimination and its clinical implications. *Clin Pharmacokinet.* 2001;40:587–603.

42. Kirchheiner J, Brockmoller J. Clinical consequences of cytochrome P450 2C9 polymorphisms. *Clin Pharmacol Ther.* 2005;77:1–16.

43. Takahashi H, Kashima T, Nomoto S, et al. Comparisons between in-vitro and in-vivo metabolism of (S)-warfarin: catalytic activities of cDNA-expressed CYP2C9, its Leu359 variant and their mixture versus unbound clearance in patients with the corresponding CYP2C9 genotypes. *Pharmacogenetics.* 1998;8:365–373.

44. Thijssen HH, Ritzen B. Acenocoumarol pharmacokinetics in relation to cytochrome P450 2C9 genotype. *Clin Pharmacol Ther.* 2003;74:61–68.

45. Ninomiya H, Mamiya K, Matsuo S, Ieiri I, Higuchi S, Tashiro N. Genetic polymorphism of the CYP2C subfamily and excessive serum phenytoin concentration with central nervous system intoxication. *Ther Drug Monit.* 2000;22:230–232.

46. Steward DJ, Haining RL, Henne KR, et al. Genetic association between sensitivity to warfarin and expression of CYP2C9*3. *Pharmacogenetics.* 1997;7:361–367.

47. Kaminsky LS, Zhang ZY. Human P450 metabolism of warfarin. *Pharmacol Ther.* 1997;73:67–74.

48. Loebstein R, Yonath H, Peleg D, et al. Interindividual variability in sensitivity to warfarin—nature or nurture? *Clin Pharmacol Ther.* 2001;70:159–164.

49. Mannucci PM. Genetic control of anticoagulation. *Lancet.* 1999;353:688–689.

50. Ogg MS, Brennan P, Meade T, Humphries SE. CYP2C9*3 allelic variant and bleeding complications. *Lancet.* 1999;354:1124.

51. Au N, Rettie AE. Pharmacogenomics of 4-hydroxycoumarin anticoagulants. *Drug Metab Rev.* 2008;40:355–375.

52. Giancarlo GM, Venkatakrishnan K, Granda BW, von Moltke LL, Greenblatt DJ. Relative contributions of CYP2C9 and 2C19 to phenytoin 4-hydroxylation in vitro: inhibition by sulfaphenazole, omeprazole, and ticlopidine. *Eur J Clin Pharmacol.* 2001;57:31–36.

53. Miners JO, Birkett DJ. Cytochrome P4502C9: an enzyme of major importance in human drug metabolism. *Br J Clin Pharmacol.* 1998;45:525–538.

54. Caraco Y, Muszkat M, Wood AJ. Phenytoin metabolic ratio: a putative marker of CYP2C9 activity in vivo. *Pharmacogenetics.* 2001;11:587–596.

55. van der Weide J, Steijns LS, van Weelden MJ, de Haan K. The effect of genetic polymorphism of cytochrome P450 CYP2C9 on phenytoin dose requirement. *Pharmacogenetics.* 2001;11:287–291.

56. Veronese ME, Miners JO, Randles D, Gregov D, Birkett DJ. Validation of the tolbutamide metabolic ratio for population screening with use of sulfaphenazole to produce model phenotypic poor metabolizers. *Clin Pharmacol Ther.* 1990;47:403–411.

57. Kirchheiner J, Brockmoller J, Meineke I, et al. Impact of CYP2C9 amino acid polymorphisms on glyburide kinetics and on the insulin and glucose response in healthy volunteers. *Clin Pharmacol Ther.* 2002;71:286–296.

58. Niemi M, Cascorbi I, Timm R, Kroemer HK, Neuvonen PJ, Kivisto KT. Glyburide and glimepiride pharmacokinetics in subjects with different CYP2C9 genotypes. *Clin Pharmacol Ther.* 2002;72:326–332.

59. Williamson KM, Patterson JH, McQueen RH, Adams KF Jr, Pieper JA. Effects of erythromycin or rifampin on losartan pharmacokinetics in healthy volunteers. *Clin Pharmacol Ther.* 1998;63:316–323.

60. Andersson T, Regardh CG, Lou YC, Zhang Y, Dahl ML, Bertilsson L. Polymorphic hydroxylation of S-mephenytoin and omeprazole metabolism in Caucasian and Chinese subjects. *Pharmacogenetics.* 1992;2:25–31.

61. Bertilsson L. Geographical/interracial differences in polymorphic drug oxidation. Current state of knowledge of cytochromes P450 (CYP) 2D6 and 2C19. *Clin Pharmacokinet.* 1995;29:192–209.

62. Helsby NA, Watkins WM, Mberu E, Ward SA. Inter-individual variation in the metabolic activation of the antimalarial biguanides. *Parasitol Today.* 1991;7:120–123.

63. Ward SA, Helsby NA, Skjelbo E, Brosen K, Gram LF, Breckenridge AM. The activation of the biguanide antimalarial proguanil co-segregates with the mephenytoin oxidation polymorphism—a panel study. *Br J Clin Pharmacol.* 1991;31:689–692.

64. Qin XP, Xie HG, Wang W, et al. Effect of the gene dosage of CgammaP2C19 on diazepam metabolism in Chinese subjects. *Clin Pharmacol Ther.* 1999;66:642–646.

65. Wan J, Xia H, He N, Lu YQ, Zhou HH. The elimination of diazepam in Chinese subjects is dependent on the mephenytoin oxidation phenotype. *Br J Clin Pharmacol.* 1996;42:471–474.

66. Sindrup SH, Brosen K, Hansen MG, Aaes-Jorgensen T, Overo KF, Gram LF. Pharmacokinetics of citalopram in relation to the sparteine and the mephenytoin oxidation polymorphisms. *Ther Drug Monit.* 1993;15:11–17.

67. Skjelbo E, Brosen K, Hallas J, Gram LF. The mephenytoin oxidation polymorphism is partially responsible for the N-demethylation of imipramine. *Clin Pharmacol Ther.* 1991;49:18–23.

68. Baumann P, Jonzier-Perey M, Koeb L, Kupfer A, Tinguely D, Schopf J. Amitriptyline pharmacokinetics and clinical response: II. Metabolic polymorphism assessed by hydroxylation of debrisoquine and mephenytoin. *Int Clin Psychopharmacol.* 1986;1:102–112.

69. Nielsen KK, Brosen K, Hansen MG, Gram LF. Single-dose kinetics of clomipramine: relationship to the sparteine and S-mephenytoin oxidation polymorphisms. *Clin Pharmacol Ther.* 1994;55:518–527.

70. Balian JD, Sukhova N, Harris JW, et al. The hydroxylation of omeprazole correlates with S-mephenytoin metabolism: a population study. *Clin Pharmacol Ther.* 1995;57:662–669.

71. Wilkinson GR, Guengerich FP, Branch RA. Genetic polymorphism of S-mephenytoin hydroxylation. *Pharmacol Ther.* 1989;43:53–76.

72. Furuta T, Ohashi K, Kamata T, et al. Effect of genetic differences in omeprazole metabolism on cure rates for *Helicobacter pylori* infection and peptic ulcer. *Ann Intern Med.* 1998;129:1027–1030.

73. Sohn DR, Kwon JT, Kim HK, Ishizaki T. Metabolic disposition of lansoprazole in relation to the S-mephenytoin 4′-hydroxylation phenotype status. *Clin Pharmacol Ther.* 1997;61:574–582.

74. Goldstein JA, Ishizaki T, Chiba K, et al. Frequencies of the defective CYP2C19 alleles responsible for the mephenytoin poor metabolizer phenotype in various Oriental, Caucasian, Saudi Arabian and American black populations. *Pharmacogenetics.* 1997;7:59–64.

75. Xie HG, Kim RB, Wood AJ, Stein CM. Molecular basis of ethnic differences in drug disposition and response. *Annu Rev Pharmacol Toxicol.* 2001;41:815–850.

76. de Morais SM, Wilkinson GR, Blaisdell J, Meyer UA, Nakamura K, Goldstein JA. Identification of a new genetic defect responsible for the polymorphism of (S)-mephenytoin metabolism in Japanese. *Mol Pharmacol.* 1994;46:594–598.

77. de Morais SM, Wilkinson GR, Blaisdell J, Nakamura K, Meyer UA, Goldstein JA. The major genetic defect responsible for the polymorphism of S-mephenytoin metabolism in humans. *J Biol Chem.* 1994;269:15419–15422.

78. Ferguson RJ, De Morais SM, Benhamou S, et al. A new genetic defect in human CYP2C19: mutation of the initiation codon is responsible for poor metabolism of S-mephenytoin. *J Pharmacol Exp Ther.* 1998;284:356–361.

79. Ibeanu GC, Blaisdell J, Ferguson RJ, et al. A novel transversion in the intron 5 donor splice junction of CYP2C19 and a sequence polymorphism in exon 3 contribute to the poor metabolizer phenotype for the anticonvulsant drug S-mephenytoin. *J Pharmacol Exp Ther.* 1999;290:635–640.

80. Ibeanu GC, Blaisdell J, Ghanayem BI, et al. An additional defective allele, CYP2C19*5, contributes to the S-mephenytoin poor metabolizer phenotype in Caucasians. *Pharmacogenetics.* 1998;8:129–135.

81. Ibeanu GC, Goldstein JA, Meyer U, et al. Identification of new human CYP2C19 alleles (CYP2C19*6 and CYP2C19*2B) in a Caucasian poor metabolizer of mephenytoin. *J Pharmacol Exp Ther.* 1998;286:1490–1495.

82. Lee SJ, Kim WY, Kim H, Shon JH, Lee SS, Shin JG. Identification of new CYP2C19 variants exhibiting decreased enzyme activity in the metabolism of S-mephenytoin and omeprazole. *Drug Metab Dispos.* 2009;37:2262–2269.

83. Morita J, Kobayashi K, Wanibuchi A, et al. A novel single nucleotide polymorphism (SNP) of the CYP2C19 gene in a Japanese subject with lowered capacity of mephobarbital 4′-hydroxylation. *Drug Metab Pharmacokinet.* 2004;19:236–238.

84. Xiao ZS, Goldstein JA, Xie HG, et al. Differences in the incidence of the CYP2C19 polymorphism affecting the S-mephenytoin phenotype in Chinese Han and Bai populations and identification of a new rare CYP2C19 mutant allele. *J Pharmacol Exp Ther.* 1997;281:604–609.

85. Desta Z, Zhao X, Shin JG, Flockhart DA. Clinical significance of the cytochrome P450 2C19 genetic polymorphism. *Clin Pharmacokinet.* 2002;41:913–958.

86. Kaneko A, Lum JK, Yaviong L, et al. High and variable frequencies of CYP2C19 mutations: medical consequences of poor drug metabolism in Vanuatu and other Pacific islands. *Pharmacogenetics.* 1999;9:581–590.

87. Pedersen RS, Brasch-Andersen C, Sim SC, et al. Linkage disequilibrium between the CYP2C19*17 allele and wildtype CYP2C8 and CYP2C9 alleles: identification of CYP2C haplotypes in healthy Nordic populations. *Eur J Clin Pharmacol.* 2010;66:1199–1205.

88. Berge M, Guillemain R, Tregouet DA, et al. Effect of cytochrome P450 2C19 genotype on voriconazole exposure in cystic fibrosis lung transplant patients. *Eur J Clin Pharmacol.* 2011;67:253–260.

89. Scordo MG, Caputi AP, D'Arrigo C, Fava G, Spina E. Allele and genotype frequencies of CYP2C9, CYP2C19 and CYP2D6 in an Italian population. *Pharmacol Res.* 2004;50:195–200.

90. Kurzawski M, Gawronska-Szklarz B, Wrzesniewska J, Siuda A, Starzynska T, Drozdzik M. Effect of CYP2C19*17 gene variant on *Helicobacter pylori* eradication in peptic ulcer patients. *Eur J Clin Pharmacol.* 2006;62:877–880.

91. Rudberg I, Mohebi B, Hermann M, Refsum H, Molden E. Impact of the ultrarapid CYP2C19*17 allele on serum concentration of escitalopram in psychiatric patients. *Clin Pharmacol Ther.* 2008;83:322–327.

92. Bravo-Villalta HV, Yamamoto K, Nakamura K, Baya A, Okada Y, Horiuchi R. Genetic polymorphism of CYP2C9 and CYP2C19 in a Bolivian population: an investigative and comparative study. *Eur J Clin Pharmacol.* 2005;61:179–184.

93. Sim SC, Risinger C, Dahl ML, et al. A common novel CYP2C19 gene variant causes ultrarapid drug metabolism relevant for the drug response to proton pump inhibitors and antidepressants. *Clin Pharmacol Ther.* 2006;79:103–113.

94. Babalola CP, Adejumo O, Ung D, et al. Cytochrome P450 CYP2C19 genotypes in Nigerian sickle-cell disease patients and normal controls. *J Clin Pharm Ther.* 2010;35:471–477.

95. Kim KA, Song WK, Kim KR, Park JY. Assessment of CYP2C19 genetic polymorphisms in a Korean population using a simultaneous multiplex pyrosequencing method to simultaneously detect the CYP2C19*2, CYP2C19*3, and CYP2C19*17 alleles. *J Clin Pharm Ther.* 2010;35:697–703.

96. Sugimoto K, Uno T, Yamazaki H, Tateishi T. Limited frequency of the CYP2C19*17 allele and its minor role in a Japanese population. *Br J Clin Pharmacol.* 2008;65:437–439.

97. Lamba JK, Dhiman RK, Kohli KK. CYP2C19 genetic mutations in North Indians. *Clin Pharmacol Ther.* 2000;68:328–335.

98. Lee SS, Lee SJ, Gwak J, et al. Comparisons of CYP2C19 genetic polymorphisms between Korean and Vietnamese populations. *Ther Drug Monit.* 2007;29:455–459.

99. Ingelman-Sundberg M, Sim SC, Gomez A, Rodriguez-Antona C. Influence of cytochrome P450 polymorphisms on drug therapies: pharmacogenetic, pharmacoepigenetic and clinical aspects. *Pharmacol Ther.* 2007;116:496–526.

100. Brosen K, Skjelbo E, Flachs H. Proguanil metabolism is determined by the mephenytoin oxidation polymorphism in Vietnamese living in Denmark. *Br J Clin Pharmacol.* 1993;36:105–108.

101. Funck-Brentano C, Becquemont L, Lenevu A, Roux A, Jaillon P, Beaune P. Inhibition by omeprazole of proguanil metabolism: mechanism of the interaction in vitro and prediction of in vivo results from the in vitro experiments. *J Pharmacol Exp Ther.* 1997;280:730–738.

102. Basci NE, Bozkurt A, Kortunay S, Isimer A, Sayal A, Kayaalp SO. Proguanil metabolism in relation to S-mephenytoin oxidation in a Turkish population. *Br J Clin Pharmacol.* 1996;42:771–773.

103. Funck-Brentano C, Bosco O, Jacqz-Aigrain E, Keundjian A, Jaillon P. Relation between chloroguanide bioactivation to cycloguanil and the genetically determined metabolism of mephenytoin in humans. *Clin Pharmacol Ther.* 1992;51:507–512.

104. Birkett DJ, Rees D, Andersson T, Gonzalez FJ, Miners JO, Veronese ME. In vitro proguanil activation to cycloguanil by human liver microsomes is mediated by CYP3A isoforms as well as by S-mephenytoin hydroxylase. *Br J Clin Pharmacol.* 1994;37:413–420.

105. Coller JK, Somogyi AA, Bochner F. Comparison of (*S*)-mephenytoin and proguanil oxidation in vitro: contribution of several CYP isoforms. *Br J Clin Pharmacol.* 1999;48:158–167.

106. Jung F, Richardson TH, Raucy JL, Johnson EF. Diazepam metabolism by cDNA-expressed human 2C P450s: identification of P4502C18 and P4502C19 as low K(M) diazepam *N*-demethylases. *Drug Metab Dispos.* 1997;25:133–139.

107. Kumana CR, Lauder IJ, Chan M, Ko W, Lin HJ. Differences in diazepam pharmacokinetics in Chinese and white Caucasians—relation to body lipid stores. *Eur J Clin Pharmacol.* 1987;32:211–215.

108. Tanaka M, Ohkubo T, Otani K, et al. Metabolic disposition of pantoprazole, a proton pump inhibitor, in relation to *S*-mephenytoin 4′-hydroxylation phenotype and genotype. *Clin Pharmacol Ther.* 1997;62:619–628.

109. Ishizaki T, Horai Y. Review article: cytochrome P450 and the metabolism of proton pump inhibitors—emphasis on rabeprazole. *Aliment Pharmacol Ther.* 1999;13(suppl 3):27–36.

110. Furuta T, Shirai N, Sugimoto M, Ohashi K, Ishizaki T. Pharmacogenomics of proton pump inhibitors. *Pharmacogenomics.* 2004;5:181–202.

111. Sibbing D, Koch W, Gebhard D, et al. Cytochrome 2C19*17 allelic variant, platelet aggregation, bleeding events, and stent thrombosis in clopidogrel-treated patients with coronary stent placement. *Circulation.* 2010;121:512–518.

112. Tiroch KA, Sibbing D, Koch W, et al. Protective effect of the CYP2C19*17 polymorphism with increased activation of clopidogrel on cardiovascular events. *Am Heart J.* 2010;160:506–512.

113. Clarke TA, Waskell LA. The metabolism of clopidogrel is catalyzed by human cytochrome P450 3A and is inhibited by atorvastatin. *Drug Metab Dispos.* 2003;31:53–59.

114. Richter T, Murdter TE, Heinkele G, et al. Potent mechanism-based inhibition of human CYP2B6 by clopidogrel and ticlopidine. *J Pharmacol Exp Ther.* 2004;308:189–197.

115. Kubica A, Kozinski M, Grzesk G, Fabiszak T, Navarese EP, Goch A. Genetic determinants of platelet response to clopidogrel. *J Thromb Thrombolysis.* 2011;32:459–466.

116. Brandt JT, Close SL, Iturria SJ, et al. Common polymorphisms of CYP2C19 and CYP2C9 affect the pharmacokinetic and pharmacodynamic response to clopidogrel but not prasugrel. *J Thromb Haemost.* 2007;5:2429–2436.

117. Hulot JS, Bura A, Villard E, et al. Cytochrome P450 2C19 loss-of-function polymorphism is a major determinant of clopidogrel responsiveness in healthy subjects. *Blood.* 2006;108:2244–2247.

118. Mega JL, Close SL, Wiviott SD, et al. Cytochrome p-450 polymorphisms and response to clopidogrel. *N Engl J Med.* 2009;360:354–362.

119. Brockmoller J, Kirchheiner J, Meisel C, Roots I. Pharmacogenetic diagnostics of cytochrome P450 polymorphisms in clinical drug development and in drug treatment. *Pharmacogenomics.* 2000;1:125–151.

120. Cascorbi I. Pharmacogenetics of cytochrome p4502D6: genetic background and clinical implication. *Eur J Clin Invest.* 2003;33(suppl 2):17–22.

121. Gardiner SJ, Begg EJ. Pharmacogenetics, drug-metabolizing enzymes, and clinical practice. *Pharmacol Rev.* 2006;58:521–590.

122. Ingelman-Sundberg M. Genetic polymorphisms of cytochrome P450 2D6 (CYP2D6): clinical consequences, evolutionary aspects and functional diversity. *Pharmacogenomics J.* 2005;5:6–13.

123. Zhou SF. Polymorphism of human cytochrome P450 2D6 and its clinical significance: part II. *Clin Pharmacokinet.* 2009;48:761–804.

124. Heim MH, Meyer UA. Evolution of a highly polymorphic human cytochrome P450 gene cluster: CYP2D6. *Genomics.* 1992;14:49–58.

125. Kimura S, Umeno M, Skoda RC, Meyer UA, Gonzalez FJ. The human debrisoquine 4-hydroxylase (CYP2D) locus: sequence and identification of the polymorphic CYP2D6 gene, a related gene, and a pseudogene. *Am J Hum Genet.* 1989;45:889–904.

126. Steen VM, Andreassen OA, Daly AK, et al. Detection of the poor metabolizer-associated CYP2D6(D) gene deletion allele by long-PCR technology. *Pharmacogenetics.* 1995;5:215–223.

127. Pai HV, Kommaddi RP, Chinta SJ, Mori T, Boyd MR, Ravindranath V. A frameshift mutation and alternate splicing in human brain generate a functional form of the pseudogene cytochrome P4502D7 that demethylates codeine to morphine. *J Biol Chem.* 2004;279:27383–27389.

128. Gaedigk A, Gaedigk R, Leeder JS. CYP2D7 splice variants in human liver and brain: does CYP2D7 encode functional protein? *Biochem Biophys Res Commun.* 2005;336:1241–1250.

129. Zanger UM, Raimundo S, Eichelbaum M. Cytochrome P450 2D6: overview and update on pharmacology, genetics, biochemistry. *Naunyn Schmiedebergs Arch Pharmacol.* 2004;369:23–37.

130. Eiermann B, Edlund PO, Tjernberg A, Dalen P, Dahl ML, Bertilsson L. 1- and 3-hydroxylations, in addition to 4-hydroxylation, of debrisoquine are catalyzed by cytochrome P450 2D6 in humans. *Drug Metab Dispos.* 1998;26:1096–1101.

131. Gonzalez FJ, Skoda RC, Kimura S, et al. Characterization of the common genetic defect in humans deficient in debrisoquine metabolism. *Nature.* 1988;331:442–446.

132. Woolhouse NM, Andoh B, Mahgoub A, Sloan TP, Idle JR, Smith RL. Debrisoquin hydroxylation polymorphism among Ghanaians and Caucasians. *Clin Pharmacol Ther.* 1979;26:584–591.

133. Dayer P, Leemann T, Striberni R. Dextromethorphan *O*-demethylation in liver microsomes as a prototype reaction to monitor cytochrome P-450 db1 activity. *Clin Pharmacol Ther.* 1989;45:34–40.

134. Jacqz-Aigrain E, Funck-Brentano C, Cresteil T. CYP2D6- and CYP3A-dependent metabolism of dextromethorphan in humans. *Pharmacogenetics.* 1993;3:197–204.

135. Schmid B, Bircher J, Preisig R, Kupfer A. Polymorphic dextromethorphan metabolism: co-segregation of oxidative *O*-demethylation with debrisoquin hydroxylation. *Clin Pharmacol Ther.* 1985;38:618–624.

136. Carcillo JA, Adedoyin A, Burckart GJ, et al. Coordinated intrahepatic and extrahepatic regulation of cytochrome p4502D6 in healthy subjects and in patients after liver transplantation. *Clin Pharmacol Ther.* 2003;73:456–467.

137. Hiroi T, Chow T, Imaoka S, Funae Y. Catalytic specificity of CYP2D isoforms in rat and human. *Drug Metab Dispos.* 2002;30:970–976.

138. Paar WD, Frankus P, Dengler HJ. The metabolism of tramadol by human liver microsomes. *Clin Investig.* 1992;70:708–710.

139. Paar WD, Poche S, Gerloff J, Dengler HJ. Polymorphic CYP2D6 mediates *O*-demethylation of the opioid analgesic tramadol. *Eur J Clin Pharmacol.* 1997;53:235–239.

140. Subrahmanyam V, Renwick AB, Walters DG, et al. Identification of cytochrome P-450 isoforms responsible for *cis*-tramadol metabolism in human liver microsomes. *Drug Metab Dispos.* 2001;29:1146–1155.

141. Eichelbaum M, Ingelman-Sundberg M, Evans WE. Pharmacogenomics and individualized drug therapy. *Annu Rev Med.* 2006;57:119–137.

142. Broly F, Marez D, Lo Guidice JM, et al. A nonsense mutation in the cytochrome P450 CYP2D6 gene identified in a Caucasian with an enzyme deficiency. *Hum Genet.* 1995;96:601–603.

143. Chida M, Yokoi T, Nemoto N, Inaba M, Kinoshita M, Kamataki T. A new variant CYP2D6 allele (CYP2D6*21) with a single base insertion in exon 5 in a Japanese population associated with a poor metabolizer phenotype. *Pharmacogenetics.* 1999;9:287–293.

144. Daly AK, Fairbrother KS, Andreassen OA, London SJ, Idle JR, Steen VM. Characterization and PCR-based detection of two different hybrid CYP2D7P/CYP2D6 alleles associated with the poor metabolizer phenotype. *Pharmacogenetics.* 1996;6:319–328.

145. Daly AK, Leathart JB, London SJ, Idle JR. An inactive cytochrome P450 CYP2D6 allele containing a deletion and a base substitution. *Hum Genet.* 1995;95:337–341.

146. Evert B, Griese EU, Eichelbaum M. Cloning and sequencing of a new non-functional CYP2D6 allele: deletion of T1795 in exon 3 generates a premature stop codon. *Pharmacogenetics.* 1994;4:271–274.

147. Gaedigk A, Blum M, Gaedigk R, Eichelbaum M, Meyer UA. Deletion of the entire cytochrome P450 CYP2D6 gene as a cause of impaired drug metabolism in poor metabolizers of the debrisoquine/sparteine polymorphism. *Am J Hum Genet.* 1991;48:943–950.

148. Gaedigk A, Bradford LD, Marcucci KA, Leeder JS. Unique CYP2D6 activity distribution and genotype–phenotype discordance in black Americans. *Clin Pharmacol Ther.* 2002;72:76–89.

149. Gaedigk A, Ndjountche L, Gaedigk R, Leeder JS, Bradford LD. Discovery of a novel nonfunctional cytochrome P450 2D6 allele, CYP2D642, in African American subjects. *Clin Pharmacol Ther.* 2003;73:575–576.

150. Gough AC, Miles JS, Spurr NK, et al. Identification of the primary gene defect at the cytochrome P450 CYP2D locus. *Nature.* 1990;347:773–776.

151. Hanioka N, Kimura S, Meyer UA, Gonzalez FJ. The human CYP2D locus associated with a common genetic defect in drug oxidation: a G1934—A base change in intron 3 of a mutant CYP2D6 allele results in an aberrant 3′ splice recognition site. *Am J Hum Genet.* 1990;47:994–1001.

152. Ji L, Pan S, Marti-Jaun J, Hanseler E, Rentsch K, Hersberger M. Single-step assays to analyze CYP2D6 gene polymorphisms in Asians: allele frequencies and a novel *14B allele in mainland Chinese. *Clin Chem.* 2002;48:983–988.

153. Kagimoto M, Heim M, Kagimoto K, Zeugin T, Meyer UA. Multiple mutations of the human cytochrome P450IID6 gene (CYP2D6) in poor metabolizers of debrisoquine. Study of the functional significance of individual mutations by expression of chimeric genes. *J Biol Chem.* 1990;265:17209–17214.

154. Klein K, Tatzel S, Raimundo S, et al. A natural variant of the heme-binding signature (R441C) resulting in complete loss of function of CYP2D6. *Drug Metab Dispos.* 2007;35:1247–1250.

155. Leathart JB, London SJ, Steward A, Adams JD, Idle JR, Daly AK. CYP2D6 phenotype–genotype relationships in African-Americans and Caucasians in Los Angeles. *Pharmacogenetics.* 1998;8:529–541.

156. Lee SJ, Lee SS, Jung HJ, et al. Discovery of novel functional variants and extensive evaluation of CYP2D6 genetic polymorphisms in Koreans. *Drug Metab Dispos.* 2009;37:1464–1470.

157. Li L, Pan RM, Porter TD, et al. New cytochrome P450 2D6*56 allele identified by genotype/phenotype analysis of cryopreserved human hepatocytes. *Drug Metab Dispos.* 2006;34:1411–1416.

158. Marez D, Legrand M, Sabbagh N, et al. Polymorphism of the cytochrome P450 CYP2D6 gene in a European population: characterization of 48 mutations and 53 alleles, their frequencies and evolution. *Pharmacogenetics.* 1997;7:193–202.

159. Marez D, Legrand M, Sabbagh N, Lo-Guidice JM, Boone P, Broly F. An additional allelic variant of the CYP2D6 gene causing impaired metabolism of sparteine. *Hum Genet.* 1996;97:668–670.

160. Marez D, Sabbagh N, Legrand M, Lo-Guidice JM, Boone P, Broly F. A novel CYP2D6 allele with an abolished splice recognition site associated with the poor metabolizer phenotype. *Pharmacogenetics.* 1995;5:305–311.

161. Marez-Allorge D, Ellis SW, Lo Guidice JM, Tucker GT, Broly F. A rare G2061 insertion affecting the open reading frame of CYP2D6 and responsible for the poor metabolizer phenotype. *Pharmacogenetics.* 1999;9:393–396.

162. Panserat S, Mura C, Gerard N, et al. An unequal cross-over event within the CYP2D gene cluster generates a chimeric CYP2D7/CYP2D6 gene which is associated with the poor metabolizer phenotype. *Br J Clin Pharmacol.* 1995;40:361–367.

163. Sachse C, Brockmoller J, Bauer S, Reum T, Roots I. A rare insertion of T226 in exon 1 of CYP2D6 causes a frameshift and is associated with the poor metabolizer phenotype: CYP2D6*15. *Pharmacogenetics.* 1996;6: 269–272.

164. Sachse C, Brockmoller J, Bauer S, Roots I. Cytochrome P450 2D6 variants in a Caucasian population: allele frequencies and phenotypic consequences. *Am J Hum Genet.* 1997;60:284–295.

165. Saxena R, Shaw GL, Relling MV, et al. Identification of a new variant CYP2D6 allele with a single base deletion in exon 3 and its association with the poor metabolizer phenotype. *Hum Mol Genet.* 1994;3:923–926.

166. Shimada T, Tsumura F, Yamazaki H, Guengerich FP, Inoue K. Characterization of (+/−)-bufuralol hydroxylation activities in liver microsomes of Japanese and Caucasian subjects genotyped for CYP2D6. *Pharmacogenetics.* 2001;11:143–156.

167. Wang SL, Lai MD, Huang JD. G169R mutation diminishes the metabolic activity of CYP2D6 in Chinese. *Drug Metab Dispos.* 1999;27:385–388.

168. Yamazaki H, Kiyotani K, Tsubuko S, et al. Two novel haplotypes of CYP2D6 gene in a Japanese population. *Drug Metab Pharmacokinet.* 2003;18:269–271.

169. Yokoi T, Kosaka Y, Chida M, et al. A new CYP2D6 allele with a nine base insertion in exon 9 in a Japanese population associated with poor metabolizer phenotype. *Pharmacogenetics.* 1996;6:395–401.

170. Yokota H, Tamura S, Furuya H, et al. Evidence for a new variant CYP2D6 allele CYP2D6J in a Japanese population associated with lower in vivo rates of sparteine metabolism. *Pharmacogenetics.* 1993;3:256–263.

171. Dahl ML, Johansson I, Palmertz MP, Ingelman-Sundberg M, Sjoqvist F. Analysis of the CYP2D6 gene in relation to debrisoquin and desipramine hydroxylation in a Swedish population. *Clin Pharmacol Ther.* 1992;51:12–17.

172. Masimirembwa C, Hasler J, Bertilssons L, Johansson I, Ekberg O, Ingelman-Sundberg M. Phenotype and genotype analysis of debrisoquine hydroxylase (CYP2D6) in a black Zimbabwean population. Reduced enzyme activity and evaluation of metabolic correlation of CYP2D6 probe drugs. *Eur J Clin Pharmacol.* 1996;51:117–122.

173. Simooya OO, Njunju E, Hodjegan AR, Lennard MS, Tucker GT. Debrisoquine and metoprolol oxidation in Zambians: a population study. *Pharmacogenetics.* 1993;3:205–208.

174. Wang SL, Huang JD, Lai MD, Liu BH, Lai ML. Molecular basis of genetic variation in debrisoquin hydroxylation in Chinese subjects: polymorphism in RFLP and DNA sequence of CYP2D6. *Clin Pharmacol Ther.* 1993;53:410–418.

175. Meyer UA, Zanger UM. Molecular mechanisms of genetic polymorphisms of drug metabolism. *Annu Rev Pharmacol Toxicol.* 1997;37:269–296.

176. Gaedigk A. Interethnic differences of drug-metabolizing enzymes. *Int J Clin Pharmacol Ther.* 2000;38:61–68.

177. Lennard MS, Iyun AO, Jackson PR, Tucker GT, Woods HF. Evidence for a dissociation in the control of sparteine, debrisoquine and metoprolol metabolism in Nigerians. *Pharmacogenetics.* 1992;2:89–92.

178. Xie HG, Xu ZH, Luo X, Huang SL, Zeng FD, Zhou HH. Genetic polymorphisms of debrisoquine and S-mephenytoin oxidation metabolism in Chinese populations: a meta-analysis. *Pharmacogenetics.* 1996;6: 235–238.

179. Johansson I, Oscarson M, Yue QY, Bertilsson L, Sjoqvist F, Ingelman-Sundberg M. Genetic analysis of the Chinese cytochrome P4502D locus: characterization of variant CYP2D6 genes present in subjects with diminished capacity for debrisoquine hydroxylation. *Mol Pharmacol.* 1994;46:452–459.

180. Lee SY, Sohn KM, Ryu JY, Yoon YR, Shin JG, Kim JW. Sequence-based CYP2D6 genotyping in the Korean population. *Ther Drug Monit.* 2006;28:382–387.

181. Nishida Y, Fukuda T, Yamamoto I, Azuma J. CYP2D6 genotypes in a Japanese population: low frequencies of CYP2D6 gene duplication but high frequency of CYP2D6*10. *Pharmacogenetics.* 2000;10:567–570.

182. Roh HK, Dahl ML, Johansson I, Ingelman-Sundberg M, Cha YN, Bertilsson L. Debrisoquine and S-mephenytoin hydroxylation phenotypes and genotypes in a Korean population. *Pharmacogenetics.* 1996;6:441–447.

183. Tateishi T, Chida M, Ariyoshi N, Mizorogi Y, Kamataki T, Kobayashi S. Analysis of the CYP2D6 gene in relation to dextromethorphan O-demethylation capacity in a Japanese population. *Clin Pharmacol Ther.* 1999;65:570–575.

184. Gaedigk A, Ndjountche L, Divakaran K, et al. Cytochrome P4502D6 (CYP2D6) gene locus heterogeneity: characterization of gene duplication events. *Clin Pharmacol Ther.* 2007;81:242–251.

185. Sistonen J, Sajantila A, Lao O, Corander J, Barbujani G, Fuselli S. CYP2D6 worldwide genetic variation shows high frequency of altered activity variants and no continental structure. *Pharmacogenet Genomics.* 2007;17:93–101.

186. Gaedigk A, Gotschall RR, Forbes NS, Simon SD, Kearns GL, Leeder JS. Optimization of cytochrome P4502D6 (CYP2D6) phenotype assignment using a genotyping algorithm based on allele frequency data. *Pharmacogenetics.* 1999;9:669–682.

187. Menoyo A, del Rio E, Baiget M. Characterization of variant alleles of cytochrome CYP2D6 in a Spanish population. *Cell Biochem Funct.* 2006;24:381–385.

188. Aynacioglu AS, Sachse C, Bozkurt A, et al. Low frequency of defective alleles of cytochrome P450 enzymes 2C19 and 2D6 in the Turkish population. *Clin Pharmacol Ther.* 1999;66:185–192.

189. Cai WM, Nikoloff DM, Pan RM, et al. CYP2D6 genetic variation in healthy adults and psychiatric African-American subjects: implications for clinical practice and genetic testing. *Pharmacogenomics J.* 2006;6:343–350.

190. Aklillu E, Herrlin K, Gustafsson LL, Bertilsson L, Ingelman-Sundberg M. Evidence for environmental influence on CYP2D6-catalysed debrisoquine hydroxylation as demonstrated by phenotyping and genotyping of Ethiopians living in Ethiopia or in Sweden. *Pharmacogenetics.* 2002;12:375–383.

191. Zhou Q, Yu XM, Lin HB, et al. Genetic polymorphism, linkage disequilibrium, haplotype structure and novel allele analysis of CYP2C19 and CYP2D6 in Han Chinese. *Pharmacogenomics J.* 2009;9:380–394.

192. Liou YH, Lin CT, Wu YJ, Wu LS. The high prevalence of the poor and ultrarapid metabolite alleles of CYP2D6, CYP2C9, CYP2C19, CYP3A4, and CYP3A5 in Taiwanese population. *J Hum Genet.* 2006;51:857–863.

193. Naveen AT, Adithan C, Soya SS, Gerard N, Krishnamoorthy R. CYP2D6 genetic polymorphism in South Indian populations. *Biol Pharm Bull.* 2006;29:1655–1658.

194. Teh LK, Ismail R, Yusoff R, Hussein A, Isa MN, Rahman AR. Heterogeneity of the CYP2D6 gene among Malays in Malaysia. *J Clin Pharm Ther.* 2001;26:205–211.

195. Sakuyama K, Sasaki T, Ujiie S, et al. Functional characterization of 17 CYP2D6 allelic variants (CYP2D6.2, 10, 14A–B, 18, 27, 36, 39, 47–51, 53–55, and 57). *Drug Metab Dispos.* 2008;36:2460–2467.

196. Gaedigk A, Simon SD, Pearce RE, Bradford LD, Kennedy MJ, Leeder JS. The CYP2D6 activity score: translating genotype information into a qualitative measure of phenotype. *Clin Pharmacol Ther.* 2008;83:234–242.

197. Baumann P, Hiemke C, Ulrich S, et al. The AGNP-TDM expert group consensus guidelines: therapeutic drug monitoring in psychiatry. *Pharmacopsychiatry.* 2004;37:243–265.

198. Kirchheiner J, Nickchen K, Bauer M, et al. Pharmacogenetics of antidepressants and antipsychotics: the contribution of allelic variations to the phenotype of drug response. *Mol Psychiatry.* 2004;9:442–473.

199. Thuerauf N, Lunkenheimer J. The impact of the CYP2D6-polymorphism on dose recommendations for current antidepressants. *Eur Arch Psychiatry Clin Neurosci.* 2006;256:287–293.

200. Brosen K, Hansen JG, Nielsen KK, Sindrup SH, Gram LF. Inhibition by paroxetine of desipramine metabolism in extensive but not in poor metabolizers of sparteine. *Eur J Clin Pharmacol.* 1993;44:349–355.

201. Brosen K, Otton SV, Gram LF. Imipramine demethylation and hydroxylation: impact of the sparteine oxidation phenotype. *Clin Pharmacol Ther.* 1986;40:543–549.

202. Dalen P, Dahl ML, Bernal Ruiz ML, Nordin J, Bertilsson L. 10-Hydroxylation of nortriptyline in white persons with 0, 1, 2, 3, and 13 functional CYP2D6 genes. *Clin Pharmacol Ther.* 1998;63:444–452.

203. Morita S, Shimoda K, Someya T, Yoshimura Y, Kamijima K, Kato N. Steady-state plasma levels of nortriptyline and its hydroxylated metabolites in Japanese patients: impact of CYP2D6 genotype on the hydroxylation of nortriptyline. *J Clin Psychopharmacol.* 2000;20:141–149.

204. Nielsen KK, Brosen K, Gram LF. Steady-state plasma levels of clomipramine and its metabolites: impact of the sparteine/debrisoquine oxidation polymorphism. Danish University Antidepressant Group. *Eur J Clin Pharmacol.* 1992;43:405–411.

205. Spina E, Gitto C, Avenoso A, Campo GM, Caputi AP, Perucca E. Relationship between plasma desipramine levels, CYP2D6 phenotype and clinical response to desipramine: a prospective study. *Eur J Clin Pharmacol.* 1997;51:395–398.

206. Spina E, Steiner E, Ericsson O, Sjoqvist F. Hydroxylation of desmethylimipramine: dependence on the debrisoquin hydroxylation phenotype. *Clin Pharmacol Ther.* 1987;41:314–319.

207. Steiner E, Spina E. Differences in the inhibitory effect of cimetidine on desipramine metabolism between rapid and slow debrisoquin hydroxylators. *Clin Pharmacol Ther.* 1987;42:278–282.

208. Yue QY, Zhong ZH, Tybring G, et al. Pharmacokinetics of nortriptyline and its 10-hydroxy metabolite in Chinese subjects of different CYP2D6 genotypes. *Clin Pharmacol Ther.* 1998;64:384–390.

209. Bondolfi G, Eap CB, Bertschy G, Zullino D, Vermeulen A, Baumann P. The effect of fluoxetine on the pharmacokinetics and safety of risperidone in psychotic patients. *Pharmacopsychiatry.* 2002;35:50–56.

210. Dahl-Puustinen ML, Liden A, Alm C, Nordin C, Bertilsson L. Disposition of perphenazine is related to polymorphic debrisoquin hydroxylation in human beings. *Clin Pharmacol Ther.* 1989;46:78–81.

211. Linnet K, Wiborg O. Steady-state serum concentrations of the neuroleptic perphenazine in relation to CYP2D6 genetic polymorphism. *Clin Pharmacol Ther.* 1996;60:41–47.

212. Nyberg S, Dahl ML, Halldin C. A PET study of D2 and 5-HT2 receptor occupancy induced by risperidone in poor metabolizers of debrisoquin and risperidone. *Psychopharmacology (Berl).* 1995;119:345–348.

213. Ozdemir V, Bertilsson L, Miura J, et al. CYP2D6 genotype in relation to perphenazine concentration and pituitary pharmacodynamic tissue sensitivity in Asians: CYP2D6-serotonin–dopamine crosstalk revisited. *Pharmacogenet Genomics.* 2007;17:339–347.

214. Ozdemir V, Naranjo CA, Herrmann N, Reed K, Sellers EM, Kalow W. Paroxetine potentiates the central nervous system side effects of perphenazine: contribution of cytochrome P4502D6 inhibition in vivo. *Clin Pharmacol Ther.* 1997;62:334–347.

215. Pollock BG, Mulsant BH, Sweet RA, Rosen J, Altieri LP, Perel JM. Prospective cytochrome P450 phenotyping for neuroleptic treatment in dementia. *Psychopharmacol Bull.* 1995;31:327–331.

216. Scordo MG, Spina E, Facciola G, Avenoso A, Johansson I, Dahl ML. Cytochrome P450 2D6 genotype and steady state plasma levels of risperidone and 9-hydroxyrisperidone. *Psychopharmacology (Berl).* 1999;147: 300–305.

217. Fjordside L, Jeppesen U, Eap CB, Powell K, Baumann P, Brosen K. The stereoselective metabolism of fluoxetine in poor and extensive metabolizers of sparteine. *Pharmacogenetics.* 1999;9:55–60.

218. Hamelin BA, Turgeon J, Vallee F, Belanger PM, Paquet F, LeBel M. The disposition of fluoxetine but not sertraline is altered in poor metabolizers of debrisoquin. *Clin Pharmacol Ther.* 1996;60:512–521.

219. Scordo MG, Spina E, Dahl ML, Gatti G, Perucca E. Influence of CYP2C9, 2C19 and 2D6 genetic polymorphisms on the steady-state plasma concentrations of the enantiomers of fluoxetine and norfluoxetine. *Basic Clin Pharmacol Toxicol.* 2005;97:296–301.

220. Sindrup SH, Brosen K, Gram LF, et al. The relationship between paroxetine and the sparteine oxidation polymorphism. *Clin Pharmacol Ther.* 1992;51:278–287.

221. Kawanishi C, Lundgren S, Agren H, Bertilsson L. Increased incidence of CYP2D6 gene duplication in patients with persistent mood disorders: ultrarapid metabolism of antidepressants as a cause of nonresponse. A pilot study. *Eur J Clin Pharmacol.* 2004;59:803–807.

222. Rau T, Wohlleben G, Wuttke H, et al. CYP2D6 genotype: impact on adverse effects and nonresponse during treatment with antidepressants—a pilot study. *Clin Pharmacol Ther.* 2004;75:386–393.

223. Kitzmiller JP, Groen DK, Phelps MA, Sadee W. Pharmacogenomic testing: relevance in medical practice: why drugs work in some patients but not in others. *Cleve Clin J Med.* 2011;78:243–257.

224. Dehal SS, Kupfer D. CYP2D6 catalyzes tamoxifen 4-hydroxylation in human liver. *Cancer Res.* 1997;57:3402–3406.

225. Jin Y, Desta Z, Stearns V, et al. CYP2D6 genotype, antidepressant use, and tamoxifen metabolism during adjuvant breast cancer treatment. *J Natl Cancer Inst.* 2005;97:30–39.

226. Jordan VC, Collins MM, Rowsby L, Prestwich G. A monohydroxylated metabolite of tamoxifen with potent antiestrogenic activity. *J Endocrinol.* 1977;75:305–316.

227. Abraham JE, Maranian MJ, Driver KE, et al. CYP2D6 gene variants: association with breast cancer specific survival in a cohort of breast cancer patients from the United Kingdom treated with adjuvant tamoxifen. *Breast Cancer Res.* 2010;12:R64.

228. Dieudonne AS, Van Belle V, Neven P. Association between CYP2D6 polymorphisms and breast cancer outcomes. *JAMA.* 2010;303:516–517.

229. Goetz MP. Tamoxifen, endoxifen, and CYP2D6: the rules for evaluating a predictive factor. *Oncology (Huntingt).* 2009;23:1233–1234, 36.

230. Madlensky L, Natarajan L, Tchu S, et al. Tamoxifen metabolite concentrations, CYP2D6 genotype, and breast cancer outcomes. *Clin Pharmacol Ther.* 2011;89:718–725.

231. Bonanni B, Macis D, Maisonneuve P, et al. Polymorphism in the CYP2D6 tamoxifen-metabolizing gene influences clinical effect but not hot flashes: data from the Italian Tamoxifen Trial. *J Clin Oncol.* 2006;24: 3708–3709.

232. Borges S, Desta Z, Li L, et al. Quantitative effect of CYP2D6 genotype and inhibitors on tamoxifen metabolism: implication for optimization of breast cancer treatment. *Clin Pharmacol Ther.* 2006;80:61–74.

233. Goetz MP, Knox SK, Suman VJ, et al. The impact of cytochrome P450 2D6 metabolism in women receiving adjuvant tamoxifen. *Breast Cancer Res Treat.* 2007;101:113–121.

234. Goetz MP, Rae JM, Suman VJ, et al. Pharmacogenetics of tamoxifen biotransformation is associated with clinical outcomes of efficacy and hot flashes. *J Clin Oncol.* 2005;23:9312–9318.

235. Lim HS, Ju Lee H, Seok Lee K, Sook Lee E, Jang IJ, Ro J. Clinical implications of CYP2D6 genotypes predictive of tamoxifen pharmacokinetics in metastatic breast cancer. *J Clin Oncol.* 2007;25:3837–3845.

236. Schroth W, Antoniadou L, Fritz P, et al. Breast cancer treatment outcome with adjuvant tamoxifen relative to patient CYP2D6 and CYP2C19 genotypes. *J Clin Oncol.* 2007;25:5187–5193.

237. Brauch H, Murdter TE, Eichelbaum M, Schwab M. Pharmacogenomics of tamoxifen therapy. *Clin Chem.* 2009;55:1770–1782.

238. Goetz MP, Suman VJ, Ingle JN, et al. A two-gene expression ratio of homeobox 13 and interleukin-17B receptor for prediction of recurrence and survival in women receiving adjuvant tamoxifen. *Clin Cancer Res.* 2006;12:2080–2087.

239. Flockhart D. CYP2D6 genotyping and the pharmacogenetics of tamoxifen. *Clin Adv Hematol Oncol.* 2008;6:493–494.

240. Goetz MP, Kamal A, Ames MM. Tamoxifen pharmacogenomics: the role of CYP2D6 as a predictor of drug response. *Clin Pharmacol Ther.* 2008;83:160–166.

241. Higgins MJ, Stearns V. CYP2D6 polymorphisms and tamoxifen metabolism: clinical relevance. *Curr Oncol Rep.* 2010;12:7–15.

242. Dalen P, Frengell C, Dahl ML, Sjoqvist F. Quick onset of severe abdominal pain after codeine in an ultrarapid metabolizer of debrisoquine. *Ther Drug Monit.* 1997;19:543–544.

243. Koren G, Cairns J, Chitayat D, Gaedigk A, Leeder SJ. Pharmacogenetics of morphine poisoning in a breastfed neonate of a codeine-prescribed mother. *Lancet.* 2006;368:704.

244. Caraco Y, Sheller J, Wood AJ. Pharmacogenetic determination of the effects of codeine and prediction of drug interactions. *J Pharmacol Exp Ther.* 1996;278:1165–1174.

245. Eckhardt K, Li S, Ammon S, Schanzle G, Mikus G, Eichelbaum M. Same incidence of adverse drug events after codeine administration irrespective of the genetically determined differences in morphine formation. *Pain.* 1998;76:27–33.

246. Lotsch J, Skarke C, Liefhold J, Geisslinger G. Genetic predictors of the clinical response to opioid analgesics: clinical utility and future perspectives. *Clin Pharmacokinet.* 2004;43:983–1013.

247. Garcia-Quetglas E, Azanza JR, Sadaba B, Munoz MJ, Gil I, Campanero MA. Pharmacokinetics of tramadol enantiomers and their respective phase I metabolites in relation to CYP2D6 phenotype. *Pharmacol Res.* 2007;55:122–130.

248. Pedersen RS, Damkier P, Brosen K. Enantioselective pharmacokinetics of tramadol in CYP2D6 extensive and poor metabolizers. *Eur J Clin Pharmacol.* 2006;62:513–521.

249. Stamer UM, Musshoff F, Kobilay M, Madea B, Hoeft A, Stuber F. Concentrations of tramadol and *O*-desmethyltramadol enantiomers in different CYP2D6 genotypes. *Clin Pharmacol Ther.* 2007;82:41–47.

250. Fliegert F, Kurth B, Gohler K. The effects of tramadol on static and dynamic pupillometry in healthy subjects—the relationship between pharmacodynamics, pharmacokinetics and CYP2D6 metaboliser status. *Eur J Clin Pharmacol.* 2005;61:257–266.

251. Poulsen L, Arendt-Nielsen L, Brosen K, Sindrup SH. The hypoalgesic effect of tramadol in relation to CYP2D6. *Clin Pharmacol Ther.* 1996;60:636–644.

252. Stamer UM, Lehnen K, Hothker F, et al. Impact of CYP2D6 genotype on postoperative tramadol analgesia. *Pain.* 2003;105:231–238.

253. Kirchheiner J, Keulen JT, Bauer S, Roots I, Brockmoller J. Effects of the CYP2D6 gene duplication on the pharmacokinetics and pharmacodynamics of tramadol. *J Clin Psychopharmacol.* 2008;28:78–83.

254. Stamer UM, Stuber F, Muders T, Musshoff F. Respiratory depression with tramadol in a patient with renal impairment and CYP2D6 gene duplication. *Anesth Analg.* 2008;107:926–929.

255. Mehvar R, Brocks DR. Stereospecific pharmacokinetics and pharmacodynamics of beta-adrenergic blockers in humans. *J Pharm Pharm Sci.* 2001;4:185–200.

256. Dayer P, Leemann T, Marmy A, Rosenthaler J. Interindividual variation of beta-adrenoceptor blocking drugs, plasma concentration and effect: influence of genetic status on behaviour of atenolol, bopindolol and metoprolol. *Eur J Clin Pharmacol.* 1985;28:149–153.

257. Otton SV, Crewe HK, Lennard MS, Tucker GT, Woods HF. Use of quinidine inhibition to define the role of the sparteine/debrisoquine cytochrome

258. Johnson JA, Burlew BS. Metoprolol metabolism via cytochrome P4502D6 in ethnic populations. *Drug Metab Dispos.* 1996;24:350–355.

259. Oldham HG, Clarke SE. In vitro identification of the human cytochrome P450 enzymes involved in the metabolism of *R*(+)- and *S*(−)-carvedilol. *Drug Metab Dispos.* 1997;25:970–977.

260. Talaat RE, Nelson WL. Regioisomeric aromatic dihydroxylation of propranolol. Synthesis and identification of 4,6- and 4,8-dihydroxy-propranolol as metabolites in the rat and in man. *Drug Metab Dispos.* 1988;16:212–216.

261. Ward SA, Walle T, Walle UK, Wilkinson GR, Branch RA. Propranolol's metabolism is determined by both mephenytoin and debrisoquin hydroxylase activities. *Clin Pharmacol Ther.* 1989;45:72–79.

262. Lennard MS, Jackson PR, Freestone S, Ramsay LE, Tucker GT, Woods HF. The oral clearance and beta-adrenoceptor antagonist activity of propranolol after single dose are not related to debrisoquine oxidation phenotype. *Br J Clin Pharmacol.* 1984;17(suppl 1):106S–107S.

263. Raghuram TC, Koshakji RP, Wilkinson GR, Wood AJ. Polymorphic ability to metabolize propranolol alters 4-hydroxypropranolol levels but not beta blockade. *Clin Pharmacol Ther.* 1984;36:51–56.

264. Sowinski KM, Burlew BS. Impact of CYP2D6 poor metabolizer phenotype on propranolol pharmacokinetics and response. *Pharmacotherapy.* 1997;17:1305–1310.

265. Volotinen M, Turpeinen M, Tolonen A, Uusitalo J, Maenpaa J, Pelkonen O. Timolol metabolism in human liver microsomes is mediated principally by CYP2D6. *Drug Metab Dispos.* 2007;35:1135–1141.

266. Heel RC, Brogden RN, Speight TM, Avery GS. Timolol: a review of its therapeutic efficacy in the topical treatment of glaucoma. *Drugs.* 1979;17:38–55.

267. Nieminen T, Lehtimaki T, Maenpaa J, Ropo A, Uusitalo H, Kahonen M. Ophthalmic timolol: plasma concentration and systemic cardiopulmonary effects. *Scand J Clin Lab Invest.* 2007;67:237–245.

268. Fux R, Morike K, Prohmer AM, et al. Impact of CYP2D6 genotype on adverse effects during treatment with metoprolol: a prospective clinical study. *Clin Pharmacol Ther.* 2005;78:378–387.

269. Zhou HH, Wood AJ. Stereoselective disposition of carvedilol is determined by CYP2D6. *Clin Pharmacol Ther.* 1995;57:518–524.

270. Zineh I, Beitelshees AL, Gaedigk A, et al. Pharmacokinetics and CYP2D6 genotypes do not predict metoprolol adverse events or efficacy in hypertension. *Clin Pharmacol Ther.* 2004;76:536–544.

271. Gonzalez FJ, Gelboin HV. Role of human cytochromes P450 in the metabolic activation of chemical carcinogens and toxins. *Drug Metab Rev.* 1994;26:165–183.

272. Guengerich FP, Shimada T. Oxidation of toxic and carcinogenic chemicals by human cytochrome P-450 enzymes. *Chem Res Toxicol.* 1991;4:391–407.

273. Omiecinski CJ, Remmel RP, Hosagrahara VP. Concise review of the cytochrome P450s and their roles in toxicology. *Toxicol Sci.* 1999;48:151–156.

274. Bozina N, Bradamante V, Lovric M. Genetic polymorphism of metabolic enzymes P450 (CYP) as a susceptibility factor for drug response, toxicity, and cancer risk. *Arh Hig Rada Toksikol.* 2009;60:217–242.

275. Zanger UM, Turpeinen M, Klein K, Schwab M. Functional pharmacogenetics/genomics of human cytochromes P450 involved in drug biotransformation. *Anal Bioanal Chem.* 2008;392:1093–1108.

276. Bondolfi G, Morel F, Crettol S, Rachid F, Baumann P, Eap CB. Increased clozapine plasma concentrations and side effects induced by smoking cessation in 2 CYP1A2 genotyped patients. *Ther Drug Monit.* 2005;27:539–543.

277. Eap CB, Bender S, Jaquenoud Sirot E, et al. Nonresponse to clozapine and ultrarapid CYP1A2 activity: clinical data and analysis of CYP1A2 gene. *J Clin Psychopharmacol.* 2004;24:214–219.

278. Ghotbi R, Christensen M, Roh HK, Ingelman-Sundberg M, Aklillu E, Bertilsson L. Comparisons of CYP1A2 genetic polymorphisms, enzyme activity and the genotype–phenotype relationship in Swedes and Koreans. *Eur J Clin Pharmacol.* 2007;63:537–546.

279. Han XM, Ouyang DS, Chen XP, et al. Inducibility of CYP1A2 by omeprazole in vivo related to the genetic polymorphism of CYP1A2. *Br J Clin Pharmacol.* 2002;54:540–543.

280. Sachse C, Brockmoller J, Bauer S, Roots I. Functional significance of a C→A polymorphism in intron 1 of the cytochrome P450 CYP1A2 gene tested with caffeine. *Br J Clin Pharmacol.* 1999;47:445–449.

281. Moonen H, Engels L, Kleinjans J, Kok T. The CYP1A2-164A→C polymorphism (CYP1A2*1F) is associated with the risk for colorectal adenomas in humans. *Cancer Lett.* 2005;229:25–31.

282. Saebo M, Skjelbred CF, Brekke Li K, et al. CYP1A2 164 A→C polymorphism, cigarette smoking, consumption of well-done red meat and risk of developing colorectal adenomas and carcinomas. *Anticancer Res.* 2008;28:2289–2295.

283. Suzuki H, Morris JS, Li Y, et al. Interaction of the cytochrome P4501A2, SULT1A1 and NAT gene polymorphisms with smoking and dietary mutagen intake in modification of the risk of pancreatic cancer. *Carcinogenesis.* 2008;29:1184–1191.

284. Xu C, Goodz S, Sellers EM, Tyndale RF. CYP2A6 genetic variation and potential consequences. *Adv Drug Deliv Rev.* 2002;54:1245–1256.

285. Kamataki T, Fujieda M, Kiyotani K, Iwano S, Kunitoh H. Genetic polymorphism of CYP2A6 as one of the potential determinants of tobacco-related cancer risk. *Biochem Biophys Res Commun.* 2005;338:306–310.

286. Malaiyandi V, Sellers EM, Tyndale RF. Implications of CYP2A6 genetic variation for smoking behaviors and nicotine dependence. *Clin Pharmacol Ther.* 2005;77:145–158.

287. Ingelman-Sundberg M, Oscarson M, McLellan RA. Polymorphic human cytochrome P450 enzymes: an opportunity for individualized drug treatment. *Trends Pharmacol Sci.* 1999;20:342–349.

288. Oscarson M, McLellan RA, Gullsten H, et al. Identification and characterisation of novel polymorphisms in the CYP2A locus: implications for nicotine metabolism. *FEBS Lett.* 1999;460:321–327.

289. Oscarson M, McLellan RA, Gullsten H, et al. Characterisation and PCR-based detection of a CYP2A6 gene deletion found at a high frequency in a Chinese population. *FEBS Lett.* 1999;448:105–110.

290. Owen A, Pirmohamed M, Khoo SH, Back DJ. Pharmacogenetics of HIV therapy. *Pharmacogenet Genomics.* 2006;16:693–703.

291. Turpeinen M, Raunio H, Pelkonen O. The functional role of CYP2B6 in human drug metabolism: substrates and inhibitors in vitro, in vivo and in silico. *Curr Drug Metab.* 2006;7:705–714.

292. Desta Z, Saussele T, Ward B, et al. Impact of CYP2B6 polymorphism on hepatic efavirenz metabolism in vitro. *Pharmacogenomics.* 2007;8:547–558.

293. Lang T, Klein K, Fischer J, et al. Extensive genetic polymorphism in the human CYP2B6 gene with impact on expression and function in human liver. *Pharmacogenetics.* 2001;11:399–415.

294. Hesse LM, He P, Krishnaswamy S, et al. Pharmacogenetic determinants of interindividual variability in bupropion hydroxylation by cytochrome P450 2B6 in human liver microsomes. *Pharmacogenetics.* 2004;14:225–238.

295. Tsuchiya K, Gatanaga H, Tachikawa N, et al. Homozygous CYP2B6 *6 (Q172H and K262R) correlates with high plasma efavirenz concentrations in HIV-1 patients treated with standard efavirenz-containing regimens. *Biochem Biophys Res Commun.* 2004;319:1322–1326.

296. Xie HJ, Yasar U, Lundgren S, et al. Role of polymorphic human CYP2B6 in cyclophosphamide bioactivation. *Pharmacogenomics J.* 2003;3:53–61.

297. Klein K, Lang T, Saussele T, et al. Genetic variability of CYP2B6 in populations of African and Asian origin: allele frequencies, novel functional variants, and possible implications for anti-HIV therapy with efavirenz. *Pharmacogenet Genomics.* 2005;15:861–873.

298. Rodriguez-Antona C, Ingelman-Sundberg M. Cytochrome P450 pharmacogenetics and cancer. *Oncogene.* 2006;25:1679–1691.

299. Telenti A, Zanger UM. Pharmacogenetics of anti-HIV drugs. *Annu Rev Pharmacol Toxicol.* 2008;48:227–256.

300. Guengerich FP. Cytochrome P-450 3A4: regulation and role in drug metabolism. *Annu Rev Pharmacol Toxicol.* 1999;39:1–17.

301. Lamba JK, Lin YS, Schuetz EG, Thummel KE. Genetic contribution to variable human CYP3A-mediated metabolism. *Adv Drug Deliv Rev.* 2002;54:1271–1294.

302. Shimada T, Yamazaki H, Mimura M, Inui Y, Guengerich FP. Interindividual variations in human liver cytochrome P-450 enzymes involved in the oxidation of drugs, carcinogens and toxic chemicals: studies with liver microsomes of 30 Japanese and 30 Caucasians. *J Pharmacol Exp Ther.* 1994;270:414–423.

303. Lee SJ, Goldstein JA. Functionally defective or altered CYP3A4 and CYP3A5 single nucleotide polymorphisms and their detection with genotyping tests. *Pharmacogenomics.* 2005;6:357–371.

304. Thummel KE, Shen DD, Podoll TD, et al. Use of midazolam as a human cytochrome P450 3A probe: II. Characterization of inter- and intraindividual hepatic CYP3A variability after liver transplantation. *J Pharmacol Exp Ther.* 1994;271:557–566.

305. Lown KS, Thummel KE, Benedict PE, et al. The erythromycin breath test predicts the clearance of midazolam. *Clin Pharmacol Ther.* 1995;57:16–24.

306. Westlind-Johnsson A, Hermann R, Huennemeyer A, et al. Identification and characterization of CYP3A4*20, a novel rare CYP3A4 allele without functional activity. *Clin Pharmacol Ther.* 2006;79:339–349.

307. Xie HG, Wood AJ, Kim RB, Stein CM, Wilkinson GR. Genetic variability in CYP3A5 and its possible consequences. *Pharmacogenomics.* 2004;5:243–272.

308. Lee SJ, Bell DA, Coulter SJ, Ghanayem B, Goldstein JA. Recombinant CYP3A4*17 is defective in metabolizing the hypertensive drug nifedipine, and the CYP3A4*17 allele may occur on the same chromosome as CYP3A5*3, representing a new putative defective CYP3A haplotype. *J Pharmacol Exp Ther.* 2005;313:302–309.

309. Kuehl P, Zhang J, Lin Y, et al. Sequence diversity in CYP3A promoters and characterization of the genetic basis of polymorphic CYP3A5 expression. *Nat Genet.* 2001;27:383–391.

310. Lee SJ, Usmani KA, Chanas B, et al. Genetic findings and functional studies of human CYP3A5 single nucleotide polymorphisms in different ethnic groups. *Pharmacogenetics.* 2003;13:461–472.

311. Hustert E, Haberl M, Burk O, et al. The genetic determinants of the CYP3A5 polymorphism. *Pharmacogenetics.* 2001;11:773–779.

312. Schroeder TJ, Shah M, Hariharan S, First MR. Increased resources are required in patients with low cyclosporine bioavailability. *Transplant Proc.* 1996;28:2151–2155.

313. Staatz CE, Tett SE. Clinical pharmacokinetics and pharmacodynamics of tacrolimus in solid organ transplantation. *Clin Pharmacokinet.* 2004;43:623–653.

314. Barry A, Levine M. A systematic review of the effect of CYP3A5 genotype on the apparent oral clearance of tacrolimus in renal transplant recipients. *Ther Drug Monit.* 2010;32:708–714.

315. Thervet E, Loriot MA, Barbier S, et al. Optimization of initial tacrolimus dose using pharmacogenetic testing. *Clin Pharmacol Ther.* 2010;87:721–726.

316. Bouamar R, Hesselink DA, van Schaik RH, et al. Polymorphisms in CYP3A5, CYP3A4, and ABCB1 are not associated with cyclosporine pharmacokinetics nor with cyclosporine clinical end points after renal transplantation. *Ther Drug Monit.* 2011;33:178–184.

317. Macphee IA, Fredericks S, Tai T, et al. Tacrolimus pharmacogenetics: polymorphisms associated with expression of cytochrome p4503A5 and P-glycoprotein correlate with dose requirement. *Transplantation.* 2002;74:1486–1489.

318. MacPhee IA, Fredericks S, Tai T, et al. The influence of pharmacogenetics on the time to achieve target tacrolimus concentrations after kidney transplantation. *Am J Transplant.* 2004;4:914–919.

319. Macphee IA, Fredericks S, Mohamed M, et al. Tacrolimus pharmacogenetics: the CYP3A5*1 allele predicts low dose-normalized tacrolimus blood concentrations in whites and South Asians. *Transplantation.* 2005;79:499–502.

6B

Phase II Drug-Metabolizing Enzymes

Michael Murray, PhD, DSc

LEARNING OBJECTIVES

- To outline the major pathways of drug biotransformation mediated by phase II enzymes.
- To define the properties and multiplicity of genes that encode phase II biotransformation enzymes.
- To emphasize the extent of genetic variation in important genes that mediate phase II drug biotransformation.
- To provide established examples of pharmacogenetic variants in phase II drug-metabolizing enzymes that influence drug therapy.
- To evaluate the evidence for additional examples of pharmacogenetic variation in drug-metabolizing enzymes that influence therapeutic outcomes with drugs.

INTRODUCTION

Role of Phase II Biotransformation in Drug Elimination

There is often a high concordance between the pharmacokinetic properties of drugs and their therapeutic actions. Serum concentrations are frequently used as surrogate markers for the likely concentrations of drugs achieved at the site of action in tissues. Rates of drug biotransformation and elimination are critical factors that influence the serum concentrations of drugs and their duration of action in the body. Rapid drug clearance may lead to subtherapeutic concentrations in tissues that diminishes efficacy. On the other hand, if clearance is impaired, drugs may accumulate and produce toxicity.

Like other xenobiotics, drugs are generally quite hydrophobic and undergo biotransformation to polar products following the concerted actions of several families of drug-metabolizing enzymes; this process enhances clearance. In phase I metabolism a functional group is introduced into the parent molecule that renders the drug more polar. However, the aqueous solubility of many phase I metabolites may be inadequate for efficient elimination. In phase II biotransformation reactions these phase I metabolites of intermediate polarity as well as parent drug

undergo conjugation with highly polar endogenous molecules. This markedly increases aqueous solubility and the resultant drug conjugates are eliminated more readily in urine or feces. Thus, phase II biotransformation pathways usually mediate the terminal phase of the removal of drugs and other foreign compounds from the body.

Enzymes of Phase II Biotransformation

There are several classes of phase II biotransformation enzymes that catalyze drug conjugation reactions (Table 6B–1 lists these enzymes and those that mediate the formation of essential cofactors). Among the most important are the UDP-glucuronosyltransferases (UGTs), sulfotransferases (SULTs), N-acetyltransferases (NATs), and glutathione S-transferases (GSTs). Together these enzymes contribute to the majority of clearance pathways that exist for most drugs. Additional phase II enzymes include thiopurine S-methyltransferase (TPMT) and the acyl-CoA synthetase medium-chain family members that act in conjunction with acyl-CoA:amino acid N-acyltransferases to generate amino acid conjugates. While not widely involved in drug biotransformation, some of these enzymes have roles in the clearance of a limited number of therapeutic agents. Finally, there is a group of enzymes such as

TABLE 6B–1 **Genes involved in phase II biotransformation: chromosomal locations, enzyme commission numbers, and typical substrates.**

	Chromosomal Location	Enzyme Commission Number	Typical Substrates
Glucuronidation enzymes			
UGT1A	2q37	EC 2.4.1.17	Irinotecan (SN-38 active metabolite)
UGT2A	4q13		Hydroxysteroids
UGT2B	4q13		NSAIDs, mycophenolate
Sulfonation enzymes			
SULT1	16p11	EC 2.8.2	Phenols, thyroid hormone, minoxidil
SULT2	19q13		Steroids
SULT4	22q13		None
Acetylation enzymes			
NAT1	8p22	EC 2.3.1.5	p-Aminobenzoylglutamate
NAT2	8p22		Isoniazid, hydralazine
Glutathione conjugation enzymes			
GSTA	6p12	EC 2.5.1.18	Busulfan, chlorambucil
GSTM	1p13		Cytotoxic drugs
GSTP	11q13		Oxaliplatin
GSTS	4q22		Prostaglandin H_2
GSTZ	14q24		Fluoroacetate
GSTO	10q25		Dehydroascorbate
GSTT	22q11		p-Nitrobenzyl chloride, propylene oxide
Amino acid conjugation enzymes			
Acyl-CoA synthetase medium-chain family member 2B	16p12	EC 6.2.1.2	Valproic acid
AcylCoA:amino acid N-acyltransferase	11q12	EC 2.3.1	
Methylation enzymes			
TPMT	6p22.3	EC 2.1.1.67	Azathioprine
COMT	22q11	EC 2.1.1.6	L-Dopa
Enzymes that regulate the production of phase II enzyme cofactors or mediate further biotransformation of conjugates			
UDP-glucose pyrophosphorylase	2p14	EC 2.7.7.9	
UDP-glucose dehydrogenase	4p15	EC 1.1.1.22	
3′-Phosphoadenosine 5′-phosphosulfate synthase	4q24 (PAPS-1)	EC 2.7.1.25	
	10q24 (PAPS-2)		
γ-Glutamylcysteine synthetase	20q11	EC 6.3.2.2	
Glutathione synthetase	20q11	EC 6.3.2.3	
GSH reductase	8p21	EC 1.8.1.7	
Cysteine conjugate β-lyase	9q34	EC 4.4.1.13	
Methionine adenosyltransferase	10q22 (MAT1A)	EC 2.5.1.6	
	2p11 (MAT2A), 5q34 (MAT2B)		

Sources: Refs.[3,23,28,33,56,58]

Website for alleles: www.ugtalleles.ulaval.ca; www.louisville.edu/medschool/pharmacology/NAT.html.

Website for GeneCards: www.genecards.org.

catechol *O*-methyltransferase (COMT) and other methyltransferases that are functionally important in the clearance of neurotransmitters or other molecules of endogenous importance. Some studies have suggested that these enzymes participate in drug clearance but the supportive clinical evidence that currently exists is inconclusive.

Biotransformation enzymes are frequently involved in pharmacokinetic drug–drug interactions because they accommodate a wide range of substrates that can compete for elimination. In addition, certain allelic variants of genes that encode biotransformation enzymes may be dysfunctional. In both of these situations drug clearance is impaired, which may lead to drug accumulation and may precipitate toxicity. Phase I enzymes typified by the cytochromes P450s (CYPs) usually catalyze the rate-limiting steps in the overall process of drug biotransformation and elimination; CYP-mediated pharmacokinetic drug–drug interactions and defective CYP gene variants are relatively common. By comparison, there are relatively few instances in which pharmacokinetic interactions and phase II pharmacogenetics affect drug clearance. This is due in part to the great reserve capacity for phase II elimination, such that drug interactions and defects in specific phase II genes may be compensated by alternate biotransformation pathways. However, there are several important examples in which the pharmacogenetics of phase II enzymes strongly influences the clearance and toxicity of specific drugs in patients.

Significance of Phase II Gene Polymorphisms

Much of the research to date on the significance of phase II gene polymorphisms has centered around the protective actions of these enzymes against toxic and reactive intermediates generated from carcinogens and aromatic amines. Thus, UGTs, SULTs, NATs, and GSTs are particularly important in the conjugation of reactive intermediates that are generated from such chemicals by the actions of phase I enzymes. Phase II biotransformation usually minimizes the toxicity of reactive species by catalyzing their conversion to stable products that are more hydrophilic and readily eliminated, for example, CYPs activate polyaromatic hydrocarbons such as benzo(*a*)pyrene to reactive epoxide intermediates that are able to bind tightly to DNA; phase II biotransformation converts these species to conjugates that are less toxic.

Drug therapy is usually initiated using a limited range of dosage regimen, with subsequent dose optimization undertaken empirically, based on observed toxicity and efficacy in individuals (although the latter may be difficult to measure). However, the desired therapeutic effects do not occur uniformly in all patients when drugs are administered according to standard regimen; many subjects are either underdosed or overdosed. Pharmacogenetic approaches, in which patient-specific factors, such as the presence of defective phase II alleles that may impact on drug pharmacokinetics, could be used to direct drug dosage and provide opportunities to tailor therapy to individuals. This chapter will focus on well-defined and emerging examples of the impact of allelic variation in genes that encode phase II drug-metabolizing enzymes that influence the clinical efficacy and safety of drugs. These factors are of greatest impact when they mediate a critical pathway of elimination of a drug or metabolite that has a major toxicity profile and for which the alternate pathways of elimination are limited.

IMPORTANT ENZYMES THAT MEDIATE PHASE II DRUG BIOTRANSFORMATION IN MAN

UGTs

Drug Glucuronidation by UGT Enzymes

UGT enzymes (EC 2.4.1.17) catalyze the glucuronidation of polar aglycones that contain phenolic, alcoholic, or carboxylic oxygen atoms and a limited number of nitrogen- and sulfur-containing molecules. The enzymes are active on a diverse range of drugs and xenobiotic substrates, as well as endobiotics such as bilirubin, steroid, and thyroid hormones. UGT activity is supported by the cofactor UDP-glucuronic acid (uridine-5′-diphospho-α-D-glucuronic acid) that is synthesized from glucose-1-phosphate and uridine triphosphate via the sequential actions of UDP-glucose pyrophosphorylase (EC 2.7.7.9) and UDP-glucose dehydrogenase (EC 1.1.1.22). Nucleophilic attack of the aglycone substrate on UDP-glucuronic acid occurs with inversion of configuration and produces the corresponding β-glucuronides. Kinetic studies have suggested that UGTs operate via an S_N2-like mechanism involving base catalysis.[1] Thus, within the active center of the UGT enzyme His and Asp residues facilitate the deprotonation or polarization of a suitable substituent in an aglycone substrate, which facilitates nucleophilic attack at C-1 of glucuronic acid. Lone electron pairs on tertiary amine substrates are sufficiently nucleophilic to generate glucuronides without the requirement for bond polarization.

UGTs are integral proteins of the endoplasmic reticulum and membrane lipid composition is a critical determinant of rates of xenobiotic glucuronidation. UGTs are oriented toward the lumen of the endoplasmic reticulum with a short C-terminal tail facing the cytoplasmic side. It has been proposed that dimerization of different UGT monomers may lead to the creation of a quasi–substrate recognition site that augments the metabolic capacity and substrate specificity of UGTs beyond that seen with the monomers.[2]

Multiplicity of the Human UGT System

Major human drug-metabolizing UGTs are encoded by three gene subfamilies: *UGT1A*, *UGT2A*, and *UGT2B*. The *UGT2B* subfamily, which comprises several genes, and the *UGT2A1* gene are located on chromosome 4. In contrast, the entire *UGT1* family is derived from a single locus of 210 kilobase (kb) on chromosome 2 (2q37). *UGT1A* genes are composed of 5 exons, with 1 of 13 alternate exons comprising exon 1 and exons 2–5 being common to all UGT1As.

A number of human UGTs have been identified to date: UGT1A1, 1A3–1A10, 2A1, 2A2 (which may be an isoform of UGT2A1), 2B4, 2B7, 2B10, 2B11, 2B15, 2B17, and 2B28.[3] All but UGT1A7, 1A8, and 1A10 are expressed in liver, while those three enzymes are expressed exclusively in the gastrointestinal tract, and UGT2A1 is expressed in the nasal epithelium where it is involved in the termination of signaling by odorant molecules.[3] UGTs 1A1, 1A3, 1A4, 1A6, 1A9, 2B7, and 2B15 contribute to hepatic drug elimination, but UGT2B7 is functionally the most important enzyme in drug glucuronidation because it accommodates a diverse range of substrates, including opioids, nonsteroidal anti-inflammatory drugs (NSAIDs), analgesics, antiepileptic agents, oncology agents, antiretrovirals, and hypolipidemic agents. UGTs 1A7, 1A8, and 1A10 may contribute to local drug biotransformation in the gastrointestinal tract.

To date many polymorphisms have been described for both UGT1 and UGT2B genes, but how UGT pharmacogenetics affects biotransformation and clearance has been defined for only a limited number of drugs (Table 6B–2). Compared with phase I CYPs there are few UGT-selective substrates that represent major toxicity concerns. Despite this general point, there remain several drugs for which defective UGT alleles are important determinants of clinical toxicity.

Role of UGT1A1 in Clearance of Bilirubin and Irinotecan

UGT1A1 has a major role in the glucuronidation of the heme degradation product bilirubin. Defects in the UGT1A1 gene impair bilirubin conjugation, leading to hyperbilirubinemias of varying severity.[4] Three levels of UGT1A1 deficiency have been identified. Crigler–Najjar syndrome type 1 is most severe and is characterized by potentially lethal hyperbilirubinemia (serum bilirubin >0.34 mM) that occurs in the absence of hemolysis or other liver disease. Crigler–Najjar syndrome type 2 is an intermediate form of hyperbilirubinemia (serum bilirubin ~0.12–0.34 mM) characterized by residual UGT1A1 activity and Gilbert syndrome is the mildest form in which serum bilirubin levels fluctuate up to 0.085 mM. In Caucasian, African American, and South Asian populations the exon sequences of the UGT1A1 gene are normal but the TATAA element in the 5′-upstream region exhibits a variable number of tandem repeat polymorphism. Thus, the UGT1A1*28 promoter variant carries the sequence A(TA)$_7$TAA in place of the wild-type A(TA)$_6$TAA (Figure 6B–1), which decreases the transcription rate of the UGT1A1 gene and results in defective bilirubin glucuronidation. Around 10% of Caucasians are homozygous and about 40% are heterozygous for the UGT1A1*28 variant. In contrast, a homozygous nonsynonymous polymorphism that encodes the Gly71Arg amino acid replacement (the *6 variant) is the common cause of the Gilbert phenotype in East Asian subjects (allele frequency ~20%).[5] Although these common UGT1A1 variants occur with differing frequency in different ethnic groups, additional UGT1A1 variants have also been detected by resequencing the UGT1A1 gene in subjects with Crigler–Najjar syndrome.

The conjugation and elimination of drugs may also be affected in individuals who carry UGT1A1 polymorphisms (Table 6B–1). Irinotecan (CPT-11 or (S)-4,11-diethyl-3,4,12,14-tetrahydro-4-hydroxy-3,14-dioxo-1H-pyrano(3′,4′:6,7)-indolizino(1,2-b) quinolin-9-yl-(1,4′-bipiperidine)-1′-carboxylate) is a topoisomerase II inhibitor that is the first-line treatment for metastatic

TABLE 6B–2 Pharmacogenetics of phase II biotransformation enzymes: impact on drug clearance and therapeutic outcomes.

Phase II Enzyme	Drug	In Vivo Consequences	References
UGT1A1	Irinotecan	Neutropenia, diarrhea	5
	Tranilast	Hyperbilirubinemia	12
UGT1A8	Mycophenolate mofetil	Diarrhea	20
UGT2B7	Mycophenolate	Clearance	19
	Diclofenac	Hepatotoxicity	18
SULT1A1	Tamoxifen	Efficacy	25
NAT2	Isoniazid	Neurotoxicity	31
	Sulfasalazine	Hemolytic anemia	32
GSTA	Busulfan	Altered clearance	46
	Cyclophosphamide	Increased survival	53
GSTM	Platinum	Toxicity	37
	Busulfan	Veno-occlusive disease	48
GSTP	Platinum	Survival	37
	Busulfan	Altered clearance	46
	Cyclophosphamide	Efficacy	52
	Adriamycin	Efficacy	52
TPMT	Azathioprine	Myelosuppression	58

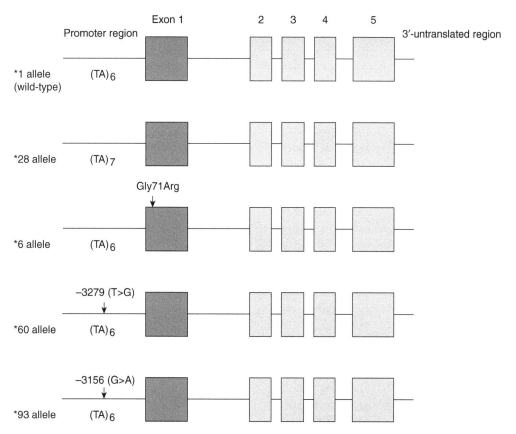

FIGURE 6B–1 Gene structure of UGT1A1 and major variants associated with impaired glucuronidation of SN-38, the pharmacologically active metabolite of irinotecan. The gene contains five exons, an important promoter sequence in the 5′-untranslated region, and intronic and 3′-untranslated regions. The *28, *60, and *93 alleles carry polymorphisms in the TATAA box or adjacent regulatory sequences, whereas the *6 allele contains a polymorphism in exon 1 that leads to the Gly71Arg amino acid substitution. (The gene structure is not drawn to scale.)

colorectal cancer. It is a prodrug that is converted by carboxylesterases to the active metabolite SN-38 (7-ethyl-10-hydroxycamptothecin; Figure 6B–2).[5] SN-38 undergoes UGT1A1-mediated glucuronidation to 10-O-glucuronyl-SN-38 (SN-38G), which limits the duration of action of the drug. Thus, UGT1A1 activity is a major factor that influences the extent of SN-38G formation and irinotecan toxicity. Indeed, the plasma ratio of SN-38G:SN-38 has been related to the incidence of neutropenia and diarrhea. In individuals with defective glucuronidation SN-38 accumulates and elicits neutropenia and diarrhea. Severe grade diarrhea induced by irinotecan does not respond to loperamide treatment and may necessitate hospitalization, as well as irinotecan

dose interruption. Mortality from irinotecan therapy is significant in up to 5% of patients who receive single-agent therapy, but some improvements have been obtained by including 5-fluorouracil and leucovorin in a combination approach.

A large number of clinical studies have shown that the *UGT1A1*28* allele confers susceptibility to irinotecan toxicity, which has led the US FDA to recommend a dose reduction for irinotecan in individuals who are homozygous for this variant (http://www.fda.gov/medwatch/SAFETY/2005/Jun_PI/Camptosar_PI.pdf).[6] This would decrease toxicity in patients who have a major glucuronidation defect, but specific guidelines on the actual dose reduction that should be applied or whether

FIGURE 6B–2 Biotransformation of irinotecan to SN-38 and SN-38 glucuronide mediated by carboxylesterases and UGTs, respectively.

heterozygotes should also receive a dose reduction are currently lacking.[5] Other *UGT1A1* allelic variants that impair SN-38 glucuronidation are more prevalent in other populations and may also necessitate irinotecan dose adjustments. In a dose-escalation study Satoh et al.[7] administered irinotecan (75, 100, or 150 mg/m²) to individuals of differing genotype: homozygous wild-type (*1/*1), heterozygous variants (*1/*6 or *1/*28), or homozygous variants (*6/*6, *28/*28, or *6/*28). In patients who progressed to the highest dose, the incidence of dose-limiting toxicities was greatest in those carrying the homozygous variant genotype. Because there is a similar incidence of the *UGT1A1*6* and *28* variants in East Asians (allele frequencies 10–25%) testing for both alleles has been approved in Japan for use in current oncology practice.[5]

The association between *UGT1A1* gene defects and impaired conjugation of both bilirubin and SN-38 suggests that hyperbilirubinemia might be a predictor of irinotecan toxicity. However, there is increasing evidence that the relationship between UGT1A1 gene function and irinotecan toxicity may be more complex. Indeed, close associations between the *UGT1A1*28* polymorphism and predisposition to irinotecan toxicity have been observed in some but not all studies. In part this may be due to the apparent capacity of other UGTs to detoxify SN-38. Thus, the affinities of the hepatic UGT1A6 and extrahepatic UGT1A7 for SN-38 are several-fold greater than that of UGT1A1.[8,9] These UGTs may also contribute to SN-38 glucuronidation and pharmacogenetic variation in UGT1A6/1A7 may influence irinotecan safety in patients.

The first haplotype analysis of a regulatory module of ~600 base pair (bp) in the *UGT1A1* 5′-flanking region that contained the *UGT1A1*28* polymorphism was conducted by Innocenti et al.[10] using samples from 55 Caucasians and 37 African Americans. This region was selected because it is implicated in basal regulation of the *UGT1A1* gene and because it was known to be highly polymorphic. Close linkages between several polymorphisms were identified, including −3279T > G (*60) and −3156G > A (*93) as well as A(TA)$_7$TA (*28), especially in Caucasians; the frequencies of inferred haplotypes varied somewhat between ethnic groups.[10,11] However, of the most common haplotypes in Caucasians and African Americans, the only major difference was in the incidence of the *60 polymorphism. Subsequently, another haplotype analysis in 195 Japanese subjects sequenced all 5 exons, the promoter and enhancer regions, and all flanking introns. Four haplotype groups based on the *1, *60, *6, and *28 alleles were identified that had similar frequencies.[11] Interestingly, all of these haplotypes were associated with a significant decrease in the serum SN-38G/SN-38 concentration ratio, which provides evidence that multiple combinations of polymorphisms in the *UGT1A1* gene are associated with decreased capacity to inactivate SN-38 by glucuronidation.

UGT Pharmacogenetics and the Incidence of Drug-Induced Hyperbilirubinemia

Several studies suggest that individuals with Gilbert syndrome who carry *UGT1A1* polymorphisms may be susceptible to drug-induced

hyperbilirubinemias. Thus, tranilast-mediated hyperbilirubinemia was more prevalent in carriers of *UGT1A1*28*[12] and plasma concentrations of the HIV-protease inhibitor atazanavir correlated directly with plasma bilirubin concentrations.[13] Indeed, there was a higher incidence of jaundice in patients who received atazanavir or indinavir and who were homozygous for *UGT1A1*28*.[14] Although atazanavir does not undergo extensive glucuronidation, it has been found to inhibit UGTs 1A1, 1A3, and 1A4.[15] This may account for clinical findings in which atazanavir-mediated inhibition of hepatic UGT activity increased serum bilirubin levels in most subjects. This was especially pronounced in the one third of individuals who carried variant *UGT1A* alleles that included *UGT1A1*28*, *UGT1A7*12* and *UGT1A7*2*, and the *UGT1A3-66C* promoter polymorphism that is found in several variant alleles of the *UGT1A3* gene.[16] Indeed, homozygous combinations of *UGT1A1*28* and one of the other single nucleotide polymorphisms significantly increased the susceptibility to drug-induced hyperbilirubinemia. From this study it was suggested that a haplotype spanning three *UGT1A* genes could predispose to atazanavir-mediated hyperbilirubinemia, and may therefore constitute a pharmacogenomic risk factor for therapy with the drug.[16] Taken together, it is emerging that potent UGT1A inhibitors may impair bilirubin glucuronidation that leads to hyperbilirubinemia. The clinical consequences seem to be most pronounced in carriers of defective *UGT1A1* alleles in whom glucuronidation capacity is already compromised. It will now be of interest to evaluate whether other HIV-protease inhibitors carry a similar risk of drug-induced hyperbilirubinemia in patients. This would provide insight into whether genotyping for *UGT1A1*28* or other *UGT1A* gene variants before initiation of antiretroviral therapy might assist in identifying HIV-infected individuals who are at risk from drug-induced jaundice.

Clinical Significance of UGT2B7 Polymorphisms

UGT2B7 is an important catalyst in the glucuronidation of a wide range of drug substrates, including NSAIDs (Table 6B–2). The common C802T polymorphism that encodes the His268Tyr amino acid substitution (the *UGT2B7*2* allele) is present in around one third of the Caucasian population; the incidence is lower in Asians.[17] The NSAID diclofenac undergoes extensive glucuronidation mediated by UGT2B7 and elicits idiosyncratic hepatotoxicity that causes significant mortality if it progresses to jaundice. Low-activity variants of *UGT2B7* appear to predispose to an increased risk of hepatotoxicity from reactive diclofenac metabolites.[18] This finding suggests that UGT2B7 plays an important protective role by mediating the conjugation and clearance of diclofenac that might otherwise undergo biotransformation to hepatotoxic reactive metabolites.

Mycophenolate mofetil is an immunosuppressive drug that prevents the rejection of transplanted organs and stem cells. The drug is an ester that undergoes esterase-mediated hydrolysis to the active metabolite mycophenolate, which is a substrate for several UGTs. In recent studies pediatric renal transplant patients who carried the *UGT2B7*2* variant (either homozygotes or heterozygotes) were found to clear mycophenolate less efficiently than wild-type subjects.[19] In that study a population pharmacokinetic model was developed that described mycophenolate dosage in individuals in terms of patient body weight, concomitant medication, and *UGT2B7* genotype.

UGT genotype may be an important determinant of gastrointestinal side effects due to mycophenolate mofetil. Diarrhea is a significant adverse effect of the drug that is reportedly less likely in patients who carry the *UGT1A8*2* variant allele.[20] The mechanism underlying this adverse effect is currently unclear but some studies suggest that it may be due to the acyl glucuronide of the drug. Because *UGT1A8* is expressed in the gastrointestinal tract, it is feasible that a decrease in the local formation of the acyl glucuronide in carriers of the low-activity allele could mediate improved tolerance to the drug. However, there are several other considerations that may be pertinent. First, mycophenolate also generates a phenol glucuronide that is inactive so that the relative formation of the acyl and phenolic glucuronides may influence the incidence of toxicity. Second, other UGTs such as UGT2B7 contribute to mycophenolate clearance and, third, ATP-binding cassette efflux transporters are important determinants of mycophenolate elimination in bile, which would deliver mycophenolate conjugates to the gastrointestinal tract. It is likely that the interplay of these factors may ultimately be found to mediate the toxicity and elimination of mycophenolate.

SULTs

Sulfonylation of Drugs by SULT Enzymes

Cytosolic SULTs (EC 2.8.2) catalyze the transfer of the sulfonyl group of 3′-phosphoadenosine 5′-phosphosulfate (PAPS) to hydroxyl, sulfhydryl, amino, or *N*-oxide substituents in suitable endobiotics and xenobiotics and generates sulfate conjugates that are readily excreted in urine. The cofactor PAPS is itself synthesized from ATP and inorganic sulfate by the bifunctional 3′-phosphoadenosine 5′-phosphosulfate synthase (PAPSS; EC 2.7.1.25) that exists as two isoforms—PAPSS-1 and PAPSS-2—that are abundant in brain and liver, respectively. Sulfation is a lower-capacity pathway than glucuronidation. Thus, many drugs and other xenobiotics are substrates for both SULTs and UGTs, but UGT-dependent pathways usually predominate.

There are two broad classes of SULTs: the membrane-bound SULTs that are located in the Golgi apparatus and that mediate the sulfonation of proteins, lipids, and glycosaminoglycans, and the cytosolic SULTs that mediate the sulfonation of drugs, other xenobiotics, and endogenous substrates that include steroids, bile acids, and neurotransmitters. Kinetic studies have suggested that sulfonation follows an ordered Bi Bi mechanism via an S_N2 nucleophilic substitution reaction in which a lone pair of electrons on the substrate oxygen attacks the activated sulfur atom in PAPS with displacement of the phosphate group.[21] Most of the cytosolic SULTs appear to exist as dimers; these may be either homodimers or heterodimers.

Multiplicity of the Human SULT System

To date, three gene families have been identified in humans: *SULT1* (located on chromosome 16), *SULT2* (chromosome 19),

and *SULT4* (chromosome 22). These families contain multiple genes that encode 13 distinct enzymes: SULT1—A1, A2, A3, A4, B1, C2, C4, and E1; SULT2—A1 and B1, and SULT4A1.[22] Both SULT2B1 and SULT4A1 encode a pair of isoforms— SULT2B1-v1 and SULT2B1-v2—that differ only in their N-terminal sequences as a result of either alternate promoter usage or alternate mRNA splicing,[22] while the SULT4A1-v1 and SULT4A1-v2 isoforms differ in their C-terminal amino acid sequences. The human SULTs that mediate the sulfonylation of endobiotics and xenobiotics containing phenolic and alcoholic hydroxyl groups belong to families 1 and 2, while the function of human SULT4A1 is currently unknown.

Quantitatively, SULT1A1 is the major SULT1A expressed in adult liver and has also been detected in numerous extrahepatic tissues. By contrast, SULT1A3 is highly expressed in extrahepatic tissues but only at low level in liver. The tissue distribution and physiological function of SULT1A2 is not well understood because although the mRNA has been detected in numerous tissues, the protein has not.[22] SULT1B1 is the principal SULT active on thyroid hormone and is detectable in cytosolic fractions from liver, small intestine, and colon, while SULT1E1 immunoreactive protein and 17β-estradiol sulfonylation is present in the soluble fraction of human liver and jejunum. SULTs 2A1, 2B1, and 2B1-v2 have been variously detected in liver and/ or hormone-responsive extrahepatic tissues.[22]

At the nucleotide level *SULT1A1* and *SULT1A2* are 93% similar, and are about 60% related to *SULT1A3*. These differences are due primarily to differences in the nucleotide sequences of the 5′-flanking and intronic regions because the exon sequences in the three genes are >90% identical. SULT1A1 contains 295 amino acids and is active toward the substrates *p*-nitrophenol and minoxidil (Table 6B–1). Together SULT1A1 and SULT1A3 are responsible for the metabolism of most phenols,[23] but the related SULT1A2 is less active in the sulfonation of such substrates. SULT1A3 also sulfonates catecholamines such as dopamine.[23]

Human SULT Gene Polymorphisms

The most polymorphic genes appear to be *SULT1A1* and *SULT1A2*, with the latter exhibiting more than 35 variants.[23,24] SULT1A1 activity varies considerably between individuals but few studies have assessed how SULTs influence drug biotransformation and clearance or how this is affected by SULT pharmacogenetics. Four common single nucleotide polymorphisms that alter transcription have been identified within a 400 bp stretch of the 5′-regulatory region of the *SULT1A1* gene. With respect to SULT1A1, the most common polymorphisms give rise to the variants SULT1A1*2 (Arg213His) and SULT1A1*3 (Met223Val). Allele frequencies vary between ethnic populations: in Caucasians, *SULT1A1*1* (frequency 66%) is the most common allele, followed by *SULT1A1*2* (33%) and *SULT1A1*3* (1%) but in Chinese subjects *SULT1A1*1* is the predominant allele (91%) and *SULT1A1*2* and *SULT1A1*3* alleles are relatively rare (8% and <1%, respectively). In African Americans, both *SULT1A1*2* and *SULT1A1*3* alleles are common (29% and 23%, respectively).[24]

Human SULT1A1 catalyzes the sulfonylation of 4-hydroxytamoxifen, which is an important active metabolite of the oncology drug tamoxifen that is used in the treatment of breast cancer patients. From in vitro studies the Arg213His substitution in SULT1A1*2 alters activity, possibly by altering the stability of the enzyme.[25] A strong association between survival and the presence of the *SULT1A1*1* allele has been described in breast cancer patients who received tamoxifen (Table 6B–2). Although not completely understood, sulfonylated 4-hydroxytamoxifen potently activated programmed cell death in breast tumor cell lines.[25] The rapid sulfonylation of active tamoxifen metabolites could stimulate tumor cell apoptosis and improve survival in individuals with the high-activity wild-type *SULT1A1* alleles. Conversely, individuals who are less competent in tamoxifen sulfonylation may also be less responsive to the drug because formation of the proapoptotic metabolite is diminished.

NATs

Acetylation of Xenobiotic Substrates by NAT Enzymes

Cytosolic NATs (EC 2.3.1.5) utilize the cofactor acetyl coenzyme A to acetylate drugs and xenobiotics that contain amino and hydrazine substituents to the corresponding amides and hydrazides, respectively. There are two NATs—NAT1 and NAT2—that mediate not only the *N*-acetylation but also the *O*-acetylation of suitable substrates. While NAT1 is widely expressed in most human tissues, NAT2 exhibits a more restricted distribution in liver, small intestine, and colon.

Both NATs possess a functional Cys–His–Asp catalytic triad.[26] In a ping-pong Bi Bi reaction mechanism the catalytic Cys68 is first acetylated by acetyl coenzyme A and then the acetyl group is transferred to the substrate. The active center of NAT1 is smaller than that of NAT2, which suggests that a more limited range of substrates is accommodated by the enzyme; the active site residues Phe125, Tyr127, and Arg129 are apparently important in substrate selectivity.[27] Substrates of NAT1 include *p*-aminobenzoic acid, *p*-aminosalicylic acid, and the folate metabolite *p*-aminobenzoylglutamate.[26,27] A wide range of drug substrates for NAT2 has been described, including sulfamethazine, procainamide, dapsone, and isoniazid, as well as many xenobiotic arylamines.

Pharmacogenetic Variation in Human NAT Genes

The *NAT1* and *NAT2* genes span 170 kb on chromosome 8 and encode 290 amino acid polypeptides that are 87% identical and that differ by only 55 amino acids. Both genes are highly polymorphic and the variant alleles occur with varying incidence in different ethnic populations. A number of *NAT2* variants, including the *5, *6, *7, *10, *14, and *17 alleles, encode defective NAT2 allozymes, whereas the *4 and *18 alleles encode active enzymes.[28]

By comparison with the *NAT2* genes, only a small number of *NAT1* variants alter phenotype[29,30] and single nucleotide polymorphisms in the NAT1 coding region are relatively uncommon. The relationship between genotype and phenotype in NAT1 is not well defined and appears to be influenced by additional factors other than exon sequences. The *4 variant is also designated as wild-type for NAT1 and the *10 and *11 alleles give rise to a "rapid" acetylator phenotype. As is the case with genes encoding other drug-metabolizing enzymes the frequency of polymorphisms in NAT1 and NAT2 varies between ethnic groups.

The "acetylation polymorphism" is probably the best established example of a genetic defect in drug biotransformation that precipitates drug toxicity. This polymorphism was initially recognized in tuberculous patients who received the hydrazine drug isoniazid that is eliminated principally by acetylation. "Rapid acetylators" were competent in isoniazid acetylation, whereas the "slow acetylators" cleared drug slowly, which led to its accumulation in serum.[31] Decreased rates of isoniazid acetylation in slow metabolizers promoted the formation of neurotoxic metabolites (Table 6B–2); this pathway is minor in rapid acetylators, but becomes more important when acetylation is deficient. In addition, hepatotoxicity is increased in slow acetylators with differences between populations due to different frequency of alleic variants (Caucasians vs. Asians). Drugs whose elimination cosegregates with the acetylation polymorphism are usually NAT2 substrates. Indeed, similar deficiencies in the clearance of certain alternate NAT2 drug substrates in slow acetylators also increase the likelihood of toxicity over that experienced by carriers of wild-type NAT2. For example, the incidence of systemic lupus erythematosus is increased in slow acetylators who received hydralazine or procainamide, and hemolytic anemia and inflammatory bowel disease were more frequent in slow acetylators who received sulfasalazine (Table 6B–2).[32]

Most of the information on the function of NAT2 allozymes encoded by allelic variants has been derived in heterologous cell-based expression systems. The approach has been to sequence *NAT2* gene exons in DNA from slow acetylators and identify new polymorphisms. Engineering and expression of variant *NAT2* cDNAs in heterologous cell systems has then enabled their functional characterization. Several NAT2 allozymes have diminished activity and/or expression as a result of decreased protein stability. However, there is little information regarding how the variant allozymes characterized in this fashion influence therapy with substrate drugs because the clinical studies are lacking.

GSTs

Multiplicity of Human GST Genes

Seven cytosolic GST families that participate in xenobiotic biotransformation have been identified in man—alpha (A), mu (M), theta (T), pi (P), sigma (S), omega (O), and zeta (Z). Individual GSTs are allocated to families based on sequence and immunochemical relatedness and substrate specificity. GST enzymes (EC 2.5.1.18) within a family are at least 40% similar at the amino acid level, while GSTs from different classes are less than 30% similar. Apart from the cytosolic GSTs other GST families are found in the mitochondrion (kappa isoforms) and the endoplasmic reticulum of the cell.[33] There are at least 16 human GSTs but heterodimerization between A- and M-class GSTs gives rise to a number of composite enzymes with differing catalytic properties. Total GST activity is greatest in liver but certain isozymes are also abundant in extrahepatic organs. GSTP1 is the predominant GST in human lung and heart, and also contributes significantly to the total GST content of brain and kidney.[33] GSTP is expressed in fetal liver and decreases rapidly after birth, but expression is upregulated during preneoplastic transformation and in tumorigenesis. GSTM1 is found in many tissues but is predominant in liver and, to a lesser extent, the testis, brain, and adrenal. GSTA1 and GSTA2 are expressed at high levels in liver, intestine, kidney, adrenal gland, and testis, while GSTA3 is expressed in steroidogenic tissues. GSTT is expressed in numerous tissues, including liver, erythrocytes, lung, kidney, brain, skeletal muscle, heart, small intestine, and spleen. By immunochemical analysis intense staining for GSTZ was observed in the liver, testis, and prostate; moderate staining was observed in the brain, heart, pancreatic islets, adrenal medulla, and the epithelial lining of the gastrointestinal tract, airways, and bladder.[33]

Roles of GSTs in Conjugation of Electrophilic Chemicals

The ability of GSTs to conjugate electrophilic chemicals is central to their importance in the detoxification of highly reactive drug metabolites.[34] Thus, GSTs catalyze the initial conjugation of electrophilic substrates with the tripeptide glutathione (GSH; γ-L-glutamyl-L-cysteinylglycine; Figure 6B–3A). Using chiral substrates the conjugation of alkyl and phenethyl halides with glutathione has been shown to occur with inversion of configuration. GSTs also catalyze reduction and isomerization reactions of oxygenated fatty acid metabolites and related substrates, and may also interact physically with certain kinases to modulate intracellular signaling pathways.[33]

The essential cofactor GSH is synthesized in consecutive ATP-dependent reactions. γ-Glutamylcysteine is generated from L-glutamate and cysteine by γ-glutamylcysteine synthetase (EC 6.3.2.2), followed by addition of glycine to the C-terminus of γ-glutamylcysteine by GSH synthetase (EC 6.3.2.3). An additional enzyme GSH reductase (EC 1.8.1.7) is important in the reduction of the oxidized form (the disulfide GSSG) back to GSH. Together these enzymes regulate the intracellular availability of GSH for GSTs and other cellular functions.

GSH conjugates formed by the action of GSTs on xenobiotic substrates are converted to the corresponding cysteine conjugates by the sequential removal of glutamate and glycine. These cysteine conjugates are then metabolized further by acetylation to form the mercapturate or are cleaved to the mercaptan by cysteine conjugate β-lyase (EC 4.4.1.13). There is an additional pathway in which thiol intermediates are first methylated and then conjugated by UGTs to form thioglucuronides. Thus, the appearance of mercapturates, CH_3S-, CH_3SO-, and CH_3SO_2 metabolites in urine is indicative of the GSH-dependent formation of conjugates of drugs and other xenobiotics in vivo.

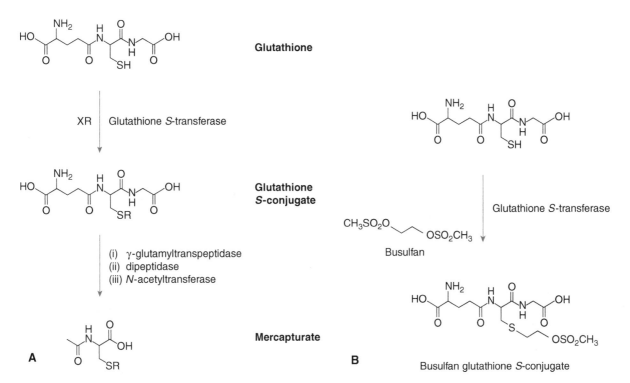

FIGURE 6B–3 **(A)** General pathway of glutathione S-transferase-mediated formation of mercapturates. In the first step the chemical substrate (XR) undergoes conjugation with glutathione, followed by further processing of the conjugate by γ-glutamyltranspeptidase, dipeptidase, and N-acetyltransferase to generate the mercapturate. **(B)** Formation of the glutathione S-conjugate of the cytotoxic drug busulfan catalyzed by glutathione S-transferase.

GST Genes and Gene Products: Polymorphisms and Allozymes

A number of polymorphic *GST* alleles have been described.[33] The *GSTP* gene is located on chromosome 11 and four allelic variants have been described to date (*GSTP1*A–D*); the wild-type form is *GSTP1*A*. *GSTP1*B* carries a single nucleotide polymorphism that encodes the amino acid substitution Ile105Val, GSTP1*C carries both the Ile105Val and Ala114Val substitutions, and the GSTP1*D allozyme carries only the Ala114Val substitution. The wild-type *GSTP1*A* exhibits a frequency of ~65–90% depending on the ethnic population. The *GSTM* gene is located on chromosome 1. The GSTM1*A enzyme is encoded by the wild-type gene, while a polymorphism in exon 7 yields the GSTM1*B variant that also retains function. However, deletion of the entire gene (*GSTM1*0*) is an important genotype in which function is abolished. Most surveyed populations have a 40–60% incidence of *GSTM1* null individuals, but this is somewhat lower in African Americans.

The *GSTA* gene is found on chromosome 6 and exhibits a number of variant alleles, including *GSTA1*B* and *GSTA2*B–*E*. GSTA is a versatile catalyst that catalyzes the GSH conjugation of the anticancer cytotoxic agents busulfan and chlorambucil, ethacrynic acid, the lipid peroxidation product 4-hydroxynonenal, and reactive diol epoxides formed from polycyclic aromatic hydrocarbons.[33] The *GSTT* gene is located on chromosome 22. The wild-type form is *GSTT1-1*, while deletion of the gene gives rise to *GSTT1* null (*GSTT1*0*) homozygotes or *GSTT1* heterozygotes (GSTT1$^{+/-}$) that have intermediate activity toward the conjugation of a range of substrates including aliphatic and aromatic halo compounds.[35] In addition to catalyzing GSH conjugation with electrophiles, GSTT1 possesses peroxidase activity toward phospholipid hydroperoxides and related intermediates. The *GSTO* gene is located on chromosome 10, with several variant alleles that enocde amino acid substitutions or deletions. GSTO supports the biotransformation of dehydroascorbate and monomethylarsonate. The *GSTZ* gene is found on chromosome 14 with four alleles having been described to date (**A–*D*). GSTZ mediates the conjugation of haloacetate and related substrates with GSH. Finally, the relatively underexplored *GSTS* gene is found on chromosome 4 and the encoded enzyme mediates the formation of prostaglandin D_2 from prostaglandin H_2.[33]

GSTs and the Conjugation of Anticancer Drugs: Clinical Significance of GST Polymorphisms

The major focus of pharmacogenetic studies to date has been on the role of GST variants in cancer risk, because defective conjugation capacity of carcinogenic chemicals has been shown to increase toxicity.[33] There have been fewer studies on how *GST* variants affect drug therapy, but several recent studies have reported relationships between the presence of variant *GST* alleles and the pharmacokinetics, safety, and efficacy of platinum drugs, busulfan, and other anticancer cytotoxic agents.

A. Platinum Drugs

Platinum drugs are among the most active and widely used agents in the treatment of a range of cancers, but toxicity is common.

Identification of genetic markers that could be used to screen patients before treatment would be beneficial in the optimization of therapy. Several aspects of platinum therapy have been correlated with *GST* gene polymorphisms in patients. Although nonenzymatic complexation of platinum by GSH occurs, GSTP enhances the rate of platinum conjugation and elimination. Indeed, the overexpression of GSTP in tumor cells could contribute to the development of drug resistance by enhancing the elimination of platinum.[36] However, from clinical studies, the GSTP1 Ile105Val polymorphism has been strongly associated with progression-free survival in ovarian cancer patients who have been treated with platinum (Table 6B–2).[37] Similarly, expression of this variant was associated with improved clinical outcomes in colorectal cancer patients who received oxaliplatin.[38]

Up to 20% of patients require a dose reduction after the cumulative dose of oxaliplatin reaches 800 mg/m^2.[39] Patients with gastrointestinal cancers who carry active *GSTP* alleles had a lower risk of developing oxaliplatin-induced cumulative neuropathy that is usually observed within 6 months of the commencement of treatment.[40] There has been controversy whether homozygosity for GSTP1 Ile105Val influences the incidence of cisplatin-related ototoxicity.[41] In patients who received the *fol*inic acid–*f*luorouracil–*ox*aliplatin (FOLFOX) regimen, homozygous carriers of the *GSTP1*B* variant were more susceptible than carriers of the wild-type allele to grade 3 neurotoxicity.[42] These findings suggest that impaired activity of GSTP1 variant allozymes decreases the clearance of platinum, which may increase toxicity. Other GSTs may also contribute to the outcome of platinum therapy. For example, survival was prolonged in patients who were homozygous for the *GSTA1-69T* variant compared with those who were homozygous for the wild-type allele (*GSTA1-69C*), although a potential mechanism to account for this has not yet been provided.[37] The toxicities of thrombocytopenia, anemia, and neuropathy were also less frequent among platinum-treated patients who carried *GSTM1* null genotypes.[37] These studies implicate several *GST* polymorphisms in clinical outcomes with platinum drugs. However, it is now important that the roles of multiple GSTs in platinum efficacy and toxicity should be clarified because not all clinical observations to date may be attributed to altered drug clearance. Such information might facilitate the rational design of dosage regimen based on *GST* genotype.

B. Busulfan

High-dose busulfan not only is used for myeloablation prior to hematopoietic stem cell transplantation but also elicits a range of serious toxicities, such as hepatic veno-occlusive disease that is associated with a significant rate of mortality. On the other hand, busulfan underexposure increases the risk of graft rejection.[43] After oral administration, large interindividual differences in busulfan AUC (the area under the busulfan serum concentration vs. time curve) of up to 10-fold have been reported.[43,44] Thus, there are particular difficulties in tailoring busulfan dosage to individual patients. At present pharmacokinetic-based dose adjustment to ensure effective drug exposure and to minimize toxicity is valuable.

GST-mediated conjugation of busulfan with GSH is the major route of biotransformation and accounts for up to 80%

of an administered dose (Figure 6B–3B). It has been proposed that genotyping for *GSTA1*, *GSTP1*, and *GSTM1* in children may facilitate dose optimization and the prediction of transplant-related toxicity. How different GST alleles influence the clearance of busulfan and therapeutic outcomes has been evaluated in several recent studies, but reaching a clear consensus is presently quite difficult. Kusama et al.[45] reported that GSTA1*A wild-type homozygotes cleared busulfan more efficiently than carriers of decreased activity alleles. In contrast, a separate study of 18 children undergoing hematopoietic stem cell transplantation found that all patients who developed graft-versus-host disease carried the *GSTM1* null genotype, while *GSTA1* and *GSTP1* genotypes were independent determinants of busulfan pharmacokinetics on prolonged dosage.[46] The potential importance of *GSTM1* genotype on busulfan therapy was also supported by findings from another study. Thus, *GSTM1* null individuals had significantly higher plasma drug concentrations and lower clearance than individuals who carried active alleles and required lower cumulative doses of busulfan for effective treatment.[47] There was also a higher incidence of veno-occlusive disease in *GSTM1* null thalassemia patients.[48] Because veno-occlusive disease is associated with higher busulfan exposure,[43,44] this is consistent with an important role for GSTM in busulfan clearance. In sharp contrast, however, two other studies did not identify relationships between first-dose pharmacokinetic variability and the *GSTM1* null genotype.[49,50] In keeping with these reports no association was found between the presence of GSTP1 variants and busulfan pharmacokinetics.[47] Together it seems likely that GST enzymes influence busulfan pharmacokinetics and a number of associations with particular *GST* gene variants have been proposed, but the findings have been inconsistent and the relationships between drug exposure, toxicity, and efficacy remain unclear. However, there are many confounders in studies of this type. Patient recruitment is extremely difficult, the test populations are often highly heterogeneous and may carry multiple *GST* gene polymorphisms, and the doses of busulfan and regimen of coadministered drugs vary widely between subjects. Ideally, larger studies with greater statistical power that combine full clinical evaluation, busulfan pharmacokinetics, and GST pharmacogenetics are now required to enable firm conclusions to be reached. If this is achieved, then GST genotyping may be useful in optimizing therapy with busulfan.

C. Other Anticancer Agents

Other important cytotoxic agents that are substrates for GSTs include adriamycin, 1,3-bis-(2-chloroethyl)-1-nitrosourea, carmustine, chlorambucil, cyclophosphamide, melphalan, etoposide, doxorubicin, mitoxantrone, and thiotepa.[33] Individuals carrying the *GSTP1*B* variant were overrepresented in cases of acute myeloid leukemia induced by the combination of cytotoxic drugs and radiotherapy.[51] This suggests that *GSTP1* may be protective against toxicity induced by chemotherapy and that toxicity is enhanced in carriers of variant alleles that are functionally less competent. However, there have also been reports that *GSTP1* variants may be associated with more favorable outcomes with certain chemotherapeutic agents, such as cyclophosphamide and adriamycin.[52] Although genotyping for *GSTP1* alleles

may assist in the prediction of adverse outcomes from cytotoxic drug therapy, it is important that the relationship between drug conjugation and cytoprotection is first clarified.

The example of cyclophosphamide illustrates how an understanding of biotransformation pathways may provide insight into the importance of pharmacogenetic variation. Cyclophosphamide undergoes CYP-mediated biotransformation (by polymorphic CYPs) to both the active metabolite phosphoramide mustard and the toxic metabolite acrolein. GSTA1 participates in cyclophosphamide biotransformation by conjugating these CYP-mediated metabolites. The defective *GSTA1*B* allele is associated with increased survival in breast cancer patients who received the drug (Table 6B–2).[53] Thus, decreased conjugation of the active phosphoramide mustard metabolite by defective GSTs prolongs the duration of action of cyclophosphamide in patients. Further study of the relationships between single nucleotide polymorphisms in GSTs and the responses to other alkylating agents could be valuable adjuncts to therapy by directing dosage prior to commencement of therapy.

Other Phase II Enzymes

Amino Acid Conjugation

Carboxylic acid moieties in a number of drugs and other xenobiotics undergo phase II conjugation with the amino acids glycine, glutamine, arginine, and taurine. The first step in this route of biotransformation is activation of the xenobiotic carboxylate to the corresponding CoA derivative by mitochondrial medium-chain:CoA ligase (EC 6.2.1.2), followed by generation of the amido linkage in the phase II metabolite by acylCoA:amino acid *N*-acyltransferase (EC 2.3.1). Two xenobiotic/medium-chain fatty acid CoA ligases were initially purified from human liver mitochondria: HXM-A and HXM-B; however, these are now believed to be isoforms of the acyl-CoA synthetase medium-chain family member 2B gene (*ACSM2B*). Subsequent cloning and heterologous expression of the corresponding cDNAs demonstrated significant activity toward benzoic, propionic, hexanoic, and octanoic acids, but otherwise substrate specificity has not been completely characterized.[54] The carboxylate drugs valproic acid and salicylic acid give rise to valproyl-CoA and salicyl-CoA conjugates prior to formation of amino acid conjugates.[54] Indeed, in humans the formation of salicyl-CoA is thought to be the rate-limiting step in clearance of salicylic acid to salicylurate.[55] Other xenobiotics that have also been shown to form their respective CoA conjugates in reactions catalyzed by mitochondrial medium-chain CoA ligases include astemizole, brompheniramine, permethrin, and triflusal.[56] It is noteworthy, however, that formation of amino acid conjugates of drugs has not been extensively explored. This is no doubt due in large part to the limited capacity of this pathway compared with alternate conjugation reactions. At present there is no evidence that gene variation alters the efficiency of amino acid conjugation pathways and impacts on therapeutic outcomes.

Enzymes that Mediate Drug Methylation

The methylation of a range of drugs and other chemicals is mediated by several enzymes that utilize the common cofactor

S-adenosylmethionine (SAM). SAM is generated by methionine adenosyltransferases (MATs; EC 2.5.1.6) in a tissue-specific manner. MAT1A and MAT2B are expressed exclusively in the liver while MAT2A is present in a number of tissues.[57] The clinical consequences of MAT1A/2B deficiency are not well understood. In some individuals, MAT deficiency is apparently benign, whereas, in others, it has been associated with neurological problems attributed to hypermethioninemia and manifests as abnormalities in gray matter and low intelligence. However, the consequences of MAT deficiency for rates of drug and chemical biotransformation have not been assessed.

A. TPMT

Thiopurines are used therapeutically as immunosuppressant and anticancer agents.[58] Thiopurines are prodrugs that require activation to 6-thioguanosine 5′-monophosphate by hypoxanthine-guanine phosphoribosyltransferase to elicit cytotoxicity (Figure 6B–4A). These are further metabolized to deoxy-6-thioguanosine 5′-triphosphate that is incorporated into DNA and triggers cell cycle arrest and apoptosis. Thus, the efficacy of thiopurine drugs is dependent on biotransformation.

Biotransformation is also important in the deactivation of thiopurines. 6-Mercaptopurine (6-MP) is S-methylated to 6-methylmercaptopurine by TPMT (EC 2.1.1.67), which is the predominant inactivation pathway of thiopurines in hematopoietic cells (Figure 6B–4A). Patients with inherited TPMT deficiency are unable to deactivate 6-MP, which leads to overproduction of cytotoxic thioguanine nucleotides in blood cells at conventional doses of these medications. Interindividual variation in toxicity or efficacy may significantly impact on therapeutic outcomes because 6-MP and azathioprine have narrow therapeutic indexes. Adverse drug reactions to azathioprine or 6-MP are observed in 15–30% of patients, due partly to pharmacogenetic variation in TPMT (Table 6B–2).

TPMT is a 27-kb gene located on chromosome 6 and has 10 exons, 8 of which encode the 28-kDa protein. The wild-type allele is designated as *TPMT*1* and common polymorphisms include *TPMT*2* (G238C; Ala80Pro), *TPMT*3A* (G460A and A719G; Ala154Thr and Tyr240Cys, respectively), *TPMT*3B* (G460A; Ala154Thr), and *TPMT*3C* (A719G; Tyr240Cys) (Figure 6B–4B).[58] Enhanced degradation of TPMT proteins encoded by *TPMT*2* and *TPMT*3A* is the likely mechanism for decreased TPMT protein and catalytic activity due to inactive alleles. Several of these variants give rise to decreased TPMT activity and elicit thiopurine toxicity.[58] The incidence of these variant TPMT alleles differs between ethnic populations. The most prevalent *TPMT* variant in Caucasians is *TPMT*3A*, whereas *TPMT*3C* is the most prevalent allele in Asians and African Americans. The *TPMT*2, *3A*, and *3B* variants are not found in Chinese populations.[58]

Erythrocyte TPMT activity reflects the expression of TPMT in tissues and can be used as a convenient surrogate marker for hepatic TPMT; the frequency distribution of erythrocyte TPMT activity is trimodal.[58] In most subjects TPMT activity is high but about 10% of subjects exhibit intermediate activity, while activity is undetectable in a small number (<1%) of individuals. Subjects with very high 6-thioguanine nucleotide concentrations in erythrocytes are at risk from drug-induced myelosuppression and require major dose reductions and close monitoring for toxicity. Conversely, patients with higher TPMT activity are at risk from undertreatment when they receive standard doses of thiopurines. Together, pharmacogenetic testing for the TPMT polymorphism prior to initiation of therapy is an important adjunct to clinical practice. Determination of *TPMT* genotype can identify homozygous individuals who should not receive a thiopurine drug because they lack the TPMT enzyme, which increases the risk of potentially fatal neutropenia. However, patients with intermediate TPMT levels can safely receive thiopurines at 30–50% of the standard dose and can undergo dose escalation safely under close monitoring.

B. Catechol O-Methyltransferase

The human *COMT* (EC 2.1.1.6) gene contains six exons and is located on chromosome 22. The *COMT* gene encodes two isoforms because it has two transcription initiation sites located in exon 3; these isoforms are the membrane-bound and soluble COMTs. The membrane-bound form of COMT contains an additional 50 amino acid sequence at the N-terminus that is absent from the cytosolic isoform. Membrane-bound COMT is highly expressed in the brain, and has an important role in neurotransmitter deactivation but expression of the soluble isoform is high in peripheral tissues, especially liver and kidney and steroid-sensitive tissues such as prostate and mammary gland. Other substrates for COMT include catechol drugs such as L-dopa, and catechol estrogens that are formed in vivo from the precursors estrone and 17β-estradiol.[59]

A major *COMT* polymorphism alters codons 108 and 158 in soluble and membrane-bound COMT, respectively; this polymorphism decreases enzyme stability.[60] Familial studies indicate that about 25% of Caucasian subjects are homozygous for the low-activity (A/A) *COMT* allele, 25% are homozygous wild-type (G/G), and 50% are heterozygotes (A/G).[60] The distribution of *COMT* genotypes differs among ethnic groups. Thus, the frequency of the wild-type allele is also 25% in individuals from South Asia but is only about 10% in Northeastern Asians and Africans.[61] As is the case with TPMT, erythrocyte COMT activity has been used as a surrogate for the activity in other tissues, including kidney, lung, and lymphocytes. Early studies suggested a relationship between erythrocyte COMT activity and the methylation of the antiparkinsonian drug L-dopa to 3-O-methyldopa and the outmoded antihypertensive agent α-methyldopa to its methyl metabolite.[62] However, more recent findings argue against a major role for the *COMT* polymorphism in L-dopa pharmacokinetics and pharmacodynamics. Thus, in a study of 104 patients, the distribution of homozygous subjects carrying the low-activity COMT allele, the heterozygous intermediate-activity subjects, and those who are homozygous for the active allele was in the ratio ~1:3:1.[63] However, the *COMT* polymorphism did not give rise to significant differences in the pharmacokinetics of L-dopa or to the incidence of dyskinesia. Similar

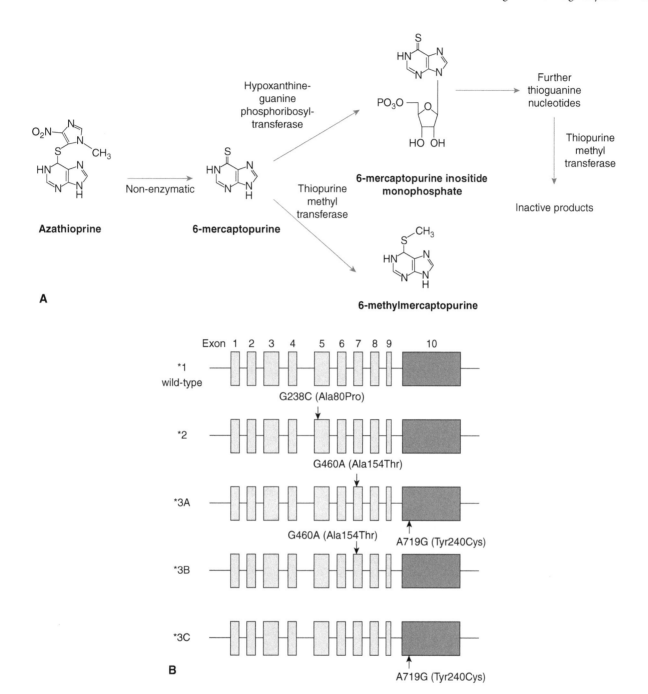

FIGURE 6B–4 (**A**) Activation of azathioprine to 6-mercaptopurine that is subsequently activated by hypoxanthine-guanine phosphoribosyltransferase to thioguanine nucleotides that are either incorporated in DNA or inactivated by TPMT. (**B**) Representation of the gene structure of TPMT. The gene contains 10 exons (not drawn to scale); the locations of the exon polymorphisms in common allelic variants are indicated.

studies have evaluated whether the *COMT* polymorphism may be a risk factor for neurological conditions as a result of impaired neurotransmitter methylation. However, again, significant associations between erythrocyte COMT activity and the incidence of such disorders have not been observed.

C. Other Methyltransferase Enzymes

Several additional enzymes are known to methylate a limited range of O-, N-, and S-containing substrates. The weight of experimental evidence to date supports roles for these enzymes in the methylation of important endobiotics but their participation in drug biotransformation is unclear. Although there is some information on the extent of polymorphism in the genes that encode these methyltransferases, whether this influences endobiotic and xenobiotic clearance is also not well understood. These enzymes are mentioned in this chapter because they resemble TPMT and COMT in a functional sense and because future studies may eventually implicate them in methylation pathways for certain drugs.

Thiol *S*-methyltransferase (EC 2.1.1.96) is a membrane-bound enzyme that catalyzes the *S*-methylation of aliphatic sulfhydryl compounds such as captopril, D-penicillamine, and 2-mercaptoethanol.[64] Histamine *N*-methyltransferase (EC 2.1.1.8) is a cytosolic SAM-dependent enzyme that catalyzes the methylation of histamine and structurally related heterocycles, but not drugs. A nonsynonymous single nucleotide polymorphism in the histamine *N*-methyltransferase gene exhibits a frequency of ~10% in Caucasians and encodes an allozyme carrying a Thr105Ile substitution; this allozyme appears to be less stable than the wild-type enzyme and undergoes rapid proteasomal degradation.[65] The phenylethanolamine *N*-methyltransferase (EC 2.1.1.28) catalyzes the *N*-methylation of the neurotransmitter norepinephrine to epinephrine. Located primarily in the adrenal medulla and central nervous system, the enzyme appears to have little involvement in drug metabolism. The cytosolic nicotinamide *N*-methyltransferase (EC 2.1.1.1) methylates pyridine-containing molecules, is highly expressed in liver, and exhibits considerable individual variation, with 25% of the population exhibiting high activity. Compared with TPMT and COMT these alternate methyltransferases have been underexplored. Greater impetus for research on these genes and the significance of their polymorphisms will be provided if their involvement in pathways of drug elimination can be established.

SUMMARY AND FUTURE PROSPECTS

This chapter has outlined the multiple pathways of drug biotransformation mediated by phase II enzymes. The multiplicity of genes that constitute each of the families of phase II biotransformation enzymes has been elaborated. Information on the gene polymorphisms and variant alleles that influence the function and expression of these genes has been provided, with emphasis on their impact on drug efficacy and toxicity. It is evident that gene variation in phase II biotransformation pathways is quite extensive but relatively underexplored compared with CYP phase I genes. This is due to difficulties in establishing the significance of such variants in therapeutic outcomes with drugs. Despite this, however, there are several important examples of phase II gene polymorphisms that are clinically important. Thus, *UGT1A1* and *TPMT* gene variants markedly influence the safety of cytotoxic drugs such as irinotecan and azathioprine. Genotyping tests that detect inactive variants of the *UGT1A1* and *TPMT* genes have been devised and approved by regulatory agencies for use in patients. Evidence is also increasing that there may be further examples of altered drug efficacy and toxicity in individuals who carry phase II gene polymorphisms. Thus, evidence is increasing for antiretroviral drug-induced hyperbilirubinemia and hepatotoxicity in individuals with diminished UGT-dependent glucuronidation capacity. Similarly, the relationships between toxicity and efficacy of busulfan and platinum drug therapy and the presence of variant GST genes are also being studied increasingly. Considered together, it is likely that we will see further examples of genotyping approaches for the analysis of phase II gene polymorphisms emerging as important adjuncts to therapy with drugs that have significant toxicity profiles.

REFERENCES

1. Patana AS, Kurkela M, Finel M, Goldman A. Mutation analysis in UGT1A9 suggests a relationship between substrate and catalytic residues in UDP-glucuronosyltransferases. *Protein Eng Des Sel.* 2008;21(9):537–543.
2. Bock KW, Köhle C. Topological aspects of oligomeric UDP-glucuronosyltransferases in endoplasmic reticulum membranes: advances and open questions. *Biochem Pharmacol.* 2009;77(9):1458–1465.
3. Mackenzie PI, Bock KW, Burchell B, et al. Nomenclature update for the mammalian UDP glycosyltransferase (UGT) gene superfamily. *Pharmacogenet Genomics.* 2005;15(10):677–685.
4. Seppen J, Bosma PJ, Goldhoorn BG, et al. Discrimination between Crigler–Najjar type I and II by expression of mutant bilirubin uridine diphosphate-glucuronosyltransferase. *J Clin Invest.* 1994;94(6):2385–2391.
5. Fujiwara Y, Minami H. An overview of the recent progress in irinotecan pharmacogenetics. *Pharmacogenomics.* 2010;11(3):391–406.
6. Hasegawa Y, Ando Y, Shimokata K. Screening for adverse reactions to irinotecan treatment using the Invader UGT1A1 Molecular Assay. *Expert Rev Mol Diagn.* 2006;6(4):527–533.
7. Satoh T, Ura T, Yamada Y, et al. A genotype-directed, dose-finding study of irinotecan in cancer patients with UGT1A1*28 and/or *6 polymorphisms. *Cancer Sci.* 2011;102(10):1868–1873.
8. Ciotti M, Basu N, Brangi M, Owens IS. Glucuronidation of 7-ethyl-10-hydroxycamptothecin (SN-38) by the human UDP-glucuronosyltransferases encoded at the UGT1 locus. *Biochem Biophys Res Commun.* 1999; 260(1):199–202.
9. Lankisch TO, Vogel A, Eilermann S, et al. Identification and characterization of a functional TATA box polymorphism of the UDP glucuronosyltransferase 1A7 gene. *Mol Pharmacol.* 2005;67(5):1732–1739.
10. Innocenti F, Grimsley C, Das S, et al. Haplotype structure of the UDP-glucuronosyltransferase 1A1 promoter in different ethnic groups. *Pharmacogenetics.* 2002;12(9):725–733.
11. Sai K, Saeki M, Saito Y, et al. UGT1A1 haplotypes associated with reduced glucuronidation and increased serum bilirubin in irinotecan-administered Japanese patients with cancer. *Clin Pharmacol Ther.* 2004;75(6):501–515.
12. Danoff TM, Campbell DA, McCarthy LC, et al. A Gilbert's syndrome UGT1A1 variant confers susceptibility to tranilast-induced hyperbilirubinemia. *Pharmacogenomics J.* 2004;4(1):49–53.
13. Rodríguez-Nóvoa S, Barreiro P, Jiménez-Nácher I, Soriano V. Overview of the pharmacogenetics of HIV therapy. *Pharmacogenomics J.* 2006;6(4): 234–245.
14. Rotger M, Taffe P, Bleiber G, et al. Swiss HIV Cohort Study. Gilbert syndrome and the development of antiretroviral therapy-associated hyperbilirubinemia. *J Infect Dis.* 2005;192(8):1381–1386.
15. Zhang D, Chando TJ, Everett DW, Patten CJ, Dehal SS, Humphreys WG. *In vitro* inhibition of UDP glucuronosyltransferases by atazanavir and other HIV protease inhibitors and the relationship of this property to *in vivo* bilirubin glucuronidation. *Drug Metab Dispos.* 2005;33(11):1729–1739.
16. Lankisch TO, Moebius U, Wehmeier M, et al. Gilbert's disease and atazanavir: from phenotype to UDP-glucuronosyltransferase haplotype. *Hepatology.* 2006;44(5):1324–1332.
17. Bhasker CR, McKinnon W, Stone A, et al. Genetic polymorphism of UDP-glucuronosyltransferase 2B7 (UGT2B7) at amino acid 268: ethnic diversity of alleles and potential clinical significance. *Pharmacogenetics.* 2000;10(8):679–685.
18. Daly AK, Aithal GP, Leathart JB, Swainsbury RA, Dang TS, Day CP. Genetic susceptibility to diclofenac-induced hepatotoxicity: contribution of UGT2B7, CYP2C8, and ABCC2 genotypes. *Gastroenterology.* 2007;132(1):272–281.
19. Zhao W, Elie V, Baudouin V, et al. Population pharmacokinetics and Bayesian estimator of mycophenolic acid in children with idiopathic nephrotic syndrome. *Br J Clin Pharmacol.* 2010;69(4):358–366.
20. Woillard JB, Rerolle JP, Picard N, et al. Risk of diarrhoea in a long-term cohort of renal transplant patients given mycophenolate mofetil: the significant role of the UGT1A8*2 variant allele. *Br J Clin Pharmacol.* 2010;69(6): 675–683.
21. Kakuta Y, Petrotchenko EV, Pedersen LC, Negishi M. The sulfuryl transfer mechanism. Crystal structure of a vanadate complex of estrogen sulfotransferase and mutational analysis. *J Biol Chem.* 1998;273(42): 27325–27330.

22. Blanchard RL, Freimuth RR, Buck J, Weinshilboum RM, Coughtrie MW. A proposed nomenclature system for the cytosolic sulfotransferase (SULT) superfamily. *Pharmacogenetics.* 2004;14(3):199–211.

23. Hempel N, Gamage N, Martin JL, McManus ME. Human cytosolic sulfotransferase SULT1A1. *Int J Biochem Cell Biol.* 2007;39(4):685–689.

24. Carlini EJ, Raftogianis RB, Wood TC, et al. Sulfation pharmacogenetics: SULT1A1 and SULT1A2 allele frequencies in Caucasian, Chinese and African-American subjects. *Pharmacogenetics.* 2001;11(1):57–68.

25. Nowell S, Sweeney C, Winters M, et al. Association between sulfotransferase 1A1 genotype and survival of breast cancer patients receiving tamoxifen therapy. *J Natl Cancer Inst.* 2002;94(21):1635–1640.

26. Sinclair JC, Sandy J, Delgoda R, Sim E, Noble ME. Structure of arylamine *N*-acetyltransferase reveals a catalytic triad. *Nat Struct Biol.* 2000;7(7):560–564.

27. Wu H, Dombrovsky L, Tempel W, et al. Structural basis of substrate-binding specificity of human arylamine *N*-acetyltransferases. *J Biol Chem.* 2007;282(41):30189–30197.

28. Sim E, Lack N, Wang CJ, et al. Arylamine *N*-acetyltransferases: structural and functional implications of polymorphisms. *Toxicology.* 2008;254(3): 170–183.

29. Butcher NJ, Ilett KF, Minchin RF. Functional polymorphism of the human arylamine *N*-acetyltransferase type 1 gene caused by C190T and G560A mutations. *Pharmacogenetics.* 1998;8(1):67–72.

30. Walraven JM, Trent JO, Hein DW. Structure–function analyses of single nucleotide polymorphisms in human *N*-acetyltransferase 1. *Drug Metab Rev.* 2008;40(1):169–184.

31. Evans DAP, White TA. Human acetylation polymorphism. *J Lab Clin Med.* 1964;63(3):394–403.

32. Chen M, Xia B, Chen B, et al. *N*-Acetyltransferase 2 slow acetylator genotype associated with adverse effects of sulphasalazine in the treatment of inflammatory bowel disease. *Can J Gastroenterol.* 2007;21(3):155–158.

33. Hayes JD, Flanagan JU, Jowsey IR. Glutathione transferases. *Annu Rev Pharmacol Toxicol.* 2005;45:51–88.

34. Reszka E, Wasowicz W, Gromadzinska J. Genetic polymorphism of xenobiotic metabolising enzymes, diet and cancer susceptibility. *Br J Nutr.* 2006;96(4):609–619.

35. Thier R, Wiebel FA, Hinkel A, et al. Species differences in the glutathione transferase GSTT1-1 activity towards the model substrates methyl chloride and dichloromethane in liver and kidney. *Arch Toxicol.* 1998;72(10):622–629.

36. Peklak-Scott C, Smitherman PK, Townsend AJ, Morrow CS. Role of glutathione *S*-transferase P1-1 in the cellular detoxification of cisplatin. *Mol Cancer Ther.* 2008;7(10):3247–3255.

37. Khrunin AV, Moisseev A, Gorbunova V, Limborska S. Genetic polymorphisms and the efficacy and toxicity of cisplatin-based chemotherapy in ovarian cancer patients. *Pharmacogenomics J.* 2010;10(1):54–61.

38. Stoehlmacher J, Park DJ, Zhang W, et al. Association between glutathione *S*-transferase P1, T1, and M1 genetic polymorphism and survival of patients with metastatic colorectal cancer. *J Natl Cancer Inst.* 2002;94(12):936–942.

39. Culy CR, Clemett D, Wiseman LR. Oxaliplatin. A review of its pharmacological properties and clinical efficacy in metastatic colorectal cancer and its potential in other malignancies. *Drugs.* 2000;60(4):895–924.

40. Lecomte T, Landi B, Beaune P, Laurent-Puig P, Loriot MA. Glutathione *S*-transferase P1 polymorphism (Ile105Val) predicts cumulative neuropathy in patients receiving oxaliplatin-based chemotherapy. *Clin Cancer Res.* 2006;12(10):3050–3056.

41. Oldenburg J, Kraggerud SM, Cvancarova M, Lothe RA, Fossa SD. Cisplatin-induced long-term hearing impairment is associated with specific glutathione *S*-transferase genotypes in testicular cancer survivors. *J Clin Oncol.* 2007;25(6):708–714.

42. Peters U, Preisler-Adams S, Hebeisen A, et al. Glutathione *S*-transferase genetic polymorphisms and individual sensitivity to the ototoxic effect of cisplatin. *Anticancer Drugs.* 2000;11(8):639–643.

43. Dix SP, Wingard JR, Mullins RE, et al. Association of busulfan area under the curve with veno-occlusive disease following BMT. *Bone Marrow Transplant.* 1996;17(2):225–230.

44. Slattery JT, Sanders JE, Buckner CD, et al. Graft-rejection and toxicity following bone marrow transplantation in relation to busulfan pharmacokinetics. *Bone Marrow Transplant.* 1995;16(1):31–42.

45. Kusama M, Kubota T, Matsukura Y, et al. Influence of glutathione *S*-transferase A1 polymorphism on the pharmacokinetics of busulfan. *Clin Chim Acta.* 2006;368(1–2):93–98.

46. Elhasid R, Krivoy N, Rowe JM, et al. Influence of glutathione *S*-transferase A1, P1, M1, T1 polymorphisms on oral busulfan pharmacokinetics in children with congenital hemoglobinopathies undergoing hematopoietic stem cell transplantation. *Pediatr Blood Cancer.* 2010;55(6):1172–1179.

47. Ansari M, Lauzon-Joset JF, Vachon MF, et al. Influence of GST gene polymorphisms on busulfan pharmacokinetics in children. *Bone Marrow Transplant.* 2010;45(2):261–267.

48. Srivastava A, Poonkuzhali B, Shaji RV, et al. Glutathione *S*-transferase M1 polymorphism: a risk factor for hepatic venoocclusive disease in bone marrow transplantation. *Blood.* 2004;104(5):1574–1577.

49. Johnson L, Orchard PJ, Baker KS, et al. Glutathione *S*-transferase A1 genetic variants reduce busulfan clearance in children undergoing hematopoietic cell transplantation. *J Clin Pharmacol.* 2008;48(9):1052–1062.

50. Zwaveling J, Press RR, Bredius RG, et al. Glutathione *S*-transferase polymorphisms are not associated with population pharmacokinetic parameters of busulfan in pediatric patients. *Ther Drug Monit.* 2008;30(4): 504–510.

51. Allan JM, Wild CP, Rollinson S, et al. Polymorphism in glutathione *S*-transferase P1 is associated with susceptibility to chemotherapy-induced leukemia. *Proc Natl Acad Sci U S A.* 2001;98(20):11592–11597.

52. Sweeney C, McClure GY, Fares MY, et al. Association between survival after treatment for breast cancer and glutathione *S*-transferase P1 Ile105Val polymorphism. *Cancer Res.* 2000;60(20):5621–5624.

53. Sweeney C, Ambrosone CB, Joseph L, et al. Association between a glutathione *S*-transferase A1 promoter polymorphism and survival after breast cancer treatment. *Int J Cancer.* 2003;103(6):810–814.

54. Vessey DA, Kelley M, Warren RS. Characterization of the CoA ligases of human liver mitochondria catalyzing the activation of short- and medium-chain fatty acids and xenobiotic carboxylic acids. *Biochim Biophys Acta.* 1999;1428(2–3):455–462.

55. Miners JO, Grgurinovich N, Whitehead AG, Robson RA, Birkett DJ. Influence of gender and oral contraceptive steroids on the metabolism of salicylic acid and acetylsalicylic acid. *Br J Clin Pharmacol.* 1986;22(2):135–142.

56. Knights KM, Sykes MJ, Miners JO. Amino acid conjugation: contribution to the metabolism and toxicity of xenobiotic carboxylic acids. *Expert Opin Drug Metab Toxicol.* 2007;3(2):159–168.

57. Kotb M, Geller AM. Methionine adenosyltransferase: structure and function. *Pharmacol Ther.* 1993;59(2):125–143.

58. Salavaggione OE, Wang L, Wiepert M, Yee VC, Weinshilboum RM. Thiopurine *S*-methyltransferase pharmacogenetics: variant allele functional and comparative genomics. *Pharmacogenet Genomics.* 2005;15(11):801–815.

59. Cavalieri EL, Stack DE, Devanesan PD, et al. Molecular origin of cancer: catechol estrogen-3,4-quinones as endogenous tumor initiators. *Proc Natl Acad Sci U S A.* 1997;94(20):10937–10942.

60. Lachman HM, Papolos DF, Saito T, Yu YM, Szumlanski CL, Weinshilboum RM. Human catechol-*O*-methyltransferase pharmacogenetics: description of a functional polymorphism and its potential application to neuropsychiatric disorders. *Pharmacogenetics.* 1996;6(3):243–250.

61. McLeod HL, Fang L, Luo X, Scott EP, Evans WE. Ethnic differences in erythrocyte catechol-*O*-methyltransferase activity in black and white Americans. *J Pharmacol Exp Ther.* 1994;270(1):26–29.

62. Reilly DK, Rivera-Calimlim L, Van Dyke D. Catechol-*O*-methyltransferase activity: a determinant of levodopa response. *Clin Pharmacol Ther.* 1980;28(2):278–286.

63. Contin M, Martinelli P, Mochi M, Riva R, Albani F, Baruzzi A. Genetic polymorphism of catechol-*O*-methyltransferase and levodopa pharmacokinetic–pharmacodynamic pattern in patients with Parkinson's disease. *Mov Disord.* 2005;20(6):734–739.

64. Keith RA, Otterness DM, Kerremans AL, Weinshilboum RM. *S*-Methylation of D- and L-penicillamine by human erythrocyte membrane thiol methyltransferase. *Drug Metab Dispos.* 1985;13(6):669–676.

65. Preuss CV, Wood TC, Szumlanski CL, et al. Human histamine *N*-methyltransferase pharmacogenetics: common genetic polymorphisms that alter activity. *Mol Pharmacol.* 1998;53(4):708–717.

Drug Transporters

Shirley M. Tsunoda, PharmD, Dallas Bednarczyk, PhD, & Hideaki Okochi, PhD

LEARNING OBJECTIVES

- Discuss the roles that membrane transporters play in drug disposition and action.

- Explain how drug transporters influence drug action in the intestine, liver, kidney, and blood–brain barrier.

- Describe how pharmacogenetic changes in P-glycoprotein may affect drug concentrations and pharmacodynamics.

- Provide examples of how pharmacogenetic variants may affect pharmacokinetics of substrate compounds for the following transporters: breast cancer resistance protein (BCRP), organic anion-transporting polypeptide 1B1 (OATP1B1), bile salt export pump (BSEP), organic cation transporter 1 (OCT1), organic cation transporter 2 (OCT2), and multidrug and toxin extrusion 1 (MATE1).

INTRODUCTION

Transporters are membrane proteins that are ubiquitous throughout the body functioning to control the influx of essential nutrients and ions and the efflux of cellular waste, toxins, and drugs. Transporters located in the liver, intestine, kidney, and blood–brain barrier (BBB) are of particular interest in drug development and utilization. Multiple transporters work in a coordinated fashion to transport endogenous and exogenous substances into and out of cells. In certain organs, such as the liver and intestine, transporters and drug-metabolizing enzymes work together to affect the pharmacokinetics of drugs.

Transporters play an important role in drug disposition, therapeutic efficacy, adverse drug reactions, and drug–drug interactions. Multiple environmental and genetic factors may affect the variability of transporter expression. Understanding the contribution of genetic variability to transporter expression and phenotype may allow clinicians to individualize drug therapy based on genetic factors. There are two major superfamilies of transporters important in drug disposition: solute carrier (SLC) transporters, a family of passive and active transporters that rely on chemical and/or electrical gradients for transport, and ATP-binding cassette (ABC) transporters, a family of primary active transporters that are ATP dependent. The following drug transporters will be discussed in this chapter with respect to the current knowledge of their pharmacogenetics: P-glycoprotein (P-gp), breast cancer resistance protein (BCRP), organic anion-transporting polypeptide (OATP1B1), bile salt export pump (BSEP), organic cation transporter 1 (OCT1), organic cation transporter 2 (OCT2), multidrug and toxin extrusion 1 (MATE1), and organic anion transporters 1 and 3 (OAT1 and OAT3). For a review of other transporters not covered in this chapter, the reader is referred to other references.[1,2] For most drug transporters, clinical evidence is sparse or, in the case of P-gp, conflicting. Due to the complex nature of drug disposition and subsequent effect on clinical outcome, isolating clinically significant drug transporter genetic variants is a challenging endeavor.

TRANSPORTERS IN THE INTESTINE

Most orally administered drugs are absorbed in the small intestine. Although the process of drug absorption is largely a passive process, transporters in the small intestine are determinants of the extent and variability of drug absorption that ultimately affect the pharmacokinetics of numerous drugs. Transporters expressed at the apical membrane of enterocytes may facilitate

Lumen

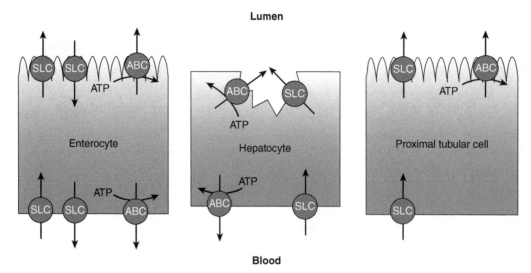

Blood

FIGURE 7–1 The transepithelial transport of drugs is facilitated by complementary transporters localized to the two membrane surfaces of polarized epithelia. Illustrated are transport processes across the enterocyte (small intestine), the hepatocyte (liver), and the cells of the renal proximal tubule (kidney). The enterocyte generally is responsible for limiting drug absorption into the blood, whereas the hepatocyte and the cells of the renal proximal tubule facilitate the excretion of drug. *Abbreviations*: solute carrier (SLC) transporter and ATP-binding cassette (ABC) transporter.

intestinal drug absorption or reduce the bioavailability of a drug. The resulting pharmacokinetic impact is dependent on the mechanism of transport. Transporters from both the ABC and SLC superfamilies are present in the apical membrane of the enterocyte (Figure 7–1). ABC transporters expressed on the apical membrane of the enterocyte act to limit drug absorption, where they transport drug from the enterocyte back into the intestinal lumen. The best characterized and apically localized efflux transporter is P-gp (ABCB1), but multidrug resistance protein 2 (MRP2/ABCC2) and BCRP (ABCG2) are also localized to the apical membrane and act to limit drug absorption. An important SLC transporter expressed on the apical membrane is PEPT1 (SLC15A1). PEPT1 is a nutrient transporter responsible for the absorption of dipeptides and tripeptides. Drugs that sufficiently resemble small peptides (peptidomimetics) may experience a faster rate of absorption than predicted because they are actively transported into the body in addition to being passively absorbed. Other SLC transporters are also localized to the apical membrane, but their role in facilitating the absorption of drugs is not established at this time. The impact of intestinal transporters on the absorption of drugs varies and depends on the passive permeability of the administered drug and the dose, among other factors. High passive permeability of drug will limit the role of transporters in drug absorption because the fraction of drug flux mediated by the transporter, either absorptive or efflux, will be small relative to the passive component. Drugs with low intrinsic passive permeability are more subject to manipulation by transporters. Similarly, a high dose of drug may saturate intestinal transport processes minimizing their impact. Because the passive component (diffusion) is not saturable, once transport is saturated absorption increases linearly with drug concentration.

Although transporters have different substrate specificities, there is overlap and redundancy in the types of substrates they transport. For example, P-gp transports a wide variety of substrates that are structurally unrelated, but are frequently either neutral or positively charged hydrophobic compounds such as antiviral agents, immunosuppressive agents, and chemotherapy agents. MRP2 also transports the chemotherapy agents methotrexate and irinotecan. BCRP (ABCG2) mediates the efflux of chemotherapy agents, antiviral drugs, HMG-CoA reductase inhibitors, calcium channel blockers, and steroid metabolites. PEPT1 mediates the absorption of beta-lactam antibiotics, angiotensin-converting enzyme inhibitors, and antiviral drugs.

TRANSPORTERS IN THE LIVER

Drugs are largely cleared by the liver, primarily by metabolic means, and also through transport mechanisms. Hepatic drug elimination through transport mechanisms, which is biliary clearance, is initiated by flux of drug into the hepatocyte across the sinusoidal membrane, by either passive diffusion or transporter-mediated uptake. Once inside the hepatocyte the drug may or may not be subject to intracellular metabolism by cytochromes P450 and/or conjugation by phase II enzymes. The metabolite, or unchanged drug, is then secreted into the bile across the canalicular membrane or back into the blood across the sinusoidal membrane by transporters that mediate the efflux of drug. The vectorial flux of drug through the hepatocyte is attributable to its polarized nature. The hepatocyte has basolateral (sinusoidal) and apical (canalicular) membranes that differ in transporter composition and consequently function (Figure 7–1). The function of the transporters localized to each membrane may be limited by the kinetic properties of the transporter, affected by the presence of a transporter inhibitor, or diminished by genetic mutations.

Drug Uptake in the Liver

The movement of drugs across the sinusoidal membrane of the hepatocyte is generally facilitated by high concentrations of drug in portal circulation following administration. The high concentrations of drug in the portal circulation create a concentration gradient that favors diffusion into the hepatocyte for drugs that are highly permeable and also favors the transporter-mediated uptake of drugs that are poorly permeable. Hepatic drug transport is primarily characterized by the translocation of large (MW greater than approximately 400 g/mol), somewhat hydrophobic organic anions and amphipathic organic molecules. The uptake of organic anions by the hepatocyte is most frequently associated with three organic anion-transporting polypeptides (OATPs), OATP1B1 (SLCO1B1), OATP1B3 (SLCO1B3), and OATP2B1 (SLCO2B1). The mechanism of organic anion transport by the OATPs is an electroneutral process; however, the associated charge-carrying ion has not been identified. Common substrates of the OATPs include pravastatin, valsartan, glyburide, and repaglinide. Complementing the OATPs is OCT1. It transports a variety of relatively small (less than approximately 400 g/mol), polar cationic molecules across the sinusoidal membrane of the hepatocyte and may facilitate the metabolism of weak bases, such as debrisoquine, by the cytochromes P450. Other substrates of OCT1 include metformin and tropisetron.

Drug Efflux from the Liver

Transporters that mediate drug efflux from the hepatocyte generally belong to the ABC subfamily. ABC transporters are localized to both the sinusoidal membrane and the canalicular membrane where they mediate drug efflux from the hepatocyte into the blood and into the bile, respectively. Transporters localized to the sinusoidal membrane include MRP3 (ABCC3), MRP4 (ABCC4), and MRP6 (ABCC6); these transporters mediate drug or drug-conjugate efflux from the hepatocyte. The transport of phase II drug conjugates into the blood by MRP3, 4, or 6 may promote the renal clearance of the more polar drug conjugates, supplementing any biliary clearance by canalicular membrane efflux transporters. ABC transporters localized to the canalicular membrane include P-gp, MRP2 (ABCC2), BCRP, and BSEP. These transporters facilitate the transport of drugs and endogenous molecules and are frequently associated with the biliary clearance of drugs. Canalicular efflux transporters demonstrate a broad range of substrate specificity that includes endogenous and exogenous molecules. Molecules transported by the canalicular ABC transporters are generally moderately lipophilic, usually >400 g/mol, and are typically differentiated by charge. For example, P-gp commonly transports cationic molecules (i.e., weak bases) such as loperamide, fexofenadine, and vinblastine, while MRP2 and BCRP frequently transport anionic compounds, including phase II conjugates, such as valsartan, methotrexate, pitavastatin, and estrone-3-sulfate. While the substrates of the canilicular transporters are often differentiated by charge, uncharged molecules, or molecules having an atypical charge, may also be transported (e.g., digoxin is transported by P-gp and prazosin is transported by BCRP). In addition to the ABC transporters, the SLC transporter, MATE1, is also expressed on the canalicular membrane and transports relatively small organic cations in exchange for a proton.

TRANSPORTERS IN THE KIDNEY

For drugs having limited or negligible metabolic or biliary clearance, the excretion of unchanged drug by the kidneys can represent a significant route of drug elimination. Additionally, renal clearance is a principal means of clearing metabolites of drugs and drug conjugates. The transepithelial translocation (secretion) of drugs from the interstitial space to the tubule lumen is a two-step process (Figure 7–1) and is additive to elimination by glomerular filtration. The proximal tubule is the primary site within the nephron for the secretion of drugs. The first step of the sequential process is the transport of drug across the epithelial cell's basolateral membrane into the cytoplasm. The second step is the transport of drug across the cell's apical membrane by a transporter whose substrate specificity is complementary to the basolateral transporter facilitating the first step in the process. Simple diffusion may substitute for one of the steps provided a drug has sufficient passive permeability. The activity of these drug transporters is characterized by Michaelis–Menten kinetics, therefore the secretory process is saturable and may be inhibited by coadministered drugs. Furthermore, the kinetic activity of these transporters may be increased or, more frequently, decreased by changes in the amino acid sequence of the protein, changes that are subsequent to changes in the genome. The transepithelial secretion of drugs therefore can be saturated, inhibited, and is subject to genetic mutations (single nucleotide polymorphisms [SNPs]). Thus, the renal clearance of drugs by transporters may be limited at high drug concentrations, restricted by coadministered drugs, or diminished by gene mutations that reduce protein function or expression.

Organic Cation Transport in Kidney

The mechanism of organic cation secretion most likely has evolutionary precedent for clearing the body of xenobiotics, such as plant alkaloids, largely acquired through dietary means, or environmental toxins, such as nicotine. However, in the modern era it plays an important role in the elimination of therapeutic drugs. As such, the secretory process is subject to clinically significant interactions with drugs. For example, the substrates metformin and procainamide show reduced renal clearances in the presence of the transporter inhibitor cimetidine. Common substrates of the processes surrounding organic cation transport in the kidney include metformin, varenicline, procainamide, and amiloride. These compounds reflect the physicochemical properties of the process, that is, they are generally ≤400 g/mol, relatively polar, and weak bases.

The secretion of organic cations is a two-step process. The first step, entry into the cell across the basolateral membrane of proximal tubule cells, is a uniport (facilitated diffusion) mechanism, driven by an electrical and chemical gradient for the substrate, and is mediated by the OCT2. The electrical component is derived from the negative membrane potential and the chemical gradient reflects the concentration gradient. An alternative means for cellular entry across the basolateral membrane is by simple diffusion. This also represents an electrically conductive means for entry and more commonly characterizes the entry step for hydrophobic organic cations.

The complementary exit step of organic cations across the luminal (apical) membrane involves an active transport process of carrier-mediated exchange (antiport) of an intracellular organic cation for one extracellular hydrogen ion (H^+), or proton, and is mediated by the multidrug and toxin extrusion family members MATE1 and MATE2-K. The electroneutral antiport is driven by the proton (pH) gradient, because the proximal tubule lumen is acidic relative to that of the cells lining the lumen.

The coordinated actions of the basolateral transport process, uniport (facilitated diffusion), and the apical transport process, antiport, result in net transepithelial secretion of organic cations. An alternative means of apical secretion of organic cations is by an ATP-dependent process, where ATP provides the energy for a mechanism of primary active transport of molecules across the apical (luminal) membrane. This mechanism of secretory flux is more frequently associated with large-molecular-weight organic cations (>400 g/mol), and is facilitated by the apically localized P-gp.

The cellular processes associated with secretion of organic cations can be summarized as follows: (1) low-molecular-weight organic cations enter proximal cells across the basolateral membrane via electrogenic process of facilitated diffusion and exit cells across the luminal/apical membrane by means of electroneutral exchange for H^+; (2) larger-molecular-weight organic cations likely diffuse into proximal tubule cells, or may be transported by an as yet to be defined transporter, across the peritubular membrane and are pumped across the apical membrane into the tubular lumen by the primary active transporter, P-gp. Notably, overlap appears to exist in the transport pathways for small and large organic cations. Furthermore, the transepithelial transport of organic cations in renal proximal tubules involves the parallel activity of multiple discrete transport processes.

Organic Anion Transport in the Kidney

The mechanism of organic anion secretion likely parallels that of organic cation transport in that it has evolutionary precedent for clearing the body of xenobiotics. However, much like the organic cation transporters, organic anion transporters play an important role in the elimination of therapeutic drugs. As such, the secretory process is subject to clinically significant interactions with drugs. For example, the clearance of adefovir and furosemide is inhibited by the presence of probenecid. Common substrates of the processes surrounding organic anion transport

in the kidney include adefovir, penicillin G, and methotrexate. Additionally, substrates of organic anion transport processes frequently include a number of products of hepatic biotransformation. These compounds reflect the physicochemical properties of the process, that is, they are generally ≤400 g/mol, relatively polar, and are weak acids.

The secretion of organic anions is also a two-step process. The coordinated actions of the basolateral transport process, anion exchange, and the apical transport processes, facilitated diffusion and active transport, result in net transepithelial secretion of organic anions. The first step, entry into the cell across the basolateral membrane of proximal tubule cells, is an active step characterized as an exchange (antiport) mechanism, where intracellular dicarboxylate ions (e.g., α-ketoglutarate, a Kreb's cycle intermediate) are exchanged for organic anions. The antiporters responsible for mediating the cellular uptake of organic anions into proximal tubule cells are the organic anion transporters OAT1 and OAT3. An alternative means for cellular entry across the basolateral membrane is by simple diffusion.

The complementary exit step of organic anions across the luminal (apical) membrane has largely been characterized as a transport process of facilitated diffusion. The process of facilitated diffusion is driven by an electrochemical and concentration gradient of the substrate inside the cell driven by the active step at the basolateral membrane. The negative membrane potential provides an electromotive force for the exit of negatively charged compounds, such as organic anions. An alternative means for exit across the apical membrane is by simple diffusion.

Organic anions, similar to organic cations, may also be secreted into the proximal tubule lumen by an ATP-dependent process, where ATP provides the energy for a mechanism of primary active transport. However, rather than being mediated by P-gp, the primary active transport of organic anions across the luminal membrane is commonly facilitated by multidrug resistance proteins, MRP2 and MRP4.

The cellular processes associated with secretion of organic anions can be summarized as follows: (1) low-molecular-weight organic cations enter proximal cells across the basolateral membrane in exchange for intracellular dicarboxylates (e.g., α-ketoglutarate) and exit cells across the luminal/apical membrane by facilitated diffusion; (2) alternatively, organic anions may also enter by the same mechanism, but may be pumped across the apical membrane into the tubular lumen by the primary active transporter, such as MRP2 or MRP4. Notably, overlap exists in the two transport pathways.

TRANSPORTERS INVOLVED IN THE BLOOD–BRAIN BARRIER

The BBB is an interface between the brain and the systemic circulation within the capillary endothelium and controls what goes in and out of the central nervous system (CNS). This barrier is known to be highly active, dynamic, and selective in mediating signals coming from the periphery and brain. The barrier function of the BBB consists of three components: tight junctions, metabolizing enzymes, and transporters. Transporters are an important component of the BBB that function as active barriers to protect the brain from drugs and other neuroactive and toxic substances. Transporters from both the SLC and ABC superfamilies are involved in the BBB. Transporters from the SLC superfamily facilitate influx of glucose, amino acids, ions, and other nutrients needed to meet the energy demands of the brain. Efflux transporters from the ABC superfamily actively clear wastes and prevent xenobiotics and other toxins from entering the brain. While the BBB transporters are an important barrier to the permeation of unwanted substances into the brain, transporters can also be an impediment when trying to get therapeutic substances into the CNS. For example, the presence of ABC transporters may limit penetration of chemotherapeutics into the CNS creating a safe harbor for brain cancers to thrive.

P-gp, BCRP, and MRP transporters are involved in limiting drug entry into BBB. P-gp is the most extensively studied with the most established examples of limiting drug penetration into the brain. The role of P-gp at the BBB was demonstrated in a study of healthy volunteers. Coadministration of the antidiarrheal agent and potent opioid, loperamide, and the P-gp inhibitor quinidine caused significant respiratory depression, a CNS side effect of opioid administration. By contrast, when loperamide was administered alone no respiratory effect was observed, because P-gp acts to prevent CNS penetration of loperamide.[3] For this reason, loperamide, while it is a potent opioid, is available over-the-counter as an antidiarrheal medication. P-gp and BCRP have overlapping substrate specificities, and are thought to cooperate in limiting drug entry into the brain. Several isoforms of MRP have been identified at the BBB: MRP1, MRP2, MRP3, MRP4, and MRP5. MRPs transport organic anions, glutathione, glucuronide- or sulfate-conjugated compounds, and nucleoside analogs.

P-GLYCOPROTEIN: ABCB1

P-gp, encoded by the gene ABCB1 (formerly known as MDR1), is a 1,280 amino acid transmembrane protein that is important in the efflux of a wide variety of drugs and endogenous compounds. In addition to the tissues previously described, P-gp is expressed at various blood–tissue barriers such as the blood–brain, blood–cerebrospinal fluid (CSF), blood–testis, and blood–placenta barriers, functioning to limit entry of xenobiotic substances into these tissues. Consistent with its ability to limit the accumulation of xenobiotics in tissues, P-gp was the first transporter identified as a facilitator of tumor cell drug resistance (multidrug resistance) by mediating efflux of chemotherapeutics from tumor cells. The role P-gp has in limiting the intestinal absorption of compounds, promoting the excretion of compounds by the liver and kidney, and limiting tissue accumulation illustrates its responsibility in the pharmacokinetics of substrate compounds.

P-gp demonstrates broad substrate diversity; P-pg substrates include analgesics, anticancer agents, HIV and HCV protease

inhibitors, immunosuppressives, corticosteroids, and antibiotics (see Table 7–1). Inhibitors and inducers of P-gp are equally diverse. Clinically this diversity is important to the underlying mechanism of drug–drug interactions. Determining drug–drug interactions involving P-gp substrates is not straightforward because P-gp has multiple drug-binding sites with different binding affinities. Therefore, determining drug interactions with P-gp substrates may require multiple drug pairs to cover the range of substrates that bind to the different binding sites.[4] Additionally, multiple substrates may be required to assess the effect of a given polymorphism if the binding pocket is altered in a way that impacts some compounds but not others. There are currently no recommendations to address the potential for multiple P-gp-binding sites.[2]

P-gp may also complement other transporters and drug-metabolizing enzymes in the intestine, liver, and kidney to affect drug concentrations in the tissue and plasma. For example, both CYP3A4 and P-gp are highly expressed in the intestine and liver and have broad overlapping substrate specificity. One hypothesis suggests that CYP3A4 and P-gp complement each other by limiting oral drug bioavailability.[5] The presence of P-gp allows a drug molecule more opportunity for CYP3A metabolism in the intestine, thus decreasing overall systemic exposure. Through repeated cycles of passive absorption and subsequent efflux by P-gp, there is an increased residence time of the drug in the enterocyte providing more opportunity for intestinal metabolism by CYP3A. Additionally, this coordinated action may play a role in drug interactions and adverse drug effects. Therefore, in order to accurately assess the mechanism of a potential drug interaction for a given P-gp substrate, the contributions from intestinal and hepatic P-gp, CYP3A4, and other transporters may need to be considered.

In addition to the diminished P-gp activity caused by drug–drug interactions, P-gp activity can be increased or decreased by a number of other factors. The expression of P-gp, and correspondingly its activity, can be inhibited or induced by drugs, disease states, or genetic polymorphisms. Many investigative studies have shown alterations in P-gp activity due to genetic polymorphisms or drug–drug interactions; however, whether these alterations are clinically significant remains unknown.

As discussed in other chapters, SNPs are one of the most important mechanisms of genetic variability. There are at least 1,200 SNPs in the ABCB1 gene with approximately 100 in the coding region.[6] Most of the human studies have focused on the three most common SNPs—rs1128503 (1236C>T, Gly412Gly), resulting in a synonymous change; rs2032582 (2677G>T/A, Ser893Ala/Thr), a nonsynonymous (or silent) SNP; and rs1045642 (3435C>T, Ile1145Ile), a synonymous SNP—which are in high linkage disequilibrium. There are thought to be four important haplotypes associated with these SNPs: 1236C/2677G/3435C (ABCB1*1), which is the reference sequence; 1236T/2677T/3435T (ABCB1*2); 1236C/2677G/3435T (also named ABCB1*2); and 1236T/2677T/3435T plus three intronic SNPs (ABCB1*13). The allelic frequency of the 3435C>T SNP varies with ethnicity with the 3435T variant allele occurring in greater frequency

TABLE 7–1 Transporters and representative substrates.

Transporter (Gene)	Organs	Selected Substrates
ABC transporters		
Pgp (ABCB1)	Brain, intestine, kidney, liver	Atorvastatin Cyclosporine Digoxin Fexofenadine Fluphenazine Irinotecan Ketoconazole Loperamide Lopinavir Rifampin Sirolimus Tacrolimus Testosterone
BCRP (ABCG2)	Brain, intestine, kidney, liver, placenta	Ciprofloxacin Erythromycin Estradiol Etoposide Irinotecan metabolite (SN-38) Methotrexate Nitrofurantoin Rosuvastatin Sirolimus Tacrolimus
BSEP (ABCB11)	Liver	Bile acids Pravastatin
SLC transporters		
OATP1B1 (SLCO1B1)	Liver	Atorvastatin Bile acids Bilirubin Caspofungin Enalapril Fexofenadine Irinotecan Methotrexate Rifampin Rosuvastatin
OCT1 (SLC22A1)	Intestine, liver	Metformin Tropisetron (not available in the United States) Oxaliplatin
OCT2 (SLC22A2)	Kidney	Cisplatin Oxaliplatin Metformin Varenicline Procainamide Amiloride
MATE1 (SLC47A1)	Kidney, liver	Metformin Cimetidine Procainamide
OAT1 and OAT3 (SLC22A6 and SLC22A8)	Kidney	Adefovir Furosemide Methotrexate Penicillin (and other β-lactam antibiotics)

in Caucasians (Caucasians; 0.52–0.57) compared with Asians (Asians; 0.41–0.47) or African blacks (0.17–0.27).[6]

The functional activity of P-gp is dependent on two major factors: (1) the gene expression of ABCB1 that controls the amount of protein available and (2) the functionality of P-gp that determines which substrates will bind and how efficiently they will bind. Amino acid changes within the P-gp protein can influence this functionality. Interestingly, one of the common ABCB1 SNPs, 3435C>T, has been shown to affect P-gp transport function in vitro even though the amino acid sequence was unchanged. This so-called silent polymorphism is thought to alter the conformation of the substrate and inhibitor interaction site, thus altering the ability of P-gp to bind to a substrate.[7]

Effect of ABCB1 Genetic Polymorphisms on Drug Pharmacokinetics

In order to determine if genetic variability in the ABCB1 gene causes changes in P-gp activity, clinical studies look for changes in the pharmacokinetics of representative drugs known to be transported primarily by P-gp. P-gp affects pharmacokinetics through its role in limiting oral absorption that can be measured by area under the concentration-versus-time curve (AUC) or maximum concentration (C_{max}). For example, if a genetic polymorphism in the ABCB1 gene causes increased P-gp expression, one would expect decreased oral bioavailability, decreased AUC, decreased C_{max}, and increased renal clearance (exemplified as apical transporter in Figure 7–2a to 7–2c). In addition, studies can investigate changes in target cell or organ tissue concentrations in which P-gp limits entry of drugs.

Studies investigating the common ABCB1 SNPs and the haplotypes have been restricted to a few compounds. Digoxin is a known P-gp substrate. Clinical studies investigating the 3435C>T and 2677G>TA with the cardiac glycoside digoxin have shown mixed results. A few studies have shown that the 3435C allele was responsible for increased P-gp activity[8,9]; however another study showed no difference in digoxin pharmacokinetics with any SNPs.[10] Additional supportive evidence of no difference in digoxin pharmacokinetics based on P-gp polymorphisms is published elsewhere.[11] Haplotype analysis has shown equally inconsistent results with digoxin pharmacokinetic parameters.[12–14] Similarly, the 3435C>T and 2677G>T/A polymorphisms have been shown not to impact the pharmacokinetics of the immunosuppressive agents cyclosporine, tacrolimus, and sirolimus, which are all P-gp substrates.[15,16] Haplotype analysis also is inconclusive for the immunosuppressive agents with the majority of studies showing no changes in the pharmacokinetics with one study suggesting that one haplotype containing T alleles for 3435 and 2677 had lower P-gp activity as measured by tacrolimus concentrations in lung transplant patients.[17] Genotype and haplotypes analyses have been conducted with other drugs such as the nonsedating antihistamine fexofenadine, the HIV protease inhibitor nelfinavir/efavirenz, and the chemotherapeutic agents vincristine and irinotecan with similar inconclusive results.

The role of ABCB1 genetic polymorphisms in drug pharmacokinetics is not clear. Possible reasons for the inconsistencies in the studies and lack of association may include the fact that multiple processes affect intestinal bioavailability, the drug substrates studied may not be measuring P-gp activity exclusively (i.e., other transporters or enzymes may be affecting the pharmacokinetics), and the studies may not have been powered adequately for the effect size.

Effect of ABCB1 Genetic Polymorphisms on Clinical Outcome

If ABCB1 genetic polymorphisms significantly affect P-gp activity such as in cell target or organ tissue concentrations (exemplified as the apical transporter in Figure 7–2a to 7–2c), then one would expect the clinical outcome of therapy with a drug that is a P-gp substrate to be altered. These clinical outcomes could manifest in either improved or worsened therapeutic effectiveness or increased or decreased adverse effects. The studies that have been conducted with P-gp substrates classified as immunosuppressives, antiretrovirals, antiepileptics, and HMG-CoA reductase inhibitors are inconclusive. Some studies have shown positive associations between the 3435C>T polymorphism, the 2677G>T polymorphism, or certain haplotypes and clinical outcome in transplant, HIV, epileptic patients, and patients treated with statins; however, many other studies have shown no differences in clinical outcomes with these polymorphisms. For example, in one prospective study of 96 HIV patients taking the P-gp substrate nelfinavir, those with the TT genotype at the 3435 locus had a significantly higher CD4 count ($P = .005$) compared with those with the CT/CC genotypes.[18] In contrast, another prospective study of 504 HIV patients showed no association with the TT genotype and CD4 counts in patients taking nelfinavir.[19] Therefore, the data are conflicting and the methodology of some of the studies is flawed. At this time, no recommendations can be made for specific P-gp genotypes and prediction of clinical outcomes.

Summary

There are many genetic variants affecting P-gp activity. However, association studies of various P-gp genetic polymorphisms have been inconclusive. Therefore, our current knowledge of the genetic variants of P-gp does not allow predictions to be made on an individual's pharmacokinetics or clinical outcome. Further research with larger numbers of subjects must be conducted before clinical practice guidelines can be implemented.[20]

BREAST CANCER RESISTANCE PROTEIN: ABCG2

The BCRP/ABCG2 is a member of the ABC transporter G-subfamily of efflux transporters. The ABCG transporter is known to be a half-size transporter (half-transporter, 6 transmembrane domains rather than the 12 common to P-gp and

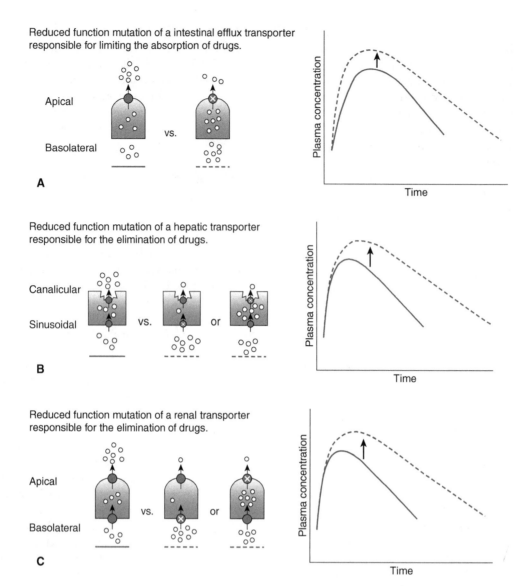

FIGURE 7–2 Illustrated mechanisms by which transporter polymorphisms mediate changes in drug plasma concentration and correspondingly drug pharmacokinetics. Examples of transporter polymorphisms and associated changes in plasma concentration for three representative tissues, small intestine (**A**), liver (**B**), and kidney (**C**), are provided. In each example the cell at the far left contains the normally functioning reference alleles. The subject's cells are illustrated to the right, and demonstrate a reduced function/loss of function allele of a transporter expressed at the basolateral/sinusoidal or apical/canalicular membranes, respectively (represented as X in transporter). Corresponding changes in the plasma concentration of drug for the reduced function alleles are represented in the graph to the right. (Adapted from Ref.[1])

the MRPs) and is expressed and functions as a homodimer or heterodimer on the apical membrane of epithelial cells. BCRP is a homodimer and is abundantly expressed in placenta, brain, intestine, liver, testis, and cancer cells. It contributes to limiting drug accumulation in tissues, expedites hepatobiliary elimination, regulates BBB, blood–testis barrier, and the maternal–fetal barrier, and controls oral bioavailability of a variety of compounds such as anticancer drugs (anthracyclines, topoisomerase I inhibitors, tyrosine kinase inhibitors), antiviral drugs, calcium channel blockers, and HMG-CoA reductase inhibitors. Physiological functions of BCRP include extrusion of

porphyrins from hematopoietic cells and hepatocytes, and secretion of vitamins (especially vitamin B_2) into breast milk. Because BCRP was originally identified from cancer cells and transports carcinogens and anticancer drugs, it is presumed to contribute to multidrug resistance, tumor development/progression, and tissue regeneration in stem cells. Recently, BCRP is considered as a possible genetic risk factor for gout because BCRP transports uric acid from the body.[21]

The ABCG2 gene is more than 66 kilobase (kb) in size, includes 16 exons, and is located on chromosome 4q22. BCRP is located on the apical membrane of intestine and acts to limit intestinal drug absorption. It is also expressed at the BBB and the blood–placental barrier and represents a barrier to entry into these tissues too. The substrate specificity and tissue localization of BCRP overlaps with that of P-gp that may consequently mask the diminished function of BCRP, whether due to drug–drug interactions or pharmacogenetic consequences. As a result, determining the significance of BCRP polymorphisms is challenging.

The ABCG2 gene has currently been reported to have 26 nonsynonymous, 5 synonymous, 3 nonsense, and 1 frameshift mutation.[22] However, most of these mutations are found from genome analysis, and the allelic frequency as well as in vitro/in vivo function has not been completed yet. Interestingly, one study suggested that there is no sex difference in intestinal BCRP in healthy human volunteers.[23] Another study suggested no effect of genetic polymorphism on intestinal BCRP protein and mRNA expression; however, BCRP protein expression was significantly higher in females.[24] The difference between the two studies could be the sites of biopsy because BCRP expression is reportedly higher in the duodenum and decreases continuously down to the colon.[25]

The nonsynonymous mutation c.421C>A (p.Q141K) is the most well studied and shows ethnic difference: allelic frequency is 2–5% in African American, 4–11% in European, 10% in Hispanic, 13% in Middle Eastern, 35% in Japanese, and 35% in Chinese descent.[24] Even if this genetic polymorphism does not clearly affect BCRP expression in the intestine, one study has reported that a carrier of this variant showed a decrease in BCRP protein expression in placenta.[26] An in vitro drug transport study using a c.421C>A ABCG2-transfected cell system suggested the c.421C>A (p.Q141K) variant decreased BCRP protein expression without altering intrinsic efflux clearance, but decreasing ATPase activity of BCRP.[27] The other well-studied ABCG2 mutation, c.34G>A (p.V12M), reported lower BCRP expression but no change of intrinsic clearance in an in vitro transfection study.[28]

Effect of ABCG2 Genetic Polymorphisms on Drug Pharmacokinetics

Two nonsynonymous (c.421C>A and c.34G>A) mutations have been extensively studied to reveal the clinical impact of BCRP (ABCG2). The c.421C>A variant was associated with increased plasma concentrations and AUCs of a variety of compounds such as sulfasalazine,[29] atorvastatin,[30] and simvastatin lactate.[31] However, this variant did not affect the pharmacokinetics of other substrate compounds such as irinotecan, SN-38,[32] SN-38 glucuronide, and pravastatin.[31]

The other common variant, c.34G>A, has also been reported in a clinical study, with patients haplotyped with the c.421C>A variant. An increased C_{max} and AUC of sulfasalazine suspension (AUC, 2.3-fold; C_{max}, 1.7-fold) was shown in patients with the 34GG/421CA haplotype compared with that in patients with the 34GG/421CC haplotype[25]; however, there was no change in any pharmacokinetic parameters of irinotecan[32] and lamivudine.[33]

Effect of ABCG2 Genetic Polymorphisms on Clinical Outcome

In contrast to the lack of pharmacokinetic changes, the c.421C>A variant contributed to decreased drug-induced adverse reactions on irinotecan administration. The variant c.421C>A might increase relative extent of glucuronidation as well as biliary elimination. The presence of both variants, c.421C>A and c.34G>A, did not affect SN-38 pharmacokinetics following irinotecan administration; however, these variants might be a predictive factor for grade 3 diarrhea.[32] Also for irinotecan administration, intronic variant, rs2622604, was associated with irinotecan-induced grade 3–4 myelosuppression.[34] The variants c.421C>A and IVS12+49G>T were moderately associated with irinotecan-induced neutropenia.[35] For gefitinib administration, the variant c.421C>A increased the prevalence of diarrhea induced by gefitinib probably due to decreased hepatobiliary elimination.[36] The variant c.421C>A was associated with grade 1–4 diarrhea with rituximab/cyclophosphamide/doxorubicin/vincristine/prednisone combination therapy.[37]

ORGANIC ANION-TRANSPORTING POLYPEPTIDE 1B1: SLCO1B1

The OATPs/SLCOs belong to the solute carrier (SLC) superfamily. They are expressed in a variety of different tissues and have a broad substrate spectrum including endogenously synthesized compounds (bile salts, steroids, hormones, and their conjugates) as well as several xenobiotics and widely prescribed drugs, such as HMG-CoA-reductase inhibitors (statins), antineoplastic agents, angiotensin II reductase inhibitors, and antibiotics. The SLCO/OATP family consists of 11 members, of which 10 are xenobiotic uptake transporters and 1 (SLCO2A1/OATP2A1) is a prostaglandin transporter. Most OATPs are expressed on the basolateral membrane of polarized cells such as brain capillary endothelial cells, kidney epithelial cells, and hepatocytes. Uptake transporters contribute to drug pharmacokinetics. For example, intestinal OATPs control absorption of weak lipophilic molecules in the body, whereas hepatic, kidney, and brain OATPs control and/or associate with tissue distribution, metabolism, and elimination of drugs. Therefore, understanding of OATP expression, function, and genetic polymorphisms is crucial in terms of suitable drug therapy management and preventing drug–drug interactions.

The SLCO1B1 gene is more that 141 kb in size, includes 15 exons, and is located on chromosome 12q. This gene is responsible for expression of OATP1B1, also known as OATP2, OATP-C, or liver-specific transporter 1 (LST-1). SLCO1B1 has been reported to have 41 nonsynonymous variants,[22] and some variants have shown decreased transport activity for estrone sulfate (ES) or estradiol-17β-D-glucuronide (E$_2$17βG) in in vitro cell studies.[38] One of the most well-known SNPs is c.521T>C (p.V174A) in exon 5 that causes a decrease in expression level of OATP1B1 on the basal membrane of hepatocytes and a decrease in hepatic uptake of ES, E$_2$17βG, rifampin, pravastatin, atorvastatin, rosuvastatin, and others. Large ethnic differences are reported in this mutation; allelic frequencies for Caucasians, African Americans, and Asians are 8–20%, 1–8%, and 8–16%, respectively.[39] Together with c.521T>C, the c.388A>G mutation in exon 4, which also has huge ethnic differences (Allelic frequency: Caucasians, 30–45%; African Americans, 72–83%; Asians, 59–86%), is also well studied as four distinct haplotypes, which are SLCO1B1*1A (c.388A–c.521T), SLCO1B1*1B (c.388G–c.521T), SLCO1B1*5 (c.388A–c.521C), and SLCO1B1*15 (c.388G–c.521C). Among these haplotypes, SLCO1B1*15 has been reported to have a decrease in drug uptake activity. On the other hand, results reported for SLCO1B1*1B are controversial. Because these 2 mutations are associated with 12 haplotypes (8 for c.388 and 4 for c.521), those contributions are significant for OATP1B1 expression and function. Other important nonsynonymous variants, which decrease transport activity, are c.217T>C (Allelic frequency: Caucasians, 0–2%), c.467A>G (Allelic frequency: Caucasians, 0–2%), c.1007C>G (Allelic frequency: Asians, 1%), c.1058T>C (Allelic frequency: Caucasians, 0–2%), c.1463G>C (Allelic frequency: African Americans, 3–9%), c.1964A>G (Allelic frequency: Caucasians, 0–2%), and c.2000A>G (Allelic frequency: Caucasians, 0–2%; African Americans, 0–34%).

Effect of SLCO1B1 Genetic Polymorphisms on Drug Pharmacokinetics

OATP1B1 (SLCO1B1) polymorphisms have been investigated in numerous clinical studies to determine their effect on substrate pharmacokinetics. Many of the clinical studies have investigated the OATP1B1*5 and *15 variants, both of which contain the c.521C>T mutation, and compared the result with OATP1B1*1A and/or *1B alleles. The c.521C>T polymorphism is associated with diminished transporter function. Consequently, individuals possessing the allele would likely transport less substrate from the blood into the hepatocyte across the sinusoidal membrane. The pharmacokinetic consequence of reduced hepatic uptake of substrate would be less hepatic clearance, by either metabolic processes or biliary transport, and a subsequent increase in the AUC (as exemplified by the basolateral transporter in Figures 7–2b and 7–3b).

Increased AUC values for repaglinide have been observed in individuals possessing reduced function OATP1B1 alleles. Niemi et al.[40] compared 521CC homozygotes with 521TT homozygotes and found that the AUC values for CC homozygotes were 188% higher than those for the TT homozygotes. Genetic polymorphisms of OATP1B1 have also been reported to lead to an increase in the AUC values for statin drugs, including pitavastatin and pravastatin. In an investigation of pitavastatin pharmacokinetics, individuals homozygous for the *15 allele demonstrated an AUC increase of 208% relative to individuals homozygous for the *1B allele.[41] Similarly, a study examining pitavastain pharmacokinetics in individuals homozygous for the OATP1B1 alleles *1A and *15 observed a 162% increase in the AUC for individuals homozygous for the *15 allele.[42] A 91% increase in the pravastatin AUC was seen in

c.521CC individuals compared with those homozygous for the *1A allele.[43] Other statins that are transported by OATP1B1, such as atorvastatin, rosuvastatin, and simvastatin, also show increases in AUC for the alleles associated with diminished transporter function.

The functional consequence of reduced function OATP1B1 alleles is not simply one of the changes in pharmacokinetics, but represents a safety issue as well. A study examining OATP1B1 variants and statin-induced myopathy found that the 521T>C mutation was associated with increased risk of statin-induced myopathy.[44] The CC homozygotes demonstrated an odds ratio for statin-induced myopathy of 16.9 relative to the TT homozygotes. Although OATP1B1 genotyping and dose adjustments have not been implemented at this time, there may be utility in doing so in the future.

Like reduced function alleles, drug interactions inhibiting OATP1B1 function would be expected to cause a decrease in the hepatic disposition and clearance, and a corresponding increase in plasma concentration and AUC of the substrate. The immunosuppressant cyclosporine A is an established perpetrator of drug–drug interactions with OATP1B1. For example, cyclosporine A increased the AUC of atorvastatin by up to 15-fold when given concomitantly.[45] However, because cyclosporine A inhibits not only OATP1B1 but also drug-metabolizing enzymes (CYPs 3A and 2C) as well as efflux transporters (P-gp, BCRP, and MRPs), the AUC increase due to concomitant dosing with cyclosporine A may not be limited to OATP1B1.

Summary

OATP1B1 is a hepatic transporter of organic anions. Because of its localization to the sinusoidal membrane of the hepatocyte, and its responsibility of translocating drugs from the blood into the hepatocyte, OATP1B1 has the potential to affect the pharmacokinetics of drugs cleared by the liver. As a consequence, for drugs that are transported by OATP1B1, OATP1B1 polymorphisms that reduce transport function may limit the cellular entry, and subsequently the metabolism or biliary clearance, of substrates.

BILE SALT EXPORT PUMP: ABCB11

The BSEP is the transporter mediating the canalicular step in the vectorial transport of bile salts from the systemic circulation into bile. Mutations in BSEP are associated with a subtype of progressive familial intrahepatic cholestasis (PFIC).[46] These mutations generally result in significantly reduced expression of BSEP leading to less efflux of bile salts into the bile canaliculus. Bile acids subsequently accumulate in the liver and systemic circulation and present as cholestasis. Similarly, reduced function of BSEP may also be associated with cholestatic drugs (cyclosporin A, troglitazone metabolites, and sulindac) that inhibit transporter function rather than reduce expression. However, BSEP has not demonstrated a significant capacity to transport therapeutic drugs and is generally not considered a significant transporter involved in the biliary clearance of drugs.

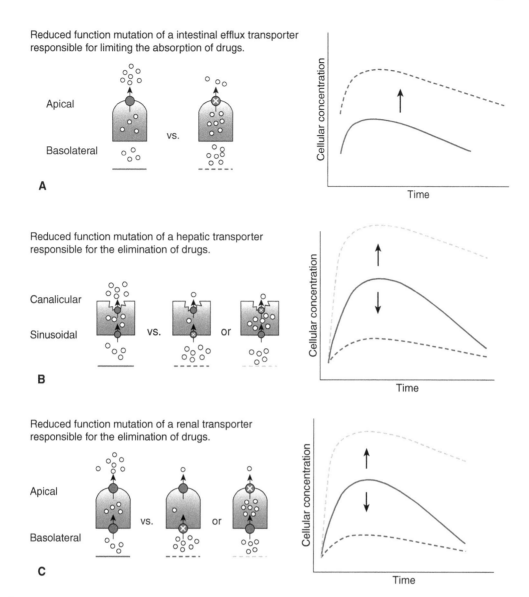

FIGURE 7–3 Illustrated mechanisms by which transporter polymorphisms mediate changes in the cellular concentration of drug. Examples of transporter polymorphisms and associated changes in plasma concentration for three representative tissues, small intestine (**A**), liver (**B**), and kidney (**C**), are provided. In each example the cell at the far left contains the normally functioning reference alleles. The subject's cells are illustrated to the right and demonstrate a reduced function/loss of function allele of a transporter expressed at the basolateral/sinusoidal or apical/canalicular membranes, respectively (represented as X in transporter). Corresponding changes in the cellular concentration of drug for the reduced function alleles are represented in the graph to the right. (Adapted from Ref.[1])

ORGANIC CATION TRANSPORTER 1: SLC22A1

OCT1 is a primary hepatic transporter of small organic cations. Because OCT1 transports a variety of therapeutic drugs, polymorphisms associated with OCT1 may have implications on the pharmacokinetics and the pharmacodyamics of drugs. An example of OCT1-associated polymorphisms being linked to the pharmacodynamics of a drug is illustrated by the drug metformin. Metformin targets a hepatic enzyme that ultimately represses hepatic glucose production. The passive cellular permeability of metformin is low; consequently, it is transported across membranes. Metformin, being of low molecular weight and weakly basic molecule (organic cation), is transported into hepatocytes by OCT1. The human OCT1 is polymorphic, a characteristic observed in ethnically diverse populations.

SLC22A1 is the gene responsible for the expression of the OCT1. It is approximately 48 kb in size; it includes 11 exons, and is located on chromosome 6q. Over 40 variants of OCT1 have been identified.[22] However, many have allelic frequencies of less than 1% and/or their impact on functional transport has not been elucidated. OCT1 variants having an allelic frequency of greater than 2% include R61C, P341L, M408V, and M420del, having allelic frequencies in the total population of 3%, 5%, 68%, and 11%, respectively.[47] Of the OCT1 variants that have been identified, the R61C, G401S, M420del, and G465R variants show reduced function in vitro and have been the most frequently studied in vivo. The G401S and G465R reduced function variants, although less frequent in the total population, occur at 1% and 4% in European Americans. Similarly, the R61C and M420del reduced function variants occur at a greater frequency in European Americans than in the population as a whole, 7–9% and 19%, respectively. These two SNPs also occur in the Mexican American population in significant numbers, 6% and 21%, respectively. By contrast, only the M420del mutation is seen with significant frequency in the African Americans population, 3%.[48]

Effect of SLC22A1 Genetic Polymorphisms on Drug Pharmacokinetics

Individuals carrying OCT1 reduced function variants (R61C, G401S, 420del, or G465R) show elevated metformin concentrations in the blood and higher AUC values.[49] Additionally, smaller volumes of distribution of metformin were seen in those with alleles associated with reduced OCT1 function when compared with those having the OCT1-reference allele. The elevated AUC value and the reduced volume of distribution stem from a compromised hepatic uptake of metformin in the individuals carrying variant alleles (as exemplified by the sinusoidal transporter in Figures 7–2b and 7–3b). The compromised function of OCT1 limits intercellular access to the liver, thus reducing volume of distribution. The increased AUC is a downstream effect of this limitation where a fraction of the metformin that would have otherwise distributed to the liver is shifted to the plasma and must be eliminated by other organs.

In addition to the relatively straightforward effect on OCT1-mediated drug disposition and pharmacokinetics seen with metformin, there can be interplay between transporters and liver metabolizing enzymes that represents more complicated mechanisms. Because entry of drug into the hepatocyte, by either transport or diffusion, must precede drug metabolism by the cytochromes P450, the localization of OCT1 to the sinusoidal membrane of the hepatocyte positions it as a gatekeeper to the metabolism of cationic drugs. For drugs that are transported by OCT1, and where the cellular accumulation of drug, by a combination of transport and diffusion, is less than its maximal rate of metabolism, transport will be the rate-limiting step. Thus, polymorphisms that result in reduced OCT1 function may correspondingly reduce the metabolic clearance of drug and change the pharmacokinetic/pharmacodynamic profile of the drug. Changes in the pharmacokinetics of tropisetron exemplify this.[50] A study investigating tropisetron demonstrated that patients possessing reduced function OCT1 variants (R61C, C88R, G401S, M420del, or G465R) have higher serum concentrations of tropisetron and coordinate improved drug efficacy. The mechanism surrounding the

increased serum concentrations was likely to be the result of decreased hepatic uptake of tropisetron and a corresponding reduction in metabolism. The cellular accumulation of tropisetron in individuals carrying reduced function OCT1 variants was limited; thus, the substrate availability to the metabolizing enzyme is correspondingly limited as well. The result was less metabolism of tropisetron, greater tropisetron plasma concentrations, and improved drug efficacy (reduced frequency of vomiting). Thus, carrier-mediated hepatic uptake of drugs by OCT1 may represent a rate-limiting step for the metabolism of some cationic drugs. The limitation may in turn lead to less metabolism and higher circulating concentrations of drug. The higher circulating concentrations may lead to end points of greater efficacy, such as those seen with tropisetron, or perhaps more deleterious end points, such as drug toxicity.

Effect of SLC22A1 Genetic Polymorphisms on Clinical Outcome

In a study investigating multiple nonsynonymous polymorphisms of OCT1 (OCT1-R61C, G401S, 420del, and G465R) a modulation of the therapeutic effect was observed.[51] In the in vivo study, human OCT1 polymorphisms investigated were associated with a diminished clinical response to metformin. The investigators measured plasma glucose concentrations in individuals homozygous for the reference OCT1 sequence and individuals possessing at least one reduced function allele following an oral glucose tolerance test prior to and after metformin treatment. The individuals homozygous for the OCT1 reference sequence had significantly lower blood glucose level compared with those with reduced function alleles when both groups were treated with metformin. In the absence of metformin treatment no difference was seen. The study provides evidence that genetic variation in OCT1 may modulate the cellular accumulation of metformin in the liver and correspondingly contribute to variation in metformin pharmacodynamics between individuals. This mechanism may extend to the pharmacodynamic variation seen in other low-molecular-weight cationic drugs requiring significant liver disposition for therapeutic response (as exemplified by the sinusoidal transporter in Figure 7–3b).

Summary

OCT1 is a primary hepatic transporter of small organic cations. Due to its localization to the liver, and its responsibility of translocating drugs from blood into the hepatocyte, OCT1 has the potential to affect the pharmacodynamics of liver-targeted drugs and the pharmacokinetics of drugs cleared by the liver. For drugs that are transported by OCT1 and targeted to the liver, where the target is intracellular, OCT1 polymorphisms that reduce transport function may limit the cellular entry and the efficacy of the drug as was demonstrated for metformin. For drugs transported by OCT1 that are predominately cleared by the liver, by either transport mechanisms or metabolism, reduced function variants of OCT1 may limit clearance like that seen with metformin and tropisetron.

ORGANIC CATION TRANSPORTER 2: SLC22A2

The OCT2 is a major renal transporter of organic cations. Because OCT2 transports a variety of therapeutic drugs, polymorphisms associated with OCT2 may have implications on drug pharmacokinetics. Similar to OCT1, OCT2 also transports metformin. Metformin is not metabolized by the body and is largely excreted in the urine as the unchanged molecule. It has a renal clearance that is substantially greater than the glomerular filtration rate suggesting that it is actively secreted by the kidney and undergoes negligible reabsorption. It has been established that OCT2 contributes to the secretion of metformin.

SLC22A2 is the gene responsible for the expression of the OCT2. It is approximately 55 kb in size; it includes 11 exons, and is located on chromosome 6q. Over 30 variants of OCT2 have been identified. However, the majority have allelic frequencies of less than 1%. Nonsynonymous OCT2 variants having an allelic frequency of greater than 1% in at least one ethnic group include 495G>A, 808G>T, 1198C>T, and 1294A>C, having allelic frequencies in the total population of 0.4%, 13%, 0.6%, and 0.6%, respectively.[52] Of these, the 495G>A, 1198C>T, and 1294A>C variants appear to be largely confined to individuals of European descent, whereas the 808G>T variant ranges in frequency from 7% to 16% and appears to be present in all ethnic backgrounds investigated. Two other unique variants have been identified in the Korean population, 596C>T and 602C>T, both at frequencies of 0.7%. The 602C>T is also found in the Vietnamese population (1.5%). All the aforementioned OCT2 variants have been associated with reduced protein function in vitro.

Effect of SLC22A2 Genetic Polymorphisms on Drug Pharmacokinetics

The renal clearance of metformin is subject to interindividual variability and genetic variation seems to contribute to this variability. Reduced function variants of OCT2 would be expected to transport less metformin from the blood into renal cells and correspondingly reduce the renal clearance of metformin (as exemplified by the basolateral transporter in Figures 7–2c and 7–3c). One study identified three genetic variants of OCT2 (596C>T, p.T199I; 602C>T, p.T201M; and 808G>T, p.A270S) that were associated with lower renal clearance of metformin.[53] The reduced renal clearance resulted in anticipated changes in the pharmacokinetic parameters of metformin—elevated peak plasma concentrations and higher area under the curve values. The in vivo function of the variants may not be completely understood at this point, however. Another study that investigated the effects of the 808G>T variant on pharmacokinetics found that the 808G>T variant was associated with greater rates of renal secretory clearance, relative to individually possessing the reference sequence.[54] The investigators attributed the increased clearance to higher levels of expression of the 808G>T variant, relative to the reference sequence. Mechanistically, higher expression levels of the variant could lead to greater rates of clearance even in the face of reduced function provided that the increase in expression was large enough to overcome the reduced function. Trials investigating OCT2 pharmacogenomics with larger numbers of patients should resolve the discrepancy observed between the two studies.

Effect of SCL22A2 Genetic Polymorphisms on Clinical Outcome

In addition to variability associated with pharmacokinetic and pharmacodynamic parameters, drug toxicity represents yet another challenge. Because transporters are able to mediate the cellular uptake of drugs, they may facilitate toxicological outcomes. Genetic differences in transporters may contribute to differences in toxicological end points seen in individuals. Because OCT2 transports a variety of therapeutic drugs, the polymorphisms associated with OCT2 may have implications on drug toxicity in the kidney.

The platinum-based anticancer therapeutic, cisplatin, is a substrate of OCT2. In vivo, OCT2 is responsible for the transport of cisplatin from the blood, across the basolateral membrane, into the cells of the renal proximal tubule. Nephrotoxicity is associated with cisplatin-based chemotherapy and doses may be limited due to the associated toxicity.

It has been demonstrated that individuals possessing a reduced function variant of OCT2 (808G>T) have a reduced risk of cisplatin-induced nephrotoxicity.[55] Cancer patients possessing the 808G>T polymorphism, a reduced function/expression variant, experienced no significant change in serum creatinine after the first cycle of cisplatin treatment. In contrast patients possessing the reference allele showed indications of renal damage, as indicated by an increase in serum creatinine. The renal damage associated with the reference allele is consistent with the transport of cisplatin. The urinary excretion of cisplatin is dependent on OCT2-mediated transport of cisplatin into the proximal tubule. Thus, an OCT2 variant associated with reduced accumulation of organic cations in the proximal tubule would be expected to transport less cisplatin into the tubule and correspondingly produce less toxicity (as exemplified by the basolateral transporter in Figure 7–3c). The role of OCT2 in cisplatin-related nephrotoxicity and the observed differences in toxicity associated with polymorphisms suggest that OCT2 contributes to the interindividual variation in cisplatin tolerability and perhaps other drugs. Furthermore, it is consistent with changes observed in the pharmacokinetic response indicated above.

Summary

OCT2 is the primary renal transporter of small organic cations. Due to its localization to the kidney, and its responsibility of translocating drugs from blood across the basolateral membrane into proximal tubule cells, OCT2 has the potential to affect the pharmacokinetics of drugs secreted by the nephron. Furthermore, for drugs that are transported by OCT2, OCT2 polymorphisms that reduce transport function may limit the cellular entry and the toxicity of substrates as was demonstrated for cisplatin.

MULTIDRUG AND TOXIN EXTRUSION 1: SLC47A1

MATE1 is the apical complement to the organic cation transporters, OCT1 and OCT2, found on the basolateral membrane of hepatocytes and proximal tubular cells, respectively. Like OCT1 and OCT2, MATE1 also transports metformin and other similar substrates and together the paired transporters contribute to the transepithelial transport of organic cations. Thus, similar to OCT1 and OCT2, MATE1 polymorphisms that reduce expression or function would be expected to result in reduced clearance of substrates, such as metformin, because of a limitation in transport from the cell into the bile canaliculus or the lumen of the proximal tubule (as exemplified by the canalicular/apical transporter in Figure 7–2b and c).

MATE1 is the gene responsible for the expression of the multidrug and toxin extruder transporter 1. It is approximately 59 kb in size; it includes 17 exons, and is located on chromosome 17p. Because MATE1 is a recently discovered transporter, relatively few MATE1 pharmacogenetic investigations have been conducted. One study identified six nonsynonymous SNPs in MATE1.[56] Of these six nonsynonymous variants, three, L125F, V338I, and C497S, had population-specific frequencies of greater than 2%. The L125F, V338I, and C497S variants were found in Mexican Americans, African Americans, and Chinese Americans at frequencies of 5%, 5%, and 2%, respectively. Additionally, the three polymorphisms demonstrated substrate-specific changes in transport function in vitro. However, the pharmacogenetic impact of L125F, V338I, and C497S polymorphisms on in vivo drug pharmacokinetics has not been investigated at this time.

Effect of MATE1 Genetic Polymorphisms on Drug Pharmacokinetics

Indirect evidence of reduced clearance associated with a MATE1 polymorphism would be an increased therapeutic response caused by elevated levels of drug. One study investigated the effects of the MATE1 polymorphism rs2289669 on HbA1c (glycosylated hemoglobin) levels in blood in patients taking metformin.[57] Patients possessing the rs2289669 polymorphism had lower HbA1c levels compared with those with the reference allele. The proposed mechanism for the decreased HbA1c levels was that the identified MATE1 polymorphism impaired metformin pharmacokinetics resulting in increased plasma, or hepatic levels of metformin. Consequently, the therapeutic effect was elevated producing better control of blood glucose and less glycosylation of hemoglobin.

The particular polymorphism investigated, rs2289669, is located in an intron and therefore does not result in an amino acid change in the MATE1 protein. Thus, the polymorphism may be associated with reduced gene expression or perhaps may be in linkage disequilibrium with a polymorphism that is associated with MATE1 function. Further pharmacokinetic studies of the pharmacogenetic impact of MATE1 are necessary to validate this study and establish its role in influencing drug pharmacokinetics.

Summary

MATE1 is a renal transporter of small organic cations. Due to its localization to the apical membrane of renal proximal tubule cells and canalicular membrane of hepatocytes, MATE1 has the potential to affect the pharmacokinetics of drugs secreted by the nephron or hepatocyte. Drugs transported by MATE1 may undergo increases in plasma concentration, AUC, and cytosolic concentrations in individuals possessing reduced function alleles when compared with those in individuals possessing active alleles (as exemplified by the canalicular/apical transporter in Figures 7–2b and c and 7–3b and c). This represents a difference between MATE1 and the corresponding basolateral organic cation transporters OCT1 and OCT2, where a reduced function polymorphism associated with MATE1 could potentially increase the cellular concentration of drug, whereas similar mutations in OCT1 or OCT2 would limit drug uptake into the cell.

ORGANIC ANION TRANSPORTERS 1 (SLC22A6) AND 3 (SLC22A8)

Both OAT1 and OAT3 mediate the basolateral transport of low-molecular-weight organic anions into cells of the renal proximal tubule. Substrates for OATs include the drugs methotrexate, penicillin, adefovir, and furosemide. Yet despite their role in the renal elimination of drugs, no OAT1 and OAT3 polymorphism that significantly impacts the clinical pharmacokinetics or pharmacodyamics of drugs has yet been identified. Polymorphisms of OAT1 have been investigated in vivo.[58] However, the single SNP identified by Fujita et al. with reduced function (a nonfunctional variant) showed no impact on the clearance of adefovir in heterozygous patients. Therefore, it remains unknown whether or not clinically significant polymorphisms of OAT1 or OAT3 exist; however, it does not eliminate the possibility that polymorphisms of OAT1 or OAT3 that affect drug pharmacokinetics will be identified.

CONCLUSION AND FUTURE PERSPECTIVES

The membrane transporters discussed in this chapter play important roles in drug disposition and response. Many genetic variants in these transporters have been discovered leading to changes in drug concentration or effect. Although no clinical guidance exists to individualize therapy for specific patient populations, our knowledge in this area has increased tremendously. Drug disposition and the resultant response to therapy are complex processes involving multiple transporters in the intestine, liver, and kidney, interplay with drug-metabolizing enzymes, drug–receptor interactions, drug–drug interactions, and environmental and genetic influences. It is critical that clinicians understand how variations in all of these processes contribute to an individual's response to therapy. Understanding these influences a priori will allow more optimal drug utilization and avoidance of adverse drug events. Future advances in this area will further enhance our ability to provide optimal therapeutic care to patients.

REFERENCES

1. Giacomini KM, Sugiyama Y. Membrane transporters and drug response. In: Brunton LL, Chabner BA, Knollman BC, eds. *Goodman & Gilman's The Pharmacological Basis of Therapeutics*. 12th ed. New York: McGraw-Hill Medical; 2011.

2. The International Transporter Consortium. Membrane transporters in drug development. *Nat Rev Drug Discov.* 2010;9:215–236.

3. Sadeque AJ, Wandel C, He H, Shah S, Wood AJ. Increased drug delivery to the brain by P-glycoprotein inhibition. *Clin Pharmacol Ther.* 2000;68:231–237.

4. Zolnerciks JK, Booth-Genthe CL, Gupta A, Harris J, Unadkat JD. Substrate- and species-dependent inhibition of p-glycoprotein-mediated transport: implications for predicting in vivo drug interactions. *J Pharm Sci.* 2011;100(8):3055–3061.

5. Wu C-Y, Benet LZ. Unmasking the dynamic interplay between efflux transporters and metabolic enzymes. *Int J Pharm.* 2004;277:3–9.

6. Cascorbi I. P-glycoprotein: tissue distribution, substrates, and functional consequences of genetic variations. *Handb Exp Pharmacol.* 2011;201:261–283.

7. Kimchi-Sarfaty C, Oh JM, Kim IW, et al. A "silent" polymorphism in the MDR1 gene changes substrate specificity. *Science.* 2007;315:525–528.

8. Hoffmeyer S, Burk O, von Richter O, et al. Functional polymorphisms of the human multidrug-resistance gene: multiple sequence variations and correlation of one allele with P-glycoprotein expression and activity in vivo. *Proc Natl Acad Sci U S A.* 2000;97:3473–3478.

9. Verstuyft C, Schwab M, Schaeffeler E, et al. Digoxin pharmacokinetics and MDR1 genetic polymorphisms. *Eur J Clin Pharmacol.* 2003;58:809–812.

10. Gerloff T, Schaefer M, Johne A, et al. MDR1 genotypes do not influence the absorption of a single oral dose of 1 mg digoxin in healthy white males. *Br J Clin Pharmacol.* 2002;54:610–616.

11. Leschziner GD, Andrew T, Pirmohamed M, Johnson MR. ABCB1 genotype and pgp expression, function and therapeutic drug response: a critical review and recommendations for future research. *Pharmacogenomics J.* 2007;7:154–179.

12. Kurata Y, Ieiri I, Kimura M, et al. Role of human MDR1 gene polymorphism in bioavailability and interaction of digoxin, a substrate of P-glycoprotein. *Clin Pharmacol Ther.* 2002;72:209–219.

13. Johne A, Köpke K, Gerloff T, et al. Modulation of steady-state kinetics of digoxin by haplotypes of the P-glycoprotein MDR1 gene. *Clin Pharmacol Ther.* 2002;72:584–594.

14. Morita N, Yasumori T, Nakayama K. Human MDR1 polymorphism: G2677T/A and C3435T have no effect on MDR1 transport activities. *Biochem Pharmacol.* 2003;65:1843–1852.

15. Haufroid V, Mourad M, Van Kerckhove V, et al. The effect of CYP3A and MDR1 (ABCB1) polymorphisms on cyclosporine and tacrolimus dose requirements and trough blood levels in stable renal transplant patients. *Pharmacogenetics.* 2004;14:147–154.

16. Anglicheau D, Le Corre D, Lechaton S, et al. Consequences of genetic polymorphisms for sirolimus requirements after renal transplant in patients on primary sirolimus therapy. *Am J Transplant.* 2005;5:595–603.

17. Zheng H, Schuetz E, Zeevi A, et al. Sequential analysis of tacrolimus dosing in adult lung transplant patients with ABCB1 haplotypes. *J Clin Pharmacol.* 2005;45:404–410.

18. Fellay J, Marzolini C, Maeden ER, et al. Response to antiretroviral treatment in HIV-1 infected individuals with allelic variants of the multidrug resistance transporter 1: a pharmacogenetics study. *Lancet.* 2002;359:30–36.

19. Haas DW, Smeaton LM, Shafer RW, et al. Pharmacogenetics of long-term responses to antiretroviral regimens containing efavirenz and/or nelfinavir: an Adult Aids Clinical Trials Group Study. *J Infect Dis.* 2005;192:1931–1942.

20. Amstutz U, Carleton BC. Pharmacogenetic testing: time for clinical practice guidelines. *Clin Pharmacol Ther.* 2011;89:924–927.

21. Woodward OM, Köttgen A, Coresh J, Boerwinkle E, Guggino WB, Köttgen M. Identification of a urate transporter, ABCG2, with a common functional polymorphism causing gout. *Proc Natl Acad Sci U S A.* 2009;106:10338–10342.

22. The International HapMap Consortium. A second generation human haplotype map of over 3.1 million SNPs. *Nature.* 2007;449:851–862.

23. Gutmann H, Hruz P, Zimmermann C, Beglinger C, Drewe J. Distribution of breast cancer resistance protein (BCRP/ABCG2) mRNA expression along the human GI tract. *Biochem Pharmacol.* 2005;70:695–699.

24. Zamber CP, Lamba JK, Yasuda K, et al. Natural allelic variants of breast cancer resistance protein (BCRP) and their relationship to BCRP expression in human intestine. *Pharmacogenetics.* 2003;13:19–28.

25. Urquhart BL, Ware JA, Tirona RG, et al. Breast cancer resistance protein (ABCG2) and drug disposition: intestinal expression, polymorphisms and sulfasalazine as an in vivo probe. *Pharmacogenet Genomics.* 2008;18:439–448.

26. Kobayashi D, Ieiri I, Hirota T, et al. Functional assessment of ABCG2 (BCRP) gene polymorphisms to protein expression in human placenta. *Drug Metab Dispos.* 2005;33:94–101.

27. Mizuarai S, Aozasa N, Kotani H. Single nucleotide polymorphisms result in impaired membrane localization and reduced atpase activity in multidrug transporter ABCG2. *Int J Cancer.* 2004;109:238–246.

28. Tamura A, Watanabe M, Saito H, et al. Functional validation of the genetic polymorphisms of human ATP-binding cassette (ABC) transporter ABCG2: identification of alleles that are defective in porphyrin transport. *Mol Pharmacol.* 2006;70:287–296.

29. Yamasaki Y, Ieiri I, Kusuhara H, et al. Pharmacogenetic characterization of sulfasalazine disposition based on NAT2 and ABCG2 (BCRP) gene polymorphisms in humans. *Clin Pharmacol Ther.* 2008;84:95–103.

30. Keskitalo JE, Zolk O, Fromm MF, Kurkinen KJ, Neuvonen PJ, Niemi M. ABCG2 polymorphism markedly affects the pharmacokinetics of atorvastatin and rosuvastatin. *Clin Pharmacol Ther.* 2009;86:197–203.

31. Keskitalo JE, Pasanen MK, Neuvonen PJ, Niemi M. Different effects of the ABCG2 c.421C>A SNP on the pharmacokinetics of fluvastatin, pravastatin and simvastatin. *Pharmacogenomics.* 2009;10:1617–1624.

32. Han JY, Lim HS, Park YH, Lee SY, Lee JS. Integrated pharmacogenetic prediction of irinotecan pharmacokinetics and toxicity in patients with advanced non-small cell lung cancer. *Lung Cancer.* 2009;63:115–120.

33. Kim HS, Sunwoo YE, Ryu JY, et al. The effect of ABCG2 V12M, Q141K and Q126X, known functional variants in vitro, on the disposition of lamivudine. *Br J Clin Pharmacol.* 2007;64:645–654.

34. Cha PC, Mushiroda T, Zembutsu H, et al. Single nucleotide polymorphism in ABCG2 is associated with irinotecan-induced severe myelosuppression. *J Hum Genet.* 2009;54:572–580.

35. Sai K, Saito Y, Meekawa K, et al. Additive effects of drug transporter genetic polymorphisms on irinotecan pharmacokinetics/pharmacodynamics in Japanese cancer patients. *Cancer Chemother Pharmacol.* 2010;66:95–105.

36. Cusatis G, Gregorc V, Li J, et al. Pharmacogenetics of ABCG2 and adverse reactions to gefitinib. *J Natl Cancer Inst.* 2006;98:1739–1742.

37. Kim IS, Kim HG, Kim DC, et al. ABCG2 Q141K polymorphism is associated with chemotherapy-induced diarrhea in patients with diffuse large B-cell lymphoma who received frontline rituximab plus cyclophosphamide/doxorubicin/vincristine/prednisone chemotherapy. *Cancer Sci.* 2008;99:2496–2501.

38. Tirona RG, Leake BF, Merino G, Kim RB. Polymorphisms in OATP-C: identification of multiple allelic variants associated with altered transport activity among European- and African-Americans. *J Biol Chem.* 2001;276:35669–35675.

39. Pasanen MK, Neuvonen M, Niemi M. Global analysis of genetic variation in SLCO1B1. *Pharmacogenomics.* 2008;9:19–33.

40. Niemi M, Backman JT, Kajosaari LI, et al. Polymorphic organic anion transporting polypeptide 1B1 is a major determinant of repaglinide pharmacokinetics. *Clin Pharmacol Ther.* 2005;77:468–478.

41. Ieiri I, Suwannakul S, Maeda K, et al. SLCO1B1 (OATP1B1, an uptake transporter) and ABCG2 (BCRP, an efflux transporter) variant alleles and pharmacokinetics of pitavastatin in healthy volunteers. *Clin Pharmacol Ther.* 2007;85:541–547.

42. Deng JW, Song IS, Shin HJ, et al. The effect of SLCO1B1*15 on the disposition of pravastatin and pitavastatin is substrate dependent: the contribution of transporting activity changes by SLCO1B1*15. *Pharmacogenet Genomics.* 2008;18:424–433.

43. Niemi M, Pasanen MK, Neuvonen PJ. SLCO1B1 polymorphism and sex affect the pharmacokinetics of pravastatin but not fluvastatin. *Clin Pharmacol Ther.* 2006;80:356–366.

44. SEARCH Collaborative Group, Link E, Parish S, et al. SLCO1B1 variants and statin-induced myopathy—a genomewide study. *N Engl J Med.* 2008;359: 789–799.

45. Lemahieu WPD, Hermann M, Asberg A, et al. Combined therapy with atorvastatin and calcineurin inhibitors: no interactions with tacrolimus. *Am J Transplant.* 2005;5:2236–2243.

46. Wang L, Soroka CJ, Boyer JL. The role of bile salt export pump mutations in progressive familial intrahepatic cholestasis type II. *J Clin Invest.* 2002; 110:965–972.

47. Shu Y, Leabman MK, Feng B, et al. Evolutionary conservation predicts function of variants of the human organic cation transporter, OCT1. *Proc Natl Acad Sci U S A.* 2003;100:5902–5907.

48. Leabman MK, Huang CC, DeYoung J, et al. Natural variation in human membrane transporter genes reveals evolutionary and functional constraints. *Proc Natl Acad Sci U S A.* 2003;100:5896–5901.

49. Shu Y, Brown C, Castro RA, et al. Effect of genetic variation in the organic cation transporter 1, OCT1, on metformin pharmacokinetics. *Clin Pharmacol Ther.* 2008;83:273–280.

50. Tzvetkov MV, Saadatmand AR, Bokelmann K, Meineke I, Kaiser R, Brockmöller J. Effects of OCT1 polymorphisms on the cellular uptake, plasma concentrations and efficacy of the 5-HT3 antagonists tropisetron and ondansetron. *Pharmacogenomics J.* 2012;12:22–29.

51. Shu Y, Sheardown SA, Brown C, et al. Effect of genetic variation in the organic cation transporter 1 (OCT1) on metformin action. *J Clin Invest.* 2007;117: 1422–1431.

52. Leabman MK, Huang CC, Kawamoto M, et al. Polymorphisms in a human kidney xenobiotic transporter, OCT2, exhibit altered function. *Pharmacogenetics.* 2002;12:395–405.

53. Song IS, Shin HJ, Shim EJ, et al. Genetic variants of the organic cation transporter 2 influence the disposition of metformin. *Clin Pharmacol Ther.* 2008; 84:559–562.

54. Chen Y, Li S, Brown C, et al. Effect of genetic variation in the organic cation transporter 2 on the renal elimination of metformin. *Pharmacogenet Genomics.* 2009;19:497–504.

55. Filipski KK, Mathijssen RH, Mikkelsen TS, Schinkel AH, Sparreboom A. Contribution of organic cation transporter 2 (OCT2) to cisplatin-induced nephrotoxicity. *Clin Pharmacol Ther.* 2009;86:396–402.

56. Chen Y, Teranishi K, Li S, et al. Genetic variants in multidrug and toxic compound extrusion-1, hMATE1, alter transport function. *Pharmacogenomics J.* 2009;9:127–136.

57. Becker ML, Visser LE, van Schaik RH, Hofman A, Uitterlinden AG, Stricker BH. Interaction between polymorphisms in the OCT1 and MATE1 transporter and metformin response. *Pharmacogenet Genomics.* 2010;20: 38–44.

58. Fujita T, Brown C, Carlson EJ, et al. Functional analysis of polymorphisms in the organic anion transporter, SLC22A6 (OAT1). *Pharmacogenet Genomics.* 2005;15:201–209.

Nongenetic Influences on Drug Metabolism

8

Shirley K. Seo, PhD, & Anne N. Nafziger, MD, PhD, MHS

LEARNING OBJECTIVES

- Understand important intrinsic and extrinsic nongenetic factors that can affect phase I and phase II drug metabolism.

- Be able to identify and recognize clinically important metabolism-based interactions.

- Understand the mechanisms of CYP inhibition and induction.

BACKGROUND

The main goal of successful drug therapy is to ensure that a patient receives safe and effective drug treatment. Therapeutic drug concentrations need to be achieved to accomplish this goal. A solid understanding of the factors that can affect drug disposition is critical in achieving appropriate drug concentrations (Figure 8–1). Drug dose or dosing frequency may need to be modified according to changes in drug biotransformation or excretion caused by intrinsic or extrinsic factors. In this chapter, intrinsic and extrinsic factors known to affect metabolism, with a particular focus on cytochromes P450 (a principal component of drug-metabolizing enzymes), will be discussed.

INTRINSIC FACTORS

Aging

A plethora of research focuses on age-based differences in drug metabolism. In pediatric patients, changes in the ontogeny of drug-metabolizing enzymes account for many of the differences in drug disposition between children and adults. Studies show differential expression patterns of CYP enzymes in neonates, infants, children, and adolescents.[1] Developmental changes such

as changes in gastric acid production, gastric emptying, renal function, pancreatic function, body composition, and total body water also play a role in the evolving absorption, distribution, metabolism, and excretion processes in infants and children. These developmental changes contribute to variability in drug disposition in the pediatric population.[2]

On the other side of the age spectrum are the elderly, who are generally described as those aged 65 years or older. In the elderly population, the aging process may involve a progressive decrease in organ and tissue function (in particular, the kidney) that can lead to altered drug disposition. Although liver size and hepatic blood flow generally decrease with age, routine clinical tests of liver function reveal that hepatic function does not change significantly.[3] In addition, in vitro studies investigating CYP enzyme activity in human hepatocytes find no differences in the activities of the 10 most predominant CYP isoforms between the age groups of 20–60 and above 60 years.[4] In clinical studies, the effect of age on CYP enzymes appears to be isoform-dependent. Plasma paroxetine concentrations were evaluated in depressed patients aged 69–95 years and no age-related changes in paroxetine disposition (metabolized by *CYP2D6*) were detected.[5] In studies involving the clearance of antipyrine (metabolized by *CYP3A4 and CYP3A5* [*collectively referred to as "CYP3A4/5" due to their high degree of homology and function*], *CYP1A2, CYP2C8, and CYP2C9*), an

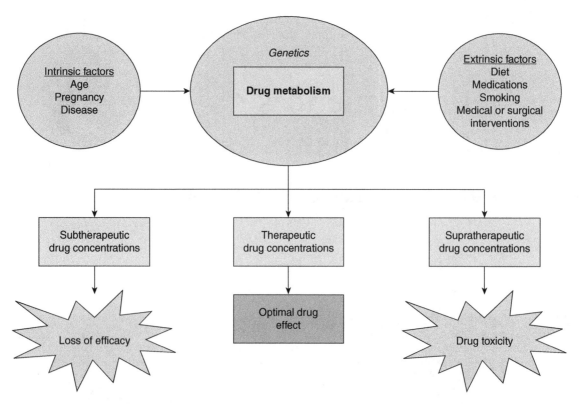

FIGURE 8–1 Intrinsic and extrinsic factors can influence the pharmacokinetics of a drug. The changes in drug clearance that occur can result in subtherapeutic, therapeutic, or supratherapeutic drug concentrations that in turn can lead to optimal drug effect or undesired drug effects.

approximate 20–25% decline in antipyrine clearance is observed between ages 25 and 76 years.[6] Therefore, although some loss of drug-metabolizing enzyme function may occur with extreme aging, the changes are not dramatic and are isoform-specific.

Pregnancy

Pregnancy results in major physiological changes in a woman's body. These include increased blood volume, increased water composition, increased urinary output, reduced intestinal motility, increased gastric pH, and changes in sex hormone concentrations. Because any of these factors can contribute to significant changes in the absorption, distribution, metabolism, and excretion of drugs, specific changes to CYP-mediated metabolism are difficult to discern. In studies measuring the ratio of excreted parent drug to metabolite, the metabolic ratio increases for *CYP1A2* and *CYP2C19* substrates, indicating lower activities for these isozymes.[47] Conversely, metabolic ratios decrease for *CYP2C9*, *CYP2D6*, and *CYP3A4/5*, indicating higher activities for these isozymes.[47] Examples of drugs that may require dose modification during pregnancy because of changes in hepatic drug metabolism include methadone, nifedipine, and lamotrigine.[48] Since potentially lifesaving drugs may be necessary during pregnancy, these changes in drug-metabolizing enzyme activities should be taken into consideration when determining appropriate drug doses. However, there are few, if any, well-controlled clinical studies that have resulted in specific product dosing recommendations for pregnancy. Additional peripartum

and postpartum changes in drug metabolism can also occur,[48] but too few data are available to make general recommendations about alteration of drug therapy in these settings.

EXTRINSIC FACTORS

Diseases

Numerous disease states can affect drug disposition. The mechanisms by which drug disposition is altered by disease can result from direct physiological changes or alterations in major drug-metabolizing enzymes. The liver and kidney are the two primary organs affecting drug metabolism and excretion, and the effects of diseases on the liver and kidney will be discussed in the next section. The reader should bear in mind that other organ systems may also be affected, although these will not be discussed in this chapter.

Inflammation and Cytokines

Infectious diseases have long been recognized to alter hepatic CYP expression and activity. In 1978, Chang et al. first described higher theophylline half-lives in asthmatic children with confirmed upper respiratory tract infection caused by influenza A or adenovirus.[7] This key report illustrated that infection can cause clinically significant alterations in drug disposition and suggested that changes in drug-metabolizing enzymes could be affected by the state of infection. Subsequent research in a mouse model showed that inflammation caused by infection causes production of a bacterial endotoxin (lipopolysaccharide [LPS]) that leads to down-regulation of CYP enzyme mRNA levels and activities that may vary during the course of infection.[8]

Inflammation is an essential component of the innate immune response to pathogens and tissue damage. The inflammatory process is mediated by cytokines, a group of secreted polypeptides that include interleukins (IL), interferons (IFN), tumor necrosis factors (TNF), and chemokines. The effect of inflammation on CYP enzymes in vitro and in vivo has been extensively reviewed.[9–11] In particular, IL-1, IL-6, IFNs, and bacterial LPS cause decreased hepatic CYP expression.[12] Coupled with the systemic release of cytokines, the liver responds to inflammation by increasing synthesis and secretion of acute-phase proteins such as fibrinogen, α1-acid glycoprotein, and C-reactive protein.[13] Cytokine cascades are known to influence inflammatory and anti-inflammatory responses in multiple disease states, can be involved in both acute and chronic inflammation, and alter the pharmacokinetics or pharmacodynamics of numerous drugs.[14] One example of a clinical impact on drug metabolism is when CYP enzyme activity is markedly decreased during allograft rejection.[15] The impairment of CYP activity in biopsy samples is attributed to an increase in the intragraft production of proinflammatory cytokines. In another example, melanoma patients treated with high-dose IFN therapy have greater than 60% suppression of CYP1A2 activity.[16]

More recently, cancer has been recognized as a disease state that can alter CYP-mediated drug metabolism. Many cancers involve the continued release of cytokines, such as TNF-α, IFN-α, IL-4, IL-6, IL-8, IL-10, IL-12, and IL-17, that are involved in tumor cell proliferation, angiogenesis, metastasis, and adaptive immunity.[17] Through the intermediate event of increased cytokine release, cancer can indirectly decrease hepatic CYP expression. Other physiological states, such as acute pain[18] and depression,[19] have also been shown to result in alterations in pharmacokinetics and pharmacodynamic responses. Since the acute-phase response involves cytokine release and inflammation, disease states with an acute-phase response may affect drug pharmacokinetics.

Chronic Liver Disease

The hallmark of chronic liver disease is gradual destruction of liver tissue that leads to fibrosis and hepatic cirrhosis. Fibrosis is the growth of scar tissue due to infection, inflammation, injury, or healing and frequently results in cirrhosis. Cirrhosis is characterized by lowered hepatic blood flow and eventual loss of liver function. Causes of liver disease include, but are not limited to, viral infections, xenobiotics, excessive alcohol consumption, metabolic disorders, and autoimmune disorders.

Although the exact mechanisms by which liver disease affects hepatic drug disposition are unknown, researchers have postulated four main mechanisms: reduced hepatocyte content and activity of metabolizing enzymes, decreased cell mass, reduced drug uptake, and diminished oxygen uptake.[20] The mechanism that affects a particular drug's disposition also depends on that drug's clearance characteristics. As blood flow can be a major determinant of drug clearance, drugs with a high extraction ratio (such as lidocaine) are most likely to have clearance affected by both decrease in metabolic activity and a decline in functional hepatic perfusion. However, in drugs with a low hepatic extraction ratio, the most likely cause of lowered hepatic clearance is decreased metabolic activity or protein binding.

Differences in drug disposition as a result of liver impairment have been demonstrated.[21] Theoretically, any chronic disease that significantly affects liver function can affect the disposition of a drug that is highly dependent on hepatic drug metabolism for elimination. However, the occurrence of impaired hepatic drug metabolism is dependent on the type and severity of liver disease. In liver cirrhosis, hepatic drug clearance is generally reduced in proportion to the degree of liver dysfunction.[20] Particular consideration should be given to drugs that target the liver, such as treatments for viral hepatitis. These drugs may be a substrate for one or more hepatic CYP enzymes as well as hepatic transporters whose function can also be affected by chronic liver disease. In patients with liver disease of varying degrees and from various etiologies, the metabolizing activities of CYP1A2, CYP2C19, CYP2D6, and CYP2E1 decrease with increasing severity of liver disease.[22] However, the degree to which activity is lowered is specific to each CYP isozyme.[22,23] Hepatic metabolic capacity usually remains intact because of multiple compensatory responses until advanced cirrhosis develops. Although there are some drugs that require dose reduction in the setting of moderate cirrhosis (e.g., morphine, verapamil, nifedipine, losartan, omeprazole), dosing adjustments are typically not required except in the setting of advanced cirrhosis.[22]

Chronic Kidney Disease

Chronic kidney disease is characterized by the gradual loss of renal function. One method of categorizing the severity of renal impairment is with creatinine clearance. Severity of renal impairment ranges from mild (creatinine clearance between 60 and 80 mL/min), moderate (creatinine clearance between 30 and 59 mL/min), and severe (creatinine clearance between 15 and 29 mL/min) to end-stage renal disease (creatinine clearance <15 mL/min or requiring dialysis).[24]

Chronic kidney disease that leads to impairment in renal function not only has consequences for drugs that are excreted by the kidneys but can also affect drugs cleared by nonrenal routes. Specifically, renal impairment causes physiological alterations such as changes in absorption, plasma protein binding, drug transport, or tissue distribution, and can affect hepatic and gut metabolism. In addition, renal dysfunction directly affects CYP-mediated metabolism and transmembrane transport of drugs in the liver. Although the exact mechanisms are unclear, it is hypothesized that systemic accumulation of uremic toxins (e.g., urea, parathyroid hormone, indoxyl sulfate, and cytokines) is responsible.[25] These solutes could contribute to transcriptional, translational, or posttranslational downregulation of drug-metabolizing enzymes and transporters. Several studies using probe CYP substrates have been conducted in humans to determine the extent of CYP enzyme inhibition. A review of these studies is presented elsewhere.[26] In brief, clinically relevant decreases in activities of CYP3A4/5, CYP2C9, CYP2D6, and CYP2C19 are demonstrated in patients with chronic kidney disease and end-stage renal disease.

Cardiac Failure

Cardiac failure is a condition in which the heart is unable to deliver sufficiently oxygenated blood throughout the body. Lower cardiac output leads to lower hepatic blood flow, and this can affect the clearance of drugs with a high extraction ratio (clearance highly dependent on blood flow).[27] Logic would dictate that a monooxygenase system such as the CYP enzyme system would be suppressed if there are inadequate oxygen levels in the systemic circulation. In fact, the activity level of hepatic CYP2C19 is significantly decreased in patients with heart failure.[27] A significant correlation between enzyme activity levels and plasma concentrations of TNF-α and IL-6 has also been demonstrated.[27] As the concentrations of these cytokines increase, CYP enzyme activities decrease. Patients with heart failure have higher circulating concentrations of TNF-α and IL-6 that correlate with the severity of heart failure. Thus, the induction of proinflammatory cytokines with consequent decreases in CYP activity likely represents another mechanism by which cardiac failure leads to alterations in drug metabolism. Although the activity of hepatic CYPs appears to be suppressed, expression of certain cardiac CYP isoforms is upregulated in a rat model of cardiac hypertrophy.[28] This indicates that the effects of cardiac failure on drug-metabolizing enzymes may be highly organ-specific.

Diet

Perhaps no extrinsic factor is more pervasive or influential on the disposition of oral medications than diet. When a solid oral drug is ingested, it is immediately vulnerable to disintegration, dissolution, and absorption in the gastrointestinal tract. Various components of diet can affect one or more of these steps as well as drug metabolism. Thus, it is essential to recognize the importance of the effect of diet on drug disposition. Meal volume, food composition (e.g., protein, fat, dairy products, presence of fortification), and food preparation techniques (e.g., charbroiling) can all play a role in the interaction between diet and drug disposition. The next section will focus on the effect of the composition of various foods on CYP enzymes, and thus factors that can influence drug metabolism.

Fruit Juices

Grapefruit juice is widely recognized to cause clinically relevant food–drug interactions, but it is only one of many juices that can do so. This recognition is often reflected by the prohibition of grapefruit juice consumption during the conduct of clinical trials. Consumption of grapefruit juice can significantly increase plasma concentrations of many drugs, including some HMG-CoA reductase inhibitors, HIV protease inhibitors, antihistamines, macrolides, cyclosporine, calcium channel antagonists, and benzodiazepines.[29] Inhibition of CYP3A4/5 in the gut wall and small intestine, leading to lower presystemic drug metabolism and higher plasma concentrations, is at least partially responsible for this effect.[30] In addition to inhibiting CYP3A4/5, grapefruit juice inhibits the intestinal efflux transporter P-glycoprotein (P-gp), which can also lead to higher plasma drug concentrations.[31] In vitro studies suggest that furanocoumarin is the component of grapefruit juice responsible for this interaction.[32] Cranberry and pomelo juice also inhibit drug metabolism via CYP3A4/5 activity and/or transporters.[33] Other fruit juices, including orange, pomegranate, carrot, tomato, wild grape, black mulberry, and black raspberry juice, have been studied in vitro but none are suggested to have clinically relevant effects on drug metabolism.[34]

Herbal Products

Herbal products are widely used and available without a prescription. Several herbs are implicated in altering drug metabolism. They include St. John's wort, garlic, ginkgo, ginseng, piperine, and echinacea. Most herbs only affect CYP enzyme in vitro tests and subsequent confirmation in human trials is lacking. However, St. John's wort, garlic, and echinacea all have clinically significant effects on drug metabolism. St. John's wort (used as a natural remedy for depression) induces CYP3A4/5, CYP2E1, and CYP2C19 activity in humans,[35,36] and results in lower plasma concentrations of drugs that are substrates for these isozymes. As further confirmation of the clinical importance of the interaction between St. John's wort and CYP3A4/5 substrates, St. John's wort is listed in the "Contraindications" section of prescribing information for drugs such as Prezista® (darunavir) and Lexiva® (fosamprenavir) or under the "Warnings" section for drugs such as Invirase® (saquinavir), Kaletra® (lopinavir), Neoral® (cyclosporine), and Prograf® (tacrolimus). Similarly, garlic supplements (used for cardioprotective effects) induce CYP3A4/5 activity in the gut and cause an approximate 50% decrease in bioavailability of CYP3A4/5 substrates with high presystemic extraction.[37] However, evidence of garlic supplementation as a CYP3A4/5 inducer has not been reproduced consistently in vivo. Echinacea (used to treat the common cold) is implicated in CYP1A2 induction and has mixed effects on CYP3A4/5 that are dependent on the organ (liver or intestine).[38]

Cruciferous Vegetables

Cruciferous vegetables belong to the Brassicaceae plant family and include cauliflower, radishes, broccoli, cabbage, and bok choy. Limited evidence from human studies shows that a diet consisting solely of cruciferous vegetables results in an 18–37% increase in CYP1A2 activity.[39] The clinical significance of this finding has yet to be demonstrated, and it is unlikely that an individual would eat a diet consisting solely of cruciferous vegetables. Nonetheless, the theoretical potential exists for cruciferous vegetables to increase the clearance of such drugs as naproxen, theophylline, and caffeine. In addition, a study investigating the effect of a cruciferous vegetable diet compared with that of a diet without vegetables showed that consumption of cruciferous vegetables resulted in an increase of up to 24% in *UGT1A1* (a major phase II metabolizing enzyme) activity in individuals with a particular *UGT1A1* genotype.[40] These data suggest that cruciferous vegetables may play an important role in altering drug-metabolizing activity in some individuals, but lack evidence for importance in most people.

Alcohol

Alcohol consumption is common and can cause extensive clinical consequences on the disposition of medications administered during or immediately after ethanol intake. Interactions with ethanol at the level of disintegration, dissolution, and absorption of a modified-release solid oral dosage form are well described.[41] In addition, CYP-mediated processes are affected by ethanol. Ethanol is both a substrate for and an inducer of *CYP2E1*. Thus, ethanol can theoretically decrease plasma concentrations of any drug that is a *CYP2E1* substrate. This is true for chlorzoxazone, a *CYP2E1* substrate used as a *CYP2E1* probe.[42] Equally as important as an interaction that could lead to loss in efficacy is one that could increase toxicity. Ethanol induction of *CYP2E1* results in higher production of its toxic metabolite, acetaldehyde. Acetaldehyde is implicated in alcohol-induced hepatotoxicity. In addition, *CYP2E1* induction is implicated in increased susceptibility to acetaminophen-induced hepatotoxicity, although the magnitude of the increased risk is a function of several factors including the amount and duration of ethanol consumption and timing of acetaminophen administration.[43]

Tobacco Smoke

Cigarette smoking and the use of other tobacco products result in the intake of chemical carcinogens that are converted to active carcinogens by CYP-mediated processes. Polycyclic aromatic hydrocarbons (PAHs, a product of incomplete tobacco combustion) are postulated to be primarily responsible for inducing drug-metabolizing enzymes and the subsequent conversion of the PAHs to active carcinogens by the induced enzymes.[44] Although PAHs are known to induce *CYP1A1* and *CYP1A2*, there are conflicting data on the effect of these compounds on *CYP2E1* activity.[45] Animal and in vitro studies show that nicotine and carbon monoxide (two major components of tobacco smoke) also modulate CYP enzymes. In several human studies, smoking is associated with clinically relevant changes in plasma drug concentrations of some psychotropic medications.[46]

Medications and Medical Interventions

Perhaps the most dramatic influences on drug metabolism occur through the use of medications. Using therapeutic doses of two drugs in combination can result in plasma concentration changes of one or both drugs that are several-fold in magnitude. In many cases, this results in subtherapeutic or toxic drug concentrations. This section discusses how the use of medications and medical interventions can directly and substantially affect drug metabolism.

Xenobiotics

Numerous studies and review articles are dedicated to elucidating and describing the mechanisms by which xenobiotics can affect drug disposition. Xenobiotics frequently alter the activities of hepatic and intestinal CYP enzymes and transporters. These alterations are often significant. Substantial clinical consequences can result when two or more drugs are administered together (discussed in more detail in the section "Drug–Drug Interactions"). When a drug is administered alone and is both a substrate for and a modifier of the key enzyme(s) or transporters involved in its metabolism, the drug can change its own rate of clearance. This is the case for drugs such as efavirenz[49] and carbamazepine[50] that exhibit autoinduction. For these medications, plasma drug concentrations decrease over time due to autoinduction of *CYP2B6*-mediated metabolism. In addition, many of examples exist for drugs that are both substrates for and inhibitors of the same CYP enzyme. Chronic dosing with these drugs results in decreased clearance, and this in turn leads to increased plasma concentrations.

Exogenous Hormones

Exogenous hormones are used to replace or augment endogenous hormone production. Common examples include estrogen and progesterone therapy for contraception, thyroid hormone for treatment of hypothyroidism, and corticosteroid use in autoimmune disorders. In most cases, the exogenous hormone functions to correct underproduction of an endogenous hormone. However, the therapeutic goal of hormones for contraception is to achieve supraendogenous concentrations of estrogen and progesterone. Combined hormonal oral contraceptives, administered to premenopausal women, decrease *CYP1A2* activity.[51,52] Additionally, the combination of ethinyl estradiol and tricyclic norgestimate decreases *CYP2C19* activity while concurrently increasing *CYP2C9* and *CYP2D6* activities.[51] No clinically significant effect on CYP3A4/5-mediated metabolism has been found.

Drug–Drug Interactions

A drug interaction resulting in subtherapeutic or toxic drug concentrations of one or more administered drugs is generally considered an unfavorable clinical event. Thus, topics surrounding drug–drug interactions have been an intense research focus in recent decades. Several probe substrates, inhibitors, and inducers are identified for each major human CYP enzyme. These probes are used to study and predict clinically important drug–drug interactions. The most commonly used probe substrates for clinically important CYP isoforms include caffeine for *CYP1A2*, warfarin for *CYP2C9*, omeprazole for *CYP2C19*, dextromethorphan for *CYP2D6*, and midazolam for *CYP3A4/5*. A drug's therapeutic index and sensitivity to PK alterations caused by known CYP modulators are particularly important characteristics of a probe substrate. Commonly used potent inhibitors of CYP isoform include ketoconazole and itraconazole for *CYP3A4/5*, fluconazole for *CYP2C19*, and buproprion for *CYP2D6*. Several of the potent inhibitors (such as fluconazole) inhibit more than one isoform and this characteristic may complicate data interpretation. Potent CYP inducers are not as common as inhibitors since not all isoforms are inducible. Rifampin is commonly used as a model inducer of *CYP3A4/5*.

Not all drug interactions are detrimental. A drug may be intentionally used as a "PK booster" to increase the plasma concentrations of a concomitantly administered drug by inhibiting CYP activity. One example of this concept is the coadministration of ritonavir with an anti-HIV protease inhibitor (e.g., lopinavir, saquinavir, darunavir, fosamprenavir). Potent *CYP3A4/5* inhibition by ritonavir allows for a lower dose and less frequent dosing of the coadministered protease inhibitor (a substrate of *CYP3A4/5*) while still achieving therapeutic concentrations.[53]

Alterations of the activity of key transporters in the gut and liver can also lead to clinically significant changes in plasma drug concentrations. Drugs that inhibit P-gp in the gut result in increased plasma concentrations of drugs that are substrates for the transporter. Since P-gp is an efflux transporter (present on the surface of enterocytes) that transports certain molecules out of cells and back into the gut lumen, inhibition of this transporter results in greater absorption and thus higher circulating drug concentrations.[54] Several key transporters are also present in the liver, such as *OATP1B1* (uptake into hepatocytes), *OATP1B3* (uptake into hepatocytes), *BCRP* (efflux into bile), *BSEP* (efflux into bile), and *MRP1* (efflux into systemic circulation).[55] Depending on the function of the particular transporter, the plasma concentrations of substrates of these transporters can either increase or decrease when these transporters are inhibited. Study of transporters, their function, and interactions with drugs and dietary components is an active area of research.

Hemodialysis and Renal Transplantation

Factors involved in nonrenal metabolism, particularly *CYP3A4/5* activity, P-gp transport, OATP transport, and phase II enzyme activity, are altered in end-stage renal disease.[56] In addition, uremic human serum downregulates CYP enzyme expression and activity in vitro, specifically *CYP1A2* and *CYP3A4/5* in the intestine and *CYP2C11* and *CYP3A1/2* in rat liver.[56] These changes are not due solely to uremia. Hemodialysis immediately corrects these alterations and results in temporary normalization of CYP activity and near-normalization of mRNA expression.[57–59] This is in contrast to renal transplantation that returns CYP activity to the levels seen in healthy volunteers.[60] Evidence suggests that hepatic *CYP3A4/5* activity is not altered in end-stage renal disease, so changes in metabolism and transport likely occur primarily in the intestine.[56]

Therapeutic Proteins

A review of in vitro and in vivo data supports a role for therapeutic proteins such as TNF-α monoclonal antibodies and IL-2 receptor antagonists in the modulation of hepatic and intestinal DMEs.[11] Proinflammatory cytokines may impair CYP enzyme activity by downregulating mRNA transcription, thereby decreasing drug clearance and leading to elevations of drug concentrations that can result in toxicity. Treatment with anticytokine drugs may limit the extent of cytokine influence and result in increased drug clearance. There is also the theoretical possibility that alterations in CYP activity might decrease conversion of prodrugs with a resultant lessening of therapeutic effect. However, this has not been demonstrated in human studies. Therapeutic IL-2 and IFNs alter drug metabolism in humans,[61] and it is likely that other therapeutic proteins may do so as well. The specificity of drug metabolizing enzyme regulation differs by the cytokine.[10]

MECHANISMS OF DRUG-METABOLIZING ENZYME INTERACTIONS

Similar to other enzyme systems throughout the body, CYP enzymes are subject to several mechanisms of inhibition and induction. Inhibition of CYPs can result in increased drug concentrations due to lower drug-metabolizing activity, and drug toxicity may occur subsequently. CYP inhibition can be either reversible (competitive, noncompetitive, uncompetitive) or irreversible (mechanism-based). Competitive inhibition results when an inhibitor interacts with the active binding site on the surface of an enzyme that then prevents a substrate from binding to the site. This type of inhibition frequently occurs for CYPs and is commonly demonstrated to have clinically significant effects with the azole family of antifungal agents (e.g., ketoconazole and itraconazole). Although the azoles have a reversible inhibitory effect on CYP3A4/5, the magnitude of effect can be extremely high (particularly for ketoconazole and itraconazole), and result in several-fold increases in substrate drug concentrations.

Noncompetitive inhibition involves the inhibitor binding to a site other than the substrate binding site and results in a conformational change to the site that prevents binding of substrate molecules. It is not observed as commonly with CYP enzymes as is competitive inhibition. There are far fewer demonstrated cases that have clinical relevance. Uncompetitive inhibition involves the inhibitor molecule binding only to the enzyme–substrate complex. The resulting inhibitor–enzyme–substrate complex is nonfunctional. Uncompetitive inhibition is infrequently observed with CYP enzymes. Mechanism-based inhibition involves inactivating an enzyme by the formation of metabolites that bind irreversibly to the enzyme. This type of inhibition often occurs with *CYP3A4/5* and results in a greater degree and longer-lasting reduction in metabolic clearance of *CYP3A4/5* substrates. Mechanism-based inhibition is both time- and NADPH-dependent.[62] An example of a clinically significant interaction resulting from mechanism-based inhibition is erythromycin inhibition of *CYP3A4/5* activity. Erythromycin is a well-described mechanism-based inhibitor and demonstrates a higher degree of CYP3A4/5 inhibition as the dosing duration lengthens.[63]

CYP enzyme induction involves a drug or chemical agent that increases the rate of enzyme synthesis, resulting in greater net enzyme activity and lower circulating substrate drug concentrations. Increasing the clearance of circulating drugs may lead to decreased clinical efficacy. In general, enzyme induction can occur through either increased gene transcription or increased stability of the mRNA or enzyme itself. CYP induction occurs most frequently through transcriptional gene activation. Because of this, the process of induction takes longer to occur than inhibition. Regulation of CYP gene transcription is achieved when the inducing agent binds to nuclear receptors (e.g., aromatic hydrocarbon receptor [AhR], constitutive androstane receptor [CAR], pregnane X receptor [PXR]). A cascade of events ultimately results in binding of the nuclear receptor to the promoter region of target CYP genes. This process upregulates transcription of these genes.[64] Compared with inhibition, there are far fewer known agents that induce CYP enzymes and only the following isoforms are generally recognized as inducible: *CYP1A1/2, CYP2B6, CYP2C9, CYP2C19, CYP2E1*, and *CYP3A4/5*. However, the clinical effect of CYP induction can be significant. For example, St. John's wort induces *CYP3A4/5* and thereby decreases midazolam (a probe *CYP3A4/5* substrate) AUC by 79% and C_{max} by 65%.[65]

One example of a potential for a detrimental effect of enzyme induction is the case of polycyclic aromatic hydrocarbons (PAHs). PAHs are both substrates for and inducers of *CYP1A1* and *CYP1A2*. Induction of *CYP1A1/2* activity leads to increased metabolic activation of PAHs as well as heterocyclic aromatic amines (HAAs).[66] Oxidation of PAHs and HAAs (present in tobacco smoke, automobile exhaust, and smoked/cooked foods) by *CYP1A1/2* is associated with the production of reactive intermediate species and known carcinogens.[67] Thus, a major consequence to this cycle of *CYP1A1/2* induction and the subsequent metabolic activation of PAHs and HAAs is the potential for the development of cancer in humans exposed to these compounds.

SUMMARY

Numerous factors can contribute to a patient's response to drug therapy. A firm understanding of the many intrinsic and extrinsic factors that can lead to toxicity or loss of efficacy of a drug is a critical tool for clinical decision making regarding drug dosing. In the real-world setting, patients often possess a combination of conditions or factors that are not genetic and can affect drug metabolism. Due to the complex interplay of conditions that can exist within an individual patient, it is not often possible to identify the magnitude of each contributing factor. Rather, modification of therapy needs to be determined by the net effect of these factors in the setting of continuous clinical observation, patient evaluation and reevaluation, and individualized decision making.

REFERENCES

1. Hines RN. The ontogeny of drug metabolism enzymes and implications for adverse drug events. *Pharmacol Ther.* 2008;118(2):250–267.
2. Kearns GL, Abdel-Rahman SM, Alander SW, Blowey DL, Leeder JS, Kauffman RE. Developmental pharmacology—drug disposition, action, and therapy in infants and children. *N Engl J Med.* 2003;349(12):1157–1167.
3. Le Couteur DG, Fraser R, Hilmer S, Rivory LP, McLean AJ. The hepatic sinusoid in aging and cirrhosis: effects on hepatic substrate disposition and drug clearance. *Clin Pharmacokinet.* 2005;44(2):187–200.
4. Parkinson A, Mudra DR, Johnson C, Dwyer A, Carroll KM. The effects of gender, age, ethnicity, and liver cirrhosis on cytochrome P450 enzyme activity in human liver microsomes and inducibility in cultured human hepatocytes. *Toxicol Appl Pharmacol.* 2004;199(3):193–209.
5. Feng Y, Pollock BG, Ferrell RE, Kimak MA, Reynolds CF 3rd, Bies RR. Paroxetine: population pharmacokinetic analysis in late-life depression using sparse concentration sampling. *Br J Clin Pharmacol.* 2006;61(5):558–569.
6. Sotaniemi EA, Arranto AJ, Pelkonen O, Pasanen M. Age and cytochrome P450-linked drug metabolism in humans: an analysis of 226 subjects with equal histopathologic conditions. *Clin Pharmacol Ther.* 1997;61(3):331–339.
7. Chang KC, Bell TD, Lauer BA, Chai H. Altered theophylline pharmacokinetics during acute respiratory viral illness. *Lancet.* 1978;1(8074):1132–1133.
8. Richardson TA, Morgan ET. Hepatic cytochrome P450 gene regulation during endotoxin-induced inflammation in nuclear receptor knockout mice. *J Pharmacol Exp Ther.* 2005;314(2):703–709.
9. Renton KW. Cytochrome P450 regulation and drug biotransformation during inflammation and infection. *Curr Drug Metab.* 2004;5(3):235–243.
10. Aitken AE, Richardson TA, Morgan ET. Regulation of drug-metabolizing enzymes and transporters in inflammation. *Annu Rev Pharmacol Toxicol.* 2006;46:123–149.
11. Morgan ET. Impact of infectious and inflammatory disease on cytochrome P450-mediated drug metabolism and pharmacokinetics. *Clin Pharmacol Ther.* 2009;85(4):434–438.
12. Morgan ET, Goralski KB, Piquette-Miller M, et al. Regulation of drug-metabolizing enzymes and transporters in infection, inflammation, and cancer. *Drug Metab Dispos.* 2008;36(2):205–216.
13. Fulop AK. Genetics and genomics of hepatic acute phase reactants: a mini-review. *Inflamm Allergy Drug Targets.* 2007;6(2):109–115.
14. Kulmatycki KM, Jamali F. Drug disease interactions: role of inflammatory mediators in disease and variability in drug response. *J Pharm Pharm Sci.* 2005;8(3):602–625.
15. Westerholt A, Himpel S, Hager-Gensch B, et al. Intragraft iNOS induction during human liver allograft rejection depresses cytochrome p450 activity. *Transpl Int.* 2004;17(7):370–378.
16. Islam M, Frye RF, Richards TJ, et al. Differential effect of IFNalpha-2b on the cytochrome P450 enzyme system: a potential basis of IFN toxicity and its modulation by other drugs. *Clin Cancer Res.* 2002;8(8):2480–2487.
17. Kacevska M, Robertson GR, Clarke SJ, Liddle C. Inflammation and CYP3A4-mediated drug metabolism in advanced cancer: impact and implications for chemotherapeutic drug dosing. *Exp Opin Drug Metab Toxicol.* 2008;4(2):137–149.
18. Kulmatycki KM, Jamali F. Drug disease interactions: role of inflammatory mediators in pain and variability in analgesic drug response. *J Pharm Pharm Sci.* 2007;10(4):554–566.
19. Kulmatycki KM, Jamali F. Drug disease interactions: role of inflammatory mediators in depression and variability in antidepressant drug response. *J Pharm Pharm Sci.* 2006;9(3):292–306.
20. Morgan DJ, McLean AJ. Clinical pharmacokinetic and pharmacodynamic considerations in patients with liver disease. An update. *Clin Pharmacokinet.* 1995;29(5):370–391.
21. Rodighiero V. Effects of liver disease on pharmacokinetics. An update. *Clin Pharmacokinet.* 1999;37(5):399–431.
22. Susla GM, Atkinson AJ. Effect of liver disease on pharmacokinetics. In: Atkinson AJ, Abernethy DR, Daniels CE, Dedrick RL, Markey SP, eds. *Principles of Clinical Pharmacology.* 2nd ed. Burlington, MA: Academic Press; 2007:73–87.
23. Frye RF, Zgheib NK, Matzke GR, et al. Liver disease selectively modulates cytochrome P450-mediated metabolism. *Clin Pharmacol Ther.* 2006;80(3):235–245.
24. KDOQI clinical practice guidelines for chronic kidney disease: evaluation, classification, and stratification. *NKF KDOQI Guidelines.* 2000. Available at: http://www.kidney.org/professionals/KDOQI/guidelines_ckd/toc.htm. Accessed April 8, 2011.
25. Guevin C, Michaud J, Naud J, Leblond FA, Pichette V. Down-regulation of hepatic cytochrome p450 in chronic renal failure: role of uremic mediators. *Br J Pharmacol.* 2002;137(7):1039–1046.
26. Nolin TD, Frye RF, Matzke GR. Hepatic drug metabolism and transport in patients with kidney disease. *Am J Kidney Dis.* 2003;42(5):906–925.

27. Frye RF, Schneider VM, Frye CS, Feldman AM. Plasma levels of TNF-alpha and IL-6 are inversely related to cytochrome P450-dependent drug metabolism in patients with congestive heart failure. *J Card Fail.* 2002;8(5):315–319.

28. Thum T, Borlak J. Testosterone, cytochrome P450, and cardiac hypertrophy. *FASEB J.* 2002;16(12):1537–1549.

29. Flockhart D. *P450 Drug Interaction Table.* 2011. Available at: http://medicine. iupui.edu/clinpharm/ddis/table.asp. Accessed April 8, 2011.

30. Lown KS, Bailey DG, Fontana RJ, et al. Grapefruit juice increases felodipine oral availability in humans by decreasing intestinal CYP3A protein expression. *J Clin Investig.* 1997;99(10):2545–2553.

31. Wang EJ, Casciano CN, Clement RP, Johnson WW. Inhibition of P-glycoprotein transport function by grapefruit juice psoralen. *Pharm Res.* 2001;18(4):432–438.

32. Guo LQ, Fukuda K, Ohta T, Yamazoe Y. Role of furanocoumarin derivatives on grapefruit juice-mediated inhibition of human CYP3A activity. *Drug Metab Dispos.* 2000;28(7):766–771.

33. Won CS, Oberlies NH, Paine MF. Influence of dietary substances on intestinal drug metabolism and transport. *Curr Drug Metab.* 2010;11(9):778–792.

34. Kim H, Yoon YJ, Shon JH, Cha IJ, Shin JG, Liu KH. Inhibitory effects of fruit juices on CYP3A activity. *Drug Metab Dispos.* 2006;34(4):521–523.

35. Wang LS, Zhou G, Zhu B, et al. St John's wort induces both cytochrome P450 3A4-catalyzed sulfoxidation and 2C19-dependent hydroxylation of omeprazole. *Clin Pharmacol Ther.* 2004;75(3):191–197.

36. Gurley BJ, Gardner SF, Hubbard MA, et al. Cytochrome P450 phenotypic ratios for predicting herb–drug interactions in humans. *Clin Pharmacol Ther.* 2002;72(3):276–287.

37. Piscitelli SC, Burstein AH, Welden N, Gallicano KD, Falloon J. The effect of garlic supplements on the pharmacokinetics of saquinavir. *Clin Infect Dis.* 2002;34(2):234–238.

38. Gorski JC, Huang SM, Pinto A, et al. The effect of echinacea (*Echinacea purpurea* root) on cytochrome P450 activity in vivo. *Clin Pharmacol Ther.* 2004;75(1):89–100.

39. Lampe JW, King IB, Li S, et al. *Brassica* vegetables increase and apiaceous vegetables decrease cytochrome P450 1A2 activity in humans: changes in caffeine metabolite ratios in response to controlled vegetable diets. *Carcinogenesis.* 2000;21(6):1157–1162.

40. Navarro SL, Peterson S, Chen C, et al. Cruciferous vegetable feeding alters UGT1A1 activity: diet- and genotype-dependent changes in serum bilirubin in a controlled feeding trial. *Cancer Prev Res (Phila).* 2009;2(4):345–352.

41. Lennernas H. Ethanol–drug absorption interaction: potential for a significant effect on the plasma pharmacokinetics of ethanol vulnerable formulations. *Mol Pharm.* 2009;6(5):1429–1440.

42. Klotz U, Ammon E. Clinical and toxicological consequences of the inductive potential of ethanol. *Eur J Clin Pharmacol.* 1998;54(1):7–12.

43. Thummel KE, Slattery JT, Ro H, et al. Ethanol and production of the hepatotoxic metabolite of acetaminophen in healthy adults. *Clin Pharmacol Ther.* 2000;67(6):591–599.

44. Conney AH. Induction of microsomal enzymes by foreign chemicals and carcinogenesis by polycyclic aromatic hydrocarbons: G. H. A. Clowes Memorial Lecture. *Cancer Res.* 1982;42(12):4875–4917.

45. Zevin S, Benowitz NL. Drug interactions with tobacco smoking. An update. *Clin Pharmacokinet.* 1999;36(6):425–438.

46. Desai HD, Seabolt J, Jann MW. Smoking in patients receiving psychotropic medications: a pharmacokinetic perspective. *CNS Drugs.* 2001;15(6):469–494.

47. Anderson GD. Pregnancy-induced changes in pharmacokinetics: a mechanistic-based approach. *Clin Pharmacokinet.* 2005;44(10):989–1008.

48. Stika CS, Frederiksen MC. Drug therapy in pregnant and nursing women. In: Atkinson AJ, Abernethy DR, Daniels CE, Dedrick RL, Markey SP, eds. *Principles of Clinical Pharmacology.* 2nd ed. Burlington, MA: Academic Press; 2007:339–357.

49. Barrett JS, Joshi AS, Chai M, Ludden TM, Fiske WD, Pieniaszek HJ Jr. Population pharmacokinetic meta-analysis with efavirenz. *Int J Clin Pharmacol Ther.* 2002;40(11):507–519.

50. Bernus I, Dickinson RG, Hooper WD, Eadie MJ. Early stage autoinduction of carbamazepine metabolism in humans. *Eur J Clin Pharmacol.* 1994;47(4):355–360.

51. Shelepova T, Nafziger AN, Victory J, et al. Effect of a triphasic oral contraceptive on drug-metabolizing enzyme activity as measured by the validated Cooperstown 5+1 cocktail. *J Clin Pharmacol.* 2005;45(12):1413–1421.

52. Granfors MT, Backman JT, Laitila J, Neuvonen PJ. Oral contraceptives containing ethinyl estradiol and gestodene markedly increase plasma concentrations and effects of tizanidine by inhibiting cytochrome P450 1A2. *Clin Pharmacol Ther.* 2005;78(4):400–411.

53. Moyle GJ, Back D. Principles and practice of HIV-protease inhibitor pharmacoenhancement. *HIV Med.* 2001;2(2):105–113.

54. Lin J, Yamazaki M. Role of p-glycoprotein in pharmacokinetics. Clinical implications. *Clin Pharmacokinet.* 2003;42:59–98.

55. Funk C. The role of hepatic transporters in drug elimination. *Exp Opin Drug Metab Toxicol.* 2008;4(4):363–379.

56. Nolin TD. Altered nonrenal drug clearance in ESRD. *Curr Opin Nephrol Hypertens.* 2008;17(6):555–559.

57. Michaud J, Nolin TD, Naud J, et al. Effect of hemodialysis on hepatic cytochrome P450 functional expression. *J Pharmacol Sci.* 2008;108(2):157–163.

58. Shi J, Montay G, Chapel S, et al. Pharmacokinetics and safety of the ketolide telithromycin in patients with renal impairment. *J Clin Pharmacol.* 2004;44(3):234–244.

59. Nolin TD, Appiah K, Kendrick SA, Le P, McMonagle E, Himmelfarb J. Hemodialysis acutely improves hepatic CYP3A4 metabolic activity. *J Am Soc Nephrol.* 2006;17(9):2363–2367.

60. Michaud J, Dube P, Naud J, et al. Effects of serum from patients with chronic renal failure on rat hepatic cytochrome P450. *Br J Pharmacol.* 2005;144(8):1067–1077.

61. Elkahwaji J, Robin MA, Berson A, et al. Decrease in hepatic cytochrome P450 after interleukin-2 immunotherapy. *Biochem Pharmacol.* 1999;57(8):951–954.

62. Zhou S, Yung Chan S, Cher Goh B, et al. Mechanism-based inhibition of cytochrome P450 3A4 by therapeutic drugs. *Clin Pharmacokinet.* 2005;44(3):279–304.

63. Okudaira T, Kotegawa T, Imai H, Tsutsumi K, Nakano S, Ohashi K. Effect of the treatment period with erythromycin on cytochrome P450 3A activity in humans. *J Clin Pharmacol.* 2007;47(7):871–876.

64. Wang H, LeCluyse EL. Role of orphan nuclear receptors in the regulation of drug-metabolising enzymes. *Clin Pharmacokinet.* 2003;42(15):1331–1357.

65. Mueller SC, Majcher-Peszynska J, Uehleke B, et al. The extent of induction of CYP3A by St. John's wort varies among products and is linked to hyperforin dose. *Eur J Clin Pharmacol.* 2006;62(1):29–36.

66. Ma Q, Lu AY. CYP1A induction and human risk assessment: an evolving tale of in vitro and in vivo studies. *Drug Metab Dispos.* 2007;35(7):1009–1016.

67. Kim D, Guengerich FP. Cytochrome P450 activation of arylamines and heterocyclic amines. *Annu Rev Pharmacol Toxicol.* 2005;45:27–49.

Public Access to Pharmacogenomic Testing and Patient Counseling

Mary W. Roederer, PharmD, BCPS,
Shanna K. O'Connor, PharmD, BCPS, &
Stefanie P. Ferreri, PharmD, BCACP, CDE

LEARNING OBJECTIVES

- Compare and contrast the patient and healthcare professional access to pharmacogenomic tests.

- Review the roles of health care professionals in patient counseling regarding pharmacogenomic tests.

- Examine the pharmacist-centered patient counseling model and the integration of pharmacogenomic information.

- Explore the application of pharmacogenomic data to patient vignettes.

INTRODUCTION

There is an eminent need for health care professionals to be prepared to integrate pharmacogenomics into clinical care. There is both growing scientific evidence and an interest of the lay press regarding individualized, tailored, or personalized medicine. As a new area of medicine, pharmacogenomics poses many challenges as well as opportunities. For health care professionals, there are challenges in obtaining a baseline understanding of the relevance of pharmacogenomics and maintaining a current understanding of the evidence supporting pharmacogenomics as it relates to patient care. For patients, there are challenges to being willing to provide genetic information for optimizing their medication therapy and to distinguish the less reputable direct-to-consumer options for genetic testing. Opportunities shared by patients and professionals include an understanding that the "one dose fits all" approach is flawed and that pharmacogenomics is one tool to improve our ability to provide the right drug in the right dose to the right patient.

Despite mounting research, the public's understanding of pharmacogenomics is not well documented. Individuals may or may not understand the benefits and risks associated with pharmacogenomics. A study published in 2009 by Kobayashi and Satoh assessed the attitudes of 1,103 Japanese adults from the general public (not a patient population) toward pharmacogenomics research and their willingness to donate samples for a DNA biobank to identify genomic markers associated with adverse drug reactions.[1] The majority of the respondents showed a positive attitude toward pharmacogenomics research (81%) and donating to a DNA biobank (70.4%). A decreased willingness to donate was significantly associated with older generations. Generally, the respondents had the following concerns regarding a DNA biobank: the confidentiality of their personal information, the manner by which research results were utilized, and the use of their own DNA for research. The authors concluded that a process of public awareness should be put into place to emphasize the beneficial aspects of identifying genomic markers associated with adverse drug reactions and to address the concerns of confidentiality and research raised in their study.[1] Although this study was conducted exclusively in Japan, the same concerns are likely to occur in other countries. Health care professionals, including physicians, nurses, pharmacists, and genetic counselors, are best positioned to play a key role in helping the public better understand and interpret pharmacogenomic information.[1]

HEALTH CARE PROFESSIONAL EDUCATION IN PHARMACOGENOMICS

Health care professionals must be exposed to pharmacogenomics during their education so they can comfortably apply this information in clinical practice and educate their patients. They must have at least a cursory knowledge of genetics and an appreciation for the benefits and limitations to pharmacogenetic tests. Currently, the curricula offered among the health care professional schools, such as schools of nursing, medicine, and pharmacy, vary, but all accredited schools must adhere to a standard group of requirements set by their accrediting body. Pharmacogenomics is not currently a required standard in all educational programs for health care professionals, but many schools offer electives or incorporate some basic concepts and theories into the curriculum.

The 2011 Secretary's Advisory Committee on Genetics, Health, and Society discovered that health care professionals generally are not comfortable with pharmacogenomics but are excited about the potential opportunities.[2] In the report, professional organizations were asked to characterize the need for integrating genetics into the curriculum and training of health care professionals. Although several organizations indicated that it was not a high priority, most felt that this integration is crucial, and several have already implemented national curricula. The 2011 SACGHS survey data found that 70% of responding health care professional organizations view genetics education and training as part of their role or responsibility.

Medical Education

An analysis of the curriculum of medical schools conducted in 2007 found that 77% of programs taught genetics in the first year of medical school, but 47% failed to incorporate any genetic content into the third and fourth years.[3] This analysis shows improvement from 2002, when many practicing physicians did not have any genetic instruction during their formal education.[4] However, these studies point to a need for medical educators to devote more time to teach pharmacogenomics.

In 2005 the International Society for Pharmacogenomics published a consensus article calling on Deans of Education in medical schools to add pharmacogenomics to their pharmacology curricula.[5] It recommended topics that focus on drug response and genetic polymorphisms linked to adverse drug reactions. This call for action spurred 46% of medical schools to offer stand-alone courses with medical genetic content while the remaining 54% embedded this content into existing courses.[3]

Nursing Education

Much like physicians, the need for education of nurses in genetics and genomics is well documented. A 2005 nursing faculty survey conducted by Prows et al. found that 29% of schools reported no genomic curriculum content.[6-8] The most common reasons were already overloaded curricula and lack of knowledge among faculty about genetics. The majority of the programs offered few (less than 5) structured hours on genetic content.[8,9] Another article by Prows and Saldana emphasized that nurses must have enough baseline knowledge in genomics to ascertain if a patient's knowledge is accurate.[10] The article lists recommended learning resources, many of which are Web-based training modules or Web sites. Although there is literature citing pharmacogenomics in nursing curricula, it is not consistent across schools.

An editorial published by Van Riper states that it is critical for family nurses to achieve basic competencies in genetics and genomics.[11] She emphasizes a leadership role for nurses in gathering genetic data from a family history rather than individual history. Therefore, nursing education must ensure their ability to assess patient knowledge, perception, and response to genomic information and provide additional information to patients with specific needs.

Genetic Counselor Education

Genetic counseling is a relatively young profession. The American Board of Medical Genetics (ABMG) began certifying genetic counselors in 1981 and in 1993 it became part of the American Board of Medical Specialties. At that time the American Board of Genetic Counseling (ABGC) formed out of the ABMG. Since 1993, according to the ABGC Web site, the number of genetic counselors recognized by the ABGC has increased from 495 to more than 2,000 and the number of accredited graduate programs has risen from 18 to 30. As medical science's understanding of genetics increases, particularly in relation to birth defects and inherited diseases, an increased need for genetic counseling is expected.

In 2006, the National Society of Genetic Counselors' Task Force Report developed a definition for genetic counseling. In this report, genetic counseling is defined as the process of helping people understand and adapt to the medical, psychological, and familial implications of genetic contributions to disease. This process integrates interpretation of family and medical histories, education about inheritance, testing, management, prevention, resources, research, and counseling.[12] The 2008–2009 National Society of Genetic Counselors' Core Skills Task Force identified six key areas of skills for a successful genetic counselor[13]:

1. Deep and broad knowledge of genetics
2. Ability to tailor, translate, and communicate complex information in a simple, relevant way for a broad range of audiences
3. Strong interpersonal skills, emotional intelligence, and self-awareness
4. Ability to dissect and analyze a complex problem
5. Research skills (self-education)
6. In-depth knowledge of health care delivery

Genetic counseling is traditionally a clinical service performed by master's degree-trained professionals educated at accredited genetic counseling training programs. A clinic-based genetic counselor will typically have patient and health care team-oriented skills including communication, critical thinking, counseling, psychosocial assessment, and professional ethics and values. Since their primary purpose is to counsel patients on genetic-related diseases or conditions, current training programs incorporate little medication-related information, pharmacology, or pharmacogenomics.

Pharmacist Education

A report published in 2002 by the Academic Affairs Committee of the American Association of Colleges of Pharmacy identified the need to include curricular outcomes relating to pharmacogenetics and pharmacogenomics in the pharmacy curriculum.[14] A literature review from 1960 to 2011 revealed that several schools have research courses, journal clubs, and application-based cases related to pharmacogenomics. Although the content is included in the curriculum, the depth of the material may be limited.[15,16]

Pharmacists must be formally educated if they are to take on future roles involving pharmacogenomics. Surveys conducted in the United States have discovered that, although some instruction in pharmacogenomics is currently provided, it needs to be enhanced and developed to keep current.[17,18]

Since pharmacists are well prepared to analyze drug issues, and are accessible to provide information to patients, they should have formal pharmacogenomics training to maximize their impact in health care.

MEDICATION THERAPY MANAGEMENT

Pharmacists are trained to be the medication expert on the health care team. Experts estimate that 1.5 million preventable adverse events occur each year, resulting in $177 billion in injury and death from medication-related problems and medication mismanagement.[19] Pharmacogenomics can be a useful tool for pharmacists to use in preventing medication-related problems and adverse events with drugs such as abacavir and warfarin. Medication therapy management is a term used to describe a broad range of health care services provided by pharmacists and other members of the health care team. As defined in a consensus statement adopted by the pharmacy profession in 2004, medication therapy management is "a service or group of services that optimize therapeutic outcomes for individual patients."[20] Medication therapy management services include, but are not limited to, medication therapy reviews, pharmacotherapy consults, anticoagulation management, immunizations, and health and wellness programs. Integration of pharmacogenomic information into these services is a logical extension of current practice. Pharmacists are the most likely professional to offer these services, but specially trained or advanced practice nurses may also provide them. Medication therapy management optimizes the benefits patients obtain from their medications by actively managing drug therapy and identifying, preventing, and resolving medication-related problems. One example of integration of pharmacogenomic data into medication therapy management would be utilizing CYP2C19 to identify patients who will not respond to clopidogrel therapy.

Medication therapy management services are offered in all care settings in which patients take medications. The goal of medication therapy management, no matter the setting, is to ensure that each medication is right for the patient and his or her health conditions and that the best possible outcomes from treatment are achieved. Integration of pharmacogenomics into the existing rubric for medication therapy management services allows the tailoring of medication therapy more precisely for the patient.

PATIENT-CENTERED MEDICAL HOME

The patient-centered medical home is an approach to providing comprehensive primary care to adults, youth, and children. It may broaden access to primary care while enhancing care coordination. Providing care to patients in this type of approach encourages clinicians to practice in a collaborative effort. This collaboration is particularly important because pharmacogenomic data do not currently have a standardized place in electronic medical records (EMRs) or pharmacy dispensing systems.

Clinicians can educate patients on preventative care utilizing environmental and genetic risk factors in the patient-centered medical home model. Working together, clinicians initiate treatment and prevention measures before costly, last-minute emergency procedures are required. Utilizing HLA-B*5701 to prevent abacavir-associated hypersensitivity reaction (HSR) is one example of integrating pharmacogenomic data to prevent patient harm. The role of the patient-centered medical home in coordinating care should result in healthier patients and using pharmacogenomic data should result in safer and more effective medication use. The consideration and evaluation of pharmacogenomic tests in this setting emphasizes the need for pharmacogenomic education for all health professionals.

Integration of Pharmacogenomics into Medication Prescribing Information or Package Inserts

When health care professionals have a question regarding the relationship between a genomic biomarker and a medication, most refer to the drug prescribing information in the package insert. In 2006, a study performed by Frueh et al. reviewed the approved drug labels in the United States to find that 121 out of approximately 1,200 drug labels contained genomic information.[21] Of the 121, only 69 contained information about normal or cancerous human genetic information. The remaining 52 labels contained viral or microbial genomic information. While the US Food and Drug Administration requires the inclusion of human genomic information in a number of drug package inserts, testing prior to prescribing is not mandated.[22] As an example, the drug label for warfarin provides a genotype-based

TABLE 9–1 Warfarin dosing based on genotype (from warfarin package insert).[a]

VKORC1	CYP2C9					
	*1/*1 (mg)	*1/*2 (mg)	*1/*3 (mg)	*2/*2 (mg)	*2/*3 (mg)	*3/*3 (mg)
GG	5–7	5–7	3–4	3–4	3–4	0.5–2
AG	5–7	3–4	3–4	3–4	0.5–2	0.5–2
AA	3–4	3–4	0.5–2	0.5–2	0.5–2	0.5–2

[a]Ranges are derived from multiple clinical studies. Other clinical factors (e.g., age, race, body weight, sex, concomitant medications, and comorbidities) are generally accounted for along with genotype in the ranges expressed in the table. VKORC1 −1639 G → A (rs9923231) variant is used in this table. Other coinherited VKORC1 variants may also be important determinants of warfarin dose. Patients with CYP2C9 *1/*3, *2/*2, *2/*3, and *3/*3 may require more prolonged time (>2–4 weeks) to achieve maximum INR effect for a given dosage regimen.

dosing using cytochrome P 450 2C9 (CYP2C9) and the vitamin K epoxide reductase subunit 1 (VKORC1) as data that may guide prescribing to achieve a therapeutic international normalized ratio (INR). (The INR is a lab value monitored to help ensure safe and effective drug therapy with warfarin.) However, the package insert does not require the prescriber to obtain, but rather describes the use of, the pharmacogenomic information "when it is available"[23] (see Table 9–1).

This lack of a provision for pharmacogenomics testing prior to dosing can be seen in at least 69 other package inserts. As more data demonstrate the value of pharmacogenomic testing prior to prescribing drugs, patients or prescribers will begin to request pharmacogenomic testing to personalize drug therapy, and pharmacists and other health care professionals will find prescribing guidance in the package inserts or on the US FDA Web site.[22]

PUBLIC ACCESS TO TESTING: TYPES OF TESTS

Direct-to-Consumer Pharmacogenomic Tests

Some pharmacogenomic tests are only available for research purposes. These tests, often referred to as "home brews," are usually specific to one particular research study and are not used in the public or clinical arena. Public access to pharmacogenomic testing typically comes in two main forms: directly to the consumer and via a health care practitioner.

As the lay press introduces pharmacogenomic applications and patients become aware of the ability to link their individual DNA with an individualized drug therapy, there will be more of a demand for genetic testing. In fact, several companies currently provide genetic testing directly to consumers. These companies often advertise via the Internet, and the number of tests and types of testing vary widely. Generally, patients ordering the tests are sent a kit to collect a buccal swab or a small blood sample from a finger stick. The kit is then mailed back to the testing location that processes the sample and provides the results of the genetic test to the consumer.

Proponents of direct-to-consumer pharmacogenomic tests claim that the provision of genetic tests directly to consumers

increases health awareness and access to genetic tests. If patients can research information and request tests on their own, they may be more likely to be active participants in their own health care. Furthermore, patient privacy may be better maintained since the results of genetic testing are not stored in a permanent medical record, and patients have the choice of sharing this information with health care professionals.

Opponents of direct-to-consumer genetic tests highlight the lack of inclusion of health care professionals in the ordering and interpretation of tests as a significant detriment. With direct-to-consumer testing, health care professionals are removed from communication with patients. Patients may be ill-equipped to understand the complex nature of genetic results but nevertheless may make their own, potentially life-altering, decisions based on these results. Without a health care professional involved in selection, interpretation, or follow-up of genetic tests, patients may misinterpret the results, which could lead to suboptimal health care choices. Although some direct-to-consumer companies offer counseling with results, a study conducted by the Government Accountability Office found that reliability of counseling services varied widely. As these companies are not regulated, the same study found wide variability between the test results from different direct-to-consumer companies.[24] This lack of regulation and standardization could put patients in danger, as the companies may not follow laws in place to protect patient privacy and may make false claims of efficacy or benefits of testing.

Although direct-to-consumer testing can increase patient access to their genetic information, this information is best conveyed by a trained health care professional. Health care professionals can support their patients by keeping current on available direct-to-consumer tests and being available for counseling. As the status of direct-to-consumer testing changes, asking patients about their use of these genetic tests may become part of routine care.

Health Care Practitioner– Ordered Lab Tests

The other mechanism for the public to access genetic testing is through health care professionals. Practitioners authorized to order genetic tests can have them completed on site, at a health center lab, or via third-party laboratory testing. The laboratories for practitioner-ordered tests are regulated by government agencies. The ordering practitioner is responsible for interpretation and follow-up of the genetic test results and the health care professionals are bound by patient privacy laws.

TYPES OF COUNSELING SERVICES FROM HEALTH CARE PROFESSIONALS

Physician Counseling

In the United States, approximately one third of physicians providing patient care are general practitioners, and two thirds are specialists. In other countries the majority of physicians are generalists, with fewer specialists. Both types of physicians may deal with genetic factors and how they affect susceptibility to disease and treatment of diseases.

The physicians are responsible for ordering studies, tests, and ancillary services and they must document all services in patient medical records, including ordering genomic tests and counseling the patient about the test results. Ultimately, physicians exercise final medical judgment and assume the most liability in all issues of health care and prescribe medical treatment, including drugs, to patients.

Nurse Counseling

Registered nurses constitute the largest health care occupation, with 2.6 million jobs in the United States. Most registered nurses in the United States, and more broadly nurses working across the world, work directly with patients and their families. They treat patients, educate patients and the public about various medical conditions, and provide advice and emotional support to patients and patients' family members. Registered nurses help collect samples for diagnostic tests and report results, operate medical machinery, administer treatment and medications, and help with patient follow-up and rehabilitation. They teach patients and their families how to manage their illnesses or injuries, explaining posttreatment home care needs, diet, nutrition, and exercise programs, and self-administration of medication and physical therapy. Because the registered nurse is on the front line with patients, the registered nurse is often the first to notice problems or raise concerns about patient progress and usually the first to counsel a patient. They may also be the first to be asked questions about pharmacogenomics by patients and must be poised to offer education and counseling appropriate to the test ordered.

Genetic Counselor Counseling

Genetic counselors work with individuals who may be at risk for a variety of inherited conditions or who have family members with birth defects or genetic disorders. Patients come to genetic counselors to understand their risks for certain diseases. The genetic counselor reviews their history and helps determine what risks exist due to genetics and medical history. Patients also come to genetic counselors to understand their risk in passing on certain birth defects or genetic disorders to their unborn children.

Genetic counselors translate technical information about inherited health disorders into language that can be understood by the average person. They explain health disorders, the available options for testing for or treatment of these disorders, and the risks associated with each option, including the risk of changes in insurability. They also help patients come to terms with the emotional and psychological aspects of having an inherited disorder or disease.

When an individual schedules an appointment, the genetic counselor usually asks the patient to gather as much specific information about the past two generations of his or her family as possible. The counselor may ask for physicians' records, photographs, and anecdotal information. If a patient is concerned about inherited cancer, for instance, the physician or genetic counselor wants to know how frequently the disease has occurred in the family, what types of cancer occurred, and at what age family members developed the disease. All of this information provides the genetic counselor with important clues about the patient's genetic probability of inheriting a disease. As with evaluating the relationship between genetics and risk of cancer, the genetic counselor's role may expand to include aspects of the relationship between genetics and medications (pharmacogenomics).

If a patient decides to proceed with testing, the genetic counselor interprets the test results, discusses treatment options, and explains the risks, both physical and emotional, associated with the various treatment options. Throughout the counseling process, the genetic counselor remains supportive of his or her patients' choices.

Pharmacist Counseling

Pharmacists are viewed as the medication experts on the health care team. They routinely utilize information found in the drug package insert or pharmacy drug databases to select, monitor, or alter drug therapy. When pharmacogenomic information is included in the package inserts, pharmacists incorporate these data to determine important counseling points and ensure safe use of medications. Pharmacists are well positioned to counsel patients on medications that are affected by pharmacogenomics. They can collect patient data, provide information about medications, and help patients understand the instructions their doctors or other health care professionals provided. In addition to advising their patients, they also serve as advisors to physicians and other health care professionals on the selection, dose, interactions, and side effects of medications, as well as monitor the health and progress of those patients to ensure that they are using their medications safely and effectively. Pharmacists must understand the composition of medicines as well as the laws that regulate their manufacture and sale. They also plan, monitor, and evaluate drug programs or regimens. Most pharmacists keep confidential computerized records of patients' drug therapies to prevent harmful drug interactions. And in all health care roles, pharmacists must impart drug information through thorough counseling to patients taking or considering taking a specific pharmacotherapy.

Pharmacist-Directed Patient Counseling and Pharmacogenomics

Basics of Pharmacist Medication Counseling

Pharmacists working in a dispensing role are required by law to counsel their patients on specific aspects of drug therapy at the time of dispensing; thus, all students who matriculate from a school of pharmacy are taught the key aspects of patient counseling. State laws differ regarding which types of prescriptions require the offer to counsel; however, one federal law typically sets the standard that all states follow. The law, referred to as OBRA '90 because it resulted from the 1990 Omnibus Budget Reconciliation Act, delineates specific points a pharmacist must review during a counseling session. The law applies to new prescriptions for certain patients but has become the standard for medication-related counseling. The points a pharmacist must include when he or she counsels are listed in Table 9–2. These counseling points reflect the minimum required information to be provided to patients on receipt of a prescription. The federal law, OBRA '90, allows for pharmacists' professional judgment to determine if all specific points need to be included in each particular counseling session. Omnibus Budget Reconciliation Act of 1990. Available from http://www.ssa.gov/OP_Home/comp2/F101-508.html. Accessed July 20, 2011.

Integrating Pharmacogenomics into Patient Counseling

Under OBRA '90, pharmacists are responsible for providing adequate information to patients in order to ensure the safe and effective use of medications. Recommendations for medications routinely take into account patient status, including renal and hepatic function, potential for drug interactions, and potential for adverse effects. The integration of pharmacogenomic data into routine counseling is a logical extension of current practice.

As discussed previously, information specific to pharmacogenomics can often be found in the drug prescribing information, or package inserts. Where drug-specific pharmacogenomic information is not available, pharmacists are trained to make clinical decisions based on key pieces of information. For example, if a patient is known to be a slow metabolizer of the CYP2D6 enzyme and two medications are available to treat a given disease, one that goes through CYP2D6 and one that does not, a pharmacist may make the recommendation for the latter. In situations where there is only one medication, a pharmacist's expertise is applied to determine monitoring parameters, dosage adjustments, and additional counseling. If the genetic variance makes the patient at increased risk for a certain side effect, the pharmacist's responsibility is to counsel the patient on monitoring for the side effect and actions to take should the adverse effect occur. This responsibility is no different from the pharmacist's usual responsibility; it is simply an integration of additional information into the usual realm of practice.

Integrating Pharmacogenomic Information into Clinical Care

Using a systematic process to evaluate the decision to order a genomic test or to apply pharmacogenomic data to the patient's unique situation is an essential component of medication therapy management for pharmacists and for the normal care provided by physicians or physician extenders. One method of systematically considering the integration of pharmacogenomic tests is to use NAVAGATE (see Table 9–3). The NAVAGATE system is not hard to understand. In fact, for clinicians, it just defines the process utilized when evaluating any new medication or laboratory test.

When considering a medication with evidence of an association with genetic variation, NAVAGATE suggests asking two important and early questions: *is the drug necessary and are there alternatives that can be substituted?* If the drug is not necessary, then there is little utility in obtaining a genetic test. Similarly, if there are alternative medications that do not require the genetic test, do not incur additional toxicities, and are available at a

TABLE 9–2   Requirements for pharmacist medication counseling as part of OBRA '90.

- Name and description of the medication
- Route of administration
- Dose, dosage form, and duration of drug therapy
- Special directions and precautions for preparation of drugs, administration, and use by the patient
- Common severe side effects or adverse effects or interactions and therapeutic contraindications that may be encountered (including their avoidance and the action required if they occur)
- Techniques for self-monitoring drug therapy
- Proper storage
- Refill information
- Appropriate action in case of a missed dose

Source: Omnibus Budget Reconciliation Act of 1990. Available from http://www.ssa.gov/OP_Home/comp2/F101-508.html. Accessed July 20, 2011.

TABLE 9–3   The NAVAGATE approach to integrating PGX into medication therapy plans.

NAVAGATE	Questions to Ask for Integrating PGX into Practice and Challenges HCPs Face
Necessary	Is the drug necessary?
Alternatives	Are there alternative treatments?
Validated Test	Is there a validated test (home brewed vs. FDA-approved test)? How do you collect the sample?
Appropriate turnaround time	Will the result return in a clinically relevant time frame?
Good evidence	Is there evidence regarding what to do with a result? Increase, decrease dose or increase monitoring for adverse effects
Acceptance	Is there provider/patient acceptance?
Test reimbursement/ payment	How will the patient pay for the test?
Evaluate results and document	How will you document it in the medical record?

reasonable cost, then the genetic test may not be required. The next important question asks: *is there a validated test available?* If no validated or commercially available test exists, then the professional will not be able to use genetic information to individualize therapy. If a test is available, *is the result obtainable in a reasonable time for the clinical scenario?* For example, in the case of a long-term maintenance medication and a concern for drug efficacy, one can start therapy and obtain the test, even waiting a few weeks for the results. However, in the case of drug toxicity and the need to initiate therapy immediately, a provider may choose to forgo the genetic test, opting to use clinical monitoring over a test that will not be available in the requisite time.

For pharmacists, the next two questions are very important: *is there good evidence to support the drug–gene relationship?* And, second, *do prescribers accept the association?* In most cases, prescribers' acceptance mirrors the amount of evidence. For example, when the relationship between abacavir HSR pointed to an association with an HLA genotype (HLA-B*5701), providers began to take note. When a prospective clinical trial evaluating the relationship discovered that abacavir HSRs could be eliminated by utilizing an HLA genotype result, the information was incorporated into the drug package insert and into the HIV treatment guidelines.[25,26] Clinical practice was changed as the evidence evolved.

Next, the evaluation of cost is an essential component of considering any new drug therapy or way to monitor drug therapy. The individual patient cost or the cost to the insurer with the rate of reimbursement is a nebulous area. Cost-effectiveness analyses, such as those using the common and systematic ACCE (analytic validity, clinical validity, clinical utility, and ethical, legal, and social implications) methodology, judge the cost-effectiveness of getting the pharmacogenomic test and the benefit to the patients.[27] In the case of abacavir, the cost-effectiveness analyses thoroughly support integrating HLA genotype results into clinical decision making. Insurance companies pay for the HLA genotype to prevent higher costs incurred from HSR. Little data exist on the rate of reimbursement for other pharmacogenomic tests.

With drugs such as clopidogrel that require a polymorphic enzyme, CYP2C19, to activate the drug to its active metabolite, the test may not be reimbursed.[28] However, the cost per month of clopidogrel is approximately one half the cost of the genetic test. With insufficient CYP2C19 activity, patients could be paying over $200 per month for a therapy that is ineffective or subtherapeutic. By having the genetic test, the patients who would benefit from alternative therapies, such as prasugrel or ticagrelor, are identified. Some might say that the use of clopidogrel as a maintenance or long-term (up to and beyond 1 year) medication supports the use of a genetic test regardless of the rate of reimbursement.

Using the pharmacogenomic data to guide the therapy of an individual is the last question. Combining the evidence and the known mechanism of action and metabolism of the drug, along with the other components of NAVAGATE, provides a useful method for the integration of pharmacogenomic data into the usual framework of therapy management. However, the most complicated component is documentation. *Where are these pharmacogenomic data input into the EMR or pharmacy dispensing system?* Few, if any, systems have a place to put pharmacogenomic data. Additionally, few, if any, pharmacy dispensing systems utilize pharmacogenomic data at the time of dispensing to identify issues with therapies. For example, CYP2C19 may be important for activating clopidogrel. CYP2C19 is also involved in the metabolism of proton pump inhibitors. Having the pharmacogenomic test result has the potential to improve therapy with a proton pump inhibitor, yet the pharmacist has no place to put the test result that will "flag" or identify future prescriptions at the time of dispensing.[29] Does the result go in as an allergy, a problem, or a laboratory result alone? Is it available by automated/computerized decision support at the time of e-prescribing? Currently, the answer to this question is "no." Developing a systematic process for each EMR or dispensing system will improve the integration of pharmacogenomic information into clinical care at each stage of prescribing and dispensing.

CLINICAL VIGNETTES

Vignette 1

GQ is a 42-year-old Caucasian female with a past medical history significant for HIV, hypertension, and end-stage renal disease requiring renal transplant. Other history and medications are as follows:

- Medical history includes HIV+ infection (CD4+ T cell count 410 cells/mm³), end-stage renal disease preparing for renal transplant, hypertension, deep vein thrombosis of the internal jugular, pericarditis, cholelithiasis.
- *Medications include:*
  - Pioglitazone 30 mg daily
  - Amitriptyline 25 mg qhs
  - Warfarin 2 mg daily
  - Glipizide 2.5 mg bid
  - Lisinopril 20 mg daily
  - Gabapentin 200 mg qhs
  - Pravachol 20 mg daily
  - Rena-vite one tablet daily
  - Sevelamer 3,200 mg ac
  - Vitamin D 50,000 IU capsule qweek
  - Oxycodone/acetaminophen 5/325 q6h prn
  - Zolpidem 6.25 mg qhs prn

As GQ returns to his infectious disease physician the decision is made to start an antiretroviral (ARV) treatment plan to prepare for the ability to do a renal transplant. See the options for treatment plans in Table 9–4. The infectious disease physician ponders the following concerns:

- For the protease inhibitor + 2 nucleoside reverse transcriptase inhibitors containing regimen, the protease inhibitors may increase the plasma concentrations of the immunosuppressives used for renal transplant and increase the risk of toxicity.[30]

TABLE 9–4 Preferred and alternative combination therapy for HIV in 2012.

NNRTI-based Regimen	Protease Inhibitor-based Regimen	INSTI-based Regimen
Efavirenz PLUS Tenofovir/embtricitabine or Abacavir/lamivudine	Atazanavir/ritonavir, or Darunavir/ritonavir, or Fosamprenavir/ritonavir or Lopinavir/ritonavir PLUS Tenofovir/embtricitabine, or Abacavir/lamivudine	Raltegravir PLUS Tenofovir/embtricitabine, or Abacavir/lamivudine
Rilpivirine PLUS Tenofovir/embtricitabine, or Abacavir/lamivudine		

NNRTI = non-nucleoside reverse transcriptase inhibitor; INSTI = integrase strand transfer inhibitor.

The preferred regimens are: efavirenz/tenofovir/emtricitabine; atazanavir or darunavir/ritonavir/tenofovir/emtricitabine; raltegravir/tenofovir/emtricitabine.

Adapted from http://www.aidsinfo.nih.gov/contentfiles/lvguidelines/adultandadolescentgl.pdf (Accessed 7/26/2012)

- The nucleoside reverse transcriptase inhibitor tenofovir is to be avoided due to the small risk of nephrotoxicity.
- The integrase strand transfer inhibitor (INSTI) containing regimen was not available to the patient at the time of the clinic visit due to the drug formulary.
- For the non-nucleoside reverse transcriptase inhibitor containing regimen, efavirenz may decrease the plasma concentrations of mycophenolate or tacrolimus (both immunosuppressives) and risk rejection.[30] However, the levels of the immunosuppressives can be monitored.

The NRTI-based regimen, containing abacavir, has the potential for an abacavir HSR. Fortunately, GQ can be genotyped for the HLA-B*5701 biomarker that helps to identify patients at risk. To assess the need for the HLA genotype and the use of abacavir, NAVAGATE (see Table 9–5) the patient scenario. The followup plan was to obtain an HLA-B*5701 genotype, liver function tests, a lipid panel, and a repeat viral load in 2 weeks. Since the HLA-B*5701 genotype was negative, a regimen of abacavir/lamivudine/efavirenz was started. The following documentation was placed in the provider note:

- Completion Date: 03/04/2008
- Test Name: **HIGH RESOLUTION HLA B**
- Test Result: HLA-B*57 IS ABSENT

Vignette 2

Allie is a 68-year-old Caucasian female (height 64 in; weight 145 lb) with a medical history significant for diabetes and hypertension controlled with medication. Allie's medications include metformin, pravastatin, aspirin 325 mg per day, and metoprolol. Atrial fibrillation was detected on her EKG during a routine evaluation and confirmed by two return visits and repeat EKGs. Allie was started on metoprolol 12.5 mg twice per day to control her heart rate (110 bpm). Her blood pressure remains controlled

with the addition of metoprolol to her regimen. Her $CHADS_2$ score is 2 and her physician recommends warfarin to prevent thromboembolic strokes secondary to her atrial fibrillation. Allie is unsure if she wants to start warfarin anticoagulation at this time. She heads home continuing her 325 mg aspirin per day and plans to return to clinic in 2 weeks with her daughter to discuss starting warfarin.

TABLE 9–5 NAVAGATE for vignette 1.

NAVAGATE	Vignette 1: Questions to Ask for Integrating PGX into Practice and Challenges HCPs Face
Necessary	ARV treatment needed prior to renal transplant
Alternatives	Other ARV combinations exist but contraindications prohibit the use
Validated test	Yes
Appropriate turnaround time	1–2 weeks; usually clinically appropriate
Good evidence	Yes; evidence proven to decrease abc-hsr (PREDICT-1 study)[25]
Acceptance	Yes; in the drug package insert
Test reimbursement/ payment	Yes
Evaluate results and document	Per the HIV Guidelines (ref#) place information in the allergy section of EHR and pharmacy dispensing system; may consider adding negative test result to document test performed.

Data from Roederer MW. NAVAGATE: from pharmacogenomics science to pharmacogenomics practice. *Pharmacogenomics*. August 2012.

Allie returns to clinic in 2 weeks with her daughter and a lab result from a direct-to-consumer warfarin panel that tests for VKORC1 and CYP2C9 genotypes. The results are as follows:

VKORC1: −1639 AA

CYP2C9: *1/*1

To evaluate the situation, Allie's physician decides to NAVAGATE (see Table 9–6).

While the information is useful if from a valid laboratory, the physician is not comfortable using the information from the direct-to-consumer company. He decides to order a warfarin genotype panel from his local approved clinical laboratory company. The results are inconsistent. The clinical lab results are: VKORC1 −1639 AA and CYP2C9*1/*2. The physician chooses to utilize the results from the clinical laboratory. Using www.warfarindosing.org and the International Warfarin Pharmacogenetics Consortium (IWPC) algorithms' prediction, along with the drug prescribing information for warfarin (see Table 9–1), Allie is begun on 3 mg daily of warfarin, a 40% lower dose of warfarin than is customarily begun based on clinical treatment guidelines (usual dose 5 mg per day) for the use of warfarin and a lower dose than is predicted using the direct-to-consumer test results.

Allie's INR, used to measure the efficacy and predict the toxicity of warfarin, is up from a baseline of 1.0–2.2 when she returns in 2 weeks, with a goal INR of 2–3 (average 2.5). Allie's physician continues Allie's dose of warfarin at 3 mg daily.

TABLE 9–6 NAVAGATE for vignette 2.

NAVAGATE	Vignette 2: Questions to Ask for Integrating PGX into Practice and Challenges HCPs Face
Necessary	For primary stroke prevention in atrial fibrillation
Alternatives	Aspirin, dabigatran
Validated test	Validated test exists; DTC test?
Appropriate turnaround time	Have a result from DTC test; results from Health System labs ~24 h
Good evidence	Yes; *New Engl J Med*, February 2009
Acceptance	Marginal
Test reimbursement/ payment	Depends, not DTC
Evaluate results and document	www.warfarindosing.org
	Documentation challenging
	Where do you put it in the EMR?
	Should this information be included in dispensing program for pharmacy?
	How is this information shared across health professions?

TABLE 9–7 NAVAGATE for vignette 3.

NAVAGATE	Vignette 3: Questions to Ask for Integrating PGX into Practice and Challenges HCPs Face
Necessary	For platelet inhibition and prevention of stent occlusion
Alternatives	Prasugrel
Validated test	Validated test exists
Appropriate turnaround time	Have a result; results in Health System labs ~2 days
Good evidence	Fair
Acceptance	Marginal
Test reimbursement/ payment	Fair in hospital, not DTC
Evaluate results and document	Results documented in hospital record under laboratory results
	Is there a capacity to document in pharmacy dispensing system?

Vignette 3

JP is a 67-year-old Caucasian male with a medical history significant for hyperlipidemia (3 years), stage 1 hypertension (4 years), and recent ST-elevation myocardial infarction (STEMI) with stent placement (8 days ago). He weighs 87 kg. His current medications include simvastatin 40 mg at bedtime, metoprolol 12.5 mg twice per day, lisinopril 20 mg daily, and clopidogrel 75 mg daily. He comes to the community pharmacy and asks to speak with the pharmacist about the lab report he just received in the mail from the hospital; his doctor ordered the test but is now on vacation. The results are as follows:

- CYP2C19: *2/*2

Through NAVAGATE (see Table 9–7), explore the results with JP and provide an explanation of the results.

The results are from a regulated lab at the hospital and are deemed reliable. JP is changed from clopidogrel 75 mg daily to prasugrel 10 mg for prevention of stent thrombosis after percutaneous coronary intervention.

CONCLUSION

Pharmacogenomics is a rapidly evolving science that improves drug use by allowing for a personalized medication therapy plan that includes matching genetics to drug choice, dose, or monitoring. While physicians, nurses, and genetic counselors are critical to evaluating and providing information to patients regarding pharmacogenomics, pharmacists are uniquely poised to counsel patients and integrate the pharmacogenomics information into a safe medication use process for patients at the pharmacy level. Utilizing a systematic process for assessing the pharmacogenomics data and using it to influence the medication therapy plan is key to bridging the gap between science and the art of medicine.

REFERENCES

1. Kobayashi E, Satoh N. Public involvement in pharmacogenomics research: a national survey on public attitudes towards pharmacogenomics research and the willingness to donate DNA samples to a DNA bank in Japan. *Cell Tissue Bank*. 2009;10:281–291.

2. Genetics education and training: a report of the Secretary's Advisory Committee on Genetics, Health, and Society. US Department of Health and Human Services. 2011. Available at: http://oba.od.nih.gov/oba/SACGHS/reports/SACGHS_education_report_2011.pdf. Accessed July 19, 2011.

3. Thurston VC, Wales PS, Bell MA, Torbeck L, Brokaw JJ. The current status of medical genetics instruction in US and Canadian medical schools. *Acad Med*. 2007;82:441–445.

4. Robertson JA, Brody B, Buchanan A, Kahn J, McPherson E. Pharmacogenetic challenges for the health care system. *Health Aff (Millwood)*. 2002; 21:155–167.

5. Gurwitz D, Lunshof JE, Dedoussis G, et al. Pharmacogenomics education: International Society of Pharmacogenomics recommendations for medical, pharmaceutical, and health schools deans of education. *Pharmacogenomics J*. 2005;5:221–225.

6. Calzone KA, Cashion A, Feetham S, et al. Nurses transforming health care using genetics and genomics. *Nurs Outlook*. 2010;58:26–35.

7. Maradiegue A, Edwards QT, Seibert D, Macri C, Sitzer L. Knowledge, perceptions, and attitudes of advanced practice nursing students regarding medical genetics. *J Am Acad Nurse Pract*. 2005;17:472–479.

8. Prows CA, Calzone KA, Jenkins J. Genetics content in nursing curriculum. In: *Proceedings of NCHPEG 2006*; Bethesda, Maryland.

9. Current Genetic/Genomic Education Priorities and Progress in Nursing. NHGRI. 2008. Available at: http://httpf//www.genome.gov/Pages/About/OD/ReportsPublications/June2008_JenkinsHoL.pdf. Accessed July 20, 2011.

10. Prows CA, Saldana SN. Nurses' genetic/genomics competencies when medication therapy is guided by pharmacogenetic testing: children with mental health disorders as an exemplar. *J Pediatr Nurs*. 2009;24:179–188.

11. Van Riper M. Family nursing in the era of genomic health care: we should be doing so much more! *J Fam Nurs*. 2006;12:111–118.

12. Resta R, Biesecker BB, Bennett RL, et al. A new definition of genetic counseling: National Society of Genetic Counselors' Task Force report. *J Genet Couns*. 2006;15:77–83.

13. National Society of Genetic Counselors' Core Skills Task Force 2008–2009. Available at: http://www.nsgc.org/Portals/0/Tools%20for%20Practice/Core SkillsSummary.pdf. Accessed July 20, 2011.

14. Johnson JA, Bootman JL, Evans WE, et al. Pharmacogenomics: a scientific revolution in pharmaceutical sciences and pharmacy practice. *Am J Pharm Educ*. 2002;66:12S–15S.

15. Murphy JE, Green JS, Adams LA, Squire RB, Kuo GM, McKay A. Pharmacogenomics in the curricula of colleges and schools of pharmacy in the United States. *Am J Pharm Educ*. 2010;74:7.

16. Vizirianakis IS. Pharmaceutical education in the wake of genomic technologies for drug development and personalized medicine. *Eur J Pharm Sci*. 2002;15:243–250.

17. Brock TP, Valgus JM, Smith SR, Summers KM. Pharmacogenomics: implications and considerations for pharmacists. *Pharmacogenomics*. 2003; 4:321–330.

18. Latif DA. Pharmacogenetics and pharmacogenomics instruction in schools of pharmacy in the USA: is it adequate? *Pharmacogenomics*. 2005;6:317–319.

19. A call to action: protecting U.S. citizens from inappropriate medication use. 2007. Available at: http://www.ismp.org/pressroom/viewpoints/CommunityPharmacy.pdf. Accessed July 20, 2011.

20. American Pharmacists Association, National Association of Chain Drug Stores Foundation. Medication therapy management in pharmacy practice: core elements of an MTM service model (version 2.0). *J Am Pharm Assoc*. 2008;48:341–353.

21. Frueh FW, Amur S, Mummaneni P, et al. Pharmacogenomic biomarker information in drug labels approved by the United States Food and Drug Administration: prevalence of related drug use. *Pharmacotherapy*. 2008; 28:992–998.

22. US FDA. Table of pharmacogenomic biomarkers in drug labels. 2011. Available at: http://www.fda.gov/Drugs/ScienceResearch/ResearchAreas/Pharmacogenetics/ucm083378.htm. Accessed July 20, 2011.

23. Coumadin (warfarin) [package insert]. Princeton, NJ: Bristol-Myers Squibb Company; 2010. Available at: http://www.accessdata.fda.gov/drugsatfda_docs/label/2010/009218s108lbl.pdf. Accessed July 20, 2011.

24. Direct-to-consumer genetic tests: misleading test results are further complicated by deceptive marketing and other questionable practices. 2010. Available at: http://www.gao.gov/new.items/d10847t.pdf. Accessed July 20, 2011.

25. Mallal S, Phillips E, Carosi G, et al. HLA-B*5701 screening for hypersensitivity to abacavir. *N Engl J Med*. 2008;358:568–579.

26. Guidelines for the use of antiretroviral agents in HIV-1-infected adults and adolescents. 2011. Available at: http://www.aidsinfo.nih.gov/Guidelines/GuidelineDetail.aspx?GuidelineID=7. Accessed July 20, 2011.

27. Gudgeon JM, McClain MR, Palomaki GE, Williams MS. Rapid ACCE: experience with a rapid and structured approach for evaluating gene-based testing. *Genet Med*. 2007;9:473–478.

28. Sangkuhl K, Klein TE, Altman RB. Clopidogrel pathway. *Pharmacogenet Genomics*. 2010;20:463–465.

29. Klotz U. Clinical impact of CYP2C19 polymorphism on the action of proton pump inhibitors: a review of a special problem. *Int J Clin Pharmacol Ther*. 2006;44:297–302.

30. Robertson SM, Penzak SR, Pau A. Drug interactions in the management of HIV infection: an update. *Expert Opin Pharmacother*. 2007;8:2947–2963.

Understanding the Use of Pharmacoeconomic Analysis to Assess the Economic Impact of Pharmacogenomic Testing

Mark Bounthavong, PharmD, Christine M. Nguyen, PharmD, BCPS, & Margaret Mendes, PharmD

LEARNING OBJECTIVES

- Define the different elements of pharmacoeconomic analysis: costs, benefits, perspective, cost-effectiveness plane, ECHO model, utility weights and quality-adjusted life years (QALYS), and discounting.

- Identify the different pharmacoeconomic analyses available: cost-minimization analysis, cost–benefit analysis, cost-effectiveness analysis, and cost–utility analysis.

- Know the elements of a decision model: decision nodes, chance nodes, and terminal nodes.

- Identify and interpret the results of a one-way sensitivity analysis, two-way sensitivity analysis, and probabilistic sensitivity analysis, and cost-effectiveness acceptability curve.

- Determine why pharmacoeconomics is needed when utilizing pharmacogenomics in clinical practice.

INTRODUCTION

Economics is the study of choosing a strategy amid limited resources or scarcity.[1] In health care, there is limited resources for all the medical needs of patients. Therefore, a formal evaluation into the costs and benefits of drugs, interventions, and programs needs to be assessed in order to efficiently and equitably distribute limited resources. Pharmacoeconomics is the quantitative assessment of the costs and benefits associated with a treatment strategy.[2] Similar to traditional economics, pharmacoeconomics assess the choices that a decision maker selects and the cascading costs and outcomes associated with that choice. What

distinguishes pharmacoeconomics from traditional economics is the assessment of health weighted by costs. In economics, decision makers are only interested in the overall costs associated with a choice or strategy, whereas, in pharmacoeconomics, costs are weighed by the benefits or outcomes associated with the treatment strategy. Treatment strategy can be a health care program to prevent chronic disease, it could represent a new molecular entity (NME) entering the market, or it can represent a new diagnostic test that can improve outcomes or avoid adverse events. In either case, pharmacoeconomics provides a scientific and quantitative method for estimating the value of a treatment strategy weighted by the costs. There are many facets

TABLE 10–1 Cost per megabyte of DNA and cost per genome, September 2001 to April 2011.

Year	Cost Per Megabyte of DNA Sequence (US$)	Cost Per Genome (US$)
2001	5292	95,263,072
2002	3,656	65,811,929
2003	2,608	46,954,619
2004	1,217	21,919,152
2005	884	15,919,004
2006	642	11,562,016
2007	479	8,632,663
2008	32	1,377,846
2009	1	141,461
2010	0	18,837

within pharmacoeconomics, of which one of the most promising is pharmacogenomic evaluation.

PHARMACOGENOMICS HISTORY

Costs of whole genome testing have decreased exponentially since 2008, 5 years after the first draft of the human genome was sequenced by the US Department of Energy and the National Institutes of Health (Table 10–1).[3] It took 13 years for the first draft to be officially completed, which cost over $13 billion.[3] It is estimated that by 2013, whole genome testing could cost as little as $100 as prices of reagents drop and the speed of sequencing technology grows.[4] Currently, it is unknown how whole genome testing will affect the application of pharmacogenomics into clinical practice. Regardless, the information due to the advancements made through the Human Genome Project (HGP) has given us a basis by which we continue to understand how genetics affects disease, traits, and metabolism of medications. Obviously it is not feasible to test every patient's genome. Therefore, methods are used to scan known areas of the genome for variations and are usually limited to scanning hundreds or thousands of base pairs. This type of technology allows for quicker and less costly method to identify mutations.

AVAILABLE PHARMACOGENOMIC TESTS

There are several pharmacogenomic tests that are commercially available today and have the major advantage of offering individualized therapy, improving clinical outcomes through advanced risk screening and disease diagnosis, and a decreased likelihood of adverse drug reactions. During the next decade, it is estimated that pharmaceutical companies will be able to develop more targeted drug therapy through new SNP discovery or improving on what is currently known. It is expected that by including only patients with known genetic variations in clinical trials there would be

decreases in adverse reactions and improvements in clinical outcomes. This may decrease drug costs and approval time by the US Food and Drug Administration (FDA), thus increasing the likelihood of survival than that in previous years. The alternative argument is that drug costs will increase if pharmacogenomic testing is included in clinical trials to determine treatment eligibility. In addition, these medications are often targeted biological agents with special handling, which are known to be more expensive as compared with small molecules. One example of a targeted biological agent developed based on a genetic test is trastuzumab (Herceptin®, Genentech). Trastuzumab targets breast cancer patients with *HER2* gene overexpression. Patients with *HER2* overexpression are more likely to respond to this medication. Testing for *HER2* is required to prevent those who are not *HER2* positive from being treated with the costly medication.

It is important to keep in mind that although costs of sequencing continue to decrease, other costs must be taken into consideration. For example, computerized patient records would need to hold billions of data points for one patient. Developing the technology to store these data in a usable manner will likely cost millions of dollars.

Pharmacoeconomics can assist decision makers in determining the cost-effectiveness of using a pharmacogenomic test versus no testing. The concept of cost-effectiveness represents the decision maker's proxy for determining if the clinical benefits of a pharmacogenomic test are worth the added costs. This is critical, especially now, when there is a scarcity of resources that need to be distributed efficiently across all elements of health care. This chapter will focus on some of the challenges that must be considered when looking at overall cost of pharmacogenomic testing in a population and implementation of testing into clinical practice.

ELEMENTS OF PHARMACOECONOMICS

Before an in-depth discussion about pharmacoeconomics application in pharmacogenomics can begin, a description of the elements of a pharmacoeconomic analysis should be introduced.

Costs

Pharmacoeconomic analysis is composed of two basic elements: costs and benefits. The costs of the analysis normally are derived from three types: direct, indirect, and intangible costs. Total direct costs represent the costs directly associated with the treatment or intervention. These costs include medication acquisition cost, resource utilization (e.g., length of stay, pharmacy filling costs, laboratory tests, and cultures), and other direct costs related to the disease (e.g., treatment failures, cost of treating adverse events, and out-of-pocket costs to the patient). Indirect costs represent the productivity value (absenteeism and presenteeism) and opportunity costs (e.g., cost of treating a family member instead of earning an income doing something else). Presenteeism is when the patient is able to work but the revenue generated is less because of limitations due to an illness,[5–7] whereas absenteeism is the loss of revenue because the patient is unable to work.[6,7] Two major approaches have been presented in literature for calculating productivity: human-capital approach and friction-cost approach. The human-capital approach assumes the monetary value of a worker in perfect health and the time worked according to the current market wage rates.[8] Friction-cost approach takes into consideration the learning period required for a replacement worker.[9] Workers who leave their job due to illness or disease may be replaced by an unemployed worker; however, mobility between workers may not be 100% and a learning period is required where the potential productivity of the replacement does not meet previous worker productivity.[9] Unlike accounting, overhead charges are not considered as indirect costs in pharmacoeconomic analyses. Intangible costs represents the cost associated with perfect health (or pain and suffering) that is difficult to measure. Depending on the perspective of the pharmacoeconomic analysis, different types of costs used will determine the type of cost analysis performed.

Benefits (Payoffs or Efficacy)

The second element of a pharmacoeconomic analysis is the benefits (also referred to as efficacy or payoffs) of the treatment strategy that includes surrogate clinical outcomes. Benefits may refer to humanistic outcomes that include patient health-related quality of life. They are the aggregate outcomes of interest that occur as a consequence of the treatment strategy. Benefits can be life years added, reduction in low-density lipoprotein (LDL), decrease in blood pressure, responder to therapy, and disease cure. Benefits can also be presented as quality-adjusted life years (QALYs), which measure morbidity and mortality of a treatment strategy and are used in cost–utility analysis (CUA). Other benefits may include the cost avoidance of preventing a chronic disease (e.g., diabetes) from occurring; however, there are methodological difficulties with estimating these types of benefits.

Perspective

The perspective of a pharmacoeconomic analysis can be from the patient, provider, health care payer, government, institution, or society. Each perspective has its own unique interest on what type of costs or benefits is important. For example, a pharmacoeconomic analysis from the perspective of the patient may focus on patient's out-of-pocket costs (direct costs) that include the copayment associated with the patient's health care, cost of travel to the clinic, and cost of deductible. In addition, pharmacoeconomic analysis from the patient's perspective may also include indirect costs. Indirect costs may include the opportunity costs of the patient spending his or her money on something he or she wants instead of spending it on his or her copay or deductible. These costs reflect the money that the patient has to pay out-of-pocket and also the costs of trade-off, opportunity costs. When a patient spends his or her resources on an intervention that he or she could have used on something else, he or she is incurring an opportunity cost. Moreover, the pharmacoeconomic analysis may also use intangible costs such as the cost of a year of perfect health or a day of suffering and emotional hazards.

Pharmacoeconomic analysis where the perspective is from the payer (institution or government) normally focuses on total direct costs. For example, in genotype-guided warfarin therapy in elderly patients who are newly diagnosed with atrial fibrillation, the payer will be focused on the costs of intracranial hemorrhaging, major bleeding, pharmacogenomic testing, warfarin and international normalized ratio (INR) monitoring, and embolic strokes.[10] These costs are directly associated with the treatment strategy and represent the resource consumed along with the costs of the outcomes in the clinical pathway. The payer is only interested in the costs that a particular treatment strategy consumes. In our example, the two strategies were to perform a pharmacogenomic test versus no testing. Based on the results of the testing, patients would have their warfarin dose adjusted in predicting the maintenance dose that can potentially decrease the incidence of bleeding due to overanticoagulation. One of the most common and dangerous side effects of warfarin is bleeding due to a supratherapeutic INR. By having a test that can predict whether a patient would be prone to high INR levels after initiating warfarin therapy, there is a potential to reduce the amount of bleeding associated with treatment. Therefore, costs associated with bleeding become an important measurement for pharmacoeconomic analysis from the payer's perspective. It is the payer who must pay for the outcomes and any associated adverse events that occur. Therefore, it is in the interest of the payer to select the strategy that will lead to reduced overall total direct costs.

According to the US Task Force on Cost-Effectiveness Analysis, the preferred perspective for pharmacoeconomic analysis is society's.[11] Societal perspective is considered to be the most comprehensive because it includes the burden of the treatment strategy and disease to society. Societal costs include direct, indirect, and intangible costs. Although direct and indirect costs are estimated using resource utilization data and worker productivity data, intangible costs are difficult and time-consuming to estimate. Emotional costs are nearly impossible to estimate and represent one of the limitations of using the societal perspective. Moreover, societal perspective is irrelevant in most pharmacoeconomic analyses because the major stakeholders usually are the payers, institutions, and patients. Previous perspectives are immediate and easily translatable with less variables and uncertainty associated with the derivation of costs compared with societal perspective. However, pharmacoeconomic analysis should strive to investigate its results using a societal perspective to provide a comprehensive estimate of the costs associated with the treatment strategy.

Cost-Effectiveness Plane

Every discussion regarding pharmacoeconomics involves understanding the cost-effectiveness plane. The cost-effectiveness plane can quickly show whether a strategy is dominant, dominated, or involves a trade-off (cost or benefits). The plane contains the *y*-axis that represents the difference in costs between intervention A and intervention B, and the *x*-axis that represents the difference in benefits between intervention A and intervention B (Figure 10–1). If a drug costs less and had more benefits

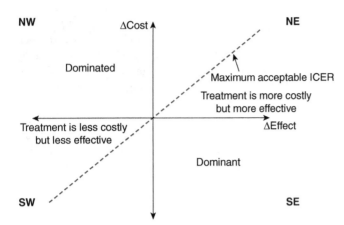

FIGURE 10-1 Cost-effectiveness (CE) plane. The CE plane consists of the incremental efficacy (ΔEffect) on the x-axis and the incremental cost (ΔCost) on the y-axis. The willingness to pay (WTP) is represented by the maximum acceptable incremental cost-effectiveness ratio (ICER). Strategies falling into the southeast (SE) quadrant are said to be in the dominant quadrant. These strategies cost less than the comparator, but yield greater benefits. Strategies that fall in the northwest (NW) quadrant are said to be in the dominated quadrant because these strategies cost more than the comparator, but yield lesser benefits. Strategies that fall in the southwest (SW) quadrant are said to be in the trade-off quadrant.

compared with its competitor, it would fall into the southeastern quadrant; in order words, it is a dominant strategy. However, if a drug costs more and had less benefits compared with its comparator, it would fall into the northwest quadrant; in order words, it is a dominated strategy. Moreover, if a drug costs more and had more benefits compared with its comparator, it would fall into the northeast quadrant where a trade-off between costs and benefits would have to be determined. A similar situation occurs when the drug costs less and had less benefits compared with its competitor (southwest quadrant). Strategies that fall into the trade-off quadrants will need to have certain thresholds for determining if it is cost-effective. In other words, what is the maximum amount of costs a decision maker is willing to pay for an increase in benefits between the two interventions?

The decision maker's willingness to pay (WTP) is the maximum incremental cost-effectiveness ratio (ICER) where a strategy would be considered cost-effective versus its competitor. Anything above the WTP would be considered not cost-effective; and anything below the WTP would be considered cost-effective or good value for money. Simply put, if the strategy is below the WTP, it is considered worth the increase in price.

The ECHO Model

The principle behind evaluating quality of interventions related to health care (e.g., drug selection, program development, and surgical intervention) is based on the ECHO model that is a framework that involves an analysis of the economic, clinical, and humanistic outcomes.[12] Clinical outcomes are common

medical objectives (e.g., mortality, cardiovascular events, and adverse events) that are measured due to the intervention or the disease. Economic outcomes quantify the direct, indirect, and intangibles costs of the consequences of the intervention and disease. Humanistic outcomes represent patient preferences, satisfaction, and quality of life as a consequence of the intervention or disease. Validated instruments that are commonly used to measure humanistic outcomes include the Euro-QOL, SF-36, and HUI-3.

Utility Scores and Quality-Adjusted Life Years

Utility scores are a measurement of patient preferences and are incorporated into CUA as quality (health-related quality of life) weights.[13] Patients are asked to rank clinical outcomes based on their preferences that are then placed on an interval scale and used to define the utility score. Quality weights are then used to define the more desirable health state versus the least desirable that are then aggregated across a time frame. The result of aggregating the quality weights over a time period is the QALYs.

The concept of QALYs was first mentioned by Klarman et al. where they used a patient's self-reported quality of life score to assess patient preferences for renal transplant versus dialysis. Preferences were then used as an adjustment factor for cost per life years gained.[14] Although they did not formally call it QALY, the concept was essentially the same. QALYs are estimated by summing up the area under the curve that is generated by the quality weight for health outcomes across time (Figure 10–2). Differences in QALYs between two interventions represent the QALYs gained or lost. QALYs provide a unique unit of

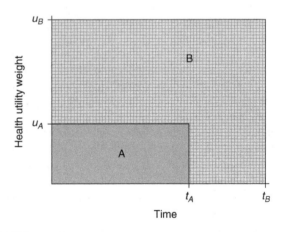

FIGURE 10-2 Estimated quality-adjusted life years (QALYs). QALYs are calculated by the product of the utility weight (u_A and u_B) and time in the health state (t_A and t_B). The QALY for strategy A is represented by the shaded region labeled "A." It is the area under the curve of the health utility (u_A) and time spent in the health state (t_A). The QALY for strategy B is represented by the larger shaded region labeled "B." It is the area under the curve of the health utility (u_B) and time spent in the health state (t_B). The incremental change in QALY gained is the difference between areas under the curves for B and A.

measurement that can be compared across different interventions and diseases. Moreover, QALY is a unit of measurement that quantifies morbidity and mortality, the quality and quantity of life. It is anchored between 0 ("death") and 1 ("perfect health"). Alternatives to the QALY include healthy-years equivalent (HYE), disability-adjusted life year (DALY), and saved-young-life equivalent (SAVE).[13]

Discounting

Discounting is a method to indicate the future cost based on the present value,[15] which should not be confused with inflation. This principle is frequently applied to direct and indirect costs that are accrued beyond 1 year. It is based on the following mathematical equation: $PV = C/(1 + r)^t$, where PV is the present discounted value, C is the future cost to be incurred, r is the constant discount rate, and t is the number of years to be discounted.[16,17] Although the rate of discounting and what parameters should be discounted are controversial, the rate of approximately 3–5% per year is generally accepted.[16,17]

Discounting is associated with cost; however, it should also be applied to benefits or efficacy.[17] There has been substantial research in applying discounting rates on efficacy as well as costs; however, the difficulty lies in determining what the discount rate for efficacy should be. Unlike costs where the discount rate remains relatively constant and for the most part predictable, benefits and efficacy do not behave that way. Delaying care for a timely procedure can reduce the efficacy without accruing costs; however, the opportunity to treat early in order to prevent an undesirable outcome is not normally accounted for in pharmacoeconomics studies where the discounting is not applied to the efficacy.

TYPES OF PHARMACOECONOMIC ANALYSIS

There are several types of pharmacoeconomics analysis that can be performed to measure the cost and effectiveness of an intervention in health care. These types of cost analysis are based on different assumptions and purposes. In this section we will examine the different types of cost analyses. Two of the most common pharmacoeconomic analyses performed are cost-effectiveness analysis (CEA) and CUA.

Cost-Minimization Analysis

Cost-minimization analysis (CMA) is a type of pharmacoeconomic analysis that focuses on the total costs of the intervention compared with its competitor when there are no differences in the benefits or efficacy.[18] CMA is the simplest to perform due to the assumption that there are no clinical differences between the two comparators. Since the benefits or efficacy are the same, the cheaper strategy is the best decision. CMA is normally applied to situations where there are equivalent generic products where the outcomes are assumed to be the same and the major differences will come from the drug acquisition costs. Several therapeutic

TABLE 10-2 Cost-minimization analysis example.

	Drug A	Drug B
Cost		
Acquisition of drug ($)	100	200
Administration fee ($)	50	50
Subtotal ($)	150	250
Efficacy		
Cure rate (%)	80	80
Cost per cure ($)	187.50	312.50

interchange studies utilize CMA to justify selection of an intervention into a drug formulary.

Suppose there were two drugs, Drug A and Drug B. The drug acquisition costs for Drug A and Drug B are $100 and $200, respectively. Both drugs require an administration by the nurse that costs $50. Moreover, the cure rates for both drugs are exactly the same at 80% (Table 10–2).

Because both drugs have the same cure rate, a decision maker will choose the intervention that costs the least. This is intuitive since the strategy that costs less is also the strategy that has the same outcomes as the comparator. In a formal analysis, investigators could determine the estimated cost per cure achieved, which is the product of the total costs of the drug and the probability of cure.

Cost–Benefit Analysis

Cost–benefit analysis (CBA) is an economic method for assessing the initial investment of an intervention versus its benefits (or efficacy) used in the development of business plans.[8,19] CBA measures both costs and benefits in the same monetary units (e.g., US dollar) by transforming benefits into costs and summarizing the return on investment for a particular strategy or intervention. For example, a benefit can be defined as the cost of a myocardial infarction avoided that is given a monetary value. This value is then considered the return on investment for the intervention. The cost of investing in the intervention is then subtracted from the total benefit. If the cost of avoiding a myocardial infarction is greater than the cost of the initial investment (total cost), then there is a net benefit to implementing the intervention. The formal expression is:

$$\text{Net benefit} = \text{total benefit} - \text{total cost}$$

Another way of evaluating the relative value of the initial investment is to perform a cost–benefit ratio (CBR). The formal expression is:

$$\text{CBR} = \frac{\text{total benefit}}{\text{total cost}}$$

The total benefit is the cost of the benefits achieved (e.g., myocardial infarction avoided, adverse reaction avoided, and prevention of a disease) divided by the cost of the initial investment (e.g., cost

TABLE 10–3 Cost–benefit analysis between Drug A and Drug B.

	Drug A	Drug B
Cost		
Acquisition ($)	100	1,000
Testing ($)	200	0
Subtotal ($)	300	1,000
Benefits		
Stevens–Johnson syndrome avoided ($)	2,000	2,000
Subtotal ($)	2,000	2,000
Net benefits ($)	1,700	1,000
Cost–benefit ratio	6.67	2

of using the pharmacogenomic tests, drug acquisition cost, and cost of the program). CBR provides a ratio that can be applied against other interventions across different treatment strategies and ranked according to the higher CBR. Technically, a CBR that is >1 is considered a good investment (total benefits outweigh the total costs), a CBR <1 is considered a bad investment (total benefits are less than the total costs), and a CBR = 1 is an investment where you will break even (total benefits equal the costs).[8,19]

Suppose there are two drugs, Drug A and Drug B. Both drugs are used to cure cancer; however, one of these drugs will cause severe Stevens–Johnson syndrome if the patient contains an allele that will react with Drug A. Drug B is an alternative; however, it costs 10 times as much as Drug A ($100). There is a pharmacogenomic test in the market that can detect this allele; however, the cost of this allele is $200. The cost of treating Stevens–Johnson syndrome is $2,000. We would like to determine if the use of the pharmacogeonomic test is worth the initial investment (Table 10–3).

In this example, we see that Drug B does not use the pharmacogenomic test; therefore, the cost is $0. However, because the test was not used, there is a potential risk for the patient to experience the adverse reaction. As a result, the provider decided to treat empirically that led to a total cost of $1,000. When the cost of choosing Drug B is subtracted from the cost of avoiding Stevens–Johnson syndrome (total benefit), the net benefit is $1,000. Conversely, if the provider chose to test, the cost is an extra $200, but the provider gets to use Drug A that costs less than Drug B. Moreover, benefit of not experiencing Stevens–Johnson syndrome is also realized. The net benefit is the total cost of using the test and treatment ($300) subtracted from the total benefit ($2,000), which is $1,700.

Cost-Effectiveness Analysis

A pragmatic approach to evaluating different interventions involves assessing the total resources consumed relative to the clinical efficacy gained from an intervention. This assessment must be performed between two or more interventions where the efficacy or benefits are different; moreover, the efficacy is measured in terms of clinical outcomes. CEA is a pharmacoeconomic method that is based on a difference in total costs between two interventions divided by their differences in total efficacy (or benefits).[20,21] CEA is commonly employed using clinical markers such as cardiovascular events avoided, responder versus nonresponder, cured versus not cured, adverse event occurrence, mortality, and laboratory outcomes. Unlike CMA, there is a difference in benefits or efficacy in CEA, and unlike CBA, the benefits are measured in clinical outcomes (physical units) instead of monetary units. In CEA, investigators are able to determine the incremental costs for each additional unit of benefit achieved, which is reported as the ICER. ICER can be calculated as follows:

$$\text{ICER} = \frac{\text{total cost of Drug A} - \text{total cost of Drug B}}{\text{total efficacy of Drug A} - \text{total efficacy of Drug B}}$$

The ICER represents the incremental costs needed in order to achieve one additional unit of benefit from the intervention of interest (Drug A) compared with its comparator (Drug B). Therefore, decision makers are able to estimate the additional funding required to realize the extra benefits of a new therapy. This is commonly seen when an NME enters the market having better clinical outcomes but also possessing a greater price than the less costly standard of therapy. Ultimately, the decision maker has to determine if the new therapy is worth the cost of the additional benefits, which is determined by their WTP.

Suppose that Drug A is a new drug that enters a market with an 85% probability of curing a disease. The cost of Drug A ($500) is higher than the cost of Drug B ($150) that has an 80% cure rate. A major advantage of Drug A is that the length of stay is less and results in a lower cost ($2,000 vs. $3000). The cost of administration for both drugs is the same ($50) (Table 10–4).

The total costs of Drug A and Drug B are $2,550 and $3,200, respectively. The cure rate is higher in Drug A versus Drug B (85% vs. 80%). The cost-effectiveness ratio is the fraction of cost per outcome and provides an independent estimate of the cost per cure. However, it does not provide a relative estimate

TABLE 10–4 Cost-effectiveness analysis example.

	Drug A	Drug B
Costs		
Acquisition ($)	500	150
Administration ($)	50	50
Length of stay ($)	2,000	3,000
Subtotal ($)	2,550	3,200
Efficacy		
Cure rate (%)	85	80
Cost-effectiveness ratio ($)	3,000	4,000
ICER ($)	Dominant (−13,000)	

of cost-effectiveness between Drug A and Drug B. This is done using the ICER. The ICER is negative because the total difference in cost is negative (numerator) and the total difference in efficacy is positive (denominator). The ICER can be plotted on the cost-effectiveness plane to illustrate the cost-effectiveness of the strategy outcome (Figure 10–1). A negative ICER means that Drug A is a dominant strategy compared with Drug B. Therefore, Drug A is a cost-effective strategy compared with Drug B.

Cost–Utility Analysis

CUA is similar in construction to the CEA except that the benefit or efficacy is based on QALYs. CUAs are appropriate when health-related quality of life is an important health outcome of the intervention. As previously discussed, quality weights (or utility scores) are assigned to different clinical outcomes of the intervention. CUAs have a broader application than CEA because the QALY allows comparisons between different interventions and diseases.[13] As a result, decision makers are able to compare the value of money between different studies and focus their budget on interventions that are cost-effective. This is useful when comparing different pharmacogenomic tests.

CEA evaluate health outcomes in physical units that cannot be compared between studies. For example, the results of a CEA on a pharmacogenomic test for *TPMT* could not be directly compared with the results of a CEA for an antibiotic for the treatment of pneumonia because the physical units would be different. CUA, on the other hand, uses the same unit, QALY, which would allow for direct comparison. Decision makers could rank the interventions using the results from a CUA to prioritize their funds.

Similar to CEA, CUAs calculate the incremental differences in costs and effect (e.g., QALY) and provide a ratio called an incremental cost–utility ratio (ICUR). The ICUR provides a quantitative analysis for the increased cost required for one additional QALY gained between two comparators. In most CUAs, researchers will still prefer to call this the ICER. However, in order to distinguish between a CUA and a CEA, the ICUR and ICER will be used, respectively.

Suppose that Drug A has an acquisition cost of $100 and is also associated with longer length of stay with a cost of $2,000. Drug B has an acquisition cost of $500 and a shorter length of stay with a cost of $1,200. Both comparators have as their physical outcome life year saved with Drug A having saved more life years than Drug B (2.5 years vs. 2 years). However, the utility weight (quality weight) assigned to a life year saved for Drug A is less than Drug B (0.43 vs. 0.67). This means that patients would rank their quality of life year saved higher with Drug B compared with Drug A. In other words, a life year saved with Drug B results in a higher quality of life even though Drug A increases an average patient's life by 0.5 years (2.5–2 years) (Table 10–5).

Using the same example in Table 10–5, suppose an investigator wanted to see the cost-effectiveness of Drug B compared with Drug A; there are two approaches that can be taken.

TABLE 10–5 Cost–utility example.

	Drug A	Drug B
Cost		
Acquisition cost ($)	100	500
Administration ($)	50	50
Length of stay ($)	2,000	1,200
Subtotal ($)	2,150	1,750
Efficacy		
Life years saved	2.5	2
Utility for each year of life saved	0.43	0.67
QALY	1.075	1.34
Cost-effectiveness ratio (cost/life year saved) ($)	860	875
ICER (cost for additional life year saved), B versus A ($)	800	
Cost–utility ratio (cost/QALY) ($)	2,000	1,306
Incremental cost–utility ratio (ICUR)	Dominant (–1509)	

A CEA could be performed. According to Table 10–5, the ICER for using Drug B versus Drug A is $800 per additional life year saved. Depending on the WTP, using Drug B may (or not) be a cost-effective strategy compared with Drug A. However, if a CUA was performed, then Drug B would be a dominant strategy compared with Drug A. The ICUR is dominant for Drug B versus Drug A; therefore, a decision maker would choose Drug B over Drug A.

The outcomes from the example demonstrate the disparity in conclusions that was based on the type of analysis performed (CUA vs. CEA). In general, the results of the CUA would be preferred because the outcomes can be used to compare treatments between diseases due to the QALY as the common denominator (or efficacy). Using the CEA will reduce its usefulness since decision makers will have a difficult time using the physical units of life year saved across all interventions and diseases.

CUAs use similar methods for calculating the incremental differences between strategies; however, their advantage is in the use of QALY, which is a universal unit of measurement that can be applied across different interventions and diseases. This becomes critical when comparing different pharmacogenomic tests across different diseases where a decision maker will need to allocate scare resources using the results of pharmacoeconomic studies.

DECISION ANALYSIS MODELS

Most pharmacoeconomic analyses are simulations that are developed using DA models where the parameters are commonly derived from the literature or other references. The simplest DA model is a decision tree model while more complex models include the Markov model and discrete event simulation (DES).[16,22–25] The appropriateness of the model selection is based

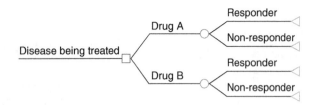

FIGURE 10–3 Decision analytic tree. The decision analytic tree provides an illustrative model of the possible clinical pathways that can occur after a strategy is chosen.

on the disease state and the intervention. Therefore, outcomes where an immediate clinical measurement can be obtained in the short run will mostly rely on the linear discrete model with a short time horizon, whereas a chronic disease where clinical outcomes are measured in months and years versus hours or days may require a complex model such as a Markov model or a DES model. Detailed information about Markov models and DES are presented elsewhere.[16,23–26]

Decision Tree Models

Decision tree models are DA models that are connected by branches that simulate a clinical pathway as a consequence of initiating an intervention.[16,22] These models normally have a short time horizon (e.g., less than 1 year), and involve two or more interventions. Usually a decision is made to initiate the intervention, and then through a series of branches (represented by chance nodes), different outcomes can occur until the tree terminates and all the costs and outcomes are calculated (Figure 10–3). The decision tree has several symbols that represent different parts of the model.[22] A square symbol represents the decision node where a decision to provide the intervention or its competitor is made. This is followed by chance nodes (circle symbol), which represents the probability that a certain outcome will occur. Several chance nodes can populate a DA model where they represent different clinical outcomes. The branch of the DA model ends at a terminal node (triangle symbol), which represents the end of that clinical pathway. Both costs and efficacy are tallied up at the end of a branch to give it a cost per event that is later incorporated into the final cost-effectiveness calculations.

According to the Modeling Good Research Practices Task Force for model design, every model must undergo face validity and content validity.[27] Experts in the subject should be consulted during the development phase of the DA model and its reasonableness must also match what is expected in clinical practice. DA models are designed to provide a realistic simulation of the clinical course of the disease; however, they should be simple enough that they can be workable and quick to perform. There is an important balance that must be maintained between complexity and simplicity where equilibrium is achieved when the question of cost-effectiveness is a concern with the appropriate amount of work and time dedicated to a project. In the place of performing randomized controlled trials (RCTs), models can be used to simulate the trials and provide quick answers to the possible cost-effectiveness of an intervention. Moreover,

models should incorporate multiple studies into developing the clinical outcome parameters that do not rely heavily on a single RCT that could lead to bias. Meta-analyses or weighted mean averages are commonly employed to estimate the probabilities of the clinical pathways (chance nodes) that provide a systematic and quantitative method that can stand the test of rigorous criticisms. In the absence of published literature, expert clinical opinions can be collected through either surveys or Delphi panel method.

STRUCTURAL AND PARAMETER UNCERTAINTY

Model uncertainty comes in two major forms: structural and parameter uncertainty.[28,29] Structural uncertainty is based on the design of the DA model. Validation of the model is critical to avoid biases or deletion of critical pathways. Moreover, it provides a good indicator for reliability of the model. Model design should always begin with a realistic impression of the possible clinical pathways. Models based on the availability of the data are discouraged because they will only focus on what is available and not on the possible gaps in the literature that are critical to measure clinical outcomes. In the absence of data, proper assumptions should be employed and tested using sensitivity analysis.

Based on the data and assumptions, the design of the model may take on different forms; these should be assessed in the sensitivity analysis. For example, if a model did not take into account the sensitivity of a pharmacogenomic test and assumed that the test was 100% sensitive and specific, an investigation should be performed to test the outcomes to determine whether there is a change in the base-case analysis if the sensitivity and specificity assumption is less than 100%. To do this, the model will need to have another branch to indicate these possible differences (Figure 10–4). The change in the model represents the structural uncertainty that occurs with model design. It is critical that researchers explore these features of the model to test their assumptions.

One-Way Sensitivity Analysis

Parameter uncertainty can be performed in several ways. One-way sensitivity analysis is the simplest method because only a single parameter is varied across a predefined range.[30] It is performed on model parameters that have the most uncertainty such as the acquisition cost of the medication, probability of clinical outcomes, probability of adverse events, and specificity and sensitivity of a pharmacogenomic test. For example, the cost of a medication may vary based on an institution's rebate or discount, which is different across several regions. By estimating a reasonable range of costs, a one-way sensitivity analysis can be performed to test the model robustness. If the range of costs changes the outcome from the base-case, then the model is said to be sensitive; however, if results do not differ from the base-case conclusions, then the model is robust, or does not change.[30]

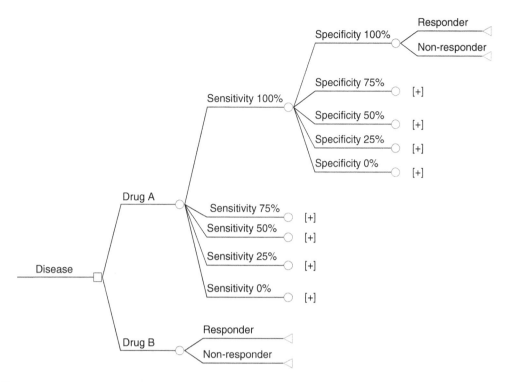

FIGURE 10–4 An example of structural uncertainty in a decision analytic (DA) model. Specificity and sensitivity are critical elements in pharmacogenomics. DA models can estimate the effect of these parameters by modifying the original diagram with sensitivity and specificity modeled into the DA tree. [+] denotes collapsed branches.

In Figure 10–5, a one-way sensitivity analysis is performed for the acquisition cost of Drug B, which was $500. The cost of Drug B was varied across a range between $100 and $700 to investigate if the cost-effectiveness ratio would be less than Drug A at some acquisition cost (represented on the *x*-axis). At a cost of $165, the cost-effectiveness ratio of Drug B is the same as Drug A. The point at which two lines intersect in a one-way sensitivity analysis is called the break-even point. The break-even point is the value at which there is no difference between Drug A and Drug B. If the cost of Drug B is less than $165, then the cost-effectiveness ratio of Drug B will be less than that of Drug A. In the base-case, the cost-effectiveness ratio of Drug A was less than that of Drug B, $429 per responder and $1,222 per responder, respectively. In the one-way sensitivity analysis, the conclusion changes when the acquisition cost of Drug B is less than $165.

The one-way sensitivity analysis provides information about the model sensitivity and identifies which variables would have changed the outcome of the base-case. However, the one-way sensitivity analysis is limited to only one variable and further investigation involving two or more variables and their relationship to each other will require more complex sensitivity analyses.

Two-Way Sensitivity Analysis

Two parameters can be varied across a reasonable range simultaneously in a model. These parameters are ones that have the most uncertainty and their relationship to each other can be

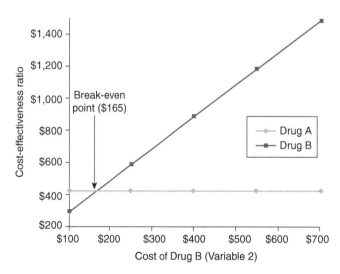

FIGURE 10–5 One-way sensitivity analysis showing a break-even point. A break-even point is observed where the acquisition cost of Drug B (Variable 2) is varied across a range ($100–700). Notice that the lines for Drug A and Drug B intersect at a drug cost for Drug B at $165. Therefore, if the price of Drug B dropped down from the base-case ($500) to $165, then there is no difference in cost-effectiveness ratio (CER) between Drug A and Drug B. In other words, if the price for Drug B is less than $165, then Drug B will have a lower CER than Drug A. Therefore, this model is considered sensitive to acquisition cost of Drug B.

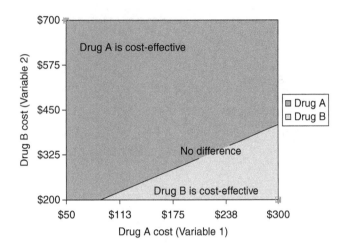

FIGURE 10-6 Two-way sensitivity analysis. In the two-way sensitivity analysis, two parameters are varied across a reasonable range (Variable 1 and Variable 2). The incremental cost-effectiveness ratio (ICER) is recalculated with the adjusted costs. The area represents all possible combinations that make up the cost-effective strategy. In this example, the acquisition cost of Drug A (Variable 1) and acquisition cost of Drug B (Variable 2) show the relationship and influence of each variable to each other.

measured using a two-way sensitivity analysis. In pharmacogenomic testing, two critical elements are necessary to evaluate the accuracy and precision of a test: sensitivity and specificity. A two-way sensitivity analysis can be performed varying the sensitivity and specificity across a reasonable range to determine the relationship between the two variables compared with the base-case. Suppose the base-case assumed that the sensitivity and specificity were 100% each; by varying each component independently, the researchers can see whether or not the sensitivity analysis results in different outcomes from the base-case.

In Figure 10–6, two variables are tested across a range of values. Variable 1 (acquisition cost of Drug A) is represented on the *x*-axis and Variable 2 (acquisition cost of Drug B) is represented on the *y*-axis. The outcome measurement is the ICER. The shaded areas represent the preferred strategy that is cost-effective. For example, the shaded area for Drug A includes a majority of the area that indicates that it is the preferred strategy over Drug B. The shaded area of Drug B contains a small area but is cost-effective when the acquisition costs of Drug A and Drug B fall into the shaded area that favors Drug B. Suppose that the acquisition cost of Drug A is changed from $120 to $250 and the acquisition cost of Drug B is changed from $500 to $250; the ICER that is calculated would fall into the shaded region that favors Drug B. Therefore, we can conclude that the model is sensitive to these two variables. Moreover, the line that separates the shaded areas from each other is considered the break-even point or the point where a combination of the two variables results in an ICER that is 0.

The two-way sensitivity analysis provides information about the relationship between two variables, in our example, the

acquisition costs for Drug A and Drug B. Unlike a one-way sensitivity analysis where one variable yields the influence of one variable on the outcome, a two-way sensitivity analysis generates more information about the influence and relationship of two separate variables. However, the two-way sensitivity analysis cannot provide information about three or more parameters. For sensitivity analyses of multivariate parameters, more complex simulations need to be performed.

Probabilistic Sensitivity Analysis

Rigorous methods for sensitivity analysis have been developed to test for the influence and relationship of multiple model parameters simultaneously. These methods require using stochastic processes for randomly selecting values based on a distribution function of the parameter.[26,28,29] In a probabilistic sensitivity analysis, multiple variables can be simultaneously varied across a distribution function and used for calculation of the ICER. Outputs from these simulations provide a distribution plot of ICER on a CE plane that can be used to estimate the probability that a strategy is cost-effective.[28,29] This method of sensitivity analysis provides decision makers with a single ICER value that also includes a description of the variance. Therefore, one could estimate the probability that selecting a strategy would be cost-effectiveness simply by looking at the CE plane and using the WTP as the maximum ICER threshold.

In Figure 10–7 the result of a probabilistic sensitivity analysis is plotted on the cost-effectiveness plane. The individual circles represent an ICER that was calculated using stochastic process. The example had a total of 1,000 simulations performed and which yielded an equal number of ICERs. These ICERs are plotted on the cost-effectiveness plane and illustrate

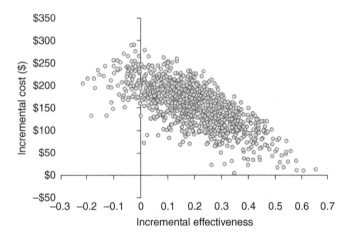

FIGURE 10-7 Probabilistic sensitivity analysis. The probabilistic sensitivity analysis is plotted on a cost-effectiveness plane (incremental effectiveness is plotted on the *x*-axis and incremental cost is plotted on the *y*-axis). Each individual point represents an incremental cost-effectiveness ratio (ICER) calculated after multiple variables are stochastically drawn from a distribution. The dispersion of ICER provides an illustration of the variance associated with the base-case ICER.

TABLE 10–6 Software that can perform probabilistic sensitivity analysis.

Software	Company/Group	Web Site
TreeAge	TreeAge Software, Inc	http://www.treeage.com/
Crystal Ball	Oracle	http://www.oracle.com/us/products/applications/crystalball/index.html
WinBUGS	MRC Biostatistics Unit, Cambridge	http://www.mrc-bsu.cam.ac.uk/bugs/winbugs/contents.shtml
Gaussian Emulation Machine (GEM)	Center for Terrestrial Carbon Dynamics	http://ctcd.group.shef.ac.uk/gem.html

the variance and distribution of the possible outcomes that can occur if multiple parameters are varied simultaneously. In Figure 10–7, the distribution of ICERs crosses two quadrants (NE and NW). A majority of the ICERs fall into the trade-off quadrant (NE); however, a small percentage falls into the dominated quadrant (NW). If the base-case result yielded an ICER that is in the trade-off quadrant (NE), then the probability sensitivity tests to see if this conclusion is maintained after multiple parameters are varied across specific ranges. Because the distribution also falls into the dominated quadrant (NW), the conclusion needs to be modified to account for this disparity. Percentages for the distribution in the different quadrant would provide quantitative information regarding the probability of the ICER being in the trade-off quadrant or the dominated quadrant. In this example, 91% of the distribution was in the trade-off quadrant (NE), whereas 9% of the distribution was in the dominated quadrant.

Probabilistic sensitivity analysis is a robust method to test for the parameter uncertainty in a DA model. The methods to perform a probabilistic sensitivity analysis are complex and time-consuming; however, the availability of software to perform these simulations allows researchers to perform thousands of simulations in a very short time. A list of software is provided in Table 10–6.

COST-EFFECTIVENESS ACCEPTABILITY CURVES

Cost-effectiveness acceptability curves (CEAC) are cumulative distribution functions that provide a probability estimate of the cost-effectiveness of a treatment strategy relative to another across a WTP threshold.[31–34] The y-axis represents the probability that the strategy is cost-effective relative to a competitor, and the x-axis represents the different levels of WTP (Figure 10–8).[32] CEAC uses different WTP to assist decision makers on the probability that the strategy they chose is cost-effective. This is an intuitive method for determining the strength of the decision by providing a probability of cost-effectiveness. Strategies where the probability of being cost-effective is less than the competitor (e.g., less than 50%) would be determined not cost-effective at the WTP. On the other hand, if the strategy was cost-effective 50% or greater, the decision maker will have to weigh either WTP against the acceptable probability. Ideally, one would want a treatment strategy that is cost-effective 100% of the time at

a WTP of $0; however, this would be considered a dominant strategy. CEAC are useful for illustrating the variability of cost-effectiveness based on the WTP if the strategy is in the trade-off quadrant. Strategies in the dominant quadrant will have a straight line that will be a value of 100% cost-effective regardless of the WTP value (Figure 10–8).[32] Conversely, for strategies where the intervention is dominated, the CEAC will be presented as a straight line at 0% for all WTP.[32]

FRAMEWORK FOR USING PHARMACOECONOMICS IN PHARMACOGENOMICS

Numerous studies have begun applying pharmacoeconomics in pharmacogenomics. Pharmacoeconomic studies have focused on the specificity and sensitivity of pharmacogenomic tests as critical variables for determining their cost-effectiveness versus the absence of pharmacogenomic tests. Investigators should be concerned with the reliability and validity of the pharmacogenomic tests and whether significant clinical outcomes occur as a result of using the results of the tests. One would theorize that the pharmacogenomic test would provide information that could increase the probability of a positive clinical outcome; however, very little evidence exists where this has been measured. Therefore, development of a pharmacoeconomics study must begin with some idea of the clinical consequence of utilizing a specific pharmacogenomic test. Clearly there will be some difficulty in finding evidence that links clinical outcomes with pharmacogenomic tests due to the limited number of literature available; however, using sensitivity analysis will provide a good approximation for the cost-effectiveness of these tests.

Cost is not the only prohibitive factor that prevents decision makers from implementing the use of pharmacogenomic tests into clinical practice. While an NME is required to go through extensive clinical trials to determine safety and efficacy prior to obtaining FDA approval,[29] such requirements for pharmacogenomic tests are lacking. In addition, health care providers may feel overwhelmed by the number of pharmacogenomic tests that are currently available, and are challenged in determining when a pharmacogenomic test should be used, and for whom would these tests be beneficial.[30] The Centers for Disease Control and Prevention (CDC) funded and supported the development of the ACCE model in order to provide a framework to systemically

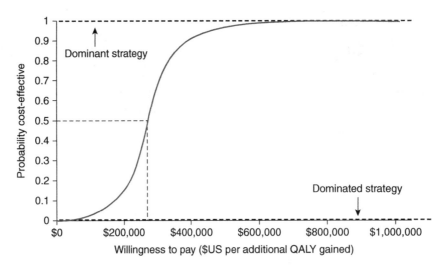

FIGURE 10–8 Cost-effectiveness acceptability curve (CEAC). The CEAC illustrates the probability that a strategy is cost-effective given different willingness to pay (WTP) thresholds. The probability that a strategy is cost-effective is plotted on the y-axis, and the WTP is plotted on the x-axis. As the WTP threshold increases, the probability that a strategy is cost-effective increases. A strategy that has a 50% probability is equivalent to an equilibrium point where the comparator also has a 50% probability of being cost-effective. If a strategy is dominant at all WTP thresholds, then the curve will be a straight line with a 100% probability of being cost-effective (denoted as Dominant strategy). However, when a strategy is dominated entirely across all WTP, then the curve will be a straight line with no fluctuations and a 0% probability of being cost-effective (as denoted by Dominated strategy).

evaluate pharmacogenomic tests in an evidence-based manner.[35] The name of this model, which consists of 44 questions, comes from the four most important components when evaluating a pharmacogenomic test: analytical validity, which represents the accuracy and reliability of the pharmacogenomic test; clinical validity, which represents the pharmacogenomic test's ability to accurately detect or predict an outcome of interest; clinical utility, which helps the decision maker determine whether the pharmacogenomic test significantly improves a patient's clinical outcomes; and, issues relating to ethnical, legal, and social implications.[35]

There are many laboratories that perform the same pharmacogenomic test using different methodologies, thus leading to variations in analytical and clinical validity. This factor may affect the cost-effectiveness of implementing a pharmacogenomic test in clinical practice, and has to be taken into consideration in the pharmacoeconomic model. As an example, a systematic review showed that eight different methods were used to perform the *TPMT* genotype test, which may have contributed to a wide range of sensitivity (55–100%), positive predictive value (PPV [67–100%]), and negative predictive values (NPV [76–100%]).[36] In this particular example, the specificity did not vary by much (94–100%); however, this is not the case with every pharmacogenomic test. While there are no guidelines on what the sensitivity, specificity, PPV, and NPV threshold should be, lower thresholds of these parameters may indicate that a pharmacogenomic test is not clinically useful. In order to fully understand the impact of wide variation on sensitivity, specificity, PPV, and NPV, sensitivity analyses should be conducted to determine the robustness of the base-case model.

APPLICATIONS OF PHARMACOECONOMICS IN PHARMACOGENOMICS

Example 1: TPMT Genotyping for Azathioprine

Hagaman et al. performed a CEA to evaluate the use of pharmacogenomic testing for the *TPMT* variant alleles.[37] TPMT is essential in the metabolism pathway of azathioprine, which is an immunosuppressant used for various conditions such as idiopathic pulmonary fibrosis (IPF). Azathioprine can lead to serious bone marrow toxicity and other side effects. A lower dose of azathioprine or an alternative agent was initiated in patients who possess a *TPMT* genotype resulting in decreased or null enzyme activity. Based on these premises, *TPMT* genotype testing should reduce or eliminate the serious bone marrow toxicity associated with azathioprine use and maximize its safety and efficacy in IPF.

The pharmacoeconomic analysis was based on a decision analytic model using references from the literature. Three study groups investigated were: azathioprine plus *N*-acetylcysteine (NAC), and steroids with or without *TPMT* testing, and conservative therapy that consisted of supportive care. In the *TPMT* testing group, *TPMT* activity was categorized as normal, intermediate, or low. Patients with the allele for normal *TPMT* activity were initiated with azathioprine, NAC, and steroids; those with intermediate *TPMT* activity were initiated on low-dose azathioprine along with normal doses of NAC and steroids; and those with low *TPMT* activity were initiated on conservative therapy. The authors do not provide information on what alleles were associated with normal, low, or high *TPMT* activity.

The decision analytic model had a time horizon of 1 year with costs presented as year 2007 US dollars. However, the cost adjustment method was not discussed. Adjustments could be performed based on the medical component of the consumer price index (CPI). Only total direct costs were evaluated. Outcome data were presented as a marginal cost-effectiveness ratio (mCER), which is essentially the ICER. Utility scores were not presented; however, QALY calculations were performed. The perspective was not stated explicitly; however, total direct costs were adjusted for year 2007 US dollars.

A critical element of the study was the prevalence of abnormal *TPMT* activity. Using a population-based study, the investigators estimated that the prevalence of *TPMT* activity was 0.5%, 11.9%, and 87.6% for patients who had low, intermediate, and normal TPMT activity in their base-case, respectively. They also assessed for the influence on these parameters in the sensitivity analysis.[37]

The authors concluded that *TPMT* testing was cost-effective if the WTP was $50,000 per QALY gained. The ICER for *TPMT* testing versus conservative therapy was $49,156 per QALY gained. The strategy to not perform *TPMT* testing was eliminated by extended dominance, meaning that the same amount of resources could be used for the more expensive strategy. The total direct costs for the *TPMT* testing strategy, no *TPMT* testing strategy, and conservative therapy were $15,818, $15,802, and $9,691, respectively. Total effectiveness (QALYs) for the *TPMT* testing strategy, no TPMT testing strategy, and conservative therapy were 2.62 QALYs, 2.61 QALYs, and 2.5 QALYs, respectively.[37]

The study performed a one-way sensitivity analysis on the prevalence of abnormal *TPMT* activity. Increasing the prevalence from 12.4% (low and intermediate *TPMT* activity) to >13.5% resulted in the *TPMT* testing strategy being dominant to the no testing strategy. A two-way sensitivity analysis was also performed on the cumulative probability of disease progression in 1 year on conservative therapy and cumulative probability of disease progression in 1 year on azathioprine, NAC, and steroid therapy. As the rate of disease progression increased with conservative therapy, *TPMT* testing is favored at higher rates of disease progression on azathioprine, NAC, and steroids. Probabilistic sensitivity analysis and CEAC were not performed or provided.

The pharmacoeconomic analysis provides information on the cost-effectiveness of *TPMT* testing prior to initiation of azathioprine in IPF. ICER reflects a cost-effective strategy with *TPMT* testing if the WTP was set at $50,000. Results from this study could be applied to different institutions to assess for the cost-effectiveness of *TPMT* testing in their IPF patient population.

Example 2: CYP2C9 and VKORC1 Testing for Warfarin

Patrick et al. performed a CUA to investigate the cost-effectiveness of using genomic testing for CYP2C9 and vitamin K epoxide reductase complex subunit 1 (VKORC1) as a method for improving warfarin dosing in achieving a targeted INR between

2 and 3 for patients newly diagnosed with atrial fibrillation.[38] Although warfarin has been shown to reduce the risk of thromboembolic risk in atrial fibrillation patients, warfarin's narrow therapeutic index range may lead to increased morbidity and mortality if the INR range is less than 2 or greater than 3.

CYP2C9 metabolizes warfarin and genetic variants of the gene that codes for CYP2C9 may affect warfarin efficacy and toxicity (e.g., excess bleeding). VKORC1 is necessary for the enzymatic activation of vitamin K that is essential to blood clotting. Patients who have a specific variant VKORC1 allele are not able to generate enough vitamin K clotting factors that may lead to excessive bleeds. Therefore, patients who possess specific CYP2C9 and VKORC1 variant alleles are at greater risk for bleeds due to overanticoagulation with warfarin therapy.

A Markov model was developed to investigate the potential impact that early identification of the variant allele would have in achieving and maintaining patients started on warfarin therapy within the INR range of 2 and 3 versus usual case. Usual care was assumed to be a patient who was seen by an anticoagulation clinic where his or her warfarin dose was adjusted periodically. A hypothetical cohort of 70-year-old patients newly diagnosed with atrial fibrillation was simulated using several health states that describe possible clinical outcomes associated with warfarin treatment. Each health status was preceded by the potential INR range a patient may find himself or herself in (e.g., <1.5, 1.5 to <2.0, 2.0–3.0, >3.0 to <4.0, and >4.0). The benefits generated by the model included life expectancy and QALYs over a lifetime horizon from a societal perspective. A discount rate of 3% was used for both costs and benefits.

Efficacy data, including mortality and INR-specific events, were derived from published literature. Costs for medication were derived from the *Red Book* and cost for warfarin genomic testing was estimated as $475. Other costs were estimated from published literature and the Medicare Current Beneficiary Survey. All costs were adjusted for inflation according to the medical component of the CPI for 2007. Utility weights were derived from published literature and applied to each health states. One-way sensitivity analyses were performed as well as probabilistic sensitivity analysis.

In their results, genomic testing that increased the time spent at INR goal increased by less than 5%, (e.g., 57.7–62.7%); the estimated ICER would be >$100,000/QALY gained. On the other hand, if the genomic testing increased the time spent at INR goal by 9%, the ICER would be <$50,000/QALY gained. The model was sensitive to several parameters that included the starting age of the hypothetical cohort, cost of the genomic tests, assumptions about the rate of bleeding, and the degree of shifts from subtherapeutic and supratherapeutic corrections into the INR goal. In the probabilistic sensitivity analysis, genomic testing did not appear to occur in the dominant quadrant (SE quadrant); however, using a threshold of $50,000/QALY and $100,000/QALY gained, there was a 42% and 70% distribution of ICERS, respectively.

The critical factor in analysis by Patrick et al. is the percentage of change from usual care that a patient spends within the INR range of 2 and 3. Changes of greater than 9% are desirable only if the payer (e.g., society) is willing to pay <$50,000 per additional QALY gained. However, none of the sensitivity analyses showed that genomic testing would be a dominant strategy compared with usual care. Therefore, an investment by society on genomic testing would be required in order to realize the benefits. Without this investment, genomic testing cannot be initiated. In their discussion, the authors admitted that the magnitude of change in the time spent within the INR range was inconsistently reported in the literature, and it is a significant variable in determining whether or not pharmacogenomic testing is cost-effective. As a consequence, the authors indicated that any generalization of their results should be used with caution.

Example 3: Serotonin 2A Receptor (HTR2A) Testing for Antidepressants

Perlis et al. performed a CUA to evaluate the cost-effectiveness of utilizing pharmacogenomic testing prior to prescribing antidepressants for patients with major depressive disorder (MDD).[39] Choosing the correct treatment would increase the likelihood of achieving remission, thus decreasing functional impairment, premature treatment discontinuation, and medical costs. The authors chose to examine a single nucleotide polymorphism in the serotonin 2A receptor (*HTR2A*) with treatment response to citalopram, a selective serotonin reuptake inhibitor (SSRI). This decision was based on the results of a single large pharmacogenomic study where patients who were homozygous for the *HTR2A* variant allele were likely to respond to citalopram therapy.

The DA was modeled for 40-year-old patients with MDD over a 3-year time horizon with a cycle length of 3 months. Although the authors indicated the analysis is from a societal perspective, indirect and intangible costs were not taken into consideration. Therefore, this analysis is more likely to be from a payer's perspective. A cohort of patients who did not receive the *HTR2A* test was compared with those who received the *HTR2A* test either prior to receiving any treatment (test-first) or after failing the initial treatment (test-second). The no-test cohort received: (a) bupropion followed by sertraline if treatment failure occurred, (b) citalopram followed by sertraline if treatment failure occurred, or (c) citalopram followed by bupropion if treatment failure occurred. In the test-first cohort, patients whose test result indicated greater likelihood of treatment response to an SSRI received citalopram, and those whose test result indicated a lesser likelihood of treatment response to an SSRI received bupropion. In the test-second cohort, patients who failed treatment with citalopram were tested and received either a second SSRI (sertraline) or bupropion. Of note, patients who failed bupropion switched to nortriptyline, followed by the combination of venlafaxine and mirtazapine; this algorithm applied to all patients regardless of the cohort stratification.

The probabilities of remission, discontinuation, and recurrence were derived from the STAR*D trial. The rate of death due to suicide among depressed patients was derived from published literature, and all-cause mortality was derived from the US life tables. Mood states that may be associated with different quality of life were derived from published literature and were used to calculate utility scores. Direct medical costs were from published literature, the Center for Medicare and Medicaid Services, and the Agency for Healthcare Research and Quality. All costs were adjusted to 2006 US dollars using the medical component of the CPI. All costs and benefits were discounted at a rate of 3% per year. One-way sensitivity analyses were performed to test the robustness of the study conclusion.

The base-case results showed that the test-first treatment strategy in which an SSRI was given as the initial treatment option followed by another SSRI trial had an ICER of $93,520 per additional QALY gained, relative to no pharmacogenomic testing. Depending on the WTP threshold, some payers may consider this treatment strategy to be cost-effective while others may not. The test-second treatment strategy was eliminated through extended dominance. One-way sensitivity analyses showed that the model is sensitive to the prevalence of genotype test results, the rate of remission for both SSRIs and bupropion, and the severity of depression.

While the authors acknowledge that race was not accounted for in the study, which may play a role in genetic variations and treatment response, there are other factors that need to be considered before a pharmacogenomic test is applied in a psychiatric practice. Decision makers need to determine whether or not the treatment algorithm analyzed in this study is similar to their clinical practice. In addition, while the variations of pharmacogenomic testing costs were accounted for, the variations in specificity and sensitivity were not. Therefore, the generalizability of the results may be dependent on the assumptions that the genomic tests are highly sensitive and specific, which may need further investigation to validate this claim.

SUMMARY

1. Pharmacoeconomic analysis should include the following elements: costs, benefits, and perspective. Additional elements may complement and enhance the results depending on the type of study performed.

2. CEA and CUA are performed more often than CMA and CBA.

3. Decision models are useful for illustrating the clinical pathways a decision can lead to. They are most useful in situations where simulation of the real world can be simplified on parameters that are critical to outcomes.

4. One-way sensitivity analysis provides an easy and intuitive test of model robustness; however, sensitivity analyses that evaluate more than one variable provide a broader perspective of the interactive effects of different variables.

5. Pharmacoeconomics is needed when there is limited resource and pharmacogenomic testing is still costly. Decision makers need to determine a WTP threshold in order to determine whether it is cost-effective to incorporate pharmacogenomic testing into clinical practice.

REFERENCES

1. O'Sullivan A, Sheffrin SM, Perez SJ. *Microeconomics: Principles, Applications, and Tools.* 5th ed. New Jersey: Pearson Prentice Hall; 2008:2–12.

2. Rascati KL. Introduction. In: *Essential of Pharmacoeconomics.* 1st ed. Philadelphia: Lippincott Williams & Wilkins; 2009:1–8.

3. Wetterstrand KA. DNA sequencing costs: data from the NHGRI Large-Scale Genome Sequencing Program. Available at: www.genome.gov/sequencingcosts. Accessed July 25, 2011.

4. The $100 genome: implications for the DoD. Available at: http://www.fas.org/irp/agency/dod/jason/. Accessed April 15, 2011.

5. Aronsson G, Gustafsson K, Dallner M. Sick but yet at work. An empirical study of sickness presenteeism. *J Epidemiol Community Health.* 2000;54(7):502–509.

6. Bergström G, Bodin L, Hagberg J, Aronsson G, Josephson M. Sickness presenteeism today, sickness absenteeism tomorrow? A prospective study on sickness presenteeism and future sickness absenteeism. *J Occup Environ Med.* 2009;51(6):629–638.

7. Aronsson G, Gustafsson K. Sickness presenteeism: prevalence, attendance-pressure factors, and an outline of a model for research. *J Occup Environ Med.* 2005;47(9):958–966.

8. Drummond MF, Sculpher MJ, Torrance GW, O'Brien BJ, Stoddart GL. Cost–benefit analysis. In: *Methods for the Economic Evaluation of Health Care Programmes.* 3rd ed. New York, NY: Oxford University Press; 2005:211–245.

9. Brouwer WBF, Koopmanschap MA. The friction-cost method: replacement for nothing and leisure for free? *Pharmacoeconomics.* 2005;23(2):105–111.

10. Leey JA, McCabe S, Koch JA, Miles TP. Cost-effectiveness of genotype-guided warfarin therapy for anticoagulation in elderly patients with atrial fibrillation. *Am J Geriatr Pharmacother.* 2009;7(4):197–203.

11. Gold MR, Siegel JE, Russell LB, et al. *Cost-Effectiveness in Health and Medicine.* New York, NY: Oxford University Press; 1996

12. Kozma CM, Reeder CE, Schulz RM. Economic, clinical, and humanistic outcomes: a planning model for pharmacoeconomic research. *Clin Ther.* 1993;15(6):1121–1132.

13. Drummond MF, Sculpher MJ, Torrance GW, O'Brien BJ, Stoddart GL. Cost utility analysis. In: *Methods for the Economic Evaluation of Health Care Programmes.* 3rd ed. New York, NY: Oxford University Press; 2005:137–196.

14. Klarman HE, Francis JO, Rosenthal GD. Cost-effectiveness analysis applied to the treatment of chronic renal disease. *Med Care.* 1968;6:48–54.

15. Brouwer WB, Niessen LW, Postma MJ, et al. Need for differential discounting of costs and health effects in cost effectiveness analyses. *Br J Med.* 2005;331(7514):446–448.

16. Sonnenberg FA, Beck JR. Markov models in medical decision making: a practical guide. *Med Decis Making.* 1993;13:322–338.

17. Drummond MF, Sculpher MJ, Torrance GW, O'Brien BJ, Stoddart GL. Cost-analysis. In: *Methods for the Economic Evaluation of Health Care Programmes.* 3rd ed. New York, NY: Oxford University Press; 2005:55–101.

18. Bootman LJ, Townsend RJ, McGhan WF. Introduction to pharmacoeconomics. In: *Principles of Pharmacoeconomics.* 3rd ed. Cincinnati: Harvey Whitney Books Co; 2005:1–18.

19. Bootman LJ, Townsend RJ, McGhan WF. Cost–benefit analysis. In: *Principles of Pharmacoeconomics.* 3rd ed. Cincinnati: Harvey Whitney Books Co; 2005:65–82.

20. Drummond MF, Sculpher MJ, Torrance GW, O'Brien BJ, Stoddart GL. Cost-effectiveness analysis. In: *Methods for the Economic Evaluation of Health Care Programmes.* 3rd ed. New York, NY: Oxford University Press; 2005:103–136.

21. Bootman LJ, Townsend RJ, McGhan WF. Cost-effectiveness analysis. In: *Principles of Pharmacoeconomics.* 3rd ed. Cincinnati: Harvey Whitney Books Co; 2005:83–116.

22. Inadomi JM. Decision analysis and economic modelling: a primer. *Eur J Gastroenterol Hepatol.* 2004;16:535–542.

23. Briggs A, Sculpher M, Claxton K. Further development in decision analytic models for economic evaluation. In: *Decision Modeling for Health Economic Evaluation.* Oxford: Oxford University Press; 2006:45–76.

24. Briggs A, Sculpher M. An introduction to Markov modelling for economic evaluation. *Pharmacoeconomics.* 1998;13:397–409.

25. Caro JJ. Pharmacoeconomic analyses using discrete event simulation. *Pharmacoeconomics.* 2005;23:323–332.

26. Briggs A, Sculpher M, Claxton K. Making decision models probabilistic. In: *Decision Modeling for Health Economic Evaluation.* Oxford: Oxford University Press; 2006:77–120.

27. Roberts M, Chambers M, Krahn M, McEwan P, Paltiel AD, Russell L. Conceptual modeling report of the ISPOR-SMDM Modeling Good Research Practices Task Force. Presented at: 16th Annual International Society for Pharmacoeconomics and Outcomes Research Meeting; May 21–25, 2011; Baltimore, MD.

28. Briggs AH. Handling uncertainty in cost-effectiveness models. *Pharmacoeconomics.* 2000;17:479–500.

29. Manning WG, Fryback DG, Weinstein MC. Reflecting uncertainty in cost-effectiveness analysis. In: Gold MR, Siegel JE, Russell LB, et al., eds. *Cost-Effectiveness in Health and Medicine.* New York, NY: Oxford University Press; 1996:247–275.

30. Rascati KL. Decision analysis. In: *Essential of Pharmacoeconomics.* 1st ed. Philadelphia: Lippincott Williams & Wilkins; 2009:135–153.

31. Briggs A, Sculpher M, Claxton K. Analyzing and presenting simulation output from probabilistic models. In: *Decision Modeling for Health Economic Evaluation.* Oxford: Oxford University Press; 2006:121–163.

32. Fenwick E, Byford S. A guide to cost-effectiveness acceptability curves. *Br J Psychiatry.* 2005;187:106–108.

33. Briggs A, Fenn P. Confidence intervals or surfaces? Uncertainty on the cost-effectiveness plane. *Health Econ.* 1998;7(8):723–740.

34. Fenwick E, O'Brien BJ, Briggs A. Cost-effectiveness acceptability curves—facts, fallacies, and frequently asked questions. *Health Econ.* 2004;13(5):405–415.

35. Centers for Disease Control and Prevention. Genomic testing: ACCE model process for evaluating genetic tests. Available at: http://www.cdc.gov/genomics/gtesting/ACCE. Accessed July 18, 2011.

36. Donnan JR. Ungar WJ, Matthews M, et al. Systematic review of thiopurine methyltransferase genotype and enzymatic testing strategies. *Ther Drug Monit.* 2011;33(2):192–199.

37. Hagaman JT, Kinder BW, Eckman MH. Thiopurine S-methyltransferase testing in idiopathic pulmonary fibrosis: a pharmacogenetic cost-effectiveness analysis. *Lung.* 2010;188:125–132.

38. Patrick AR, Avorn J, Choudhry NK. Cost-effectiveness of genotype-guided warfarin dosing for patients with atrial fibrillation. *Circ Cardiovasc Qual Outcomes.* 2009;2:429–436.

39. Perlis RH, Patrick A, Smoller JW, et al. When is pharmacogenomic testing for antidepressant response ready for the clinic? A cost-effectiveness analysis based on data from the STAR*D study. *Neuropsychopharmacology.* 2009;34:2227–2236.

C H A P T E R

11

Cardiovascular Pharmacogenomics

Christina L. Aquilante, PharmD, &
Robert Lee Page II, PharmD, MSPH, FCCP, FAHA, BCPS

LEARNING OBJECTIVES

- Identify key candidate genes and polymorphisms that influence the pharmacokinetics, clinical response, and toxicity of cardiovascular medications.

- Describe, in depth, how key polymorphisms affect the pharmacokinetics, clinical response, and toxicity of cardiovascular medications such as clopidogrel, statins, and β-blockers.

- Discuss the role of genome-wide association studies in identifying genes and polymorphisms associated with response to cardiovascular medications.

- Weigh the evidence of available pharmacogenomic literature to determine the clinical utility of genetic testing in the management of cardiovascular diseases.

- Using a case-based approach, illustrate how genomic information may be used to guide drug selection and management of clopidogrel and statins.

INTRODUCTION

Over the past decade, significant progress has been made in the field of cardiovascular pharmacogenomics. Pharmacogenomic literature is now available for most major cardiovascular disease states and includes medications that are at various stages in the pharmacogenomic research process. In some cases, the use of a patient's genetic makeup to individualize drug therapy is far from being used in the clinic. However, in other cases, genetic information is included in prescribing information, and published guidelines exist to facilitate the use of genotype-guided drug therapy in clinical practice. This chapter will cover major cardiovascular disease states for which there exists a moderate to high amount of pharmacogenomic research. Within this framework, each disease state will highlight one or two genes of interest in which there are well-documented associations between genetic polymorphisms and variability in drug disposition, response, toxicity, or clinical outcomes. In addition, other pharmacokinetic and pharmacodynamic genes of interest will be presented in each section.

ACUTE CORONARY SYNDROMES

Acute coronary syndromes (ACS) describe a group of cardiovascular disorders including unstable angina (UA), non-ST-segment elevation myocardial infarction (NSTEMI), and ST-segment elevation myocardial infarction (STEMI).[1] The common theme underlying these disorders is the rupture of a vulnerable atherosclerotic plaque followed by partial or complete thrombotic occlusion of an artery. Platelets play a key role in the pathophysiology of ACS and thrombus formation. As such, most ACS pharmacotherapy is geared toward inhibition of platelet adhesion, activation, and aggregation. Pharmacologic antiplatelet agents that are routinely used in the treatment of ACS include aspirin, thienopyridines (e.g., clopidogrel and prasugrel), and glycoprotein IIb/IIIa inhibitors (e.g., abciximab, eptifibatide, tirofiban).[2] Recently, the Food and Drug Administration approved ticagrelor, a cyclopentyltriazolopyrimidine, to reduce the rate of thrombotic cardiovascular events in patients with ACS. The goal of antiplatelet therapy in ACS is to decrease ischemia, limit the extent of infarction, and decrease the risk of death and recurrent cardiovascular events. To date, clopidogrel is the agent that has been studied most extensively in antiplatelet pharmacogenomics and is the focus of this discussion.

Clopidogrel

Clopidogrel, typically used in combination with aspirin, is indicated for the treatment of UA and NSTEMI, including patients who undergo percutaneous coronary interventions (PCI) and those who are managed medically.[3] Clopidogrel is also indicated for patients with STEMI, and patients with recent myocardial infarction, recent stroke, or established peripheral arterial disease.[3] Despite being an effective antiplatelet agent, marked interindividual differences exist in the ability of clopidogrel to inhibit platelet aggregation, which is partly due to variability in clopidogrel pharmacokinetics.[4] Of an absorbed clopidogrel dose, 85% is hydrolyzed by esterases to inactive metabolites. The remaining 15% of the dose undergoes a sequential two-step oxidative process in the liver to form an intermediate metabolite (2-oxo-clopidogrel), and then an active metabolite (R-130964). It is this active metabolite that irreversibly inhibits the $P2Y_{12}$ receptor on platelets, thereby inhibiting adenosine diphosphate–mediated platelet aggregation. As shown in Figure 11–1, several cytochrome P450 (CYP) enzymes mediate clopidogrel bioactivation, and the CYP2C19 isoenzyme plays a major role in both oxidative steps of this process.[5] Importantly, CYP2C19 genetic polymorphisms contribute to variability in clopidogrel pharmacokinetics that has translated into differences in clopidogrel pharmacodynamics and clinical outcomes.

Pharmacogenetic Focus: CYP2C19

The CYP2C19 alleles most often studied in clopidogrel pharmacogenetics are CYP2C19*1, CYP2C19*2, CYP2C19*3, and CYP2C19*17. CYP2C19*1 is the normal function (wild-type) allele, CYP2C19*2 (c.681G>A) and CYP2C19*3 (c.636G>A) are loss-of-function alleles, and CYP2C19*17 is a gain-of-function allele.[6,7] These alleles result in different CYP2C19 metabolic phenotypes including ultrarapid, extensive, intermediate, and poor metabolizers (Table 11–1). Polymorphic CYP2C19 allele frequencies vary considerably by race. For example, the CYP2C19*2 allele frequency is 27% in Asians, 18% in African Americans, and 14% in Caucasians.[8] The CYP2C19*3 allele frequency is 9% in Asians, but virtually nonexistent in African Americans and Caucasians.[8] In contrast, the CYP2C19*17 allele is common in Caucasians (18%) and African Americans (18%), but less common in Asians (4%).[9]

In relation to clopidogrel pharmacokinetics, CYP2C19 loss-of-function alleles, primarily CYP2C19*2, have been associated with decreased active metabolite plasma exposure in healthy volunteers and in patients with ACS.[10–12] For example, in healthy volunteers who received a 300 mg loading dose of clopidogrel, active metabolite plasma exposure was 55% lower in poor metabolizers compared with that in extensive metabolizers, and 26% lower in intermediate metabolizers compared with that in extensive metabolizers.[12] This pharmacokinetic difference resulted in smaller absolute reductions in platelet aggregation in poor and intermediate metabolizers as compared with those in extensive metabolizers.[12] Importantly, the link between CYP2C19 genetics and clopidogrel pharmacokinetics and pharmacodynamics has been replicated in over 20 studies in healthy volunteers and patients with ACS.[7,13,14] For example, a genome-wide association study in an Amish population found 13 polymorphisms within the CYP2C18–CYP2C19–CYP2C9–CYP2C8 cluster on chromosome 10q24 to be associated with poor clopidogrel pharmacodynamic response.[15] The most significant polymorphism in this cluster was in strong linkage disequilibrium with the CYP2C19*2 allele. On further analysis, the CYP2C19*2 allele was significantly associated with clopidogrel-mediated inhibition of platelet aggregation in a gene dose-dependent manner (i.e., *1*/1 > *1/*2 > *2/*2).[15] Furthermore, platelet response to clopidogrel was highly heritable, and about 12% of the variation in clopidogrel response was explained by the CYP2C19*2 allele.[15] Taken together, it is clear that CYP2C19 genotype-mediated differences in clopidogrel metabolism result in differential effects on platelet aggregation.

Beyond pharmacokinetics and pharmacodynamics, the CYP2C19*2 loss-of-function allele has been consistently associated with an increased risk of adverse cardiovascular outcomes (e.g., cardiovascular death, myocardial infarction, and stent thrombosis) in ACS/PCI patients treated with clopidogrel.[12,15–23] Similar findings have been observed for CYP2C19*3, although this allele is rare in non-Asian populations.[12,17,20,21,23] A meta-analysis of 9,685 patients treated with clopidogrel, predominantly for PCI, showed an increased risk of the composite end point of cardiovascular death, myocardial infarction, or stroke in carriers of one CYP2C19 loss-of-function allele (HR, 1.55;

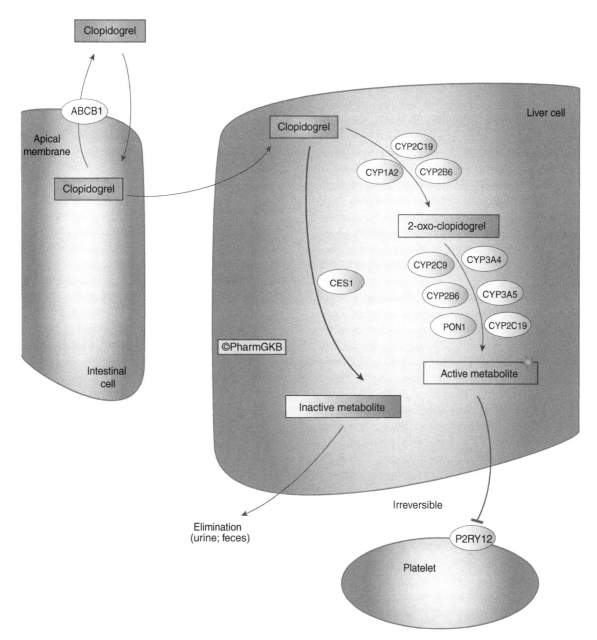

FIGURE 11-1 Clopidogrel pharmacokinetic and pharmacodynamic pathway. ABCB1: efflux transporter; CYP2C19, CYP1A2, CYP2B6, CYP2C9, CYP3A4, CYP3A5, CYP2B6, and PON1: metabolizing enzymes; CES1: esterase; P2RY12: drug receptor. Figure copyright PharmGKB; reprinted with permission from PharmGKB and Stanford University.[24]

TABLE 11-1 Relationship between *CYP2C19* genotypes and phenotypes.

CYP2C19 Phenotype Classification	CYP2C19 Genotype	CYP2C19 Activity
Ultrarapid metabolizer	Two gain-of function alleles (*17/*17), or one wild-type allele plus one gain-of-function allele (*1/*17)	Normal or increased
Extensive metabolizer	Two wild-type alleles (*1/*1)	Normal
Intermediate metabolizer	One wild-type allele plus one loss-of-function allele[a] (e.g., *1/*2, *1/*3)	Intermediate
Poor metabolizer	Two loss-of-function alleles (e.g., *2/*2, *2/*3, *3/*3)	Decreased or absent

[a]Other CYP2C19 loss-of-function alleles exist such as *4, *5, *6, *7, and *8; however, these alleles occur at a low frequency (<1%) in the population. Although it has not been extensively investigated, individuals with a loss-of-function allele plus a gain-of-function allele (e.g., *2/*17) are assigned the provisional classification of intermediate metabolizer.[7,33]

Reprinted by permission from Macmillan Publishers Ltd. Scott SA, Sangkuhl K, Gardner EE, et al. Clinical pharmacogenetics implementation consortium guidelines for cytochrome P450-2C19 (CYP2C19) genotype and clopidogrel therapy. *Clin Pharmacol Ther.* 2011;90(2):328–332.

95% CI, 1.11–2.17) or two *CYP2C19* loss-of-function alleles (HR, 1.76; 95% CI, 1.24–2.50) as compared with that in noncarriers.[25] In addition, the risk of stent thrombosis was substantially increased in carriers of one loss-of-function allele (HR, 2.67; 95% CI, 1.69–4.22) or two loss-of-function alleles (HR, 3.97; 95% CI, 1.75–9.02) as compared with that in noncarriers. In contrast, *CYP2C19* loss-of-function alleles have not been associated with an increased risk of cardiovascular events in studies with a low incidence of PCIs or in patients taking clopidogrel for other reasons such as atrial fibrillation.[26,27] The wealth of clinical outcome data shows that *CYP2C19* loss-of-function alleles, particularly *CYP2C19**2, are important determinants of major adverse cardiovascular events in clopidogrel-treated patients with ACS/PCI.[25,28–30] Perhaps even more concerning, the risk of stent thrombosis is substantially increased in clopidogrel-treated individuals with genetically mediated *CYP2C19* poor metabolism.

While much of the focus of clopidogrel pharmacogenetics has been on *CYP2C19* loss-of-function alleles, recent data suggest that the *CYP2C19**17 gain-of-function allele is a determinant of clopidogrel pharmacodynamics.[12,31–33] Specifically, this allele has been associated with enhanced clopidogrel-mediated inhibition of platelet aggregation, presumably due to increased formation of the active metabolite.[12,31–33] Clinical outcome studies have reported lower cardiovascular event rates and an increased risk of bleeding in carriers of the *CYP2C19**17 allele.[32,34] However, these associations have not been consistently replicated across clinical studies.[15,20,35] Therefore, the exact role of *CYP2C19**17 in clopidogrel response and clinical outcomes remains to be determined.

Other Pharmacokinetic and Pharmacodynamic Genes of Interest

Figure 11–1 shows the CYP enzymes, drug transporters, and drug targets that are involved in clopidogrel clinical pharmacology. In terms of drug metabolism, studies have evaluated the impact of *CYP3A4/5*, *CYP2B6*, *CYP1A2*, and *CYP2C9* polymorphisms on clopidogrel disposition and/or response.[10,12,35–39] However, there are conflicting results regarding the impact of polymorphisms within each of these genes on clopidogrel clinical pharmacology. Recently, the esterase paraoxonase-1 (*PON1*) was identified as an enzyme involved in the second step of the clopidogrel bioactivation process, and the *PON1* Q192R polymorphism was shown to affect clopidogrel metabolism.[40] Specifically, the 192R allele was associated with increased enzyme efficiency, and was correlated with clopidogrel active metabolite concentrations and clopidogrel-mediated inhibition of platelet aggregation.[40] Furthermore, in clopidogrel-treated ACS patients, the risk of stent thrombosis was substantially higher in patients with the Q/Q and Q/R genotypes as compared with that in patients with the R/R genotype.[40] Although these findings are intriguing, subsequent studies have not replicated these associations.[41–43] In terms of drug transporters, P-glycoprotein (*ABCB1*) mediates clopidogrel efflux in the gastrointestinal tract. The *ABCB1* 3435T variant allele was associated with decreased clopidogrel

bioavailability, diminished pharmacodynamic platelet effects, and worse patient outcomes.[20,44,45] However, other studies have found no association between *ABCB1* 3435 genotype and clopidogrel response.[15,21,34] Some data suggest that the combination of *CYP2C19* and *ABCB1* polymorphisms may provide complementary information regarding clopidogrel pharmacodynamics and clinical outcomes.[20,45] Lastly, polymorphisms in *P2RY12*, the gene which encodes the drug target of clopidogrel, have not been consistently associated with clopidogrel response in clinical studies.[20,46–48]

Clinical Implications

Owing to the accumulation of clopidogrel *CYP2C19* pharmacogenetic and clinical outcome data, the Food and Drug Administration updated the clopidogrel prescribing information in March 2010 to include a boxed warning regarding the reduced effectiveness of clopidogrel in patients who are CYP2C19 poor metabolizers.[49] The warning advised, but did not mandate, the use of other antiplatelet agents or alternative clopidogrel dosing strategies in these individuals. The warning also informed health care professionals that genetic tests are available to identify differences in CYP2C19 function; however, genetic testing prior to clopidogrel use was not mandated. Following this revision of clopidogrel prescribing information, the American College of Cardiology Foundation (ACCF) and American Heart Association (AHA) published a report to provide guidance on how to approach the boxed warning.[50] The task force acknowledged that clinicians should be aware of the effects of *CYP2C19* polymorphisms on clopidogrel metabolism and response; however, the task force found the evidence base to be insufficient to recommend routine genetic testing. In this regard, the task force highlighted the following issues and gaps in knowledge regarding clopidogrel pharmacogenetics: (1) available data suggest that the positive predictive value of *CYP2C19* genotyping for adverse clinical events in ACS/PCI patients is low (12–20%);[12,17] (2) *CYP2C19* polymorphisms account for only a small portion of variability in clopidogrel response (~12%);[15] and (3) there is a lack of clinical trial data showing that routine *CYP2C19* genetic testing improves clinical outcomes. Nonetheless, the task force suggested that *CYP2C19* genotyping may be warranted before initiating clopidogrel in certain ACS/PCI patients, such as those with a moderate or high risk of poor outcomes (e.g., patients undergoing complex or high-risk PCI procedures).

More recently, the Clinical Pharmacogenetics Implementation Consortium of the National Institutes of Health's Pharmacogenomics Research Network published guidelines for *CYP2C19* genotype-directed antiplatelet therapy.[7] These guidelines acknowledge the absence of randomized trials documenting that *CYP2C19* genotype-guided antiplatelet therapy improves clinical outcomes. However, the guidelines put forth that the strength and scope of existing studies, along with the availability of potentially more effective antiplatelet agents, supports the use of *CYP2C19* genotyping in clinical practice. The guidelines recommend two options for patient genotyping:

(1) genotype all patients who undergo PCI or (2) genotype only those patients who are at moderate or high risk for poor outcomes (e.g., patients undergoing high-risk PCI procedures or who have prior stent thrombosis or diabetes). In ACS/PCI patients, standard clopidogrel doses are recommended in ultra-rapid or extensive metabolizers. In ACS/PCI patients who are intermediate or poor metabolizers (i.e., defined as carriers of the CYP2C19*2 allele), either prasugrel (which is metabolized by multiple CYP isoenzymes) or alternative drug therapies that do not require metabolic activation (e.g., ticagrelor, ticlopidine, cilostazol) are recommended, assuming no contraindications to therapy. Another potential option is to increase the clopidogrel dose in intermediate or poor metabolizers, although additional clinical outcome data in ACS/PCI patients are needed in this regard.[51,52] In terms of alternative ACS/PCI drug therapies, prasugrel is a newer thienopyridine that does not undergo extensive CYP2C19 metabolism, and whose disposition is not affected by CYP2C19 polymorphisms.[53] In ACS patients, prasugrel was superior to clopidogrel on clinical outcomes, but with an increased risk of major bleeding.[54] Ticagrelor is a non-thienopyridine reversible inhibitor of the P2Y$_{12}$ receptor that was approved by the FDA in July 2011. It does not undergo CYP2C19 metabolism, and was superior to clopidogrel in decreasing the risk of cardiovascular death, myocardial infarction, or stroke in patients with ACS, irrespective of CYP2C19 or ABCB1 polymorphisms.[26] In addition, ticagrelor was effective in patients who were nonresponsive to clopidogrel.[55] Beyond drug therapy, clinical factors (e.g., diabetes, increased body mass index, use of proton pump inhibitors) and possibly other genetic variants (e.g., CYP2C19*3) should be considered in patient care decisions.

Clopidogrel pharmacogenetics has made significant strides in the last 5 years, and it is one of the more well-developed areas in cardiovascular pharmacogenomics. However, there remain a number of issues regarding the implementation of prospective CYP2C19 genotyping in clinical practice. The most pressing need is for prospective, randomized trials to assess whether genotype-guided antiplatelet drug selection will improve clinical outcomes compared with standard of care approaches. While the simple solution may be to prescribe non-CYP2C19-dependent medications such as prasugrel or ticagrelor to all ACS/PCI patients, these agents are not without limitations including cost (both are brand name products), specific contraindications, limited approved indications, and bleeding risks.[8] Further complicating the issue, clopidogrel became generic in 2011, resulting in major cost savings and additional use. Therefore, more studies are needed to determine the cost effectiveness of generic clopidogrel plus CYP2C19 genotyping versus alternative brand-name antiplatelet agents. Other issues that will need to be addressed in the future include payer reimbursement for genetic tests, availability of point-of-care genotyping assays, clarification of the role of platelet responsiveness testing in drug therapy selection and management, and the development of algorithms that incorporate genetic and nongenetic factors into the decision-making process.[8,50,51]

Clinical Case: Clopidogrel

JS is a 68-year-old, 59-kg female who is being admitted to the emergency department after experiencing an episode of sustained, "crushing," substernal chest pain that radiates down her left arm. She has a past medical history significant for uncontrolled type 2 diabetes, depression, hypertension, and hyperlipidemia. She has no known drug allergies, has excellent medication coverage through her health insurance, and takes lisinopril, aspirin, glipizide, simvastatin, sertraline, and ranitidine. Based on her presenting symptoms, increased cardiac biomarkers, and electrocardiographic changes, she is diagnosed with STEMI and sent immediately for coronary angiography and subsequent PCI. Prior to PCI, JS is given 325 mg of aspirin and 300 mg of clopidogrel along with abciximab. During PCI, the patient is found to have 95% occlusion of her left anterior descending artery in which a drug-eluting stent (e.g., paclitaxel-eluting stent) is deployed. After 1 week of medical therapy, the patient is stabilized and discharged on the following medications: clopidogrel 75 mg daily, aspirin 325 mg daily, lisinopril 20 mg daily, metoprolol succinate 25 mg daily, ranitidine 75 mg twice daily, Lantus insulin 35 U at bedtime, atorvastatin 80 mg daily, and sertraline 75 mg daily. Four weeks after discharge, JS is readmitted with sustained chest pain, elevated cardiac biomarkers, and electrocardiographic changes suggestive of STEMI. Again, she is immediately sent for coronary angiography in which she is given 325 mg of aspirin and 600 mg of clopidogrel along with abciximab. JS is found to have thrombosed her drug-eluting stent. Pharmacogenetic testing indicates that JS has the CYP2C19*2/*2 genotype. JS's medication adherence is also assessed and she is found to have missed only one dose of clopidogrel since her admission.

Question: Based on the case and her pharmacogenetic results, what should be done with this patient's long-term antiplatelet regimen?

Answer: When assessing stent thrombosis that is possibly due to clopidogrel failure, many patient-related factors should be taken into consideration. First, medication adherence is one of the major causes of clopidogrel failure. Data suggest that one in six patients may delay filling his or her index clopidogrel after hospital discharge for drug-eluting stent implantation. Such delay has been associated with a significant increase in the risk of both death and myocardial infarction. Second, a patient's medication regimen should be evaluated for potential drug–drug interactions that could impede metabolic activation of clopidogrel because of CYP2C19 inhibition. In the case of JS, she has excellent medication adherence, adequate drug coverage through her health insurance, and no major drug–drug interactions with clopidogrel. Based on the recommendations from the Clinical Pharmacogenetics Implementation Consortium of the National Institutes of Health's Pharmacogenomics Research Network, JS would warrant CYP2C19 genotype testing as she possesses risk factors that increase the possibility of poor outcomes (e.g., diabetes and stent thrombosis). Based on her testing, JS has the CYP2C19*2/*2 genotype (i.e., poor metabolizer) meaning that she may lack the ability to metabolically convert clopidogrel to its active metabolite. What then would be the best long-term antiplatelet therapy for JS in addition to her aspirin? Options would consist of increasing her maintenance dose of clopidogrel to 150 mg daily or consider changing to ticlopidine, prasugrel, or ticagrelor. For higher dose clopidogrel, recent data from the GRAVITAS study suggest that patients with either one or two *CYP2C19* loss-of-function alleles (*2) do not generally respond to double-dose clopidogrel. Ticlopidine is also not a therapeutic option for JS as it has limited data in patients with drug-eluting stents and is associated with significant adverse effects such as neutropenia, rash, and severe diarrhea. As JS has medication coverage through her health insurance, changing to either prasugrel or ticagrelor is an option. However, prasugrel is not recommended in patients with a body weight of 60 kg or less, age of 75 years or greater, or a propensity to bleed, as each of these risk factors increases the risk for major bleed. Since JS weighs less than 60 kg, prasugrel may not be an option. Compared with clopidogrel and prasugrel, ticagrelor is a twice-daily medication, so the potential exists for medication nonadherence. The aspirin dose will also need to be changed to 81 mg daily, as doses above 100 mg daily may reduce the effectiveness of ticagrelor. Nonetheless, based on the clinical evidence, ticagrelor may be the most optimal long-term antiplatelet therapy for this patient.

DYSLIPIDEMIA

Statins

Statins are the most commonly prescribed medications for the treatment of dyslipidemia.[56] They lower LDL cholesterol by 18–55%, lower triglycerides by 7–30%, and raise HDL cholesterol by 5–15%.[57] More importantly, statins reduce the risk of cardiovascular morbidity and mortality in patients with and without existing coronary heart disease.[57,58] The statin drug class includes atorvastatin, fluvastatin, lovastatin, pitavastatin, pravastatin, rosuvastatin, and simvastatin. Statins competitively inhibit HMG CoA-reductase, the rate-limiting step in hepatic cholesterol biosynthesis. They also have pleiotropic effects including attenuation of endothelial dysfunction, inhibition of vascular inflammation, immunomodulation, and antithrombotic actions.[59] Genetic polymorphisms have been shown to influence interindividual variability in statin pharmacokinetics, pharmacodynamics, and the risk of adverse effects.[60] To date, a plethora of genes and polymorphisms has been investigated as potential predictors of statin response. However, in many cases, the pharmacogenetic associations are inconsistent and the clinical relevance is unclear. As such, the following section will focus on the more well-developed statin pharmacogenetic examples, namely, the role of solute carrier organic anion transporter family member 1B1 (*SLCO1B1*) drug transporter polymorphisms in statin clinical pharmacology, and the role of *KIF6* genetics in the risk of cardiovascular disease and statin response. In addition, a brief overview of other genes involved in statin pharmacokinetics and pharmacodynamics will be presented.

Pharmacogenetic Focus: SLCO1B1

Organic anion-transporting polypeptide 1B1 (OATP1B1) is a sodium-independent uptake transporter expressed on the basolateral surface of hepatocytes. OAPT1B1 mediates the active uptake of drugs and endogenous compounds from portal blood into the liver.[61,62] All of the statins are OATP1B1 substrates, and hepatic uptake of statins via OATP1B1 is the first step in their subsequent hepatic metabolism and biliary elimination (Figure 11–2).[63] Owing to the key role of OATP1B1 in statin transport, alterations in OATP1B1 transporter function due to genetic polymorphisms may influence statin pharmacokinetics and pharmacodynamics.[64]

SLCO1B1 is the gene that encodes OATP1B1. The *SLCO1B1* polymorphisms most often studied in relation to drug disposition are c.521 T>C (Val174Ala) and c.388 A>G (Asn130Asp). The frequency of the c.521C allele is 8–20% in Caucasians, 1–8% in those of African descent, and 8–16% in Asians.[63] The frequency of the c.388G allele is 30–45% in Caucasians, 72–83% in those of African descent, and 59–86% in Asians.[63] These polymorphisms are often studied in haplotype form (Table 11–2). The c.521C allele is associated with decreased OATP1B1 transporter activity, and the *5 and *15 haplotypes that contain this allele are referred to as low-activity haplotypes.[65] The c.388G allele has been associated with increased transporter activity, and the *1B haplotype that contains this allele is referred to as a high-activity haplotype.[66–68] In clinical studies, the c.521C allele (present in the *5 and *15 haplotypes) has been associated with decreased hepatic uptake and increased plasma exposure of atorvastatin, pitavastatin, pravastatin, rosuvastatin, and simvastatin.[67,69–81] For example, the plasma exposure of simvastatin acid was 221% higher in healthy individuals with the variant c.521 C/C genotype compared with that in individuals with the wild-type T/T genotype.[80] Of note, the c.521 T>C polymorphism does not affect the pharmacokinetics of fluvastatin, most likely due to the lipophilic nature of this statin.[77] In some studies, the c.388G allele (present in the *1B haplotype) has been associated with increased hepatic uptake and decreased plasma concentrations of pravastatin and pitavastatin.[63,67,82,83]

Statins inhibit cholesterol biosynthesis in the liver. Therefore, it might be expected that changes in the hepatic uptake of statins due to *SLCO1B1* polymorphisms would result in variability in the lipid-lowering efficacy of these drugs. However, *SLCO1B1* polymorphisms have not been consistently associated with the lipid-lowering effects of statins in clinical studies.[74,84,85] In contrast, *SLCO1B1* polymorphisms appear to play a greater role in mediating the risk of statin-associated adverse effects, namely, myopathy and rhabdomyolysis. The *SLCO1B1* c.521 T>C polymorphism is associated with increased statin plasma concentrations, and statin-induced myopathy is a concentration-dependent toxicity.[63] In this regard, a genome-wide association study showed that the *SLCO1B1* c.521 T>C polymorphism was significantly associated with severe myopathy in a case–control study of patients treated with simvastatin 80 mg.[84] Specifically, the odds ratio for myopathy was 16.9 (95% CI, 4.7–61.1) in patients with the c.521 C/C genotype as compared with the

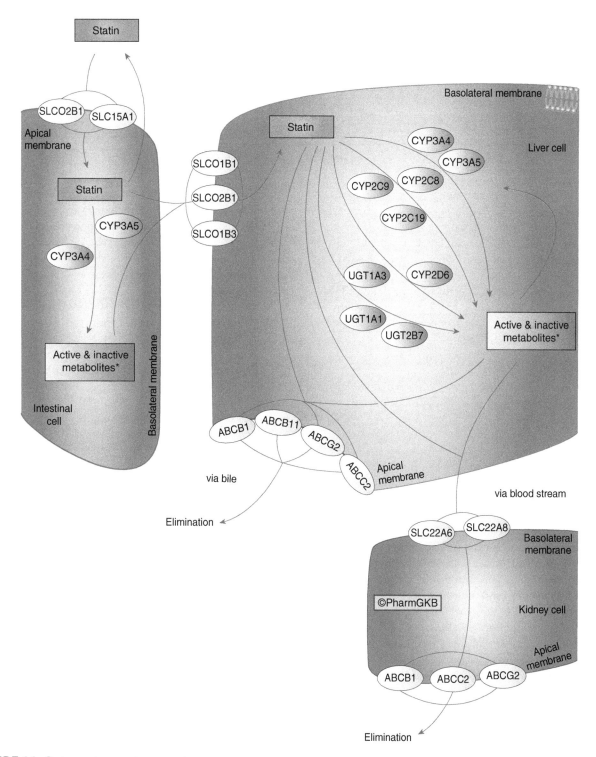

FIGURE 11–2 Statin pharmacokinetic pathway. SLCO1B1, SLCO2B1, SLCO1B3, SLC15A1, SLC22A6, and SLC22A8: uptake transporters; CYP3A4, CYP3A5, CYP2C9, CYP2C8, CYP2C19, CYP2D6, UGT1A3, UGT1A1, and UGT2B7: metabolizing enzymes; ABCB1, ABCB11, ABCG2, and ABCC2: efflux transporters. Figure copyright PharmGKB; reprinted with permission from PharmGKB and Stanford University.[86]

TABLE 11-2 Description of *SLCO1B1* haplotypes.

Haplotype Designation	c.388 A>G (Asn130Asp)	c.521 T>C (Val174Ala)	Effect on OATP1B1 Activity
*1A (reference)	A	T	Normal
*1B	**G**	T	Increased or no change
*5	A	**C**	Decreased
*15	**G**	**C**	Decreased

The bold font in table represents the polymorphic alleles in the respective haplotypes.

wild-type T/T genotype. Furthermore, over 60% of myopathy cases in this study were attributed to the c.521C allele.[84] This study highlights the utility of genome-wide association studies in identifying genetic predictors of less common adverse events, such as statin myopathy. Another study showed that the *SLCO1B1**5 haplotype was associated with milder forms of simvastatin- and atorvastatin-induced muscle side effects.[85] Taken together, the *SLCO1B1* c.521 T>C polymorphism has been proven to be a significant predictor of both mild and severe statin-induced muscle side effects.

Clinical Implications

Currently, *SLCO1B1* genotyping to identify patients who may be at risk for statin-induced myopathy is not routinely used in clinical practice. However, in the future, prospective *SLCO1B1* genotyping could potentially serve as a risk assessment tool. Genotype-based risk stratification may be most applicable during the first year of statin therapy, when the risk of myopathy is the highest. *SLCO1B1* genotyping may be most relevant for patients with an increased risk for myopathy such as those with kidney or liver disease, muscle disease, advanced age, low body weight, on high-dose statin therapy, or on concomitant interacting medications (e.g., transplant and HIV populations).[63,84] In patients with *SLCO1B1* low-activity polymorphisms, potential alternative treatment options may include the use of low-dose statin therapy, use of other statins with a lower risk of myopathy (e.g., pravastatin), use of statins that do not appear to be affected by *SLCO1B1* polymorphisms (e.g., fluvastatin), use of nonstatin lipid-lowering agents, or enhanced safety monitoring.[63,87,88] *SLCO1B1* genotyping may also serve as a useful tool to understand the etiology of severe myopathy or rhabdomyolysis when other clinical risk factors do not exist or are ruled out.

Pharmacogenetic Focus: KIF6

The *KIF6* gene encodes the kinesin-like protein 6. This protein mediates the intracellular transport of organelles, protein complexes, and mRNA along microtubules.[89] A nonsynonymous polymorphism, Trp719Arg, exists in *KIF6*. The 719Arg allele is common in the population, with frequencies of 37% in Caucasians, 84–90% in Africans/African Americans, and 48–57% in Asians.[90] The *KIF6* Trp719Arg polymorphism has been associated with an increased risk of coronary events in the placebo arms of two large clinical trials, the Cholesterol and Recurrent Events (CARE) trial and the West of Scotland Coronary Prevention Study (WOSCOPS).[91] In the CARE trial,

carriers of the *KIF6* 719Arg allele (i.e., Trp/Arg and Arg/Arg) had a 50% increased risk of recurrent myocardial infarction compared with noncarriers (i.e., Trp/Trp genotype). In WOSCOPS, carriers of the *KIF6* 719Arg allele had 55% increased odds of coronary heart disease compared with noncarriers.[91] Further analysis of WOSCOPS revealed that carriers of the 719Arg allele derived a greater benefit from pravastatin therapy as compared with noncarriers. Specifically, pravastatin therapy resulted in a 5.49% absolute risk reduction in 719Arg carriers compared with a 0.09% absolute risk reduction in noncarriers. Along the same lines, in the Pravastatin or Atorvastatin Evaluation and Infection Therapy: Thrombolysis in Myocardial Infarction 22 (PROVE IT-TIMI 22) trial, 719Arg carriers had a greater benefit from high-dose statin therapy (atorvastatin 80 mg daily) compared with that from moderate-dose statin therapy (pravastatin 40 mg daily) than did 719Trp homozygotes.[92] Taken together, these studies suggest that 719Arg carriers have an increased risk of coronary heart disease, and may derive greater benefit from statin therapy.

Clinical Implications

The *KIF6* findings from large clinical cohorts spurred much excitement about the potential use of *KIF6* Trp719Arg genotyping in cardiovascular disease risk assessment and the prediction of relative statin efficacy.[89,92–97] Along these lines, a *KIF6* genetic test was developed and marketed to health care practitioners. It is estimated that over 150,000 *KIF6* genetic tests have been performed to date.[98,99] However, recent studies have begun to refute the initial associations between *KIF6* genotype and coronary event risk. These studies have found no increased risk of coronary events in carriers of the 719Arg allele, and no interaction between *KIF6* genotype and statin risk reduction.[100–103] For example, a meta-analysis of 17,000 cases and over 39,000 controls found that the *KIF6* Trp719Arg polymorphism was not associated with the risk of clinical coronary artery disease.[100] The reasons for the discrepancies in the literature are unclear, but false-positive results in the early studies may be a factor.[104] Another concerning factor is that the biological relationship between *KIF6* and cardiovascular disease and statin response has not been fully elucidated.[104] For example, *KIF6* genotype does not appear to mediate the LDL-lowering effects of statin therapy.[92,95,102] In light of the conflicting reports and the unclear biological plausibility of this gene, many experts have begun to question the clinical utility of *KIF6* genetic testing. Furthermore, some experts have put forth that KIF6 genotyping is not warranted at this time.[99,100,102,104] Additional analyses of large-scale clinical trials, and the execution of genome-wide association studies, will be needed to ascertain the definitive role of *KIF6* Trp719Arg genotyping in cardiovascular disease risk assessment and statin efficacy.

Other Pharmacokinetic Genes of Interest

The CYP3A family plays a major role in the phase 1 metabolism of atorvastatin, lovastatin, and simvastatin (Figure 11–2). A few studies have investigated the impact of *CYP3A4* and *CYP3A5* gene polymorphisms on statin pharmacokinetics and pharmacodynamics. In this regard, the *CYP3A4**1B (−392A>G) polymorphism, which results in increased CYP3A4 expression, was associated with higher LDL cholesterol levels following atorvastatin treatment. This finding was hypothesized to be due to increased metabolism and lower systemic atorvastatin concentrations.[105] The *CYP3A5**3/*3 genotype, which results in no CYP3A5 protein expression (i.e., nonexpressor phenotype), was associated with increased simvastatin plasma exposure, and enhanced lipid-lowering effects of atorvastatin, lovastatin, and simvastatin in clinical studies.[106,107] Along these lines, the *CYP3A5**3/*3 genotype was associated with more severe muscle damage compared with *CYP3A5**1/*3 heterozygotes (i.e., expressor phenotype) in atorvastatin-treated patients.[108] Additional studies are needed to confirm these above findings, and to determine whether *CYP3A4* and *CYP3A5* polymorphisms affect clinical outcomes in patients receiving statin therapy.

P-glycoprotein (encoded by *ABCB1*) and breast cancer resistance protein (encoded by *ABCG2*) are important efflux transporters that play a role in statin disposition (Figure 11–2). Three polymorphisms in the *ABCB1* gene, c.1236C>T, c.2677G>A/T, and c.3435 C>T, have been studied in relation to statin pharmacokinetics and lipid-lowering effects. For example, the *ABCB1* 1236T/2677T/3435T diplotype was associated with higher plasma exposure of atorvastatin and simvastatin compared with the wild-type 1236C/2677G/3435C diplotype.[109] In another study, carriers of the c.1236T allele experienced a greater reduction in total and LDL cholesterol following treatment with simvastatin, as compared with wild-type homozygotes.[110] Of note, the effects of *ABCB1* polymorphisms on statin pharmacokinetics may be statin-specific, as one study showed that *ABCB1* 1236/2677/3435 haplotypes were not associated with the pharmacokinetics of fluvastatin, pravastatin, lovastatin, and rosuvastatin.[111] In terms of *ABCG2*, the c.421C>A has been shown to influence statin pharmacokinetics and pharmacodynamics. Specifically, the c.421A allele was associated with increased plasma concentrations of atorvastatin, fluvastatin, rosuvastatin, and simvastatin lactone.[112–114] Interestingly, the effect of the c.421A allele on plasma exposure appears to be greatest for rosuvastatin.[113–115] The c.421 A/A genotype has been associated with enhanced reductions in LDL cholesterol compared with the C/C genotype following rosuvastatin treatment in Chinese and Caucasian populations.[116–118] Taken together, *ABCB1* and *ABCG2* polymorphisms affect statin pharmacokinetics and pharmacodynamics, and the effects appear to be statin-specific.

Additional studies are needed to determine whether these drug transporter polymorphisms translate into differences in clinical outcomes and adverse effects in patients treated with statins.

Other Pharmacodynamic Genes of Interest

Although the mechanism of action of the statins is to directly inhibit the HMG-CoA reducase enzyme, their subsequent effects on lipid homeostasis are complex. As such, identifying polymorphisms that predict statin pharmacodynamics is a challenging task. Traditionally, a candidate gene approach has been used to elucidate statin drug target pharmacogenomics. As a result, over 40 genes have been implicated in statin response.[119] However, many of these initial genetic associations have a small effect on lipid homeostasis, and many examples have failed to be replicated in subsequent studies.

One of the genes most commonly associated with statin response in candidate gene analyses is apolipoprotein E (*APOE*). APOE is a component of chylomicrons and very-low-density lipoprotein cholesterol, and mediates chylomicron remnant removal. The three alleles most commonly studied in *APOE* include ε2, ε3 (wild-type), and ε4. The ε2 allele is associated with enhanced HMG-CoA activity, while the ε4 allele is associated with decreased HMG-CoA activity.[119] Some, but not all, studies suggest that LDL-lowering response following statin treatment is greatest for the ε2 allele and smallest for the ε4 allele.[119] For example, LDL-lowering following atorvastatin therapy was 3.5% greater in carriers of the ε2 allele compared with wild-type.[120] Another candidate gene that has been variably associated with LDL response following statin therapy is *HMGCR*, which encodes HMG-CoA reductase (the target of statin action). Two polymorphisms in *HMGCR* have been associated with smaller reductions in total and LDL cholesterol following pravastatin therapy.[121] However, this finding has not been consistently replicated in the literature. As previously mentioned, a large number of polymorphisms in other genes (e.g., *CETP*, *PCSK9*, *ADAMTS1*) have been implicated in statin response, but the effect sizes tend to be small, and the associations have not been consistently replicated between studies.

Recently, two genome-wide association studies have been conducted in the field of statin pharmacogenomics. The genome-wide approach allows for a comprehensive interrogation of the human genome, and potential identification of novel proteins involved in drug response.[122] Participants from the Treating to New Targets (TNT) trial, who had received atorvastatin 10 mg daily for 8 weeks, were genotyped using whole genome and candidate gene approaches.[123] Over 290,000 polymorphisms were evaluated; however, none were significantly associated with atorvastatin-induced changes in LDL, HDL, or triglyceride at the whole genome level. In a subsequent candidate gene analysis of this clinical population, only the *APOE* rs7412 polymorphism, which is contained in the ε2 allele, was associated with LDL cholesterol response after correction for multiple statistical tests.[123] This is consistent with previous studies showing associations between the *APOE* ε2 variant and greater LDL-lowering following statin therapy. A recent genome-wide association study evaluated 3,936 patients who had participated in three different statin trials.[124] The polymorphism that was most significantly associated with total cholesterol response at the whole genome level was located in the calmin (*CLMN*) gene. The function of *CLMN*, and its relationship to lipid homeostasis, is not known. This association remains to be replicated in additional cohorts.

Given the state of research in the field, polymorphisms related to statin pharmacodynamics are not ready for use in the clinical setting. In the future, genome-wide association studies will likely shed more light on genetic predictors of statin response and cardiovascular disease risk. Since many polymorphisms have a small effect on lipid response, it may be that a combination of polymorphisms (e.g., a genetic risk score) will be used to help guide statin therapy. Studies assessing the impact of genetics on cardiovascular outcomes will also be needed to move statin pharmacogenomics closer to the clinic.

Clinical Case: Statins

DT is a 55-year-old white male of normal weight who is admitted to the coronary care unit for a STEMI. The patient has a past medical history significant for hypertension and atrial fibrillation. DT has no known drug allergies, and does not smoke or consume alcohol. Prior to admission he was taking metoprolol succinate 150 mg twice daily, warfarin 5 mg daily, and lisinopril 20 mg daily. After receiving medical management, the patient was discharged 7 days later on the following medications: aspirin 325 mg daily, sotalol 160 mg twice daily, metoprolol succinate 25 mg daily, dabigatran 150 mg twice daily, lisinopril 40 mg daily, simvastatin 40 mg at bedtime, clopidogrel 75 mg daily, and sublingual nitroglycerin as needed. Three months after discharge, DT began passing dark colored urine with complaints of severe muscular thigh pain, confusion, nausea and vomiting, and significant dehydration. DT was readmitted to the hospital where his serum creatinine was 3.4 mg/dL (baseline, 1 mg/dL), serum potassium was 5.9 mEq/L (baseline, 3.5 mEq/L), and creatine kinase was 100,000 U/L (baseline, 60 U/L). DT is diagnosed with rhabdomyolysis. In order to address potential causes of his rhabdomyolysis, *SLCO1B1* genetic testing is performed. DT is found to have the *SLCO1B1 *5/*15* genetic makeup.

Question: Based on the case and his genetic results, what is the potential cause of DT's rhabdomyolysis?

Answer: After ruling out potential medical causes for rhabdomyolysis (e.g., extreme physical exertion, muscle crush from a car accident, alcohol intoxication, metabolic abnormalities, hyperthermia, or infection), drug-induced etiologies should be evaluated. A drug class that is often associated with rhabdomyolysis is the statins. Rhabdomyolysis associated with statin therapy has an incidence of 3.4 per 100,000 patient-years of treatment. Unfortunately, the etiology of statin-induced rhabdomyolysis is poorly understood. Theoretically, decreased mevalonate production may disrupt small regulatory proteins required for myocyte cell membrane maintenance leading to the disorder. The risk of statin-induced myotoxicity is multifactorial, and varies with the pharmacokinetic properties of the individual statins and with the clinical factors of the individual patient. Transport of statins into the liver is an active process via OATP1B1, which is located on the basolateral side of hepatocytes. The majority of statins, such as simvastatin, are metabolized in the liver by the CYP enzymes, particularly CYP3A4. In the myocytes, the transport is dependent on passive diffusion; thus, statin concentrations and dose have been shown to increase the risk of rhabdomyolysis, although in a nonlinear fashion. Predisposing risks for statin-induced rhabdomyolysis consist of any factors affecting statin volume of distribution or metabolism (e.g., advanced age or renal and hepatic dysfunction), recent surgery, heavy exercise, and certain comorbidities (e.g., hypothyroidism and diabetes). Medically, DT has no obvious predisposing medical risk factors. From the standpoint of drug–drug interactions that could increase concentrations of simvastatin, none exist. While multiple medications are known to significantly increase concentrations of simvastatin (e.g., amiodarone, dronedarone, verapamil, diltiazem, amlodipine, ranolazine, cyclosporine, gemfibrozil, macrolides, azole antifungals, and protease inhibitors), none of DT's medications are metabolized by CYP3A4. Therefore, this patient remains a clinical conundrum, thus warranting genetic testing.

In this case, DT has the *SLCO1B1 *5/*15* diplotype. Recent studies have identified common variants in *SLCO1B1*, such as c.521 T>C, to alter OATP1B1 activity. The *5/*15 diplotype, which contains two variant c.521C alleles, is associated with decreased OATP1B1 transporter function. Such a variant could significantly increase simvastatin systemic concentrations and possibly lead to rhabdomyolysis. As this patient is post-MI, he warrants a statin for overall reduction in morbidity and mortality. After an episode of potential statin-induced rhabdomyolysis, many clinicians would dismiss the idea of reconsidering statin administration. However, in the case of DT, the benefits of a statin may outweigh the risks. Using the genetic data provided, this can steer potential therapeutic recommendations. For DT, potential treatment options include a more water-soluble statin with less myopathy (e.g., pravastatin or low-dose rosuvastatin), a statin that does not appear to be affected by *SLCO1B1* polymorphisms (e.g., fluvastatin), or an alternative lipid-lowering agent such as niacin or ezetimibe. However, it is important to note that ezetimibe may lack the pleiotropic cardiovascular effects that statins and niacin seem to possess. Taken together, *SLCO1B1* genotyping may be useful in this case to elucidate potential etiologies of statin-induced rhabdomyolysis.

HYPERTENSION

Hypertension is a highly prevalent disease, affecting 34% of adults in the United States.[125] It results in numerous adverse clinical consequences such as cardiovascular morbidity and mortality, stroke, and chronic kidney disease. A variety of pharmacologic agents exist for the treatment of hypertension, and current guidelines recommend the following drug classes as potential first-line

TABLE 11–3 Examples of putative pharmacogenes in hypertension.

Drug Class	Gene Name	Protein	Role in Clinical Pharmacology
β-Blockers	ADRB1	β_1-Adrenergic receptor	Drug target; adrenergic signaling pathway
	ADRB2	β_2-Adrenergic receptor	Drug target; adrenergic signaling pathway
	GNAS1	Gs protein α-subunit	Adrenergic signaling pathway
	GNB3	G protein β_3-subunit	Adrenergic signaling pathway
	GRK5	G protein–coupled receptor kinase 5	Adrenergic signaling pathway
	CYP2D6	Cytochrome P450 2D6	Drug metabolism
Thiazide diuretics	ADD1	α-Adducin 1	Sodium homeostasis and signal transduction
	SCNN1G	Sodium channel γ-subunit promoter	Potentially sodium homeostasis
	NOS3	Endothelial nitric oxide synthase	Nitric oxide production and vasodilation
	WNK1	Lysine-deficient protein kinase 1	Sodium homeostasis
	GNB3	G protein β_3-subunit	Adrenergic signaling pathway
	NPPA	Atrial natriuretic precursor A	Sodium homeostasis
	NEDD4L	Neural precursor cell expressed, developmentally downregulated 4-like	Sodium homeostasis
	SCNN1A	α-Subunit of the amiloride-sensitive epithelial sodium channel	Metabolic side effects
	LYZ	Lysozyme	Unknown
	YEATS4	YEATS domain containing 4	Unknown
RAAS modulators	ACE	Angiotensin-converting enzyme	Drug target; RAAS effector protein
	AGT	Angiotensinogen	RAAS effector protein
	REN	Renin	Drug target; RAAS effector protein
	AGTR1	Angiotensin II type 1 receptor	Drug target; RAAS effector protein
Calcium channel blockers	CACNA1C	α_{1C}-Subunit of the L-type calcium channel	Drug target
	CACNA1D	α_{1D}-Subunit of the L-type calcium channel	Potential drug target
	CACNB2	β_2-Subunit of the L-type calcium channel	Potential drug target
	CYP3A4	Cytochrome P450 3A5	Drug metabolism
	ABCB1	P-glycoprotein	Drug transport
	KCNMB1	β_1-Subunit of the large-conductance calcium and voltage-dependent potassium channel	Contractile pathway of vascular smooth muscle
	RGS2	Regulator of G protein signaling-2	Contractile pathway of vascular smooth muscle
	NPPA	Atrial natriuretic precursor A	Sodium homeostasis
	NOS1AP	Nitric oxide synthase 1 adaptor protein	Nitric oxide pathway

treatment options: angiotensin-converting enzyme (ACE) inhibitors, angiotensin receptor blockers, β-blockers, calcium channel blockers, and thiazide diuretics.[126] Data from large clinical trials show that these drug classes reduce the risk of adverse clinical outcomes in patients with hypertension.[126] However, it is estimated that 52% of hypertensive patients do not achieve adequate blood pressure control following pharmacologic therapy.[125] Clinical, environmental, and adherence factors certainly play a role in blood pressure response rates. However, over the last decade, the field of hypertension pharmacogenomics has shown that genetic

polymorphisms can account for some of the interindividual variability in antihypertensive agent disposition, response, and toxicity.[127] A summary of putative pharmacogenes in hypertension is shown in Table 11–3. To date, hypertension pharmacogenomics has focused most extensively on β-blockers and thiazide diuretics, which will be the focus of this section. In addition, the pharmacogenomics of renin–angiotensin–aldosterone system (RAAS) modulators (i.e., ACE inhibitors, angiotensin receptor blockers, direct renin inhibitors) and calcium channel blockers will be briefly reviewed.

β-Blockers

β-Blockers are used extensively for the treatment of hypertension, particularly in high-risk conditions with compelling indications such as heart failure, postmyocardial infarction, high coronary disease risk, and diabetes.[126] They work by antagonizing the actions of catecholamines on β_1- and β_2-adrenergic receptors. Over a dozen oral β-blockers are available worldwide, and they differ primarily in their selectivity for β-adrenergic receptors (e.g., β_1-selective, nonselective, or mixed β_1-, β_2-, and α_1-selectivity).[128] Unfortunately, 30–60% of patients have an inadequate antihypertensive response following β-blocker therapy.[128] Therefore, potential genetic determinants of interindividual variability in β-blocker response have garnered considerable interest in the last decade. Given that β-blockers act on adrenergic receptors, primarily β_1, the logical starting point for pharmacogenetic investigations is polymorphisms in the gene encoding the β_1-adrenergic receptor.

Pharmacogenetic Focus: ADRB1

The β_1-adrenergic receptor is encoded by *ADRB1*. The two most commonly studied polymorphisms in *ADRB1* are c.1165 C>G (Arg389Gly) and c.145 A>G (Ser49Gly). The frequency of the Gly389 allele is 24–34% in Caucasians, 39–46% in blacks, and 20–30% in Asians.[129] The frequency of the Gly49 allele is 12–16% in Caucasians, 23–28% in blacks, and 14% in Asians.[129] The Arg389Gly and Ser49Gly polymorphisms have undergone extensive evaluations of their functional consequences. For example, at codon 389, the Arg allele is associated with greater basal and agonist-promoted adenylyl cyclase activation than the Gly allele.[130] At codon 49, the Gly allele is associated with enhanced agonist-promoted downregulation of receptor expression than the wild-type Ser allele.[131,132] Interestingly, these in vitro findings are associated with variable cardiovascular phenotypes in humans. For example, the Arg389Gly polymorphism was significantly associated with systolic and diastolic blood pressure in a genome-wide association meta-analysis of about 86,000 individuals.[133]

It has been hypothesized that individuals carrying the Arg389 and/or Ser49 alleles may have an enhanced response to β-adrenergic receptor blockers in the clinical setting.[128,134] Studies have largely supported this hypothesis, particularly for the β_1-selective blocker, metoprolol.[128,134–136] For example, in a prospective study of metoprolol-treated hypertensive patients, those with the codon 389 Arg/Arg genotype experienced a 6.5 mm Hg greater reduction in diastolic blood pressure than Gly389 carriers.[134] Furthermore, when codons 49 and 389 were considered together, patients with two copies of the Ser49/Arg389 haplotype had a significantly greater decrease in diastolic blood pressure than those with the Gly49Arg389/Ser49Gly389 combination (−14.7 mm Hg vs. −0.5 mm Hg, respectively).[134] These findings have been confirmed in some prospective studies;[135–137] however, other retrospective and prospective studies have not found consistent associations between *ADRB1* polymorphisms and antihypertensive response to β-blocker

therapy.[138–144] Beyond antihypertensive effects, the relationship between *ADRB1* polymorphism and hard clinical outcomes has been evaluated in large studies.[145,146] For example, in approximately 6,000 hypertensive coronary artery disease patients who participated in the INternational VErapamil SR/Trandolapril STudy (INVEST), participants with one or two copies of the Ser49/Arg389 haplotype had an increased risk of all-cause mortality compared with noncarriers.[145] Furthermore, patients with the Ser49/Arg389 risk haplotype derived a survival benefit from atenolol treatment as compared with those assigned to a calcium channel blocker (verapamil) strategy. In contrast, the risk of death in noncarriers of the Ser49/Arg389 haplotype was not influenced by beta-blocker versus calcium channel blocker therapy.[145] Taken together, these data suggest that *ADRB1* genetics influences the risk of adverse clinical outcomes, and attenuation of this risk depends on the type of antihypertensive drug class selected for treatment.

Although many β-blockers are selective for the β_1-adrenergic receptor, some agents also have actions at the β_2-adrenergic receptor (e.g., carvedilol, labetalol, propranolol). The β_2-adrenergic receptor is encoded by *ADRB2*, and the two most commonly studied polymorphisms in *ADRB2* are c.46 G>A (Gly16Arg) and c.79 C>G (Gln27Glu). The frequency of the Arg16 allele is 39% in Caucasians, 49% in blacks, and 51% in Asians.[128] The frequency of the Glu27 allele is 25% in Caucasians, 19% in blacks, and 9% in Asians.[128] In vitro, the Gly16 allele results in enhanced agonist-promoted downregulation, while the Glu27 allele is resistant to receptor downregulation.[128,147] The *ADRB2* codon 16 and codon 27 polymorphisms have not been associated with blood pressure lowering responses to β-blocker therapy.[138,142,143,148] In studies that evaluated clinical outcomes, an interaction was observed between *ADRB2* haplotypes and atenolol versus verapamil treatment on the outcome of all-cause mortality, nonfatal myocardial infarction, or stroke.[145] However, in a different study, no interaction between *ADRB2* polymorphisms, β-blocker use, and the risk of myocardial infarction or stroke was observed.[146] Additional studies are needed to make definitive conclusions regarding the influence of *ADRB2* polymorphisms on β-blocker antihypertensive response and clinical outcomes.

Clinical Implications

Small prospective studies have shown that antihypertensive response to β-blockers differs by *ADRB1* genetic makeup, namely, increased blood pressure lowering with the Arg389 and/or Ser49 forms of the receptor. However, other studies have found no association between *ADRB1* polymorphisms and antihypertensive response to β-blockers, which makes the role of *ADRB1* genotyping in clinical practice unclear at this time. Ongoing, large, prospective, randomized pharmacogenomic trials (e.g., Pharmacogenomic Evaluation of Antihypertensive Responses [PEAR]) will certainly shed light on this topic.[149] Potential reasons for discrepancies in the literature include differences in study design (e.g., prospective vs. retrospective), type of β-blocker and dosing scheme, and methods to assess blood pressure.[128,150] Importantly, clinical outcome data suggest that *ADRB1* Ser49/Arg389 is a risk allele, and that β-blocker use (as compared with treatment with an alternative drug class) is associated with a decrease in the risk of adverse clinical outcomes.[150] Along these lines, additional studies are needed to compare the relative benefit/risk of different antihypertensive treatment strategies in patients with these risk alleles.[149] In the future, pharmacogenetic information such as this may be used to tailor antihypertensive drug selection (e.g., β-blocker vs. calcium channel blocker strategy) based on blood pressure response and those most likely to gain benefit based on their genetic risk profile.

Other Pharmacodynamic and Pharmacokinetic Genes of Interest

Following blockade of the β-receptor, the downstream actions of β-blockers within the cell are diverse and complex. The relationship between polymorphisms in adrenergic receptor response pathways and β-blocker pharmacodynamics/outcomes has been investigated in several studies. The most commonly studied genes in adrenergic receptor response pathways are *GNAS1*, *GNB3*, and *GRK5*. *GNAS1* encodes the Gs protein α-subunit that mediates signal transduction for the $β_1$- and $β_2$-adrenergic receptors. A synonymous polymorphism (Ile131Ile) in *GNAS1* results in the presence (+) or absence (−) of a *Fok*I restriction site.[151] A retrospective study found that the frequency of the *Fok*I+ allele was higher in responders versus nonresponders following β-blocker therapy.[151] *GNB3* encodes the G protein $β_3$-subunit, which is also involved in adrenergic receptor signal transduction pathways. In one study, the *GNB3* 825 C>T polymorphism was associated with a greater reduction in blood pressure following β-blocker therapy.[138] G protein–coupled receptor kinases (GRKs), such as *GRK5*, help regulate β-adrenergic receptor signaling. The *GRK5* Gln41Leu polymorphism was not associated with blood pressure response to atenolol in the PEAR Study.[152] However, in a genetic substudy of INVEST, the Leu41 allele was associated with a decreased risk of death, nonfatal myocardial infarction, or stroke, which was independent of beta-blocker or calcium channel blocker treatment.[152] Given that most of the associations for *GNAS1*, *GNB3*, and *GRK5* have not been replicated, these findings all warrant evaluation in other cohorts. Genome-wide association studies in large patient cohorts will be essential to help elucidate polymorphisms in adrenergic receptor response pathways, and perhaps other pathways, that influence interindividual variability in β-blocker response.

In terms of pharmacokinetics, CYP2D6 is involved in the metabolism of some β-blockers (e.g., metoprolol). Polymorphisms, gene deletions, and gene duplications in the *CYP2D6* gene result in four metabolic phenotypes including ultrarapid, extensive, intermediate, and poor metabolizers.[153] *CYP2D6* polymorphisms have been shown to significantly influence the pharmacokinetics of β-blockers that are extensively metabolized by CYP2D6, such as metoprolol.[154] For example, CYP2D6 poor metabolizers had 6-fold higher metoprolol plasma concentrations than extensive metabolizers.[155] It is reasonable to hypothesize that higher β-blocker plasma exposure will result in increased blood pressure lowering response and/or risk of adverse events with β-blocker therapy. Along these lines, a population-based cohort study found that diastolic blood pressure was lower in CYP2D6 poor metabolizers compared with that in extensive metabolizers treated with metoprolol.[156] However, several prospective studies have shown that *CYP2D6*-mediated differences in β-blocker plasma exposure are not associated with antihypertensive efficacy or adverse effects.[157–159] Taken together, *CYP2D6* genotyping likely does not have clinical utility for prediction of efficacy or adverse events during β-blocker treatment.

Thiazide Diuretics

The thiazide diuretics (e.g., hydrochlorothiazide, chlorthalidone) are a cornerstone of antihypertensive therapy. Thiazides are recommended as initial therapy for most patients with hypertension, either as monotherapy or in combination with other drug classes.[126] The mechanism of action of thiazides is to inhibit the sodium–chloride transporter in the distal tubule, thereby promoting sodium and chloride excretion.

Pharmacogenetic Focus: ADD1

The gene most commonly studied in thiazide pharmacogenetics is α-adducin (*ADD1*). Adducin consists of α-, β-, and γ-subunits, and regulates signal transduction within the cell. The *ADD1* Gly460Trp polymorphism has been associated with renal sodium retention and salt-sensitive hypertension.[160,161] In turn, the *ADD1* Trp460 allele has been associated with an enhanced blood pressure lowering response to thiazide diuretics in some studies.[162] Furthermore, in a population-based case–control study in individuals who carried a Trp460 allele, the risk of myocardial infarction or stroke was lower in individuals who received either thiazide or loop diuretics compared with that in individuals who used other antihypertensive medications. Conversely, individuals who had the wild-type Gly/Gly genotype and received diuretics did not have a reduction in the risk of myocardial infarction or stroke.[163] These findings suggest that *ADD1* Gly460Trp may help predict which patients will derive benefit from diuretic therapy. However, other studies have failed to consistently replicate these findings in regards to blood pressure response and clinical outcomes.[164–167] Therefore, given these conflicting reports, it does not appear that prospective screening for the *ADD1* Gly460Trp polymorphism is warranted in the clinical setting at this time.

Other Pharmacodynamic Genes of Interest

Beyond *ADD1*, numerous genes in multiple pathways (e.g., sodium homeostasis, adrenergic signaling) have been evaluated in thiazide pharmacogenomic studies. In many of these cases, the findings have yielded conflicting results, or have not been replicated. Nonetheless, some of the largest candidate gene studies are presented for consideration. In a study of 19 candidate genes, sodium channel γ-subunit promoter (*SCNN1G*) and endothelial nitric oxide synthase (*NOS3*) gene polymorphisms were associated with differences in diastolic blood pressure response to hydrochlorothiazide.[168] The role of *SCNN1G* in thiazide pharmacodynamics is unclear, but this gene has previously been associated with hypertension.[169] The *NOS3* polymorphism, Glu298Asp, is associated with decreased nitric oxide production, and has been associated with hydrochlorothiazide response in a previous report.[164] A different study evaluated 16 candidate genes and found polymorphisms in lysine-deficient protein kinase 1 (*WNK1*) to be associated with interindividual differences in hydrochlorothiazide blood pressure response.[170] *WNK1* regulates thiazide-sensitive renal sodium transport, and is therefore mechanistically relevant. In terms of adrenergic signaling pathways, a study of 387 adults with hypertension found the G protein β₃-subunit (*GNB3*) 825 T/T genotype to be a significant predictor of greater systolic and diastolic blood pressure responses to hydrochlorothiazide therapy.[171] Of note, genotype accounted for <5% of interindividual differences in blood pressure response. Another gene implicated in thiazide response is atrial natriuretic precursor A (*NPPA*), which is involved in fluid and electrolyte homeostasis. In the Genetics of Hypertension Associated Treatment (GenHAT) study, which evaluated over 38,000 patients, the *NPPA* 2238 T>C polymorphism was associated with better cardiovascular outcomes in those assigned to chlorthalidone versus calcium channel blocker (amlodipine) therapy.[172] Conversely, the T/T genotype was associated with better cardiovascular outcomes in those assigned to calcium channel blocker therapy. These findings illustrate how genetic polymorphisms can interact with the type of antihypertensive treatment to influence the risk of clinical outcomes.[172] Another protein, NEDD4L, plays an important role in sodium homeostasis, encoding a ligase that mediates the expression of epithelial sodium channels in the kidney.[173,174] A study found that the *NEDD4L* rs4149601 G>A polymorphism was a predictor of antihypertensive response to hydrochlorothiazide, with greater blood pressure reduction in A carriers compared with the G/G genotype.[174] A subsequent study showed that the patients on diuretic or β-blocker therapy who carried the *NEDD4L* G allele had greater blood pressure reduction and protection from cardiovascular events than those with the A/A genotype.[175]

In complex physiological systems, such as those involving renal sodium transport and homeostasis, the interaction between genes cannot be ignored. This paradigm has recently been applied to thiazide diuretic therapy. For example, a combination of common alleles in *ADD1*, *WNK1*, and *NEDD4L* was significantly associated with antihypertensive response to hydrochlorothiazide.[173] In the future, evaluation of gene–gene interactions will likely yield greater insight into genetic predictors of antihypertensive drug response. Another potential role of pharmacogenomics is to predict the likelihood for thiazide-associated metabolic adverse events. It is known that thiazide diuretics result in metabolic abnormalities such as elevated plasma glucose.[176] The extent to which genetic variation modulates metabolic risk in patients receiving antihypertensive

therapy is an evolving area of research.[177] For example, a recent study of GenHAT participants found that the 663T>A polymorphism in the α-subunit of the amiloride-sensitive epithelial sodium channel (*SCNN1A*) was associated with differential effects on fasting glucose based on chlorthalidone versus amlodipine treatment.[178] Specifically, in participants with the G/G genotype, fasting glucose levels were significantly higher in those assigned to chlorthalidone versus amlodipine. Thus, pending additional research, pharmacogenomics may be used in the future to identify metabolic risk associated with diuretic therapy.[177,179]

While all of the thiazide studies described above used a candidate gene approach, in the future, genome-wide association studies will likely play an integral role in identifying predictors of thiazide response and cardiovascular disease risk. For example, a recent genome-wide association study found polymorphisms in lysozyme (*LYZ*) and YEATS domain containing 4 (*YEATS4*) to be associated with diastolic blood pressure response following hydrochlorothiazide therapy.[180] Although the role of these genes in hypertension pathophysiology and/or thiazide pharmacology is not known, this example illustrates how genome-wide association studies can be used to identify novel disease and drug response pathways.

In sum, the above candidate gene and genome-wide association examples highlight the burgeoning amount of research in the field; however, in most cases, the polymorphisms explained only a small percentage of interindividual variability in thiazide response. This brings up an important point in hypertension pharmacogenomics; while genotype may be a significant predictor of response, oftentimes the overall contribution to response is small. Therefore, genotype-guided thiazide prescribing does not have clinical utility at this time.

Renin–Angiotensin–Aldosterone System Modulators

The RAAS plays a pivotal role in blood pressure regulation and electrolyte homeostasis. ACE inhibitors, ARBs, and direct renin inhibitors effectively block the RAAS and improve cardiovascular and renal outcomes.[181] The *ACE* gene is often studied in RAAS pharmacogenomics. A 267 base pair deletion (D)/insertion (I) polymorphism exists in intron 16 of *ACE*, and the D allele is associated with increased plasma levels of ACE.[182,183] Thus, it can be hypothesized that therapeutic response to ACE inhibitors may be greater for the D allele as compared with that for the I allele. However, collective data suggest that the *ACE* D/I polymorphism does not influence ACE inhibitor response.[181] For example, in the GenHAT study, neither was the *ACE* D/I polymorphism associated with the antihypertensive effects of the ACE inhibitor, lisinopril, nor was the polymorphism a predictor of coronary heart disease in this population.[184] This polymorphism also does not appear to influence blood pressure response or clinical outcomes following ARB therapy.[181,185] In terms of other RAAS proteins, renin (*REN*) catalyzes the first and rate-limiting step of the RAAS (i.e., conversion of angiotensinogen to angiotensin I). The *REN*−5312 C>T polymorphism has been shown to increase gene transcription.[186] In one clinical study, this polymorphism was associated with variability in blood pressure response to the direct renin inhibitor, aliskiren, and the ARB, losartan. Given this single report, these data merit replication in additional studies.[187] Angiotensinogen (*AGT*) is another important RAAS effector protein. In most clinical studies, *AGT* polymorphisms (e.g., M235T) have not been significant predictors of the antihypertensive effects of ACE inhibitors or ARBs.[181] ARBs inhibit the angiotensin II type 1 receptor (*AGTR1*). The *AGTR1* 1166 A>C polymorphism has not been associated with the blood pressure lowering effects of ARBs in clinical studies[181] Taking RAAS effector proteins together, the data do not support the use of routine genotyping to guide treatment decisions regarding ACE inhibitors, ARBs, or direct renin inhibitors in hypertension.

Calcium Channel Blockers

Over the last 5 years, studies have begun to shed light on the contribution of genetics to calcium channel blocker disposition and response. One of the first genes identified was *CACNA1C*, which encodes the α_{1C}-subunit of the voltage-dependent, L-type calcium channel (the drug target of calcium channel blockers). Polymorphisms in *CACNA1C* have been associated with antihypertensive response and clinical outcomes following calcium channel blocker therapy.[188–190] For example, in a genetic substudy of INVEST, the rs1051375 A>G (Thr1835Thr) polymorphism significantly interacted with calcium channel blocker versus β-blocker treatment strategy. Specifically, participants with the wild-type A/A genotype who received verapamil had a lower risk of death, nonfatal myocardial infarction, or nonfatal stroke than those who received atenolol.[189] In contrast, participants with the variant G/G genotype who received verapamil had a greater risk for the primary outcome than those who received atenolol. These findings have yet to be replicated in other studies; however, they suggest that *CACNA1C* polymorphisms may be useful in predicting which patients might benefit from calcium channel blocker versus β-blocker antihypertensive treatment strategies. In addition to *CACNA1C*, other pharmacokinetic and pharmacodynamic pathway genes have emerged as potential predictors of calcium channel blocker response and/or cardiovascular outcomes. Some of these genes include the CYP3A5 metabolizing enzyme, P-glycoprotein (*ABCB1*), α_{1D}-subunit of the voltage-dependent L-type calcium channel (*CACNA1D*), the β_2-subunit of the voltage-dependent L-type calcium channel (*CACNB2*), the β_1-subunit of the large-conductance calcium and voltage-dependent L-type potassium channel (*KCNMB1*), the regulator of G protein signaling-2 (*RGS2*), atrial natriuretic precursor A (*NPPA*), and nitric oxide synthase 1 adaptor protein (*NOS1AP*).[172,190–199] Additional studies of polymorphisms in *CACNA1C*, and other calcium channel response pathways, are needed to better understand if genotyping has a potential role in calcium channel blocker therapy.

HEART FAILURE

Heart failure affects over 5 million adults in the United States, and remains the leading discharge diagnosis for patients 65 years of age and older.[125,200] This syndrome is associated with high rates of mortality and morbidity, including frequent hospital readmissions and reduced quality of life.[200] According to the Heart Failure Society of America, the goals of management of heart failure patients with reduced left ventricular ejection fraction are to: (1) improve symptoms and quality of life; (2) slow or reverse the progression of cardiac dysfunction; and (3) reduce mortality.[201] The backbone of heart failure pharmacotherapy includes β-blockers and ACE inhibitors. Other agents that are often used in chronic heart failure treatment regimens include diuretics, aldosterone antagonists, ARBs (if intolerant of ACE inhibitors), digoxin, and/or the combination of isosorbide dinitrate and hydralazine. Given the complexity of heart failure treatment regimens, pharmacogenomics has the potential to improve the management of this syndrome by accounting for some of the interindividual variability in pharmacologic disposition, response, and toxicity. A summary of putative pharmacogenes in heart failure is shown in Table 11–4. To date, heart failure pharmacogenomics has focused mostly on β-blockers, which will be the focus of this section. In addition, the pharmacogenetics of RAAS modulators (i.e., ACE inhibitors, ARBs, and aldosterone antagonists) and isosorbide dinitrate/hydralazine will be briefly discussed.

β-Blockers

β-Blockers significantly reduce morbidity and mortality in heart failure, and are standard of care in this population.[201] They inhibit the deleterious effects of sympathetic nervous system activation (e.g., norepinephrine) on cardiac adrenergic receptors, thereby improving the ejection fraction.[200] The β-blockers that are currently approved for the treatment of heart failure (i.e., metoprolol succinate, bisoprolol, and carvedilol) differ in their selectivity for β-adrenergic receptors. Metoprolol succinate and bisoprolol are β_1-selective agents, while carvedilol has mixed β_1-, β_2-, and α_1-selectivity. It is well known that interindividual variability exists in β-blocker response in heart failure.[202,203] As such, the field of pharmacogenomics has sought to better understand genetic mechanisms underlying these response differences between patients. The primary focus of these investigations has been receptors and kinases in adrenergic signaling pathways.[150]

Pharmacogenetic Focus: ADRB1

The β_1-adrenergic receptor (*ADRB1*) is the primary target for β-blockers. As previously discussed in the section "Hypertension," the two most commonly studied polymorphisms in *ADRB1* are c.1165 C>G (Arg389Gly) and c.145 A>G (Ser49Gly). Pharmacogenetic studies have investigated the relationship between *ADRB1* polymorphisms and various clinical end points in heart failure.[150,202] Although not entirely consistent in the literature, a few studies have shown

TABLE 11–4 Examples of putative pharmacogenes in heart failure.

Drug Class	Gene Name	Protein	Role in Clinical Pharmacology
β-Blockers	ADRB1	β$_1$-Adrenergic receptor	Drug target; adrenergic signaling pathway
	ADRB2	β$_2$-Adrenergic receptor	Drug target; adrenergic signaling pathway
	ADRA2C	α$_{2C}$-Adrenergic receptor	Adrenergic signaling pathway
	GRK5	G protein–coupled receptor kinase 5	Adrenergic signaling pathway
	CYP2D6	Cytochrome P450 2D6	Drug metabolism
RAAS modulators	ACE	Angiotensin-converting enzyme	Drug target; RAAS effector protein
	AGT	Angiotensinogen	RAAS effector protein
	AGTR1	Angiotensin II type 1 receptor	Drug target; RAAS effector protein
Isosorbide dinitrate and hydralazine	CYP11B2	Aldosterone synthase	Aldosterone production
	NOS3	Endothelial	Nitric oxide production and vasodilation

differential effects of β-blockers on left ventricular remodeling based on *ADRB1* genotype.[204–206] For example, heart failure patients with the *ADRB1* codon 389 Arg/Arg genotype had greater improvements in left ventricular ejection fraction and remodeling in response to metoprolol succinate than Gly389 carriers.[205] In addition, the codon 49 Ser/Ser and codon 389 Arg/Arg genotypes were significant predictors of end-of-study left ventricular end-diastolic diameter, a measure of ventricular remodeling.[205] *ADRB1* genetics has also been shown to influence β-blocker tolerability, particularly the need to increase concomitant heart failure medications during metoprolol succinate dose titration.[207] Successful dose titration during β-blocker therapy is crucial as higher doses have been associated with greater reductions in mortality.[201] In terms of hard clinical outcomes (e.g., death, hospitalization, or heart transplantation), risk appears to differ within *ADRB1* genotype groups according to the treatment to which patients are assigned (e.g., high-dose β-blocker vs. low-dose or no β-blocker).[208–210] For example, Arg389 carriers on high-dose β-blockers had better heart failure survival than Arg389 carriers on low-dose or no β-blockers.[209] In another study, heart failure patients with the codon 49 Ser/Ser genotype treated with high-dose β-blockers had better survival than patients with the Ser/Ser genotype who were treated with low-dose β-blockers.[210] In contrast, patients who carried the Gly49 allele had similar survival benefits regardless of whether they were treated with either high-dose or low-dose β-blockers.[210]

Clinical Implications

The examples above suggest that Arg389 and/or Ser49 are adverse risk alleles in heart failure that may influence surrogate and hard clinical outcomes. However, *ADRB1* genotyping is not currently utilized in clinical practice. Given the scope of evidence showing that β-blockers have mortality benefits in heart failure, it is unlikely that patients would be denied a β-blocker based

solely on their *ADBR1* genetic makeup.[203] However, the examples above suggest that patients who possess the Arg389 and/or Ser49 alleles may need tailored therapy (e.g., higher β-blocker doses) for optimal clinical benefit. Additional studies are needed to evaluate the utility and outcomes of this type of approach in heart failure. Along these lines, bucindolol is an investigational, nonselective β-blocker that has been studied for use in heart failure. Although it is not yet approved by the Food and Drug Administration, the evaluation of bucindolol in the β-Blocker Evaluation of Survival Trial (BEST) is an excellent example of the potential clinical utility of pharmacogenetics in heart failure and drug development. Specifically, heart failure patients with the codon 389 Arg/Arg genotype who received bucindolol had better survival rates than those treated with placebo.[208] In contrast, heart failure patients who carried a Gly389 allele had similar survival rates in the bucindolol and placebo groups.[208] This information is consistent with Arg389 functioning as an adverse risk allele in heart failure. With this in mind, should bucindolol be prescribed only to patients with the codon 389 Arg/Arg genotype? The manufacturers of bucindolol are in the process of answering this question by conducting a study that will compare the efficacy of bucindolol with that of metoprolol succinate in heart failure patients who are codon 389 Arg/Arg homozygotes (i.e., the genotype which responded most favorably to bucindolol in BEST). This study will be one of the first to investigate the prospective use of genetics to target pharmacologic therapy in heart failure.

Other Pharmacodynamic and Pharmacokinetic Genes of Interest

Other adrenergic signaling molecules implicated in heart failure pharmacogenomics include the α$_{2C}$-adrenergic receptor, the β$_2$-adrenergic receptor, and *GRK5*. The α$_{2C}$-adrenergic receptor, which is encoded by *ADRA2C*, is an important regulator of the sympathetic nervous system. It mediates the release of norepinephrine from cardiac presynaptic sympathetic nerve terminals, which then exerts a stimulatory effect on β_1-adrenergic receptors in the heart. In terms of genetic polymorphisms, *ADRA2C* contains a four amino acid deletion, Del322-325, that causes receptor dysregulation and increased norepinephrine release.[211,212] Given the physiological interplay between the α_{2C}- and β_1-adrenergic receptors, studies have evaluated whether a synergistic relationship exists between polymorphisms in *ADRA2C* and *ADRB1*.[213] In this regard, black patients who were homozygous for both the *ADRA2C* Del322-325 and *ADRB1* 389Arg alleles had a marked increase in the risk of heart failure.[213] This suggests that the combination of these risk alleles results in greater activation of the sympathetic nervous system, and potentially a greater likelihood for beneficial response to β-blockers. A clinical study evaluated this theory and found that patients who were *ADRA2C* Del322-325 carriers and *ADRB1* Arg homozygotes had the largest increase in left ventricular ejection fraction following metoprolol therapy compared with other genotype combinations.[214] The synergistic effects of these polymorphisms on clinical outcomes remain to be determined in larger studies. The association between β_2-adrenergic receptor (*ADRB2*) polymorphisms and carvedilol response has been evaluated in patients with heart failure. Carvedilol has been the focus of these investigations because it has β_2-adrenergic receptor inhibitory properties. In most studies, the *ADRB2* Gln27Glu polymorphism has been associated with interindividual variability in carvedilol response.[215-217] Specifically, codon 27 Glu homozygotes appear to have greater improvements in left ventricular ejection fraction following carvedilol treatment than Gln27 carriers.[203] However, the extent to which the *ADRB2* Gln27Glu polymorphism influences the effect of carvedilol on clinical outcomes in heart failure has not yet been studied. GRKs, such as *GRK5*, help regulate β-adrenergic receptor signaling. The *GRK5* Gln41Leu polymorphism is associated with suppressed β_1-adrenergic receptor signaling and, in essence, the Leu41 allele acts as a "genetic β-blocker."[150] Of note, the frequency of the Leu41 allele frequency is more common in African Americans (23%) versus Caucasians (~2%).[218] As such, racial differences in the Leu41 allele frequency may explain, in part, racial differences in heart failure phenotypes and clinical outcomes. The Gln41Leu polymorphism has been shown to influence survival and β-blocker outcomes in heart failure patients.[218,219] For example, African American patients with the codon 41 Gln/Gln genotype who were treated with a β-blocker had better survival rates than those with the same genotype who did not receive a β-blocker.[219] Conversely, African American patients who carried a protective Leu41 allele had similar survival rates regardless of whether or not they received a β-blocker.[219] These data suggest that *GRK5* Gln41Leu genotype may help identify African American patients who will derive the greatest survival benefit from β-blocker therapy. However, additional studies are needed before this genetic test can be used in the clinic setting.

Beyond pharmacodynamics, the relationship between polymorphisms in genes related to β-blocker pharmacokinetics has also been evaluated in patients with heart failure. As discussed in the section "Hypertension," *CYP2D6* polymorphisms influence β-blocker pharmacokinetics, particularly agents that are extensively metabolized by CYP2D6, such as metoprolol.[154] However, in hypertension, *CYP2D6*-mediated differences in β-blocker plasma exposure did not influence antihypertensive efficacy or adverse effects. Similar results have been found in the setting of heart failure. For example, in heart failure patients, metoprolol plasma concentrations differed significantly between CYP2D6 metabolic phenotypes.[207] However, the risk of cardiac decompensation and the need for adjustment of background heart failure medications were not significantly different between CYP2D6 phenotype groups.[207] Other metoprolol heart failure studies have shown similar findings.[220,221] In addition, no association between CYP2D6 phenotype and carvedilol response has been observed.[221] Therefore, *CYP2D6* genotyping likely has limited clinical utility for the prediction of β-blocker tolerability in heart failure.

Renin–Angiotensin–Aldosterone System Modulators

Activation of the RAAS is a major player in the pathophysiology of heart failure.[200] ACE inhibitors block the conversion of angiotensin I to angiotensin II, thereby decreasing the detrimental effects of angiotensin II–mediated vasoconstriction on the cardiovascular system. ACE inhibitors reduce morbidity and mortality in heart failure, and are an essential component of pharmacotherapy in this patient population.[201,222] Compared with other cardiovascular disease states (e.g., hypertension), the impact of RAAS polymorphisms on heart failure pharmacotherapy has not been studied to a great extent.[223] However, the 287 base pair deletion (D)/insertion (I) polymorphism in the *ACE* gene appears to be a potential genetic target in this population. As previously discussed in the section "Hypertension," the *ACE* D allele has been associated with increased plasma levels of ACE.[182,183] Thus, in the setting of heart failure, it is reasonable to hypothesize that a pharmacogenetic interaction may exist between the *ACE* D/I polymorphism and ACE inhibitor therapy. This idea was investigated in a clinical study, and it was found that the *ACE* D allele was associated with worse clinical outcomes (e.g., poorer transplant-free survival) in heart failure patients.[224] More importantly, adverse risk associated with the *ACE* D allele was greatest in patients who received low-dose ACE inhibitor versus high-dose ACE inhibitor therapy.[224] This study also noted an interaction with β-blocker therapy, whereby the benefit of high-dose ACE inhibitors plus β-blockers was greatest in patients with the *ACE* D/D genotype. These findings suggest that the *ACE* D/I polymorphism may be useful in identifying heart failure patients who may benefit from aggressive ACE inhibitor and β-blocker treatment strategies. However, this genetic paradigm has not yet been developed for clinical use.

In regards to other RAAS modulators, ARBs are recommended for the treatment of heart failure in patients who are intolerant of ACE inhibitors.[201,222] ARBs block the action of angiotensin II at the AT_1 receptor. Few studies have examined the effects of RAAS polymorphisms on ARB response and outcomes in heart failure. However, a small, proof-of-concept study found an association between the *AGTR1* 1166 A>C polymorphism and reductions in blood pressure and N-terminal proB-type natriuretic peptide (a neurohormonal biomarker) following add-on candesartan treatment in heart failure patients receiving ACE inhibitors. Given the small size of this study, the association between *AGTR1* polymorphisms and response to ARBs in heart failure needs to be evaluated in larger populations.[225] Aldosterone also plays an important role in the pathophysiology of heart failure. As such, aldosterone antagonists (i.e., spironolactone and eplerenone) are often used to treat heart failure patients, particularly those with advanced symptoms.[200,201,222] There is limited pharmacogenetic information on aldosterone antagonists to date, but one small study showed that the effects of spironolactone treatment on left ventricular function and remodeling may be influenced by the *ACE* D/I polymorphism.[226] Taken together, a few genetic associations have been observed for RAAS modulators in heart failure; however, none of these examples are at the stage where they could be implemented in the clinical practice setting.

Isosorbide Dinitrate and Hydralazine

The combination of isosorbide dinitrate and hydralazine can be used as either an adjunct treatment option in black patients with heart failure already receiving background therapy or a background therapy to replace ACE inhibitors in patients who are intolerant.[201,222] This race-based indication came primarily from the African American Heart Failure Trial (A-HeFT), which found that a fixed-dose combination of isosorbide dinitrate and hydralazine, in addition to standard background therapy, was better than placebo in black patients with advanced heart failure.[227] Subsequently, a fixed-dose tablet containing both agents was approved by the Food and Drug Administration and specifically indicated for self-identified blacks.[228] This approval caused much controversy regarding race-based therapeutics. However, it has led to researchers to evaluate the extent to which genetic polymorphisms may underlie racial differences in heart failure phenotype and race-based effects of isosorbide dinitrate/hydralazine. The aldosterone synthase (*CYP11B2*) gene has been studied in this regard. Specifically, in a genetic substudy of A-HeFT, the *CYP11B2* −344T>C polymorphism was associated with higher aldosterone levels and worse outcomes in black patients with heart failure.[229] Interestingly, patients with the T/T genotype appeared to derive the greatest benefit from isosorbide dinitrate/hydralazine therapy. These findings are consistent with the knowledge that heart failure phenotypes differ between African Americans and Caucasians, and that the T allele is more prevalent in the black population.[229] Another gene that has been studied in a genetic substudy of A-HeFT is endothelial nitric oxide synthase (*NOS3*). Three *NOS3* polymorphisms, −786T>C, a repeat polymorphism in intron 4, and Glu298Asp, were found to have genotype frequencies that differed significantly between blacks and whites.[230] Additionally, in blacks, isosorbide dinitrate/hydralazine therapy was more effective in patients with the Glu/Glu genotype.[230] The *CYP11B2* and *NOS3* findings merit additional study. However, these data suggest that genetic differences underlying heart failure

phenotypes and drug response may help guide pharmacologic treatment strategies in heart failure.

CONCLUSION

Over the past decade, significant strides have been made in the field of cardiovascular pharmacogenomics. Clopidogrel is a good example of the development and potential application of pharmacogenomics in clinical medicine. In addition, genome-wide association studies of hypertension and statin pharmacotherapy illustrate the power of an exploratory approach to identify novel pathways in drug response and less common adverse effects. Given the continual evolution of genomic technologies, the field of cardiovascular pharmacogenomics will undoubtedly expand at a rapid pace. In the years to come, opportunities and challenges facing the field will include the identification and replication of polymorphisms underlying drug response in large clinical cohorts and genome-wide association studies, the elucidation of the predictive value of genetic testing for a given cardiovascular medication, and the translation of cardiovascular pharmacogenomic information to clinical practice.

REFERENCES

1. Anderson JL, Adams CD, Antman EM, et al. ACC/AHA 2007 guidelines for the management of patients with unstable angina/non-ST-elevation myocardial infarction: a report of the American College of Cardiology/American Heart Association Task Force on Practice Guidelines (Writing Committee to Revise the 2002 Guidelines for the Management of Patients with Unstable Angina/Non-ST-Elevation Myocardial Infarction) developed in collaboration with the American College of Emergency Physicians, the Society for Cardiovascular Angiography and Interventions, and the Society of Thoracic Surgeons endorsed by the American Association of Cardiovascular and Pulmonary Rehabilitation and the Society for Academic Emergency Medicine. *J Am Coll Cardiol.* 2007;50(7):e1–e157.
2. Wright RS, Anderson JL, Adams CD, et al. 2011 ACCF/AHA focused update of the guidelines for the management of patients with unstable angina/non-ST-elevation myocardial infarction (updating the 2007 guideline): a report of the American College of Cardiology Foundation/American Heart Association Task Force on Practice Guidelines. *Circulation.* 2011;123(18):2022–2060.
3. Plavix (clopidogrel) prescribing information. Bridgewater, NJ: Bristol-Myers Squibb/Sanofi Pharmaceuticals Partnership; February 2011. Available at: http://products.sanofi.us/plavix/plavix.html.
4. Gurbel PA, Bliden KP, Hiatt BL, O'Connor CM. Clopidogrel for coronary stenting: response variability, drug resistance, and the effect of pretreatment platelet reactivity. *Circulation.* 2003;107(23):2908–2913.
5. Kazui M, Nishiya Y, Ishizuka T, et al. Identification of the human cytochrome P450 enzymes involved in the two oxidative steps in the bioactivation of clopidogrel to its pharmacologically active metabolite. *Drug Metab Dispos.* 2010;38(1):92–99.
6. http://www.cypalleles.ki.se/.
7. Scott SA, Sangkuhl K, Gardner EE, et al. Clinical pharmacogenetics implementation consortium guidelines for cytochrome P450-2C19 (CYP2C19) genotype and clopidogrel therapy. *Clin Pharmacol Ther.* 2011;90(2):328–332.
8. Beitelshees AL, Horenstein RB, Vesely MR, Mehra MR, Shuldiner AR. Pharmacogenetics and clopidogrel response in patients undergoing percutaneous coronary interventions. *Clin Pharmacol Ther.* 2011;89(3):455–459.
9. Sim SC, Risinger C, Dahl ML, et al. A common novel CYP2C19 gene variant causes ultrarapid drug metabolism relevant to the drug response to proton pump inhibitors and antidepressants. *Clin Pharmacol Ther.* 2006;79(1):103–113.

10. Brandt JT, Close SL, Iturria SJ, et al. Common polymorphisms of CYP2C19 and CYP2C9 affect the pharmacokinetic and pharmacodynamic response to clopidogrel but not prasugrel. *J Thromb Haemost*. 2007;5(12):2429–2436.

11. Umemura K, Furuta T, Kondo K. The common gene variants of CYP2C19 affect pharmacokinetics and pharmacodynamics in an active metabolite of clopidogrel in healthy subjects. *J Thromb Haemost*. 2008;6(8):1439–1441.

12. Mega JL, Close SL, Wiviott SD, et al. Cytochrome p-450 polymorphisms and response to clopidogrel. *N Engl J Med*. 2009;360(4):354–362.

13. Ellis KJ, Stouffer GA, McLeod HL, Lee CR. Clopidogrel pharmacogenomics and risk of inadequate platelet inhibition: US FDA recommendations. *Pharmacogenomics*. 2009;10(11):1799–1817.

14. Yin T, Miyata T. Pharmacogenomics of clopidogrel: evidence and perspectives. *Thromb Res*. 2011;128(4):307–316.

15. Shuldiner AR, O'Connell JR, Bliden KP, et al. Association of cytochrome P450 2C19 genotype with the antiplatelet effect and clinical efficacy of clopidogrel therapy. *JAMA*. 2009;302(8):849–857.

16. Trenk D, Hochholzer W, Fromm MF, et al. Cytochrome P450 2C19 681G>A polymorphism and high on-clopidogrel platelet reactivity associated with adverse 1-year clinical outcome of elective percutaneous coronary intervention with drug-eluting or bare-metal stents. *J Am Coll Cardiol*. 2008;51(20):1925–1934.

17. Collet JP, Hulot JS, Pena A, et al. Cytochrome P450 2C19 polymorphism in young patients treated with clopidogrel after myocardial infarction: a cohort study. *Lancet*. 2009;373(9660):309–317.

18. Giusti B, Gori AM, Marcucci R, et al. Relation of cytochrome P450 2C19 loss-of-function polymorphism to occurrence of drug-eluting coronary stent thrombosis. *Am J Cardiol*. 2009;103(6):806–811.

19. Sibbing D, Stegherr J, Latz W, et al. Cytochrome P450 2C19 loss-of-function polymorphism and stent thrombosis following percutaneous coronary intervention. *Eur Heart J*. 2009;30(8):916–922.

20. Simon T, Verstuyft C, Mary-Krause M, et al. Genetic determinants of response to clopidogrel and cardiovascular events. *N Engl J Med*. 2009;360(4):363–375.

21. Harmsze AM, van Werkum JW, Ten Berg JM, et al. CYP2C19*2 and CYP2C9*3 alleles are associated with stent thrombosis: a case–control study. *Eur Heart J*. 2010;31(24):3046–3053.

22. Malek LA, Przyluski J, Spiewak M, et al. Cytochrome P450 2C19 polymorphism, suboptimal reperfusion and all-cause mortality in patients with acute myocardial infarction. *Cardiology*. 2010;117(2):81–87.

23. Yamamoto K, Hokimoto S, Chitose T, et al. Impact of CYP2C19 polymorphism on residual platelet reactivity in patients with coronary heart disease during antiplatelet therapy. *J Cardiol*. 2011;57(2):194–201.

24. Sangkuhl K, Klein TE, Altman RB. Clopidogrel pathway. *Pharmacogenet Genomics*. 2010; 20(7):463–465.

25. Mega JL, Simon T, Collet JP, et al. Reduced-function CYP2C19 genotype and risk of adverse clinical outcomes among patients treated with clopidogrel predominantly for PCI: a meta-analysis. *JAMA*. 2010;304(16):1821–1830.

26. Wallentin L, James S, Storey RF, et al. Effect of CYP2C19 and ABCB1 single nucleotide polymorphisms on outcomes of treatment with ticagrelor versus clopidogrel for acute coronary syndromes: a genetic substudy of the PLATO trial. *Lancet*. 2010;376(9749):1320–1328.

27. Pare G, Mehta SR, Yusuf S, et al. Effects of CYP2C19 genotype on outcomes of clopidogrel treatment. *N Engl J Med*. 2010;363(18):1704–1714.

28. Hulot JS, Collet JP, Silvain J, et al. Cardiovascular risk in clopidogrel-treated patients according to cytochrome P450 2C19*2 loss-of-function allele or proton pump inhibitor coadministration: a systematic meta-analysis. *J Am Coll Cardiol*. 2010;56(2):134–143.

29. Jin B, Ni HC, Shen W, Li J, Shi HM, Li Y. Cytochrome P450 2C19 polymorphism is associated with poor clinical outcomes in coronary artery disease patients treated with clopidogrel. *Mol Biol Rep*. 2011;38(3):1697–1702.

30. Sofi F, Giusti B, Marcucci R, Gori AM, Abbate R, Gensini GF. Cytochrome P450 2C19*2 polymorphism and cardiovascular recurrences in patients taking clopidogrel: a meta-analysis. *Pharmacogenomics J*. 2011;11(3):199–206.

31. Frere C, Cuisset T, Gaborit B, Alessi MC, Hulot JS. The CYP2C19*17 allele is associated with better platelet response to clopidogrel in patients admitted for non-ST acute coronary syndrome. *J Thromb Haemost*. 2009;7(8):1409–1411.

32. Sibbing D, Koch W, Gebhard D, et al. Cytochrome 2C19*17 allelic variant, platelet aggregation, bleeding events, and stent thrombosis in clopidogrel-treated patients with coronary stent placement. *Circulation*. 2010;121(4):512–518.

33. Sibbing D, Gebhard D, Koch W, et al. Isolated and interactive impact of common CYP2C19 genetic variants on the antiplatelet effect of chronic clopidogrel therapy. *J Thromb Haemost*. 2010;8(8):1685–1693.

34. Tiroch KA, Sibbing D, Koch W, et al. Protective effect of the CYP2C19 17 polymorphism with increased activation of clopidogrel on cardiovascular events. *Am Heart J*. 2010;160(3):506–512.

35. Geisler T, Schaeffeler E, Dippon J, et al. CYP2C19 and nongenetic factors predict poor responsiveness to clopidogrel loading dose after coronary stent implantation. *Pharmacogenomics*. 2008;9(9):1251–1259.

36. Angiolillo DJ, Fernandez-Ortiz A, Bernardo E, et al. Contribution of gene sequence variations of the hepatic cytochrome P450 3A4 enzyme to variability in individual responsiveness to clopidogrel. *Arterioscler Thromb Vasc Biol*. 2006;26(8):1895–1900.

37. Hulot JS, Bura A, Villard E, et al. Cytochrome P450 2C19 loss-of-function polymorphism is a major determinant of clopidogrel responsiveness in healthy subjects. *Blood*. 2006;108(7):2244–2247.

38. Frere C, Cuisset T, Morange PE, et al. Effect of cytochrome p450 polymorphisms on platelet reactivity after treatment with clopidogrel in acute coronary syndrome. *Am J Cardiol*. 2008;101(8):1088–1093.

39. Giusti B, Gori AM, Marcucci R, et al. Cytochrome P450 2C19 loss-of-function polymorphism, but not CYP3A4 IVS10 + 12G/A and P2Y12 T744C polymorphisms, is associated with response variability to dual antiplatelet treatment in high-risk vascular patients. *Pharmacogenet Genomics*. 2007;17(12):1057–1064.

40. Bouman HJ, Schomig E, van Werkum JW, et al. Paraoxonase-1 is a major determinant of clopidogrel efficacy. *Nat Med*. 2011;17(1):110–116.

41. Sibbing D, Koch W, Massberg S, et al. No association of paraoxonase-1 Q192R genotypes with platelet response to clopidogrel and risk of stent thrombosis after coronary stenting. *Eur Heart J*. 2011;32(13):1605–1613.

42. Trenk D, Hochholzer W, Fromm MF, et al. Paraoxonase-1 Q192R polymorphism and antiplatelet effects of clopidogrel in patients undergoing elective coronary stent placement. *Circ Cardiovasc Genet*. 2011;4(4):429–436.

43. Fontana P, James R, Barazer I, et al. Relationship between paraoxonase-1 activity, its Q192R genetic variant and clopidogrel responsiveness in the ADRIE study. *J Thromb Haemost*. 2011;9(8):1664–1666.

44. Taubert D, von Beckerath N, Grimberg G, et al. Impact of P-glycoprotein on clopidogrel absorption. *Clin Pharmacol Ther*. 2006;80(5):486–501.

45. Mega JL, Close SL, Wiviott SD, et al. Genetic variants in ABCB1 and CYP2C19 and cardiovascular outcomes after treatment with clopidogrel and prasugrel in the TRITON-TIMI 38 trial: a pharmacogenetic analysis. *Lancet*. 2010;376(9749):1312–1319.

46. Fontana P, Dupont A, Gandrille S, et al. Adenosine diphosphate-induced platelet aggregation is associated with P2Y12 gene sequence variations in healthy subjects. *Circulation*. 2003;108(8):989–995.

47. Angiolillo DJ, Fernandez-Ortiz A, Bernardo E, et al. Lack of association between the P2Y12 receptor gene polymorphism and platelet response to clopidogrel in patients with coronary artery disease. *Thromb Res*. 2005;116(6):491–497.

48. Smith SM, Judge HM, Peters G, et al. Common sequence variations in the P2Y12 and CYP3A5 genes do not explain the variability in the inhibitory effects of clopidogrel therapy. *Platelets*. 2006;17(4):250–258.

49. http://www.fda.gov/drugs/drugsafety/PostmarketDrugSafetyInformation forPatientsandProviders/ucm203888.htm.

50. Holmes DR Jr, Dehmer GJ, Kaul S, Leifer D, O'Gara PT, Stein CM. ACCF/AHA clopidogrel clinical alert: approaches to the FDA "boxed warning": a report of the American College of Cardiology Foundation Task Force on clinical expert consensus documents and the American Heart Association endorsed by the Society for Cardiovascular Angiography and Interventions and the Society of Thoracic Surgeons. *J Am Coll Cardiol*. 2010;56(4):321–341.

51. Simon T, Bhatt DL, Bergougnan L, et al. Genetic polymorphisms and the impact of a higher clopidogrel dose regimen on active metabolite exposure and antiplatelet response in healthy subjects. *Clin Pharmacol Ther*. 2011;90(2):287–295.

52. Collet JP, Hulot JS, Anzaha G, et al. High doses of clopidogrel to overcome genetic resistance: the randomized crossover CLOVIS-2 (Clopidogrel and Response Variability Investigation Study 2). *JACC Cardiovasc Interv*. 2011;4(4):392–402.

53. Effient (prasugrel) prescribing information. Daiichi Sankyo Inc/Eli Lilly and Company; December 2010. Available at: http://pi.lilly.com/us/effient.pdf.

54. Wiviott SD, Braunwald E, McCabe CH, et al. Prasugrel versus clopidogrel in patients with acute coronary syndromes. *N Engl J Med.* 2007;357(20):2001–2015.

55. Gurbel PA, Bliden KP, Butler K, et al. Response to ticagrelor in clopidogrel nonresponders and responders and effect of switching therapies: the RESPOND study. *Circulation.* 2010;121(10):1188–1199.

56. Li M, Ong KL, Tse HF, Cheung BM. Utilization of lipid lowering medications among adults in the United States 1999–2006. *Atherosclerosis.* 2010;208(2):456–460.

57. National Cholesterol Education Program (NCEP) Expert Panel on Detection, Evaluation, and Treatment of High Blood Cholesterol in Adults (Adult Treatment Panel III). Third report of the National Cholesterol Education Program (NCEP) Expert Panel on Detection, Evaluation, and Treatment of High Blood Cholesterol in Adults (Adult Treatment Panel III) final report. *Circulation.* 2002;106(25):3143–3421.

58. Grundy SM, Cleeman JI, Merz CN, et al. Implications of recent clinical trials for the National Cholesterol Education Program Adult Treatment Panel III guidelines. *Circulation.* 2004;110(2):227–239.

59. Blum A, Shamburek R. The pleiotropic effects of statins on endothelial function, vascular inflammation, immunomodulation and thrombogenesis. *Atherosclerosis.* 2009;203(2):325–330.

60. Zineh I. Pharmacogenetics of response to statins. *Curr Atheroscler Rep.* 2007;9(3):187–194.

61. Ho RH, Kim RB. Transporters and drug therapy: implications for drug disposition and disease. *Clin Pharmacol Ther.* 2005;78(3):260–277.

62. Shitara Y, Horie T, Sugiyama Y. Transporters as a determinant of drug clearance and tissue distribution. *Eur J Pharm Sci.* 2006;27(5):425–446.

63. Niemi M, Pasanen MK, Neuvonen PJ. Organic anion transporting polypeptide 1B1: a genetically polymorphic transporter of major importance for hepatic drug uptake. *Pharmacol Rev.* 2011;63(1):157–181.

64. Oshiro C, Mangravite L, Klein T, Altman R. PharmGKB very important pharmacogene: SLCO1B1. *Pharmacogenet Genomics.* 2010;20(3):211–216.

65. Tirona RG, Leake BF, Merino G, Kim RB. Polymorphisms in OATP-C: identification of multiple allelic variants associated with altered transport activity among European- and African-Americans. *J Biol Chem.* 2001;276(38):35669–35675.

66. Michalski C, Cui Y, Nies AT, et al. A naturally occurring mutation in the SLC21A6 gene causing impaired membrane localization of the hepatocyte uptake transporter. *J Biol Chem.* 2002;277(45):43058–43063.

67. Mwinyi J, Johne A, Bauer S, Roots I, Gerloff T. Evidence for inverse effects of OATP-C (SLC21A6) 5 and 1b haplotypes on pravastatin kinetics. *Clin Pharmacol Ther.* 2004;75(5):415–421.

68. Kameyama Y, Yamashita K, Kobayashi K, Hosokawa M, Chiba K. Functional characterization of SLCO1B1 (OATP-C) variants, SLCO1B1*5, SLCO1B1*15 and SLCO1B1*15 + C1007G, by using transient expression systems of HeLa and HEK293 cells. *Pharmacogenet Genomics.* 2005;15(7):513–522.

69. Choi JH, Lee MG, Cho JY, Lee JE, Kim KH, Park K. Influence of OATP1B1 genotype on the pharmacokinetics of rosuvastatin in Koreans. *Clin Pharmacol Ther.* 2008;83(2):251–257.

70. Chung JY, Cho JY, Yu KS, et al. Effect of OATP1B1 (SLCO1B1) variant alleles on the pharmacokinetics of pitavastatin in healthy volunteers. *Clin Pharmacol Ther.* 2005;78(4):342–350.

71. Deng JW, Song IS, Shin HJ, et al. The effect of SLCO1B1*15 on the disposition of pravastatin and pitavastatin is substrate dependent: the contribution of transporting activity changes by SLCO1B1*15. *Pharmacogenet Genomics.* 2008;18(5):424–433.

72. Ho RH, Choi L, Lee W, et al. Effect of drug transporter genotypes on pravastatin disposition in European- and African-American participants. *Pharmacogenet Genomics.* 2007;17(8):647–656.

73. Ieiri I, Suwannakul S, Maeda K, et al. SLCO1B1 (OATP1B1, an uptake transporter) and ABCG2 (BCRP, an efflux transporter) variant alleles and pharmacokinetics of pitavastatin in healthy volunteers. *Clin Pharmacol Ther.* 2007;82(5):541–547.

74. Igel M, Arnold KA, Niemi M, et al. Impact of the SLCO1B1 polymorphism on the pharmacokinetics and lipid-lowering efficacy of multiple-dose pravastatin. *Clin Pharmacol Ther.* 2006;79(5):419–426.

75. Lee E, Ryan S, Birmingham B, et al. Rosuvastatin pharmacokinetics and pharmacogenetics in white and Asian subjects residing in the same environment. *Clin Pharmacol Ther.* 2005;78(4):330–341.

76. Lee YJ, Lee MG, Lim LA, Jang SB, Chung JY. Effects of SLCO1B1 and ABCB1 genotypes on the pharmacokinetics of atorvastatin and 2-hydroxyatorvastatin in healthy Korean subjects. *Int J Clin Pharmacol Ther.* 2010;48(1):36–45.

77. Niemi M, Pasanen MK, Neuvonen PJ. SLCO1B1 polymorphism and sex affect the pharmacokinetics of pravastatin but not fluvastatin. *Clin Pharmacol Ther.* 2006;80(4):356–366.

78. Niemi M, Schaeffeler E, Lang T, et al. High plasma pravastatin concentrations are associated with single nucleotide polymorphisms and haplotypes of organic anion transporting polypeptide-C (OATP-C, SLCO1B1). *Pharmacogenetics.* 2004;14(7):429–440.

79. Pasanen MK, Fredrikson H, Neuvonen PJ, Niemi M. Different effects of SLCO1B1 polymorphism on the pharmacokinetics of atorvastatin and rosuvastatin. *Clin Pharmacol Ther.* 2007;82(6):726–733.

80. Pasanen MK, Neuvonen M, Neuvonen PJ, Niemi M. SLCO1B1 polymorphism markedly affects the pharmacokinetics of simvastatin acid. *Pharmacogenet Genomics.* 2006;16(12):873–879.

81. Nishizato Y, Ieiri I, Suzuki H, et al. Polymorphisms of OATP-C (SLC21A6) and OAT3 (SLC22A8) genes: consequences for pravastatin pharmacokinetics. *Clin Pharmacol Ther.* 2003;73(6):554–565.

82. Maeda K, Ieiri I, Yasuda K, et al. Effects of organic anion transporting polypeptide 1B1 haplotype on pharmacokinetics of pravastatin, valsartan, and temocapril. *Clin Pharmacol Ther.* 2006;79(5):427–439.

83. Wen J, Xiong Y. OATP1B1 388A>G polymorphism and pharmacokinetics of pitavastatin in Chinese healthy volunteers. *J Clin Pharm Ther.* 2010;35(1):99–104.

84. Link E, Parish S, Armitage J, et al. SLCO1B1 variants and statin-induced myopathy—a genomewide study. *N Engl J Med.* 2008;359(8):789–799.

85. Voora D, Shah SH, Spasojevic I, et al. The SLCO1B1*5 genetic variant is associated with statin-induced side effects. *J Am Coll Cardiol.* 2009;54(17):1609–1616.

86. McDonagh EM, Whirl-Carrillo M, Garten Y, Altman RB, Klein TE. From pharmacogenomic knowledge acquisition to clinical applications: the PharmGKB as a clinical pharmacogenomic biomarker resource. *Biomarkers Med.* 2011;5(6):795–806.

87. Peters BJ, Klungel OH, Visseren FL, de Boer A, Maitland-van der Zee AH. Pharmacogenomic insights into treatment and management of statin-induced myopathy. *Genome Med.* 2009;1(12):120.

88. Rossi JS, McLeod HL. The pharmacogenetics of statin therapy: when the body aches, the mind will follow. *J Am Coll Cardiol.* 2009;54(17):1617–1618.

89. Li Y, Iakoubova OA, Shiffman D, Devlin JJ, Forrester JS, Superko HR. KIF6 polymorphism as a predictor of risk of coronary events and of clinical event reduction by statin therapy. *Am J Cardiol.* 2010;106(7):994–998.

90. http://www.ncbi.nlm.nih.gov/projects/SNP/snp_ref.cgi?rs=20455.

91. Iakoubova OA, Tong CH, Rowland CM, et al. Association of the Trp719Arg polymorphism in kinesin-like protein 6 with myocardial infarction and coronary heart disease in 2 prospective trials: the CARE and WOSCOPS trials. *J Am Coll Cardiol.* 2008;51(4):435–443.

92. Iakoubova OA, Sabatine MS, Rowland CM, et al. Polymorphism in KIF6 gene and benefit from statins after acute coronary syndromes: results from the PROVE IT-TIMI 22 study. *J Am Coll Cardiol.* 2008;51(4):449–455.

93. Morrison AC, Bare LA, Chambless LE, et al. Prediction of coronary heart disease risk using a genetic risk score: the Atherosclerosis Risk in Communities Study. *Am J Epidemiol.* 2007;166(1):28–35.

94. Shiffman D, Chasman DI, Zee RY, et al. A kinesin family member 6 variant is associated with coronary heart disease in the Women's Health Study. *J Am Coll Cardiol.* 2008;51(4):444–448.

95. Iakoubova OA, Robertson M, Tong CH, et al. KIF6 Trp719Arg polymorphism and the effect of statin therapy in elderly patients: results from the PROSPER study. *Eur J Cardiovasc Prev Rehabil.* 2010;17(4):455–461.

96. Shiffman D, O'Meara ES, Bare LA, et al. Association of gene variants with incident myocardial infarction in the Cardiovascular Health Study. *Arterioscler Thromb Vasc Biol.* 2008;28(1):173–179.

97. Bare LA, Morrison AC, Rowland CM, et al. Five common gene variants identify elevated genetic risk for coronary heart disease. *Genet Med.* 2007;9(10):682–689.

98. http://www.kif6-statincheck.com/.

99. Musunuru K. Current role of pharmacogenomics in cardiovascular medicine. *Curr Treat Options Cardiovasc Med.* 2011;13(4):302–312.

100. Assimes TL, Holm H, Kathiresan S, et al. Lack of association between the Trp719Arg polymorphism in kinesin-like protein-6 and coronary artery disease in 19 case–control studies. *J Am Coll Cardiol.* 2010;56(19):1552–1563.

101. Ridker PM, Macfadyen JG, Glynn RJ, Chasman DI. Kinesin-like protein 6 (KIF6) polymorphism and the efficacy of rosuvastatin in primary prevention. *Circ Cardiovasc Genet.* 2011;4(3):312–317.

102. Hopewell JC, Parish S, Clarke R, et al. No impact of KIF6 genotype on vascular risk and statin response among 18,348 randomized patients in the heart protection study. *J Am Coll Cardiol.* 2011;57(20):2000–2007.

103. Stewart AF, Dandona S, Chen L, et al. Kinesin family member 6 variant Trp719Arg does not associate with angiographically defined coronary artery disease in the Ottawa Heart Genomics Study. *J Am Coll Cardiol.* 2009;53(16):1471–1472.

104. Topol EJ, Damani SB. The KIF6 collapse. *J Am Coll Cardiol.* 2010; 56(19):1564–1566.

105. Kajinami K, Brousseau ME, Ordovas JM, Schaefer EJ. CYP3A4 genotypes and plasma lipoprotein levels before and after treatment with atorvastatin in primary hypercholesterolemia. *Am J Cardiol.* 2004;93(1):104–107.

106. Kim KA, Park PW, Lee OJ, Kang DK, Park JY. Effect of polymorphic CYP3A5 genotype on the single-dose simvastatin pharmacokinetics in healthy subjects. *J Clin Pharmacol.* 2007;47(1):87–93.

107. Kivisto KT, Niemi M, Schaeffeler E, et al. Lipid-lowering response to statins is affected by CYP3A5 polymorphism. *Pharmacogenetics.* 2004;14(8):523–525.

108. Wilke RA, Moore JH, Burmester JK. Relative impact of CYP3A genotype and concomitant medication on the severity of atorvastatin-induced muscle damage. *Pharmacogenet Genomics.* 2005;15(6):415–421.

109. Keskitalo JE, Kurkinen KJ, Neuvoneni PJ, Niemi M. ABCB1 haplotypes differentially affect the pharmacokinetics of the acid and lactone forms of simvastatin and atorvastatin. *Clin Pharmacol Ther.* 2008;84(4):457–461.

110. Fiegenbaum M, da Silveira FR, Van der Sand CR, et al. The role of common variants of ABCB1, CYP3A4, and CYP3A5 genes in lipid-lowering efficacy and safety of simvastatin treatment. *Clin Pharmacol Ther.* 2005;78(5):551–558.

111. Keskitalo JE, Kurkinen KJ, Neuvonen M, Backman JT, Neuvonen PJ, Niemi M. No significant effect of ABCB1 haplotypes on the pharmacokinetics of fluvastatin, pravastatin, lovastatin, and rosuvastatin. *Br J Clin Pharmacol.* 2009;68(2):207–213.

112. Keskitalo JE, Pasanen MK, Neuvonen PJ, Niemi M. Different effects of the ABCG2 c.421C>A SNP on the pharmacokinetics of fluvastatin, pravastatin and simvastatin. *Pharmacogenomics.* 2009;10(10):1617–1624.

113. Keskitalo JE, Zolk O, Fromm MF, Kurkinen KJ, Neuvonen PJ, Niemi M. ABCG2 polymorphism markedly affects the pharmacokinetics of atorvastatin and rosuvastatin. *Clin Pharmacol Ther.* 2009;86(2):197–203.

114. Zhang W, Yu BN, He YJ, et al. Role of BCRP 421C>A polymorphism on rosuvastatin pharmacokinetics in healthy Chinese males. *Clin Chim Acta.* 2006;373(1–2):99–103.

115. Hu M, To KK, Mak VW, Tomlinson B. The ABCG2 transporter and its relations with the pharmacokinetics, drug interaction and lipid-lowering effects of statins. *Expert Opin Drug Metab Toxicol.* 2011;7(1):49–62.

116. Tomlinson B, Hu M, Lee VW, et al. ABCG2 polymorphism is associated with the low-density lipoprotein cholesterol response to rosuvastatin. *Clin Pharmacol Ther.* 2010;87(5):558–562.

117. Hu M, Lui SS, Mak VW, et al. Pharmacogenetic analysis of lipid responses to rosuvastatin in Chinese patients. *Pharmacogenet Genomics.* 2010;20(10):634–637.

118. Bailey KM, Romaine SP, Jackson BM, et al. Hepatic metabolism and transporter gene variants enhance response to rosuvastatin in patients with acute myocardial infarction: the GEOSTAT-1 Study. *Circ Cardiovasc Genet.* 2010;3(3):276–285.

119. Nieminen T, Kahonen M, Viiri LE, Gronroos P, Lehtimaki T. Pharmacogenetics of apolipoprotein E gene during lipid-lowering therapy: lipid levels and prevention of coronary heart disease. *Pharmacogenomics.* 2008;9(10):1475–1486.

120. Thompson JF, Man M, Johnson KJ, et al. An association study of 43 SNPs in 16 candidate genes with atorvastatin response. *Pharmacogenomics J.* 2005;5(6):352–358.

121. Chasman DI, Posada D, Subrahmanyan L, Cook NR, Stanton VP Jr, Ridker PM. Pharmacogenetic study of statin therapy and cholesterol reduction. *JAMA.* 2004;291(23):2821–2827.

122. Daly AK. Genome-wide association studies in pharmacogenomics. *Nat Rev Genet.* 2010;11(4):241–246.

123. Thompson JF, Hyde CL, Wood LS, et al. Comprehensive whole-genome and candidate gene analysis for response to statin therapy in the Treating to New Targets (TNT) cohort. *Circ Cardiovasc Genet.* 2009;2(2): 173–181.

124. Barber MJ, Mangravite LM, Hyde CL, et al. Genome-wide association of lipid-lowering response to statins in combined study populations. *PLoS One.* 2010;5(3):e9763.

125. Roger VL, Go AS, Lloyd-Jones DM, et al. Heart disease and stroke statistics—2011 update: a report from the American Heart Association. *Circulation.* 2011;123(4):e18–e209.

126. Chobanian AV, Bakris GL, Black HR, et al. The seventh report of the Joint National Committee on Prevention, Detection, Evaluation, and Treatment of High Blood Pressure: the JNC 7 report. *JAMA.* 2003; 289(19):2560–2572.

127. Johnson JA. Pharmacogenomics of antihypertensive drugs: past, present and future. *Pharmacogenomics.* 2010;11(4):487–491.

128. Shin J, Johnson JA. Pharmacogenetics of beta-blockers. *Pharmacotherapy.* 2007;27(6):874–887.

129. Pacanowski MA, Johnson JA. PharmGKB submission update: IX. ADRB1 gene summary. *Pharmacol Rev.* 2007;59(1):2–4.

130. Mason DA, Moore JD, Green SA, Liggett SB. A gain-of-function polymorphism in a G-protein coupling domain of the human beta1-adrenergic receptor. *J Biol Chem.* 1999;274(18):12670–12674.

131. Rathz DA, Brown KM, Kramer LA, Liggett SB. Amino acid 49 polymorphisms of the human beta1-adrenergic receptor affect agonist-promoted trafficking. *J Cardiovasc Pharmacol.* 2002;39(2):155–160.

132. Levin MC, Marullo S, Muntaner O, Andersson B, Magnusson Y. The myocardium-protective Gly-49 variant of the beta 1-adrenergic receptor exhibits constitutive activity and increased desensitization and down-regulation. *J Biol Chem.* 2002;277(34):30429–30435.

133. Johnson AD, Newton-Cheh C, Chasman DI, et al. Association of hypertension drug target genes with blood pressure and hypertension in 86,588 individuals. *Hypertension.* 2011;57(5):903–910.

134. Johnson JA, Zineh I, Puckett BJ, McGorray SP, Yarandi HN, Pauly DF. Beta 1-adrenergic receptor polymorphisms and antihypertensive response to metoprolol. *Clin Pharmacol Ther.* 2003;74(1):44–52.

135. Liu J, Liu ZQ, Tan ZR, et al. Gly389Arg polymorphism of beta1-adrenergic receptor is associated with the cardiovascular response to metoprolol. *Clin Pharmacol Ther.* 2003;74(4):372–379.

136. Liu J, Liu ZQ, Yu BN, et al. Beta1-adrenergic receptor polymorphisms influence the response to metoprolol monotherapy in patients with essential hypertension. *Clin Pharmacol Ther.* 2006;80(1):23–32.

137. Sofowora GG, Dishy V, Muszkat M, et al. A common beta1-adrenergic receptor polymorphism (Arg389Gly) affects blood pressure response to beta-blockade. *Clin Pharmacol Ther.* 2003;73(4):366–371.

138. Filigheddu F, Reid JE, Troffa C, et al. Genetic polymorphisms of the beta-adrenergic system: association with essential hypertension and response to beta-blockade. *Pharmacogenomics J.* 2004;4(3):154–160.

139. O'Shaughnessy KM, Fu B, Dickerson C, Thurston D, Brown MJ. The gain-of-function G389R variant of the beta1-adrenoceptor does not influence blood pressure or heart rate response to beta-blockade in hypertensive subjects. *Clin Sci (Lond).* 2000;99(3):233–238.

140. Karlsson J, Lind L, Hallberg P, et al. Beta1-adrenergic receptor gene polymorphisms and response to beta1-adrenergic receptor blockade in patients with essential hypertension. *Clin Cardiol.* 2004;27(6):347–350.

141. Mahesh Kumar KN, Ramu P, Rajan S, Shewade DG, Balachander J, Adithan C. Genetic polymorphisms of beta1 adrenergic receptor and their influence on the cardiovascular responses to metoprolol in a South Indian population. *J Cardiovasc Pharmacol.* 2008;52(5):459–466.

142. Suonsyrja T, Donner K, Hannila-Handelberg T, Fodstad H, Kontula K, Hiltunen TP. Common genetic variation of beta1- and beta2-adrenergic receptor and response to four classes of antihypertensive treatment. *Pharmacogenet Genomics.* 2010;20(5):342–345.

143. Filigheddu F, Argiolas G, Degortes S, et al. Haplotypes of the adrenergic system predict the blood pressure response to beta-blockers in women with essential hypertension. *Pharmacogenomics*. 2010;11(3):319–325.

144. Lee J, Aziz H, Liu L, et al. Beta(1)-adrenergic receptor polymorphisms and response to beta-blockade in the African-American study of kidney disease and hypertension (AASK). *Am J Hypertens*. 2011;24(6):694–700.

145. Pacanowski MA, Gong Y, Cooper-Dehoff RM, et al. Beta-adrenergic receptor gene polymorphisms and beta-blocker treatment outcomes in hypertension. *Clin Pharmacol Ther*. 2008;84(6):715–721.

146. Lemaitre RN, Heckbert SR, Sotoodehnia N, et al. Beta1- and beta2-adrenergic receptor gene variation, beta-blocker use and risk of myocardial infarction and stroke. *Am J Hypertens*. 2008;21(3):290–296.

147. Green SA, Turki J, Innis M, Liggett SB. Amino-terminal polymorphisms of the human beta 2-adrenergic receptor impart distinct agonist-promoted regulatory properties. *Biochemistry*. 1994;33(32):9414–9419.

148. Jia H, Sharma P, Hopper R, Dickerson C, Lloyd DD, Brown MJ. Beta2-adrenoceptor gene polymorphisms and blood pressure variations in East Anglian Caucasians. *J Hypertens*. 2000;18(6):687–693.

149. Johnson JA, Boerwinkle E, Zineh I, et al. Pharmacogenomics of anti-hypertensive drugs: rationale and design of the Pharmacogenomic Evaluation of Antihypertensive Responses (PEAR) study. *Am Heart J*. 2009;157(3):442–449.

150. Johnson JA, Liggett SB. Cardiovascular pharmacogenomics of adrenergic receptor signaling: clinical implications and future directions. *Clin Pharmacol Ther*. 2011;89(3):366–378.

151. Jia H, Hingorani AD, Sharma P, et al. Association of the G(s)alpha gene with essential hypertension and response to beta-blockade. *Hypertension*. 1999;34(1):8–14.

152. Lobmeyer MT, Wang L, Zineh I, et al. Polymorphisms in genes coding for GRK2 and GRK5 and response differences in antihypertensive-treated patients. *Pharmacogenet Genomics*. 2011;21(1):42–49.

153. Owen RP, Sangkuhl K, Klein TE, Altman RB. Cytochrome P450 2D6. *Pharmacogenet Genomics*. 2009;19(7):559–562.

154. Zhou SF. Polymorphism of human cytochrome P450 2D6 and its clinical significance: part I. *Clin Pharmacokinet*. 2009;48(11):689–723.

155. Rau T, Heide R, Bergmann K, et al. Effect of the CYP2D6 genotype on metoprolol metabolism persists during long-term treatment. *Pharmacogenetics*. 2002;12(6):465–472.

156. Bijl MJ, Visser LE, van Schaik RH, et al. Genetic variation in the CYP2D6 gene is associated with a lower heart rate and blood pressure in beta-blocker users. *Clin Pharmacol Ther*. 2009;85(1):45–50.

157. Zineh I, Beitelshees AL, Gaedigk A, et al. Pharmacokinetics and CYP2D6 genotypes do not predict metoprolol adverse events or efficacy in hypertension. *Clin Pharmacol Ther*. 2004;76(6):536–544.

158. Fux R, Morike K, Prohmer AM, et al. Impact of CYP2D6 genotype on adverse effects during treatment with metoprolol: a prospective clinical study. *Clin Pharmacol Ther*. 2005;78(4):378–387.

159. Sehrt D, Meineke I, Tzvetkov M, Gultepe S, Brockmoller J. Carvedilol pharmacokinetics and pharmacodynamics in relation to CYP2D6 and ADRB pharmacogenetics. *Pharmacogenomics*. 2011;12(6):783–795.

160. Cusi D, Barlassina C, Azzani T, et al. Polymorphisms of alpha-addu-cin and salt sensitivity in patients with essential hypertension. *Lancet*. 1997;349(9062):1353–1357.

161. Manunta P, Cusi D, Barlassina C, et al. Alpha-adducin polymorphisms and renal sodium handling in essential hypertensive patients. *Kidney Int*. 1998;53(6):1471–1478.

162. Manunta P, Citterio L, Lanzani C, Ferrandi M. Adducin polymorphisms and the treatment of hypertension. *Pharmacogenomics*. 2007;8(5):465–472.

163. Psaty BM, Smith NL, Heckbert SR, et al. Diuretic therapy, the alpha-adducin gene variant, and the risk of myocardial infarction or stroke in persons with treated hypertension. *JAMA*. 2002;287(13):1680–1689.

164. Turner ST, Chapman AB, Schwartz GL, Boerwinkle E. Effects of endo-thelial nitric oxide synthase, alpha-adducin, and other candidate gene polymorphisms on blood pressure response to hydrochlorothiazide. *Am J Hypertens*. 2003;16(10):834–839.

165. Davis BR, Arnett DK, Boerwinkle E, et al. Antihypertensive therapy, the alpha-adducin polymorphism, and cardiovascular disease in high-risk hypertensive persons: the Genetics of Hypertension-Associated Treatment Study. *Pharmacogenomics J*. 2007;7(2):112–122.

166. Gerhard T, Gong Y, Beitelshees AL, et al. Alpha-adducin polymorphism associated with increased risk of adverse cardiovascular outcomes: results from GENEtic Substudy of the INternational VErapamil SR-trandolapril STudy (INVEST-GENES). *Am Heart J*. 2008;156(2):397–404.

167. van Wieren-de Wijer DB, Maitland-van der Zee AH, de Boer A, et al. Interaction between the Gly460Trp alpha-adducin gene variant and diuret-ics on the risk of myocardial infarction. *J Hypertens*. 2009;27(1):61–68.

168. Maitland-van der Zee AH, Turner ST, Schwartz GL, Chapman AB, Klungel OH, Boerwinkle E. A multilocus approach to the antihyperten-sive pharmacogenetics of hydrochlorothiazide. *Pharmacogenet Genomics*. 2005;15(5):287–293.

169. Iwai N, Baba S, Mannami T, et al. Association of sodium channel gamma-sub-unit promoter variant with blood pressure. *Hypertension*. 2001;38(1):86–89.

170. Turner ST, Schwartz GL, Chapman AB, Boerwinkle E. WNK1 kinase polymorphism and blood pressure response to a thiazide diuretic. *Hypertension*. 2005;46(4):758–765.

171. Turner ST, Schwartz GL, Chapman AB, Boerwinkle E. C825T polymor-phism of the G protein beta(3)-subunit and antihypertensive response to a thiazide diuretic. *Hypertension*. 2001;37(2 part 2):739–743.

172. Lynch AI, Boerwinkle E, Davis BR, et al. Pharmacogenetic association of the NPPA T2238C genetic variant with cardiovascular disease outcomes in patients with hypertension. *JAMA*. 2008;299(3):296–307.

173. Manunta P, Lavery G, Lanzani C, et al. Physiological interaction between alpha-adducin and WNK1-NEDD4L pathways on sodium-related blood pressure regulation. *Hypertension*. 2008;52(2):366–372.

174. Luo F, Wang Y, Wang X, Sun K, Zhou X, Hui R. A functional variant of NEDD4L is associated with hypertension, antihypertensive response, and orthostatic hypotension. *Hypertension*. 2009;54(4):796–801.

175. Svensson-Farbom P, Wahlstrand B, Almgren P, et al. A functional vari-ant of the NEDD4L gene is associated with beneficial treatment response with beta-blockers and diuretics in hypertensive patients. *J Hypertens*. 2011;29(2):388–395.

176. Elliott WJ, Meyer PM. Incident diabetes in clinical trials of antihyperten-sive drugs: a network meta-analysis. *Lancet*. 2007;369(9557):201–207.

177. Duarte JD, Cooper-DeHoff RM. Mechanisms for blood pressure lower-ing and metabolic effects of thiazide and thiazide-like diuretics. *Expert Rev Cardiovasc Ther*. 2010;8(6):793–802.

178. Irvin MR, Lynch AI, Kabagambe EK, et al. Pharmacogenetic association of hypertension candidate genes with fasting glucose in the GenHAT Study. *J Hypertens*. 2010;28(10):2076–2083.

179. Padmanabhan S. Antihypertensive pharmacogenetics: missed opportunity. *J Hypertens*. 2010;28(10):2007–2009.

180. Turner ST, Bailey KR, Fridley BL, et al. Genomic association analysis sug-gests chromosome 12 locus influencing antihypertensive response to thia-zide diuretic. *Hypertension*. 2008;52(2):359–365.

181. Konoshita T, Genomic Disease Outcome Consortium (G-DOC) Study Investigators. Do genetic variants of the renin–angiotensin system predict blood pressure response to renin–angiotensin system-blocking drugs? A systematic review of pharmacogenomics in the renin–angiotensin system. *Curr Hypertens Rep*. 2011;13(5):356–361.

182. Thorn CF, Klein TE, Altman RB. PharmGKB summary: very impor-tant pharmacogene information for angiotensin-converting enzyme. *Pharmacogenet Genomics*. 2010;20(2):143–146.

183. Rigat B, Hubert C, Alhenc-Gelas F, Cambien F, Corvol P, Soubrier F. An insertion/deletion polymorphism in the angiotensin I-converting enzyme gene accounting for half the variance of serum enzyme levels. *J Clin Invest*. 1990;86(4):1343–1346.

184. Arnett DK, Davis BR, Ford CE, et al. Pharmacogenetic association of the angiotensin-converting enzyme insertion/deletion polymorphism on blood pressure and cardiovascular risk in relation to antihypertensive treat-ment: the Genetics of Hypertension-Associated Treatment (GenHAT) study. *Circulation*. 2005;111(25):3374–3383.

185. Nordestgaard BG, Kontula K, Benn M, et al. Effect of ACE insertion/dele-tion and 12 other polymorphisms on clinical outcomes and response to treatment in the LIFE study. *Pharmacogenet Genomics*. 2010;20(2):77–85.

186. Fuchs S, Philippe J, Germain S, et al. Functionality of two new poly-morphisms in the human renin gene enhancer region. *J Hypertens*. 2002;20(12):2391–2398.

187. Moore N, Dicker P, O'Brien JK, et al. Renin gene polymorphisms and haplotypes, blood pressure, and responses to renin–angiotensin system inhibition. *Hypertension*. 2007;50(2):340–347.

188. Bremer T, Man A, Kask K, Diamond C. CACNA1C polymorphisms are associated with the efficacy of calcium channel blockers in the treatment of hypertension. *Pharmacogenomics.* 2006;7(3):271–279.

189. Beitelshees AL, Navare H, Wang D, et al. CACNA1C gene polymorphisms, cardiovascular disease outcomes, and treatment response. *Circ Cardiovasc Genet.* 2009;2(4):362–370.

190. Kamide K, Yang J, Matayoshi T, et al. Genetic polymorphisms of L-type calcium channel alpha1C and alpha1D subunit genes are associated with sensitivity to the antihypertensive effects of L-type dihydropyridine calcium-channel blockers. *Circ J.* 2009;73(4):732–740.

191. Langaee TY, Gong Y, Yarandi HN, et al. Association of CYP3A5 polymorphisms with hypertension and antihypertensive response to verapamil. *Clin Pharmacol Ther.* 2007;81(3):386–391.

192. Jin Y, Wang YH, Miao J, et al. Cytochrome P450 3A5 genotype is associated with verapamil response in healthy subjects. *Clin Pharmacol Ther.* 2007;82(5):579–585.

193. Kim KA, Park PW, Park JY. Effect of ABCB1 (MDR1) haplotypes derived from G2677T/C3435T on the pharmacokinetics of amlodipine in healthy subjects. *Br J Clin Pharmacol.* 2007;63(1):53–58.

194. Zhao LM, He XJ, Qiu F, Sun YX, Li-Ling J. Influence of ABCB1 gene polymorphisms on the pharmacokinetics of verapamil among healthy Chinese Han ethnic subjects. *Br J Clin Pharmacol.* 2009;68(3):395–401.

195. Kelley-Hedgepeth A, Peter I, Kip K, et al. The protective effect of KCNMB1 E65K against hypertension is restricted to blood pressure treatment with beta-blockade. *J Hum Hypertens.* 2008;22(7):512–515.

196. Beitelshees AL, Gong Y, Wang D, et al. KCNMB1 genotype influences response to verapamil SR and adverse outcomes in the INternational VErapamil SR/Trandolapril STudy (INVEST). *Pharmacogenet Genomics.* 2007;17(9):719–729.

197. Niu Y, Gong Y, Langaee TY, et al. Genetic variation in the beta2 subunit of the voltage-gated calcium channel and pharmacogenetic association with adverse cardiovascular outcomes in the INternational VErapamil SR-Trandolapril STudy GENEtic Substudy (INVEST-GENES). *Circ Cardiovasc Genet.* 2010;3(6):548–555.

198. Sugimoto K, Katsuya T, Kamide K, et al. Promoter polymorphism of RGS2 gene is associated with change of blood pressure in subjects with antihypertensive treatment: the Azelnidipine and Temocapril in Hypertensive Patients with Type 2 Diabetes Study. *Int J Hypertens.* 2010;2010:196307.

199. Becker ML, Visser LE, Newton-Cheh C, et al. A common NOS1AP genetic polymorphism is associated with increased cardiovascular mortality in users of dihydropyridine calcium channel blockers. *Br J Clin Pharmacol.* 2009;67(1):61–67.

200. Jessup M, Brozena S. Heart failure. *N Engl J Med.* 2003;348(20):2007–2018.

201. Lindenfeld J, Albert NM, Boehmer JP, et al. HFSA 2010 comprehensive heart failure practice guideline. *J Card Fail.* 2010;16(6):e1–e194.

202. Shin J, Johnson JA. Beta-blocker pharmacogenetics in heart failure. *Heart Fail Rev.* 2010;15(3):187–196.

203. Davis HM, Johnson JA. Heart failure pharmacogenetics: past, present, and future. *Curr Cardiol Rep.* 2011;13(3):175–184.

204. Mialet Perez J, Rathz DA, Petrashevskaya NN, et al. Beta 1-adrenergic receptor polymorphisms confer differential function and predisposition to heart failure. *Nat Med.* 2003;9(10):1300–1305.

205. Terra SG, Hamilton KK, Pauly DF, et al. Beta1-adrenergic receptor polymorphisms and left ventricular remodeling changes in response to beta-blocker therapy. *Pharmacogenet Genomics.* 2005;15(4):227–234.

206. Chen L, Meyers D, Javorsky G, et al. Arg389Gly-beta1-adrenergic receptors determine improvement in left ventricular systolic function in nonischemic cardiomyopathy patients with heart failure after chronic treatment with carvedilol. *Pharmacogenet Genomics.* 2007;17(11):941–949.

207. Terra SG, Pauly DF, Lee CR, et al. Beta-adrenergic receptor polymorphisms and responses during titration of metoprolol controlled release/extended release in heart failure. *Clin Pharmacol Ther.* 2005;77(3):127–137.

208. Liggett SB, Mialet-Perez J, Thaneemit-Chen S, et al. A polymorphism within a conserved beta(1)-adrenergic receptor motif alters cardiac function and beta-blocker response in human heart failure. *Proc Natl Acad Sci U S A.* 2006;103(30):11288–11293.

209. Biolo A, Clausell N, Santos KG, et al. Impact of beta1-adrenergic receptor polymorphisms on susceptibility to heart failure, arrhythmogenesis, prognosis, and response to beta-blocker therapy. *Am J Cardiol.* 2008;102(6):726–732.

210. Magnusson Y, Levin MC, Eggertsen R, et al. Ser49Gly of beta1-adrenergic receptor is associated with effective beta-blocker dose in dilated cardiomyopathy. *Clin Pharmacol Ther.* 2005;78(3):221–231.

211. Small KM, Forbes SL, Rahman FF, Bridges KM, Liggett SB. A four amino acid deletion polymorphism in the third intracellular loop of the human alpha 2C-adrenergic receptor confers impaired coupling to multiple effectors. *J Biol Chem.* 2000;275(30):23059–23064.

212. Neumeister A, Charney DS, Belfer I, et al. Sympathoneural and adrenomedullary functional effects of alpha2C-adrenoreceptor gene polymorphism in healthy humans. *Pharmacogenet Genomics.* 2005;15(3):143–149.

213. Small KM, Wagoner LE, Levin AM, Kardia SL, Liggett SB. Synergistic polymorphisms of beta1- and alpha2C-adrenergic receptors and the risk of congestive heart failure. *N Engl J Med.* 2002;347(15):1135–1142.

214. Lobmeyer MT, Gong Y, Terra SG, et al. Synergistic polymorphisms of beta1 and alpha2C-adrenergic receptors and the influence on left ventricular ejection fraction response to beta-blocker therapy in heart failure. *Pharmacogenet Genomics.* 2007;17(4):277–282.

215. Metra M, Covolo L, Pezzali N, et al. Role of beta-adrenergic receptor gene polymorphisms in the long-term effects of beta-blockade with carvedilol in patients with chronic heart failure. *Cardiovasc Drugs Ther.* 2010;24(1):49–60.

216. Kaye DM, Smirk B, Williams C, Jennings G, Esler M, Holst D. Beta-adrenoceptor genotype influences the response to carvedilol in patients with congestive heart failure. *Pharmacogenetics.* 2003;13(7):379–382.

217. Troncoso R, Moraga F, Chiong M, et al. Gln(27)→Glubeta(2)-adrenergic receptor polymorphism in heart failure patients: differential clinical and oxidative response to carvedilol. *Basic Clin Pharmacol Toxicol.* 2009;104(5):374–378.

218. Cresci S, Kelly RJ, Cappola TP, et al. Clinical and genetic modifiers of long-term survival in heart failure. *J Am Coll Cardiol.* 2009;54(5):432–444.

219. Liggett SB, Cresci S, Kelly RJ, et al. A GRK5 polymorphism that inhibits beta-adrenergic receptor signaling is protective in heart failure. *Nat Med.* 2008;14(5):510–517.

220. Sharp CF, Gardiner SJ, Jensen BP, et al. CYP2D6 genotype and its relationship with metoprolol dose, concentrations and effect in patients with systolic heart failure. *Pharmacogenomics J.* 2009;9(3):175–184.

221. Baudhuin LM, Miller WL, Train L, et al. Relation of ADRB1, CYP2D6, and UGT1A1 polymorphisms with dose of, and response to, carvedilol or metoprolol therapy in patients with chronic heart failure. *Am J Cardiol.* 2010;106(3):402–408.

222. Jessup M, Abraham WT, Casey DE, et al. 2009 focused update: ACCF/AHA guidelines for the diagnosis and management of heart failure in adults: a report of the American College of Cardiology Foundation/American Heart Association Task Force on Practice Guidelines: developed in collaboration with the International Society for Heart and Lung Transplantation. *Circulation.* 2009;119(14):1977–2016.

223. Beitelshees AL, Zineh I. Renin–angiotensin–aldosterone system (RAAS) pharmacogenomics: implications in heart failure management. *Heart Fail Rev.* 2010;15(3):209–217.

224. McNamara DM, Holubkov R, Postava L, et al. Pharmacogenetic interactions between angiotensin-converting enzyme inhibitor therapy and the angiotensin-converting enzyme deletion polymorphism in patients with congestive heart failure. *J Am Coll Cardiol.* 2004;44(10):2019–2026.

225. de Denus S, Zakrzewski-Jakubiak M, Dube MP, et al. Effects of AGTR1 A1166C gene polymorphism in patients with heart failure treated with candesartan. *Ann Pharmacother.* 2008;42(7):925–932.

226. Cicoira M, Rossi A, Bonapace S, et al. Effects of ACE gene insertion/deletion polymorphism on response to spironolactone in patients with chronic heart failure. *Am J Med.* 2004;116(10):657–661.

227. Taylor AL, Ziesche S, Yancy C, et al. Combination of isosorbide dinitrate and hydralazine in blacks with heart failure. *N Engl J Med.* 2004;351(20):2049–2057.

228. BiDil (isosorbide dinitrate and hydralazine) prescribing information. Charlotte, NC: NitroMed Inc; 2009. Available at: http://www.nitromed.com/PI.pdf.

229. McNamara DM, Tam SW, Sabolinski ML, et al. Aldosterone synthase promoter polymorphism predicts outcome in African Americans with heart failure: results from the A-HeFT Trial. *J Am Coll Cardiol.* 2006;48(6):1277–1282.

230. McNamara DM, Tam SW, Sabolinski ML, et al. Endothelial nitric oxide synthase (NOS3) polymorphisms in African Americans with heart failure: results from the A-HeFT trial. *J Card Fail.* 2009;15(3):191–198.

Pharmacogenomics and Pharmacogenetics for Infectious Diseases

Shashi Amur, PhD, & Lawrence Lee Soon-U, MD, PhD

LEARNING OBJECTIVES

- Outline how pharmacogenomics of the virus and host affect the response to drug therapy.
- Discuss individualized medicine with pharmacogenomics as it relates to HIV therapy.
- Review pharmacogenomics pertinent to therapy for other viral illnesses.

INTRODUCTION

The concept of "chemical individuality" was developed in 1908 by Sir Archibald Garrod in 1908. He described the incidence of toxicity in a small proportion of individuals with a dose of a drug that had no toxic effects in the majority of the patients. The first example of a pharmacogenetic study probably is an observation that "taste blindness" was inherited in an autosomal recessive manner and that the characteristic varied in different ethnic groups.[1]

The recognition of pharmacogenomics as a distinct discipline occurred in the 1950s in the context of antimalarial dugs. Treatment with antimalarial drugs such as primaquine resulted in development of a hemolytic crisis in a high proportion of African American soldiers. Variants in glucose 6-phosphate dehydrogenase (G6PD) were identified to be responsible for this toxicity. The term "pharmacogenetics" was coined by Friedrich Vogel in 1959.

INFLUENCE OF VIRAL GENETICS ON DRUG RESPONSE

Drug response can be influenced by the viral genome as well as the host genome. Thus, both viral and host genome considerations are important in optimizing therapy in viral diseases.

Viral Genotype as Predictor of Response

Viral genotype can be a predictor of response. An example is that of treatment of chronic hepatitis C infection with peginterferon (PEG-IFN) and ribavirin (RBV). Response rates to PEG-IFN and RBV vary depending on HCV genotype: about 40–50% of the patients infected with genotype 1 virus treated for 48 weeks with PEG-IFN and RBV reach sustained virologic response (SVR), whereas 70–80% of patients with genotype 2 or 3 virus attain SVR after only 24 weeks of PEG-IFN and RBV therapy.[2]

Viral Genetics and Resistance to Antiviral Treatments

Viral genome also is an important consideration in antiretroviral therapy. Certain sequences in the viral genome confer resistance to antiretroviral treatments. In addition, resistance to an antiretroviral drug can develop during treatment causing treatment failure in patients infected with agents such as HIV. Contributors to the development of antiretroviral drug resistance are errors in copying viral RNA into DNA that include base substitutions, coupled with high rate of replication of HIV viruses. In addition, multiple variants of the virus might be present in HIV-infected patients and these could have differing sensitivities to antiretroviral therapy that make successful treatment of HIV infection challenging. Thus, an understanding of the mechanisms leading to resistance and development of strategies to identify and avoid/overcome drug resistance can lead to successful therapy. HIV drug resistance testing is one of the powerful tools that is currently being used to help clinicians tailor combination therapy to HIV patients.[3,4]

Viral Genetics, HIV Tropism, and Selection of Patients for Antiviral Therapy

The tropism of HIV viruses is important in determining whether a targeted therapeutic, such as maraviroc, should be prescribed to HIV patients. The European Consensus Group on clinical management recently recommended V3 (HIV third hypervariable loop) population genotyping as one of the methods for tropism testing based on recent data.[5]

INFLUENCE OF HOST GENETICS ON DRUG RESPONSE

Drugs are absorbed, distributed, metabolized, and eliminated in the host and mechanisms involved in these steps are likely to influence the outcome. This is particularly true for drugs with narrow therapeutic indices and for drugs that are metabolized and/or transported by polymorphic proteins that can differentially influence the rate at which the drug is metabolized or transported. Several antiretroviral drugs fit this description.[6]

Pharmacogenomics and Disease Progression

Variations in the host genome could influence disease progression through impacting viral–host interaction, which is the first step in viral infections. An example is that of a mutation (Δ32, deletion of 32 base pair) in the CCR5 receptor that results in formation of a truncated protein that is not transported to the cell surface. A strong, but incomplete, resistance to HIV infection has been reported in individuals who are homozygous for the Δ32 allele and delayed progression to disease has been reported in individuals heterozygous for the allele.[7] In addition, several genetic polymorphisms in the CCR5 promoter region have been reported to affect HIV transmission or disease progression.[8]

PHARMACOGENOMICS CAN ALTER PHARMACOKINETICS AND IMPACT DRUG DISPOSITION AND THERAPY OF DRUGS

Interindividual differences in patient response to treatment make it difficult to predict the safety and efficacy with standard doses of drugs. Most of the drugs appear to have the expected therapeutic effect in only 50% of the patients treated with the standard regimen. The patients who do not have the expected response are either underdosed with less/no therapeutic benefit or overdosed with associated drug toxicity. This poses a serious concern, particularly with drugs that have narrow therapeutic indexes.[9]

Genetic variations in the drug-metabolizing enzymes or transporter proteins are reflected in the enzyme activities or in the transporter activities, respectively.[10] Four major phenotypes of drug-metabolizing enzymes can be identified by phenotyping or genotyping as extensive metabolizer (EM), poor metabolizer (PM), intermediate metabolizer (IM), and ultrarapid metabolizer (UM). Rapid clearance rates caused by patients with UM genotype could result in suboptimal concentrations of drugs leading to lower efficacious response to drugs. On the other hand, slower clearance due to PM or IM genotype may lead to drug accumulation and toxicity. With a prodrug, the effect of the metabolizer genotype will be reversed, where the PM genotype is associated with lower efficacy and the UM genotype is associated with toxicity. Knowledge of the identity of the metabolizing enzyme(s) and transporter(s) associated with the drug in combination with the knowledge of genetic variations in these proteins in an individual can help identify the appropriate dose required by the individual.

Examples showing impact of genetic variations in drug-metabolizing enzymes and transporters are described below.

PHASE 1 ENZYMES (CYTOCHROME P450)

Cytochrome P450 2B6 (CYP2B6)

CYP2B6 was initially not thought to be important in drug metabolism, but recent studies revealed the relevance of this enzyme in the metabolism of the anticancer drugs cyclophosphamide and ifosfamide, and the anti-HIV drugs efavirenz (EFV) and nevirapine (NVP).

The human CYP2B6 gene is highly polymorphic. Variant alleles are associated with lower expression such as CYP2B6*6, CYP2B6*16, and CYP2B6*18. Of these, CYP2B6*6 is common in several different populations including Chinese (20–30% frequency), whereas CYP2B6*16 and CYP2B6*18 are common in black subjects where the allele frequency is relatively high (7–9%).

In clinical studies, subjects homozygous for the alleles CYP2B6*6, CYP2B6*16, and CYP2B6*18 exhibit lower capacity for metabolism of CYP2B6 substrates such as EFV.[11] In addition, the CYP2B6*6 allele appears to cause both high and low activity of CYP2B6 in different studies. It is possible that the 516G>T and 785A>G mutations, causing the amino acid substitutions Q172H and K262R, are linked to other mutations, giving rise to specific haplotypes that are associated with high or low activity of CYP2B6. Also, the CYP2B6*4 allele can cause higher V_{max} values in vivo.[12]

Overall, there is a marked interindividual variability in the CYP2B6 activity. These interindividual differences in CYP2B6 expression may lead to variable systemic exposure, and perhaps response, to drugs metabolized by CYP2B6.

CYP2B6 and Efavirenz

The antiretroviral drug EFV is a non-nucleoside reverse transcriptase inhibitor (NNRTI) and an integral part of the combination therapy for HIV patients. EFV has a relatively narrow therapeutic index and its plasma concentration displays large interindividual variability. CYP2B6 is primarily responsible for EFV metabolism, to the major metabolite 8-hydroxy-EFV.[13] Therefore, pharmacogenetics has great potential to influence the clinical use of this drug.

Elevated plasma concentrations of EFV cause CNS-related side effects such as dizziness and depression. This can contribute to discontinuation, poor adherence, and eventual therapeutic failure. Among the identified polymorphic alleles, CYP2B6*6, predominantly the 516G>T mutation, is associated with elevated EFV plasma concentrations and CNS-related side effects in several studies.[14]

The high frequency of the 2B6*6 allelic expression in a variety of ethnic populations suggests that CYP2B6 genotyping be used as a tool for EFV dose choice and adjustment. Genotype-specific dosing of EFV, in a Japanese cohort study, led to a decrease in EFV dose by 33% or 66% and a decrease in plasma concentrations proportionate to the reduction in dose. Patients maintained therapeutic effectiveness and their CNS-related symptoms improved.[15]

Although the role of CYP2B6 polymorphisms in EFV metabolism is now firmly established, data regarding drug–drug interactions between EFV and concomitant therapeutics are limited. Of particular concern is the interaction between EFV and rifampicin, where it appears that induction of EFV metabolism by rifampicin may be abrogated or even reversed by CYP2B6 polymorphisms, therefore leading to a paradoxical increase in EFV in patients with these polymorphisms.[16] Increasing the dose of EFV as recommended in some treatment guidelines may therefore be disastrous in these patients.

CYP2B6 and Nevirapine

NVP is another NNRTI used to treat HIV infection in combination with other anti-HIV drugs. In human liver microsomes, NVP is oxidized to 2, 3-, 8-, and 12-hydroxynevirapine. In cDNA-expressed human CYPs, 2- and 3-hydroxynevirapine were exclusively formed by CYP3A4/3A5 and 2B6, respectively. Multiple cDNA-expressed CYPs produced 8- and 12-hydroxynevirapine, although CYP2D6 and 3A4 primarily catalyzed their formation, respectively. For the formation of 12-OH-nevirapine, CYP3A5, 2D6, and 2C9 (minor) also play a role, while CYP2A6, 2B6, and 3A4 catalyzed 8-OH-nevirapine formation with a low activity. Overall, NVP is principally metabolized by CYP3A4 and 2B6,[17] and this complicated metabolism is reflected in the equivocal results for the role of CYP2B6 in NVP metabolism.

CYP2B6 516T/T genotype was associated with greater (1.7- and 1.8-fold) plasma levels of NVP in HIV-infected patients.[18] No association was observed between the other polymorphisms in MDR1 3435C>T and 2677G>T, CYP3A4*1B and CYP3A5*3, and NVP concentrations in these patients.[19]

The 983T>C SNP, part of the CYP2B6*18 allele, was also associated with NVP plasma concentration. However, 1459C>T was not associated with plasma concentrations of NVP.[20] However, other studies showed that CYP2B6 516/983 metabolizer status was not associated with NVP levels.[21,22]

Pharmacogenetics may also affect anti-HIV treatment outcomes. Children with the 516T/T genotype had decreased

clearance and significant increase in CD4+ T-cell percentage, compared with those with the G/G and G/T genotypes, from baseline to week 12.[23]

Pharmacogenetics may also affect NVP toxicities. Haas et al. studied the association between MDR1, CYP2B6, and cytochrome P450 3A (CYP3A) polymorphisms and NVP hepatotoxicity in a randomized study in South Africa. Among the polymorphisms studied, only MDR1 3435C>T was significantly associated with decreased risk of hepatotoxicity (risk ratio = 0.30).[24] This polymorphism was also found to correlate with hepatotoxicity in Mozambique. Four other SNPs in CYP2B6 and CYP3A5 correlated with transaminase levels.[25] In a case–control study, cutaneous reactions were associated with CYP2B6 516G>T (OR 1.66), HLA-Cw*04 (OR 2.51), and HLA-B*35 (OR 3.47). Hepatic AEs were associated with HLA-DRB*01 (OR 3.02), but not CYP2B6 genotypes. Associations differed by population, at least in part reflecting allele frequencies.[26] While promising, the effect size is much smaller than other recognized associations such as HLA-B*5701 and abacavir.

Cytochrome P450 2C19 (CYP2C19)

CYP2C19 is responsible for the metabolism of approximately 10% of commonly used drugs. These include proton pump inhibitors, tricyclic antidepressants, selective serotonin reuptake inhibitors, moclobemide, benzodiazepines, barbiturates, phenytoin, bortezomib, voriconazole, selegiline, nelfinavir, and proguanil.

CYP2C19 is a highly polymorphic enzyme with wide variation of distribution in various ethnic groups. The Asian population has a much greater frequency of CYP2C19 PMs (12–23%), when compared with Caucasians (1–6%) and black Africans (1–7.5%). The frequency of PMs in African, African American, and Middle Eastern populations is very similar to Caucasians. Indigenous populations, such as the Canadian Indians and the Australian Aboriginals, have a high frequency of PMs, which is similar to that of the Asian population. Further details about CYP2C19 are available in other chapters of this textbook.

CYP2C19 and Voriconazole

Voriconazole is a second-generation broad-spectrum triazole antifungal agent, exhibiting potent activity against a broad range of significant pathogens, including *Aspergillus, Candida, Scedosporium*, and *Fusarium* species. Voriconazole is extensively metabolized by the liver, with less than 2% of the dose excreted unchanged. N-oxidation of the fluoropyrimidine ring, its hydroxylation, and hydroxylation of the adjacent methyl group are known pathways of voriconazole oxidative metabolism, with the N-oxide being the major circulating metabolite in humans. Voriconazole is mainly metabolized by CYP2C19 and 2C9 and, to a lesser extent, by CYP3A4 and FMO1.

The considerable interindividual variability in the pharmacokinetics of voriconazole is partially due to CYP2C19 polymorphism, with PMs having 2- to 6-fold higher AUCs than EMs.[27] In a study with 28 pediatric patients, heterozygous EMs and

PMs had a 46% lower clearance of voriconazole than homozygous EMs.[28] Therefore, PMs may be predisposed to concentration-dependent side effects such as hepatotoxicity. However, there was no significant relationship between CYP2C19 polymorphisms and serum liver enzyme levels in patients treated with voriconazole.[29] On the other hand, UMs had significantly lower voriconazole concentrations.[30] This may lead to treatment failure in patients with these genotypes. However, this has not been proven to date.

CYP2C19 genotype appears to affect the interaction of voriconazole with St. John's wort. The baseline clearance of voriconazole and the absolute increase in clearance with St. John's wort were smaller in carriers of one or two deficient CYP2C19*2 alleles, compared with wild-type individuals.[31] These results demonstrate that long-term treatment of St. John's wort leads to prolonged extensive reduction in voriconazole exposure, with CYP2C19 wild-type individuals being at higher risk for potential treatment failure. Similar effects on voriconazole could be seen with induction of CYP2C19 by other drugs. This could have major clinical significance as patients on voriconazole are often on other drugs at the same time.

Cytochrome P450 3A

CYP3As are the most abundant CYPs in human liver and participate in the metabolism of about 60% of drugs. Overall CYP3A4 is the most important contributor to drug oxidation, with significant contribution from CYP3A5 and CYP3A7. Important substrates in the anti-infective area include most HIV protease inhibitors and macrolide antibiotics.

Many variants have been described for CYP3A4, but their low allelic frequencies do not seem to be able to account for the high observed phenotypic variability. Genetic variation is also not well understood for CYP3A4 and haplotype analysis may be more useful. Nevertheless, the CYP3A4*1B polymorphism was found to influence the pharmacokinetics and hyperlipidemic effects of indinavir.[32]

Unlike CYP3A4, the hepatic expression of CYP3A5 is distributed bimodally due to a significant gene polymorphism. The active enzyme is encoded by the wild-type allele CYP3A5*1 that has a low frequency of 5–7% in Caucasians, but 40% in Africans and African Americans, and 25% in Asians.

The CYP3A5*1 genotype was associated with increased saquinavir clearance, probably from the effect of the contribution of hepatic rather than intestinal CYP3A5.[33] However, the effect of CYP3A5 polymorphisms was found to be small for atazanavir[34] and indinavir.[35]

Genetic variation in the regulatory nuclear receptors CAR and PXR that mediate induction of CYPs 3A by drugs may also contribute to antiretroviral pharmacokinetics. For example, the PXR 63396C>T (rs2472677) SNP was found to increase unboosted atazanavir clearance.[36]

CYP3A is induced by rifampin, NVP, EFV, dexamethasone, carbamazepine, phenytoin, and St. John's wort that act via the PXR and CAR nuclear receptors. Rifampin and rifabutin are commonly coadministered with antiretroviral drugs because of the increased incidence of tuberculosis in HIV patients. The reduction of HIV protease inhibitor concentrations may reduce its efficacy and result in treatment failure or resistance. However, this phenomenon does not seem to be mediated by genetic factors.[37] Similarly coadministering EFV or NVP with HIV protease inhibitors may reduce their efficacy. However, this effect may also be overcome by adjusting doses.[38]

CYP3A is inhibited by inhibitors including ketoconazole, troleandomycin, ritonavir, and bergamottin, which is the active inhibitor in grapefruit juice. Low-dose ritonavir is now used to boost other protease inhibitors. It is unclear if genetics can modify this boosting effect.

PHASE 2 ENZYMES

N-acetyltransferase Type 2 (NAT2)

The role of NAT2 in the metabolism of the antituberculosis drug isoniazid is one of the earliest and most well-known examples of the role of pharmacogenetics in infectious diseases. When isoniazid was introduced as an antituberculosis agent nearly 50 years ago, investigators found that a significant proportion of patients (up to 17%) experienced serious side effects, that is, progressive damage to the nervous system, or peripheral neuropathy. Interindividual differences were found in the ability to acetylate drugs; patients who were less able to acetylate isoniazid (catalyzed by the NAT2 enzyme) had mean elimination half-lives of 180 minutes compared with 80 minutes for rapid acetylators. These slow acetylators were more likely to experience the observed neurological adverse effects if not given pyridoxine. Further studies showed that antituberculosis drug-induced hepatotoxicity was also linked to slow NAT2 activity.[39]

The wild-type NAT2 allele is designated NAT2*4 and is associated with the fast acetylation phenotype. NAT2 alleles containing G191A, T341C, A434C, and/or G590A were associated with slow acetylator phenotypes. The most common slow acetylator alleles in human populations contain one or more of these polymorphisms, identified as NAT2*5, NAT2*6, NAT2*7, and NAT2*14 and their subtypes.

NAT2*4 makes up 20–25% of alleles in Caucasians. The wild-type allele occurs at a somewhat higher frequency in African Americans (36–41%) and in Hispanics (41%). The frequency of wild-type alleles was highest in Asians, ranging from approximately 50% in Chinese to nearly 70% in Japanese. Wild-type NAT2 was least prevalent (6%) in the African Gabonese population. NAT2*5 and its subtypes were most frequent among Caucasians (44%), Gabonese (41%), Hispanics, and those of African descent (26%). NAT2*6 was found to be fairly evenly distributed across ethnic groups, while NAT2*7 was more prevalent among Asians. A unique class of slow acetylator variants, NAT2*14, was identified in Gabonese and in African Americans and makes up about 8–9% of alleles studied in these groups. These alleles have not yet been identified in Caucasians.[40]

To achieve similar isoniazid exposure, it has been suggested that doses may be decreased or increased by approximately 50%

for patients with no or two such slow acetylator alleles, respectively.[41] However, this approach has not been widely adopted.

UDP-Glucuronosyltransferase 1A1 (UGT1A1)

Despite the widespread participation of UDP-glucuronosyltransferases (UGTs) and glucuronidation in the fate of endogenous and foreign compounds, the impact of UGT pharmacogenetics on drug biotransformation has generally been relatively underexplored. However, there are now an increasing number of drugs metabolized by UGTs including a few antiretroviral drugs such as raltegravir, zidovudine, and abacavir.

UGT isoform 1A1 (UGT1A1) is the isoform involved in the clearance of bilirubin to its glucuronide and in the pathogenesis of bilirubin disorders such as Gilbert syndrome. The most common UGT1A1 variant is the UGT1A1*28 allele or a TA insertion in the UGT1A1 promoter region. Up to 33% of Caucasians carry the *28 variant. In Asians the UGT1A1*6 variant (211 G>A) is common as well.

Raltegravir is predominantly cleared by UGT isoform 1A1. Raltegravir concentrations are higher in patients with the UGT1A1*28 polymorphism,[42] although the increase is small and unlikely to be clinically significant, possibly due to the wide therapeutic index of the drug.

Atazanavir is a known inhibitor of UGT1A1 and this causes an increase in unconjugated bilirubin. Mutations in UGT1A1 and other UGT isoforms have been associated with increased risk of unconjugated hyperbilirubinemia.[43] Although this is generally regarded to be harmless, this phenomenon may cause treatment discontinuation in patients who are distressed by looking jaundiced.

TRANSPORTERS

P-Glycoprotein (MDR1, ABCB1)

ABCB1 (MDR1) is one of many adenosine triphosphate (ATP)–binding cassette (ABC) genes that is responsible for cellular homeostasis. ABC genes encode transporter proteins possessing multiple membrane-spanning domains that form pores, and intracellular nucleotide-binding domains for ATP-dependent translocation of substrates across the cell membrane.

The ABCB1 gene is highly polymorphic. The number and frequency of SNPs observed varies by ethnicity. In 2002, Fellay et al. reported that HIV-infected patients with the C3435T allelic variant (TT) in the MDR1 gene had a greater increase in CD4 cells count 6 months after initiating therapy when they were homozygous, even though they had lower concentrations of EFV and nelfinavir.[44] The C3435T mutation is a synonymous mutation and the mechanism for this could not be found. Eventually this study could not be replicated.[45] Further studies were conflicting and the significance of this mutation remains unknown.

Data have also been conflicting about the effect of MDR1 polymorphisms on atazanavir concentrations.[46,47] Therefore, the clinical application of these polymorphisms remains uncertain.

Organic Anion-Transporting Polypeptide 1B1 (OATP1B1)

OATP1B1 is a genetically polymorphic influx transporter expressed on the sinusoidal membrane of human hepatocytes, and it mediates the hepatic uptake of many xenobiotics. Recent studies have demonstrated that OATP1B1 plays a major, clinically important role in the hepatic uptake of many drugs. A common single-nucleotide variation (coding DNA c.521T>C, protein p.V174A, rs4149056) in the SLCO1B1 gene encoding OATP1B1 decreases the transporting activity of OATP1B1.

A number of anti-infective agents have also been identified as OATP1B1 substrates. For example, rifampin is a substrate of OATP1B1. Interestingly, the SLCO1B1 c.463C>A SNP was associated with a 42% reduced AUC of rifampin but there was no effect of c.521T>C.[48]

In addition, certain HIV protease inhibitors, but not NNRTIs, are OATP1B1 substrates. The c.521T>C polymorphism was associated in markedly increased plasma concentrations of lopinavir.[49]

Penicillins as well as certain cephalosporins are OATP1B1 as well as OATP1B3 substrates.[50] The antifungal drug caspofungin is also an OATP1B1 substrate.[51] It remains to be seen if polymorphisms in transporter genes will affect the pharmacokinetics or pharmacodynamics of these drugs.

HOST GENETICS AND ANTIMALARIALS

Although antimalarial drugs have been in use since the 1930s, few data are available on the absorption–distribution–metabolism–excretion parameters of these drugs in humans. Recently, there have been more methodological developments in the area of antimalarial pharmacokinetics. Through these advancements, pharmacokinetics and the major metabolic pathways of a number of antimalarial drugs have been found. However, little emphasis has been placed on understanding basic mechanisms responsible for the pharmacogenetics of major antimalarial drugs classes.

Studies suggest that noticeable interindividual variability can occur in the blood concentrations of chloroquine and its metabolite desethylchloroquine, and this variability may affect the parasitological treatment outcome. However, whether genetic variability in the chloroquine metabolism also contributed to the variability was not addressed in these studies. Chloroquine is metabolized by cytochromes 2C8, 3A4/5, and 2D6, and polymorphisms in these enzymes could contribute to the variability observed.

Interethnic differences exist in the concentrations of primaquine and carboxyprimaquine (the active metabolite of the drug), which may cause treatment failures in those with low concentrations, especially in Caucasians and Indians who have lower concentrations. Primaquine is metabolized by cytochromes CYP3A4 and CYP1A2. However, no attempt has yet been made to link the primaquine pharmacokinetics and treatment outcome to genetic variation in the primaquine metabolism.[36]

Unfortunately similar gaps in knowledge exist for possible other pharmacogenetic interactions for other antimalarial drugs such as amodiaquine (metabolized by CYP2C8), proguanil (metabolized by CYP2C19), artemisinin (metabolized by CYP2B6 and 2A6), and quinine (metabolized by CYP3A4/5).

GENETICS CAN INFLUENCE PHARMACODYNAMICS AND IMPACT RESPONSE TO DRUGS

One of the major challenges in drug development as well as in the practice of medicine is interindividual variation in responding to a given medication. Factors responsible for the variation in response include environmental and genetic factors. Genetic factors are believed to account for 15–30% of the interindividual differences in drug response. However, genetic factors can account for up to 95% of the variability between individuals in drug effects for some drugs.[52–54]

The influence of the genetic factors could be on efficacy or safety. Thus, a subgroup of individuals with a specific genotype may have a higher response to a specific drug compared with the group with a different genotype. Also, toxicity to certain drugs may be observed in a small number of individuals with genotypes that confer increased risk of adverse events. Some examples are provided below to illustrate the impact of genetics on pharmacodynamics and drug response.

IL28B Polymorphism and Response to Anti-HCV Therapy

Peginterferon alfa and ribavirin (PR) have been the standard of care for treatment of chronic HCV infection. Recently, the results from four different genome-wide association studies (GWAS) showed that a genetic variant near the IL28B gene (rs12979860, C to T change) is a strong predictor of response to PR therapy in patients with chronic hepatitis C infection.[55–57] Many publications have since confirmed this finding and the IL28B polymorphism is now recognized as one of the strongest predictors of response to PR therapy. The mechanism by which the response is impacted due to this genetic variant is not yet understood, especially since the variant is not located near, but not in the IL28B gene. However, it is interesting to note that the IL28B gene encodes interferon-lambda-3 (IFN-λ3), which is a cytokine produced by immune cells in response to viral infection. It has been suggested, but not demonstrated, that the IL28B gene variant exerts its effects through regulation of IL28B gene.

The response rates to PR therapy were higher in subjects with the IL28B C/C genotype than in those with the C/T or T/T genotype. A similar pattern was observed in Caucasians, Hispanics, and African Americans, even though SVR rates were higher in Caucasians (69%) than in Hispanics (56%) or African Americans (48%) in subjects with the IL28B C/C genotype.[58] It is possible that additional alleles may impact the response to PR in the ethnic subgroups. Also, the IL28B variant may not be a causative allele, but may be in linkage disequilibrium with the causative allele and this relationship could be different in the ethnic groups studied. The allele frequency of the C allele was found to be highest in Asians, followed by Caucasians, Hispanics, and African Americans.[55] The differences in the allele frequency offer a partial explanation to the differences in the response rates observed in the different ethnicities (46% in Caucasians, 41% in Hispanics, and 19% in African Americans).[58]

HLA-B*5701 and Abacavir Hypersensitivity Reactions (ABC-HSR)

Abacavir, which is used alone or in combination with other drugs, is a nucleoside reverse transcriptase inhibitor, an antiretroviral drug used in the treatment of HIV-1 infection. An abacavir hypersensitivity reaction (ABC-HSR) was observed in about 5–8% of patients in the phase 3 clinical trials of abacavir. The clinical manifestations of the ABC-HSR included fever and/or rash, and, to a lesser degree, gastrointestinal (nausea, vomiting, diarrhea, and stomach pain) and/or respiratory (cough, shortness of breath, and sore throat) symptoms that emerged within the first 6 weeks of treatment in more than 90% of patients with ABC-HSR. Symptoms worsened with continued therapy but usually resolved on discontinuation of the drug. If the therapy was not discontinued, this adverse event could be life-threatening, Clinical diagnosis was imprecise because of the patients' concurrent illness or drug treatments that caused similar symptoms.

Pharmacogenomic research identified that HLA-B*5701, an allele in the HLA-B region, to be associated with the ABC-HSRs. A prospective randomized controlled trial (PREDICT-1)[59] was carried out to assess the clinical utility of HLA-B*5701 screening before beginning abacavir treatment. The trial design consisted of two arms: one was an abacavir-containing regimen with ABC-HSR monitoring according to standard of care (control arm) and the other an abacavir-containing regimen with ABC-HSR monitoring preceded by prospective HLA-B*5701 screening (pharmacogenetics arm). The PGx arm excluded patients who screened for HLA-B*5701 and tested positive. The incidence of clinically suspected ABC-HSR was 7.8% and 3.4% in the control and PGx arms, respectively ($P < .001$). A research tool, patch test, was used to confirm the clinically suspected ABC-HSR. Using this research tool the rates for immunologically confirmed ABC-HSR were 2.7% for the control arm and 0% for the PGx arm ($P < .001$). A point to note is that all patients who test positive for the HLA-B*5701 will not develop abacavir ABC-HSR suggesting that additional alleles or nongenetic risk factors could be involved. Also, abacavir ABC-HSRs have been shown to occur in very few individuals who tested negative for HLA-B*5701.

The HIV treatment guidelines recommended testing for HLA-B*5701 prior to prescribing abacavir to HIV patients and this test has been well accepted in clinical practice. Also, several publications have shown the usefulness of testing for HLA-B*5701 in different regions of the world.[60]

Other Antiretroviral Drugs and Metabolic Toxicities

Genetics may affect Metabolic Toxicities of Antiretroviral Drugs. Variants of ABCA1, APOA5, APOC3, APOE, and CETP contributed to plasma triglyceride levels, particularly while on ritonavir-containing antiretroviral therapy. Variants of APOA5 and CETP contributed to high-density lipoprotein-cholesterol levels. Variants of CETP and LIPG contributed to non-high-density lipoprotein-cholesterol levels.[61]

INDIVIDUALIZED MEDICINE WITH PHARMACOGENOMICS IN ANTIVIRAL THERAPY

It is a well-accepted fact that response rates to drugs vary in individuals and that interindividual variability presents a challenge to physicians. Identification of responders to medications would avoid unnecessary exposure of patients to drugs that have no beneficial effects and might have adverse events. Also, identification of individuals likely to develop serious adverse events could help in reducing risk of adverse drug reactions (ADRs) and providing alternative therapy to patients. These goals of individualized or personalized medicine definitely apply to antiviral therapy also. Examples are given below.

Maraviroc-CCR5

HIV utilizes CD4 as the receptor on host cells to gain entry into the cells and infect them. Even though CD4 is essential, it is not sufficient to gain entry into the cells. Coexpression of a chemokine receptor with CD4 on the cell surface is needed for HIV entry and infection. CCR5 and CXCR4 are the major chemokine receptors involved in HIV infection.

CCR5 receptor is expressed on macrophages and on some populations of T cells and appears to be the most physiologically important coreceptor during natural infection. M-tropic HIV isolates (R5 viruses) appear to use CCR5 as their coreceptor for infection both of macrophages and of some T cells. Maraviroc is a selective, reversible, small-molecule CCR5 receptor antagonist that blocks the entry of CCR5-tropic HIV into host cells. A tropism test that determines whether the HIV strains in HIV patients are CCR5-tropic or CXCR4-tropic or mixed needs to be performed prior to prescribing maraviroc. Only those patients whose isolates show CCR5 tropism qualify for treatment with maraviroc. Thus, patient selection for efficacy in HIV treatment with a targeted therapeutic is achieved with a tropism test.

Abacavir Hypersensitivity and HLA-B*5701

Association of HLA-B*5701 to abacavir hypersensitivity has been shown in a large, prospective, postmarketing study, PREDICT-1. The study provided demonstration of clinical usefulness and influenced the inclusion of strong recommendations for HLA-B*5701 screening in professional guidelines and prescribing information in the United States. This provides an example of patient selection for drug safety in HIV treatment using a genetic test.

DRUG DEVELOPMENT IN ANTIVIRAL THERAPY AND PHARMACOGENOMICS

If a PGx biomarker is known to impact the efficacy of the drugs as could be the case with targeted therapeutics, where the drug being developed is likely to work only in either biomarker-positive or biomarker-negative population, the trial design will have different inclusion/exclusion criteria. If the efficacy is expected to be higher in a population that carries a particular genetic variant (e.g., IL28B C/C genotype in chronic HCV-infected patients) than in the population with the alternative variants (e.g., IL28B C/T and T/T genotypes), stratification by the genotype may be needed to ensure accurate results.

In the adverse events scenario in drug development, PGx studies could contribute either during early clinical trials where adverse events can occur or in the postmarketing stage when adverse events are rare and are detected only after thousands of patients have used the drugs. If the adverse events that occur in the early clinical trials are serious, PGx studies can help understand the cause for adverse events if an association of the ADRs to genetics exists and help in the design of a modified drug.

CASE STUDIES

Efavirenz-Polymorphism of 2B6

A 28-year-old HIV-infected Asian woman with a CD4 count of 325 cells/mm³ was started on her first antiretroviral regimen consisting of a recommended first-line antiretroviral regimen tenofovir–emtricitabine–EFV (Atripla®). Her past history is notable for goiter with normal thyroid function. She was asked to take her antiretroviral medication on an empty stomach at night before going to bed in order to reduce initial drug concentrations. Despite this, 1 week after starting this regimen, she calls to complain that she is feeling very dizzy and is having difficulty concentrating at work. Her primary physician tells her to continue her medications as the symptoms should get better in 2–4 weeks.

Unfortunately 2 weeks after starting her medications, her dizziness had not improved and the symptoms were really affecting her work. She came back for further counseling and was advised to continue her medications and speak to her employer about changing the intensity of her work. A mid-dose concentration was drawn at that time.

Three weeks after starting her medications, she developed abdominal discomfort and nausea. These symptoms worsened and at 4 weeks a full comprehensive workup was done. At that stage the patient was found to have severe hepatitis with ALT and AST about 10 times upper limit of normal. Her medications were stopped immediately.

Drug concentrations done earlier had come back with a mid-dose concentration of 7,324 ng/mL (recommended range 1,000–4,000 ng/mL). Genotyping for the CYP2B6 was done and that showed homozygous mutations at the 516 (TT) and 785 (GG) loci. The subject was considered to be too high risk to consider EFV rechallenge even at low dose. She was eventually started on a raltegravir-containing regimen to reduce the risk of further hepatotoxicity.

Anti-HCV Therapy and IL28B Polymorphism

A 51-year-old Japanese male afflicted with chronic hepatitis C (genotype 1b) infection had failed two courses of Pegylated interferon-α2b (PEG-IFN α2b) and ribavirin (PR). Living donor liver transplantation (LDLT) was performed on this patient using grafts from two donors. The left lobe was from his 21-year-old son and the right lobe from his 42-year-old wife. The grafts were implanted by anastomosis of hepatic veins, portal veins, and arteries from each side. Mycophenolate mofetil with basiliximab was the immunosuppressant used and tacrolimus was used for maintenance.

HCV infection was detected 4 weeks after LDLT and the HCV viral load increased sharply to 6.7 log IU/mL at 9 weeks after LDLT. He was started on PR therapy 15 weeks post-LDLT with a weekly dose of 60 μg PEG-IFN α2b and 600 mg ribavirin daily. The viral load decreased steadily for 60 weeks. However, 24 weeks later, HCV RNA was detected again and PEG-IFN α2b was switched to PEG-IFN α2a. However, his liver function gradually worsened and PR therapy was terminated 96 weeks after commencement. Although the HCV viral load increased up to 6.0 log IU/mL, his liver function did not worsen with liver supporting therapy alone. Liver biopsies were performed on each graft.

The recipient's and the donors' DNA was extracted from the liver biopsies at transplantation. The recipient carried the minor IL28B allele, T/G (rs8099917), his son carried the major genotype (T/T), and his wife carried the minor genotype (T/G). The patient's left lobe from the donor with the major genotype (T/T) displayed mild hepatitis and no fibrosis with a metavir grading of A1F0. In contrast, the right lobe from the donor with the minor genotype (T/G) showed moderate inflammation and bridging fibrosis (A2F2). Moreover, no HCV RNA was detected in the left lobe, whereas 15.3 copies/μg of HCV RNA were detected in the right lobe using qRT-PCR. These findings can possibly be explained by the different genotypes of IL28B.

PRACTICAL LIMITATIONS OF APPLYING PHARMACOGENOMIC CONCEPTS TO ROUTINE THERAPY

Translational Studies for Bench to Bedside

Numerous GWAS have appeared in recent years that show genetic associations to disease and to ADRs and some of these are likely to be applied to clinical practice. Since the GWAS approach is powered to detect common variants with modest effects, but not powered to detect rare variants, some of the important variants may not be detected by this technology. Some of the other limitations of the technology problems include reproducibility, false positives, sample size issues, and effect size. Novel technologies such as next-generation sequencing may help resolve some of the issues.

After a significant genetic association has been identified and reproduced, the next step is to develop a test. Generally, a different platform/technology such as PCR is used for the development of the test that could consist of one gene variant or a panel of variants from multiple genes. Analytical validation of the test follows the development of a test.

For a test to be taken up in clinical practice, sufficient data and concurrence by the thought leaders in the antiviral field that the test has clinical utility are very important. This can be achieved through publication of the data followed by confirmation by another research group and presentation of the data in national/international conferences. Oftentimes, this results in recommendation for use of the test in treatment guidelines. In addition, information regarding genetic associations and associated test(s) provided in the drug labels by regulatory authorities, such as US FDA, also helps the clinical practitioners in deciding to use the test in clinical practice.

Universal Availability of Diagnostic Tests and Associated Costs

Availability of the diagnostic tests could be a challenge, particularly in rural areas. In addition to the costs of developing the tests, the cost of the tests/kits as well as reimbursements for the tests plays a major role in the acceptability of the test by the clinicians in their practice.

Availability of Drugs for Which Pharmacogenomics May Not Play a Critical Role

One of the problems encountered in antiviral therapy is development of resistance to the drugs. Sometimes, resistance develops to a drug in a class (NRTIs), but not to other drugs in the same class. Thus, multiple antiviral drugs in the same class are developed to provide alternative treatments to patients who develop resistance to a drug. If one of these drugs needs a genetic test prior to prescribing the drug, the clinician may prefer to choose another drug from the same class to avoid the additional expense or time delay in prescribing the drug that needs a test.

Challenge of Keeping Up with New Information and Technologies

In order to make the appropriate decision (to get the test done or not to get the test done), the clinical practitioner needs to keep up with the new developments in the antiviral arena. This is generally accomplished mostly by keeping up with the literature and by attending conferences related to the therapeutic area. The novel/emerging technologies also bring up the need to understand the capability/limitations of these technologies and to develop the skills needed for interpretation of complex test results.

CONCLUSIONS

Pharmacogenomics plays a significant role in influencing the pharmacokinetics and pharmacodynamics of drugs. Exploratory pharmacogenetics studies could help in understanding the mechanisms underpinning disease and assist in identifying novel drug targets. In clinical trials, pharmacogenomic biomarkers can be used to identify responder populations and employ enrichment strategies. PGx studies could also help identify individuals at risk of developing adverse reaction either due to increased exposure caused by the poor metabolism/transport of the drugs or due to association of the adverse events to specific genotypes. The significant findings would lead to application of pharmacogenomics in developing tests that can either help adjust the dose to correct for exposure or treat patients with alternative therapies if individuals with a particular genotype are at risk of developing ADRs with the specific therapeutic product.

Some examples of application of PGx in clinical practice are known in antiviral therapy. However, there are many challenges in identifying the pharmacogenomic biomarker associated with efficacy or safety. Platforms used, size of samples, and reproducibility of findings are some of the limitations. After a test employing a pharmacogenomic biomarker is found to be useful, challenges of availability, costs of development, and reimbursement of the tests need to be faced. It is also a challenge for the clinical practitioner to keep up with the fast growing information and technologies.

REFERENCES

1. Meyer UA. Pharmacogenetics—five decades of therapeutic lessons from genetic diversity. *Nat Rev Genet.* 2004;5(9):669–676.
2. Afdhal NH, McHutchison JG, Zeuzem S, et al. Hepatitis C pharmacogenetics: state of the art in 2010. *Hepatology.* 2011;53(1):336–345.
3. Zdanowicz MM. The pharmacology of HIV drug resistance. *Am J Pharm Educ.* 2006;70(5):1–9.
4. Dunn DT, Coughlin K, Cane PA. Genotypic resistance testing in routine clinical care. *Curr Opin HIV AIDS.* 2011;6(4):251–257.
5. Vandekerckhove LP, Wensing AM, Kaiser R, et al. European guidelines on the clinical management of HIV-1 tropism testing. *Lancet Infect Dis.* 2011;11(5):394–407.
6. Pirmohamed M, Back DJ. The pharmacogenomics of HIV therapy. *Pharmacogenomics J.* 2001;1(4):243–253.
7. Hogan CM, Hammer SM. Host determinants in HIV infection and disease. Part 2: genetic factors and implications for antiretroviral therapeutics. *Ann Intern Med.* 2001;134(10):978–996.
8. Mummidi S, Ahuja SS, McDaniel BL, Ahuja SK. The human CC chemokine receptor 5 (CCR5) gene. Multiple transcripts with 5'-end heterogeneity, dual promoter usage, and evidence for polymorphisms within the regulatory regions and noncoding exons. *J Biol Chem.* 1997;272(49):30662–30671.
9. Crettol S, Petrovic N, Murray M. Pharmacogenetics of phase I and phase II drug metabolism. *Curr Pharm Des.* 2010;16(2):204–219.
10. Amur S, Zineh I, Abernethy DR, Huang S, Lesko LJ. Pharmacogenomics and adverse drug reactions. *Personalized Med.* 2010;7(6):633–642.

11. Rotger M, Tegude H, Colombo S, et al. Predictive value of known and novel alleles of CYP2B6 for efavirenz plasma concentrations in HIV-infected individuals. *Clin Pharmacol Ther.* 2007;81(4):557–566.
12. Kirchheiner J, Klein C, Meineke I, et al. Bupropion and 4-OH-bupropion pharmacokinetics in relation to genetic polymorphisms in CYP2B6. *Pharmacogenetics.* 2003;13(10):619–626.
13. Desta Z, Saussele T, Ward B, et al. Impact of CYP2B6 polymorphism on hepatic efavirenz metabolism in vitro. *Pharmacogenomics.* 2007;8(6):547–558.
14. Gounden V, van Niekerk C, Snyman T, George JA. Presence of the CYP2B6 516G>T polymorphism, increased plasma efavirenz concentrations and early neuropsychiatric side effects in South African HIV-infected patients. *AIDS Res Ther.* 2010;7:32.
15. Gatanaga H, Hayashida T, Tsuchiya K, et al. Successful efavirenz dose reduction in HIV type 1-infected individuals with cytochrome P450 2B6 *6 and *26. *Clin Infect Dis.* 2007;45(9):1230–1237.
16. Kwara A, Lartey M, Sagoe KW, Court MH. Paradoxically elevated efavirenz concentrations in HIV/tuberculosis-coinfected patients with CYP2B6 516TT genotype on rifampin-containing antituberculous therapy. *AIDS.* 2010;25(3):388–390.
17. Erickson DA, Mather G, Trager WF, Levy RH, Keirns JJ. Characterization of the in vitro biotransformation of the HIV-1 reverse transcriptase inhibitor nevirapine by human hepatic cytochromes P-450. *Drug Metab Dispos.* 1999;27(12):1488–1495.
18. Penzak SR, Kabuye G, Mugyenyi P, et al. Cytochrome P450 2B6 (CYP2B6) G516T influences nevirapine plasma concentrations in HIV-infected patients in Uganda. *HIV Med.* 2007;8(2):86–91.
19. Mahungu T, Smith C, Turner F, et al. Cytochrome P450 2B6 516G→T is associated with plasma concentrations of nevirapine at both 200 mg twice daily and 400 mg once daily in an ethnically diverse population. *HIV Med.* 2009;10(5):310–317.
20. Wyen C, Hendra H, Vogel M, et al. Impact of CYP2B6 983T>C polymorphism on non-nucleoside reverse transcriptase inhibitor plasma concentrations in HIV-infected patients. *J Antimicrob Chemother.* 2008;61(4):914–918.
21. Haas DW, Gebretsadik T, Mayo G, et al. Associations between CYP2B6 polymorphisms and pharmacokinetics after a single dose of nevirapine or efavirenz in African Americans. *J Infect Dis.* 2009;199(6):872–880.
22. Chen J, Sun J, Ma Q, et al. CYP2B6 polymorphism and nonnucleoside reverse transcriptase inhibitor plasma concentrations in Chinese HIV-infected patients. *Ther Drug Monit.* 2010;32(5):573–578.
23. Saitoh A, Sarles E, Capparelli E, et al. CYP2B6 genetic variants are associated with nevirapine pharmacokinetics and clinical response in HIV-1-infected children. *AIDS.* 2007;21(16):2191–2199.
24. Haas DW, Bartlett JA, Andersen JW, et al. Pharmacogenetics of nevirapine-associated hepatotoxicity: an Adult AIDS Clinical Trials Group collaboration. *Clin Infect Dis.* 2006;43(6):783–786.
25. Ciccacci C, Borgiani P, Ceffa S, et al. Nevirapine-induced hepatotoxicity and pharmacogenetics: a retrospective study in a population from Mozambique. *Pharmacogenomics.* 2009;11(1):23–31.
26. Yuan J, Guo S, Hall D, et al. Toxicogenomics of nevirapine-associated cutaneous and hepatic adverse events among populations of African, Asian, and European descent. *AIDS.* 2011;25(10):1271–1280.
27. Mikus G, Schowel V, Drzewinska M, et al. Potent cytochrome P450 2C19 genotype-related interaction between voriconazole and the cytochrome P450 3A4 inhibitor ritonavir. *Clin Pharmacol Ther.* 2006;80(2):126–135.
28. Walsh TJ, Karlsson MO, Driscoll T, et al. Pharmacokinetics and safety of intravenous voriconazole in children after single- or multiple-dose administration. *Antimicrob Agents Chemother.* 2004;48(6):2166–2172.
29. Levin MD, den Hollander JG, van der Holt B, et al. Hepatotoxicity of oral and intravenous voriconazole in relation to cytochrome P450 polymorphisms. *J Antimicrob Chemother.* 2007;60(5):1104–1107.
30. Wang G, Lei HP, Li Z, et al. The CYP2C19 ultra-rapid metabolizer genotype influences the pharmacokinetics of voriconazole in healthy male volunteers. *Eur J Clin Pharmacol.* 2009;65(3):281–285.
31. Rengelshausen J, Banfield M, Riedel KD, et al. Opposite effects of short-term and long-term St John's wort intake on voriconazole pharmacokinetics. *Clin Pharmacol Ther.* 2005;78(1):25–33.

32. Bertrand J, Treluyer JM, Panhard X, et al. Influence of pharmacogenetics on indinavir disposition and short-term response in HIV patients initiating HAART. *Eur J Clin Pharmacol.* 2009;65(7):667–678.

33. Mouly SJ, Matheny C, Paine MF, et al. Variation in oral clearance of saquinavir is predicted by CYP3A5*1 genotype but not by enterocyte content of cytochrome P450 3A5. *Clin Pharmacol Ther.* 2005;78(6):605–618.

34. Shin J, Pauly DF, Pacanowski MA, Langaee T, Frye RF, Johnson JA. Effect of cytochrome P450 3A5 genotype on atorvastatin pharmacokinetics and its interaction with clarithromycin. *Pharmacotherapy.* 2011;31(10):942–950.

35. Solas C, Simon N, Drogoul MP, et al. Minimal effect of MDR1 and CYP3A5 genetic polymorphisms on the pharmacokinetics of indinavir in HIV-infected patients. *Br J Clin Pharmacol.* 2007;64(3):353–362.

36. Schipani A, Siccardi M, D'Avolio A, et al. Population pharmacokinetic modeling of the association between 63396C→T pregnane X receptor polymorphism and unboosted atazanavir clearance. *Antimicrob Agents Chemother.* 2010;54(12):5242–5250.

37. Floyd MD, Gervasini G, Masica AL, et al. Genotype–phenotype associations for common CYP3A4 and CYP3A5 variants in the basal and induced metabolism of midazolam in European- and African-American men and women. *Pharmacogenetics.* 2003;13(10):595–606.

38. Soon GH, Shen P, Yong EL, Pham P, Flexner C, Lee L. Pharmacokinetics of darunavir at 900 milligrams and ritonavir at 100 milligrams once daily when coadministered with efavirenz at 600 milligrams once daily in healthy volunteers. *Antimicrob Agents Chemother.* 2010;54(7):2775–2780.

39. Sun F, Chen Y, Xiang Y, Zhan S. Drug-metabolising enzyme polymorphisms and predisposition to anti-tuberculosis drug-induced liver injury: a meta-analysis. *Int J Tuberc Lung Dis.* 2008;12(9):994–1002.

40. Walker K, Ginsberg G, Hattis D, Johns DO, Guyton KZ, Sonawane B. Genetic polymorphism in *N*-acetyltransferase (NAT): population distribution of NAT1 and NAT2 activity. *J Toxicol Environ Health B Crit Rev.* 2009;12(5–6):440–472.

41. Kinzig-Schippers M, Tomalik-Scharte D, Jetter A, et al. Should we use *N*-acetyltransferase type 2 genotyping to personalize isoniazid doses? *Antimicrob Agents Chemother.* 2005;49(5):1733–1738.

42. Wenning LA, Petry AS, Kost JT, et al. Pharmacokinetics of raltegravir in individuals with UGT1A1 polymorphisms. *Clin Pharmacol Ther.* 2009;85(6):623–627.

43. Lankisch TO, Moebius U, Wehmeier M, et al. Gilbert's disease and atazanavir: from phenotype to UDP-glucuronosyltransferase haplotype. *Hepatology.* 2006;44(5):1324–1332.

44. Fellay J, Marzolini C, Meaden ER, et al. Response to antiretroviral treatment in HIV-1-infected individuals with allelic variants of the multidrug resistance transporter 1: a pharmacogenetics study. *Lancet.* 2002;359(9300):30–36.

45. Nasi M, Borghi V, Pinti M, et al. MDR1 C3435T genetic polymorphism does not influence the response to antiretroviral therapy in drug-naive HIV-positive patients. *AIDS.* 2003;17(11):1696–1698.

46. Ma Q, Brazeau D, Zingman BS, et al. Multidrug resistance 1 polymorphisms and trough concentrations of atazanavir and lopinavir in patients with HIV. *Pharmacogenomics.* 2007;8(3):227–235.

47. Rodriguez-Novoa S, Martin-Carbonero L, Barreiro P, et al. Genetic factors influencing atazanavir plasma concentrations and the risk of severe hyperbilirubinemia. *AIDS.* 2007;21(1):41–46.

48. Weiner M, Peloquin C, Burman W, et al. Effects of tuberculosis, race, and human gene SLCO1B1 polymorphisms on rifampin concentrations. *Antimicrob Agents Chemother.* 2010;54(10):4192–4200.

49. Hartkoorn RC, Kwan WS, Shallcross V, et al. HIV protease inhibitors are substrates for OATP1A2, OATP1B1 and OATP1B3 and lopinavir plasma concentrations are influenced by SLCO1B1 polymorphisms. *Pharmacogenet Genomics.* 2010;20(2):112–120.

50. Nakakariya M, Shimada T, Irokawa M, Maeda T, Tamai I. Identification and species similarity of OATP transporters responsible for hepatic uptake of beta-lactam antibiotics. *Drug Metab Pharmacokinet.* 2008;23(5):347–355.

51. Sandhu P, Lee W, Xu X, et al. Hepatic uptake of the novel antifungal agent caspofungin. *Drug Metab Dispos.* 2005;33(5):676–682.

52. Evans WE, Relling MV. Moving towards individualized medicine with pharmacogenomics. *Nature.* 2004;429(6990):464–468.

53. Evans WE, McLeod HL. Pharmacogenomics—drug disposition, drug targets, and side effects. *N Engl J Med.* 2003;348(6):538–549.

54. Weinshilboum R, Wang L. Pharmacogenomics: bench to bedside. *Nat Rev Drug Discov.* 2004;3(9):739–748.

55. Ge D, Fellay J, Thompson AJ, et al. Genetic variation in IL28B predicts hepatitis C treatment-induced viral clearance. *Nature.* 2009;461(7262):399–401.

56. Suppiah V, Moldovan M, Ahlenstiel G. IL28B is associated with response to chronic hepatitis C interferon-α and ribavirin therapy. *Nat Genet.* 2009;41(10):1100–1105.

57. Tanaka Y, Nishida N, Sugiyama M. Genome-wide association of IL28B with response to pegylated interferon-α and ribavirin therapy for chronic hepatitis C. *Nat Genet.* 2009;41(10):1105–1111.

58. Thompson AJ, Muir AJ, Sulkowski MS, et al. Interleukin-28B polymorphism improves viral kinetics and is the strongest pretreatment predictor of sustained virologic response in genotype 1 hepatitis C virus. *Gastroenterology.* 2010;139(1):120–129.e18.

59. Mallal S, Phillips E, Carosi G. HLA-B*5701 screening for hypersensitivity to abacavir. *N Engl J Med.* 2008;358:568–579.

60. Hughes CA, Foisy MM, Dewhurst N, et al. Abacavir hypersensitivity reaction: an update. *Ann Pharmacother.* 2008;42(3):387–396.

61. Arnedo M, Taffe P, Sahli R, et al. Contribution of 20 single nucleotide polymorphisms of 13 genes to dyslipidemia associated with antiretroviral therapy. *Pharmacogenet Genomics.* 2007;17(9):755–764.

Pharmacogenomics in Oncology

Ogechi Ikediobi, PharmD, PhD, Julie Nangia, MD, & Meghana V. Trivedi, PharmD, PhD

LEARNING OBJECTIVES

- Define and explain carcinogenesis and cancer genetics.
- Identify the most common germline variants and describe how these can modulate treatment outcome.
- Describe how somatic variants can predict drug response.
- Discuss pharmacogenomics in oncology clinical trials.

INTRODUCTION

Most types of cancer show considerable variability in their response to chemotherapy. In addition, anti-cancer therapies for treatment of a particular type of cancer, although significantly different in their mechanism of action, show only a marginal difference in outcome when compared with one another. This variability is thought to be due to inter-tumor and intra-tumor heterogeneity and host-specific factors and may reflect the lack of knowledge on how the molecular abnormalities in cancer cells affect responsiveness to anti-cancer therapies. In this aspect, pharmacogenomics can play an important role in predicting efficacy and toxicities of anti-cancer drugs.

Currently, there are over 100 drugs approved for treating cancer,[1] and over 800 more in clinical development.[2] Compared with other non-neoplastic diseases, selection of an anti-cancer treatment regimen is more critical since the mortality in patients increases significantly with the progression of disease.[3] Due to a large number of therapeutic options, low response rates, high incidence of de novo and acquired resistance to therapies, and severe toxicities associated with anti-cancer agents, pharmacogenomic applications to develop predictive markers for drug response or toxicity are essential in oncology therapeutics.

Traditionally, most cytotoxic chemotherapy dosing is calculated with the use of weight, body surface area, or area under the curve. However, patients with inherited deficiencies in enzymes responsible for drug metabolism and disposition can have severe toxicities at these traditional doses. Patients who have a deficiency in thiopurine S-methyltransferase (TPMT) can have greatly elevated concentrations of active drug metabolites and are at risk for life-threatening, drug-induced myelosuppression. On the other hand, patients with increased enzymatic activity may be at risk for treatment failure resulting in cancer progression. Other examples of enzyme deficiencies and the drugs they metabolize include uridine diphosphate glucuronosyltransferase 1A1 (UGT1A1) and irinotecan, cytochrome P450 2D6 (CYP2D6) and tamoxifen, and dihydropyrimidine dehydrogenase (DPD) and 5-fluorouracil (5-FU).

In addition to pharmacogenomics of drug-metabolizing enzymes, there are mutations in drug targets that influence treatment outcome by conferring either sensitivity or resistance to therapy. One classical example is trastuzumab, a monoclonal antibody targeting human epidermal growth factor receptor 2 (ERBB2/HER2), which is overexpressed in some of the breast tumors. Trastuzumab resistance is seen in tumors that express p95, a truncated form of HER2, with no extracellular domain containing the trastuzumab binding site. In these cases, it is suggested that lapatinib may be a more effective treatment choice. Another example is breakpoint cluster region–v-abl Abelson murine leukemia viral oncogene homolog 1 (BCR-ABL)–targeted therapy in the treatment of chronic myeloid leukemia (CML). Treatment resistance to all the currently available BCR-ABL inhibitors (imatinib, dasatinib, and nilotinib) is seen when there is a T315I mutation.

Pharmacogenomic markers that predict response to treatment will allow clinicians to individualize treatment regimens based on patients' genetic makeup. In the last decade there have been many advances and a variety of tests have been developed to see if a patient will respond to specific cancer therapies or will have a higher risk of toxicities. Examples include the K-RAS mutation test, where expression of the wild-type protein is associated with benefit from treatment with cetuximab, and the epidermal growth factor receptor (EGFR) mutation test, where gefitinib is only effective in those with activating mutations in the EGFR gene. In this chapter we provide a brief overview of cancer, present pertinent clinical cases demonstrating the importance of pharmacogenomics in oncology, and discuss the pharmacogenomics of cancer therapy and its role in clinical trials.

Cancer

In order to truly understand the importance of pharmacogenomics in cancer therapy, one must have a good understanding of carcinogenesis and cancer genetics. The current view of cancer is that a malignancy arises from a transformation of the genetic material of a normal cell, followed by successive mutations, ultimately leading to the uncontrolled proliferation of progeny cells.[4] Tumorigenesis is thought to require four to six rate-limiting mutation events to occur in the lineage of a single cell.[4–6] Based on this working theory of cancer progression, newer genetic models of tumorigenesis have emerged and enhanced our current understanding of cancer genetics. One of these models is the first genetic model for colorectal tumorigenesis by Fearon and Vogelstein (Figure 13–1).[7]

The principles of Fearon and Vogelstein's genetic model for colorectal tumorigenesis are as follows[7]: first, colorectal tumors arise as a result of the mutational activation of oncogenes coupled with the mutational inactivation of tumor suppressor genes (TSG); the latter changes predominate. Second, mutations in at least four to five genes are required for the formation of a malignant tumor. Third, although the genetic alterations often occur according to a preferred sequence, the total accumulation of changes, rather than their order, is responsible for determining the tumor's biological properties. Fourth, in some cases, mutant TSG appear to exert a phenotypic effect even when present in the heterozygous state; thus, some TSG may not be "recessive" at the cellular level. V-Ki-ras2 Kirsten rat sarcoma viral oncogene homolog (KRAS) is an oncogene involved in this process, and EGFR signal transduction results in *KRAS* activation. If *KRAS* is wild type, targeted therapies such as cetuximab (which is an EGFR inhibitor) are effective in the treatment of colon cancer. The general features of this model may be applicable to other common epithelial neoplasms.[7]

It is thought that alterations of cancer genes, resulting from gain-of-function mutations, can lead to overly active growth-promoting genes, which appear in cancerous cells as activated oncogenes.[8] The precursors to these oncogenes, known as proto-oncogenes, are usually dominantly acting genes at the cellular level.[9] The somatic mutations that cause activation of oncogenes are characterized by mutations that cause structural changes to

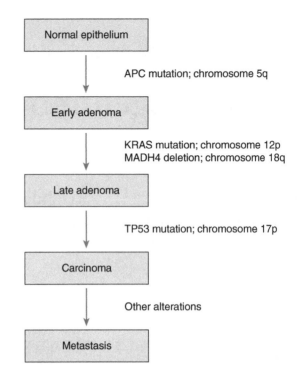

FIGURE 13–1 A genetic model for colorectal tumorigenesis. Tumorigenesis proceeds through a series of genetic alterations involving oncogenes (e.g., *KRAS*) and tumor suppressor genes (e.g., TP53 particularly those on chromosomes 5q, 17p, and 18q). (Adapted from Fearon ER, Vogelstein B. A genetic model for colorectal tumorigenesis. *Cell*. Jun 1 1990;61(5):759–767. Copyright 1990, with permission from Elsevier.)

the encoded protein, such as point mutations and chromosomal translocations.[8] Proto-oncogenes can also be transformed to oncogenes by elevated expression through gene amplification or chromosomal translocations.[10]

In addition to the oncogenes, there are also TSG. These TSG operate to suppress cell proliferation through many biochemical mechanisms, and are often inactivated in various ways in cancer cells.[11] An inherited mutant copy of a TSG increases susceptibility to specific types of cancer.[10] The Knudson hypothesis of TSG inactivation postulates that mutant alleles of TSG are recessive at the cellular level.[12] Therefore, both alleles of a TSG must be inactivated by loss-of-function mutations in the transformation of normal cells to cancerous cells. The loss of TSG function can occur by either genetic mutation or epigenetic silencing of genes via promoter methylation.[13] Inactivation of TSG by mutation or methylation of one allele may be followed by other mechanisms that facilitate loss of the second copy,[14] such as loss of heterozygosity (LOH) at the TSG locus.[15]

A census from the literature of reported cancer genes was recently compiled, which indicated that mutations in more than 1% of genes contribute to human cancer.[9] Of the 291 reported cancer genes, 90% show somatic mutations that are acquired in cancer, 20% show germline mutations that predispose to cancer, and 10% show both (Figure 13–2). According to the census, the most common mutation class among the known cancer genes is a chromosomal translocation. Seventy percent of the cancer

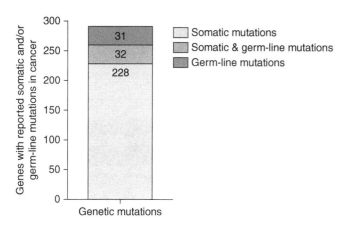

FIGURE 13–2 Schematic of the relative number of cancer genes with reported germline and somatic mutations in cancer. Adapted from *The Biology of Cancer* (© Garland Science 2007).[10]

TABLE 13–1 Examples of germline variants reported to modulate treatment outcomes.

Gene Product	Minor Allele	Drug	Treatment Outcome
TPMT	*3A, *3C, *2	6-Mercaptopurine	Increased toxicity
DPYD	*2A	5-Fluorouracil	Increased toxicity
UGT1A1	*28	Irinotecan	Increased toxicity
CYP2D6	*4	Tamoxifen	Decreased efficacy

TPMT, thiopurine methyltransferase; *DPYD*, dihydropyrimidine dehydrogenase; *UGT1A1*, uridine 5'-diphosphate-glucuronosyl-transferase; *CYP2D6*, cytochrome P450 2D6.

genes, altered by chromosomal translocations, are implicated in leukemias, lymphomas, and sarcomas but only represent 10% of human cancers.[9] This bias is likely due to the fact that non-solid tumors such as leukemias are easier to analyze with cytogenetic techniques compared with solid tumors. Solid tumors have many translocations but few have been analyzed in great detail, except for sarcomas. The remaining 90% of cancers of epithelial origin have been shown to be altered by other types of mutations: base substitutions that lead to missense amino acid changes, nonsense changes, alterations in conserved splice site positions, and insertions or deletions in coding sequences or splice sites that may cause in-frame or frameshift alterations of the protein.

GERMLINE VARIANTS AS PREDICTORS OF DRUG RESPONSE

Genetic variations are inherited DNA sequence mutations that typically cause minor physiologic changes, if any. Even with a complete loss of gene function due to a polymorphism, the biological impact is often modest. However, rare inherited DNA mutations known as germline mutations have shown to impact the risk of cancer, cancer prognosis, as well as treatment response

and toxicity. Many of the first examples from pharmacogenomics in cytotoxic chemotherapy focus on understanding the inherited (germline) inter-individual differences involved in drug metabolism. Examples are described in Table 13–1.

TPMT and 6-Mercaptopurine

Thiopurine drugs, such as 6-mercaptopurine (6-MP), are purine antimetabolites used clinically to treat leukemias and are metabolized by the enzyme TPMT.[16] Inter-individual variability in TPMT activity in red blood cells (RBCs) has been demonstrated to be a heritable autosomal co-dominant trait in exploratory studies.[16] Over 11% of the population is found to have a coding nucleotide polymorphism, which is associated with low TPMT activity. More than 10% of the patients are heterozygous and only 0.3% of the population is homozygous for TPMT.[16,17] The clinical importance of this variation was realized when patients who experienced severe hematological toxicity from thiopurine therapy were found to have low TPMP activity and elevated concentrations of mercaptopurine metabolites.[18,19]

TPMT is a cytosolic enzyme that preferentially catalyzes the *S*-methylation of aromatic and heterocyclic thio compounds such as 6-MP. 6-MP is an inactive prodrug and requires metabolism to 6-thioguanine (6-TG), which exerts cytotoxicity by incorporation into DNA and RNA[20] (Figure 13–3). Alternatively, 6-MP undergoes inactivation by TPMT to thiouric acid and oxidation to 6-methylmercaptopurine by xanthine oxidase. However, hematopoietic cells (such as RBCs and leukocytes) do not have

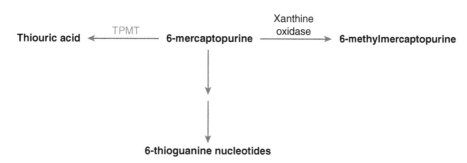

FIGURE 13–3 Metabolism of 6-mercaptopurine (6-MP). 6-MP is metabolically activated to form 6-thioguanine nucleotides. It undergoes metabolism catalyzed by xanthine oxidase or *TPMT*.

measurable xanthine oxidase activity, leaving TPMT as the major enzyme responsible for 6-MP inactivation.[21] In the absence of or decreased TPMT enzyme activity, 6-MP is metabolized preferentially to 6-TG, which has potent bone marrow suppressive activity.

It is important to recognize such individuals both to avoid fatal bone marrow failure through inadvertent overdose and to ensure that an adequate drug effect can be achieved at a desirable dose.[19,22] The potential benefit of testing TPMT activity to adjust the dose of 6-MP was demonstrated in a 6-year-old acute lymphoblastic leukemia (ALL) patient.[23] After receiving a standard dose of 6-MP for post-remission therapy, the patient developed severe myelosuppression requiring a discontinuation of her treatment regimen. Interestingly, she was found to have 7× the population median value of 6-TG in her RBCs. Subsequent therapy with 6% of the standard 6-MP dosage allowed her to complete the potentially curative regimen without further toxicity.

Since assays measuring TPMT activity and RBC 6-TG concentrations are not clinically feasible, genetic testing has been developed to provide greater convenience and better reproducibility. This test evaluates three variant alleles known as *TPMT*2*, *TPMT*3A*, and *TPMT*3C* (Table 13–1), which accounts for 95% of the detected variant *TPMT* alleles. Importantly, there is also a high concordance between measured TPMT activity and the incidence of these polymorphisms.[24,25] Genotyping for common *TPMT* alleles has shown to identify patients at risk of severe 6-MP toxicity such that *TPMT* genotyping can be integrated into the clinical management of patients undergoing 6-MP treatment.[26] In July 2003, an advisory subcommittee of the FDA Center for Drug Evaluation and Research met to consider the role of *TPMT* genotyping in the administration of 6-MP treatment to pediatric leukemia patients. Even though comprehensive evaluation of the clinical benefit and cost-effectiveness of screening strategies with this test was not completed, the FDA decided that the evidence was sufficient to indicate benefit and to warrant informing prescribers, pharmacists, and patients of the availability of *TPMT* genotyping tests and their possible role in the selection and dosing of 6-MP.

There is now an FDA-approved genetic test (DNA-based) to determine which patients will be likely to experience severe myelosuppression prior to administration of 6-MP.[27] However, in a recent cost-effectiveness analysis from a health care system perspective, screening for *TPMT* mutations via genotyping prior to the administration of 6-MP was not found to be cost-effective.[28] In addition, some patients who developed severe myelosuppression possessed normal TPMT activity. This suggests additional pathways are responsible for this toxicity.

In summary, measurement of *TPMT* genotypes and/or TPMT enzyme activity before instituting 6-MP may help prevent toxicity by identifying individuals with low or absent TPMT enzyme activity. Despite the usefulness of the *TPMT* genotyping test, it is recommended that clinicians monitor complete blood count (CBC) and liver function tests as well as clinical status routinely in patients undergoing 6-MP therapy. In addition, a normal TPMT enzyme activity in the screening test should not preclude this routine clinical assessment.

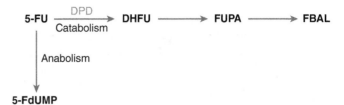

FIGURE 13–4 Metabolism of 5-FU. 5-Fluoro-2'-deoxyuridine-5'-monophosphate (5-FdUMP) is the active cytotoxic product resulting from a multistep 5-FU activation route. The initial and rate-limiting step is the catabolism of 5-FU by dihydropyrimidine dehydrogenase (DPD), catalyzing the reduction of 5-FU into 5,6-dihydrofluorouracil (DHFU). Subsequently, DHFU is degraded into fluoro-β-ureidopropionic acid (FUPA) and fluoro-β-alanine (FBAL).

DPD and 5-Fluorouracil

5-FU is widely used as a part of combination chemotherapy regimen for the treatment of breast, colorectal, and head & neck cancers. Inside the tumor cells, 5-FU is bioconverted into cytotoxic nucleotides (Figure 13–4). The main mechanism of cytotoxicity is thought to be inhibition of thymidylate synthase by the metabolite 5-fluoro-2'-deoxyuridine-5'-monophosphate (5-FdUMP).[29] Only a small part of the administered 5-FU dose exerts cytotoxicity since the majority of 5-FU is rapidly metabolized into inactive metabolites. The rate-limiting step is catabolism of 5-FU by DPD, which catalyzes the reduction of 5-FU into 5,6-dihydrofluorouracil (DHFU) (Figure 13–4). DPD plays a major role in the regulation of 5-FU metabolism and thus in the amount of 5-FU available for cytotoxicity.[30–33]

In patients with DPD enzyme deficiency, 5-FU chemotherapy is associated with severe, life-threatening toxicity.[34] Moreover, a markedly prolonged elimination half-life of 5-FU has been observed in a patient with complete deficiency of DPD enzyme activity.[35] Several mutations in the dihydropyrimidine dehydrogenase gene (*DPYD*), which encodes for the DPD enzyme, have recently been identified.[34,36] Population studies have suggested that 4–7% of the American population that exhibit a 5-FU dose-limiting toxicity might be associated with a genetic defect in the *DPYD* gene.[37] Although complete DPD deficiency is rare, reduced levels of enzyme activity are more common, particularly in African Americans and women. These demographic differences have been illustrated in an analysis of enzyme levels from 258 normal volunteers. Partial DPD deficiency is present in 12.3% of black women, 4.0% of black men, 3.5 of white women, and 1.9% of white men.[38]

Many polymorphisms in the *DPYD* gene have been identified that may result in partial or total loss of DPD activity. A few alleles are associated with a marked decrease in DPD activity and enhanced fluoropyrimidine toxicity, the most important of which is *DPYD*2A*. In one series, at least one of three variants (*DPYD*2A*, *DPYD*9B*, or *DPYD*13*) has been found in 30% of 5-FU-treated patients (13 of 44) who developed grade 3 or 4 toxicities.[39] This study demonstrated that patients with inherited high-risk *DPYD* variants have a 7-fold increased risk of severe toxicity with 5-FU. Other studies have found that *DPYD*2A* is present in less than 10% of patients with severe 5-FU toxicity. In one of these prospective studies of 683 patients receiving 5-FU monotherapy, genotyping has revealed the *DPYD*2A* allele in only 5% of those with treatment-related toxicities.[40] Furthermore, less than one half of those with the *DPYD*2A* allele had grade 3 or 4 toxicity. Interestingly, the presence of *DPYD*2A* has been shown to be a stronger predictive factor for severe toxicity in men than in women.[40]

Inheritance of one of these alleles does not account for all cases of DPD deficiency. Impaired DPD activity has been detected in some patients with wild-type *DPYD*, presumably due to epigenetic mechanisms that regulate enzyme activity.[41] To avoid the risk of severe and potentially fatal reactions, the manufacturers of both IV 5-FU and the oral form of fluoropyrimidine (e.g., capecitabine) recommend that these drugs be contraindicated in patients with known DPD deficiency. However, preemptive testing of all patients scheduled to receive 5-FU in order to identify those with a DPD deficiency is controversial and not widely practiced.

UGT1A1 and Irinotecan

Irinotecan is a topoisomerase I inhibitor used in combination with 5-FU as first-line therapy for the treatment of metastatic colorectal cancer.[42] It is metabolized to its active metabolite, SN-38, which is 1,000× more potent than the parent drug (Figure 13–5).[43] SN-38 is inactivated by a polymorphic hepatic enzyme UGT1A1.[44] It has been observed that human liver samples harboring a seven dinucleotide TA repeat sequence (e.g., *UGT1A1*28*) in the UGT1A1 promoter have reduced SN-38 metabolism.[44] Patients with the *UGT1A1*28* allele have an increased risk for severe neutropenia, severe diarrhea, and death compared with patients without the *UGT1A1*28* polymorphism.[45]

Approximately 10% of the North American population is homozygous for the *UGT1A1*28* allele (which is responsible for

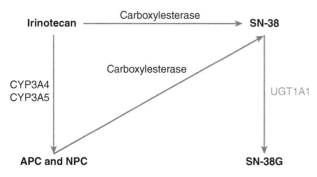

FIGURE 13–5 Metabolism of irinotecan. Irinotecan is primarily metabolized by human carboxylesterase 2 (hCE2) to the active metabolite, SN-38. SN-38 is glucuronidated by uridine diphosphate glucuronyl transferase (UGT1A1) to the inactive metabolite SN-38G, which is subsequently excreted. Other irinotecan metabolism pathways include oxidation by cytochrome P450 3A (CYP3A) into 7-ethyl-10[4-*N*-(5-aminopentanoic acid)-1-piperidino]-carbonyloxycamptothecin (APC) and 7-ethyl-10[4-(1-piperidino)-1-amino]-carbonyloxycamptothecin (NPC); SN-38 = 7-ethyl-10-hydroxy-camptothecin. In turn, NPC can also be converted into SN-38 by carboxylesterase.

Gilbert syndrome); an additional 40% of the North Americans are heterozygotes (Camptosar package insert). In November 2004, the FDA Advisory Committee on Pharmaceutical Sciences considered the findings of several pharmacogenetic trials that had assessed the association between irinotecan-induced toxicities in patients who were homozygous with the *UGT1A1*28/*28* genotype.[45–48] These studies suggested that the *UGT1A1*28/*28* genotype is associated with a decreased conversion of SN-38 to SN-38G, thus resulting in an increased severity of irinotecan-induced diarrhea and neutropenia.[42,45,46] Based on these findings, the FDA advised an amendment of the product information to include information regarding the *UGT1A1*28* polymorphism and hematological toxicity. In addition, the FDA recommended that patients with the *UGT1A1*28/*28* genotype receive a lower starting dose of irinotecan. A pharmacogenomic test (i.e., Invader UGT1A1 Molecular Assay; Third Wave Technologies, Inc, Madison, WI) was FDA-approved to test for the *UGT1A1*28* allele.

Recent data indicate that the association between *UGT1A1*28* and irinotecan-induced neutropenia is dose-dependent. A meta-analysis showed that even though the inheritance of the *UGT1A1*28/*28* genotype was associated with an increased risk of neutropenia at all doses, the relative risk for neutropenia at doses ≥250 mg/m² was significantly higher (RR 7.0, 95% CI 3.10–16.78) than that for the lower doses (80–145 mg/m² weekly, RR 2.43, 95% CI 1.34–4.39).[49,50] This dose dependency on the risk of neutropenia could be explained by the relative extent of SN-38 glucuronidation. Similarly, the risk of severe diarrhea at medium and high doses of irinotecan was higher among patients with a *UGT1A1*28/*28* genotype than among those with *UGT1A1*1/*1* or *UGT1A1*1/*28* genotypes.[49] This increased risk of diarrhea in patients carrying *UGT1A1*28* alleles was not apparent with lower doses (<125 mg/m²). In an evidence-based review, the quality of evidence on the analytical as well as clinical validity of current *UGT1A1* testing methods was found to be adequate for severe toxicities such as neutropenia and diarrhea as stratified by *UGT1A1* genotypes.[51] The strongest association for a clinical end point was severe neutropenia since the patients homozygous for the *UGT1A1*28* allele were 3.5 times more likely to develop severe neutropenia compared with individuals with the wild-type *UGT1A1* genotype (risk ratio 3.51, 95% confidence interval 2.03–6.07). The cost-effectiveness of *UGT1A1*28* genotyping has also been demonstrated primarily for Caucasian and African populations.[52] These results show that *UGT1A1* testing may be particularly useful in patients who are considered for medium- to high-dose irinotecan therapy to avoid severe neutropenia.

Despite strong evidence to support the use of *UGT1A1* testing, routine use of this assay in all patients who are to receive irinotecan is not widely accepted. Even though such testing has been suggested to be cost-effective, the study lacked the assessment of the clinical relevance of identifying homozygotes. In addition, there are no current guidelines on how to dose the homozygous and heterozygous patients for the *UGT1A1*28* allele(s). Additional clinical studies focusing on these key questions will facilitate implementation of *UGT1A1* testing into clinical practice.

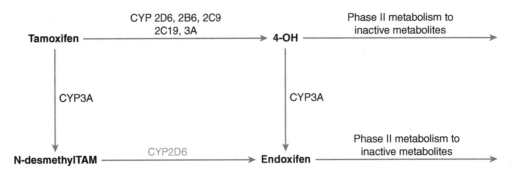

FIGURE 13-6 Biotransformation of tamoxifen to endoxifen. Tamoxifen is predominantly *N*-demethylated by the CYP3A enzyme to *N*-desmethyltamoxifen, which is the major primary metabolic pathway. This metabolite undergoes multiple oxidations including 4-hydroxylation by *CYP2D6* to endoxifen. Tamoxifen 4-hydroxylation is metabolized by multiple CYPs to 4-hydroxytamoxifen (minor metabolic pathway). A small portion of endoxifen plasma concentrations appears to result from CYP3A-catalyzed *N*-demethylation of 4-hydroxytamoxifen. The hydroxylated metabolites undergo conjugation by phase II enzymes.

CYP2D6 and Tamoxifen

Tamoxifen is an anti-estrogenic drug used for the treatment of estrogen receptor–positive breast cancer.[53] Although the estrogen receptor is a predictive marker of response to tamoxifen, not all women with estrogen receptor–positive breast cancer benefit from tamoxifen.[54] Tamoxifen undergoes sequential biotransformation by several metabolic pathways (Figure 13–6).[55,56] Endoxifen (4-hydroxy-*N*-desmethyl tamoxifen) is a more potent antiestrogen compared with tamoxifen as well as another active metabolite 4-hydroxytamoxifen (4-OH) in terms of relative contribution to the overall anti-cancer effect of tamoxifen. Tamoxifen to 4-OH is catalyzed by multiple enzymes. Cytochrome P-450 2D6 (CYP2D6) mediates oxidation of *N*-desmethyltamoxifen to endoxifen, which is also the most abundant tamoxifen metabolite.

Initial clinical studies demonstrated that women on tamoxifen therapy who possessed genetic variants of *CYP2D6* associated with low or no enzymatic activity or who received concomitant CYP2D6 inhibitors have significantly decreased endoxifen concentrations.[57,58] Women possessing *CYP2D6* variants responsible for decreased enzyme activity were found to have a higher risk of relapse and lower incidence of hot flashes.[53,59] In addition, CYP2D6 metabolism was found to be an independent predictor of breast cancer outcome.[53] Additional studies to confirm these results found that CYP2D6 poor and intermediate metabolizers had higher recurrence rates, all-cause mortality rates, and decreased event-free survival. Overall survival was not affected.[58] Despite the positive findings in terms of the association between the *CYP2D6* genotype and the effectiveness of tamoxifen in some studies, there are several studies that have not found a similar association.

This controversy was resolved by the recent retrospective analyses from two large clinical studies,[60,61] which did not find an association between the *CYP2D6* genotype and the effectiveness of tamoxifen in preventing breast cancer recurrence. In the Arimidex, Tamoxifen, Alone or in Combination (ATAC) trial, subjects who were genotyped (588 out of 3,116 women; 18%) and categorized into poor, intermediate, or extensive metabolizers of tamoxifen showed that the breast cancer recurrence rates were not significantly different in any of the groups in either the tamoxifen or the anastrozole (control) group.[61] In addition, approximately 9% of women who were concomitantly taking potent CYP2D6 inhibitors (e.g., selective serotonin reuptake inhibitors [SSRIs]) did not have a significantly different clinical outcome compared with other women. Similarly, the analysis of the Breast International Group (BIG) 1-98 trial, involving 48% of the original study subjects (1,243 of 2,459 women) who were *CYP2D6* genotyped and categorized into poor, intermediate, and extensive metabolizer groups, did not find any significant difference in event-free survival between groups.[60] In addition, the incidence of hot flashes, which was previously associated with response, was not significantly different between groups. Although these studies were retrospective analyses and did not consider adherence to tamoxifen or the concomitant use of over-the-counter drugs, the conclusions provide evidence not to routinely recommend *CYP2D6* testing in patients being considered for tamoxifen therapy. Even though the use of tamoxifen and strong CYP2D6 inhibitors such as SSRIs is controversial, the current recommendations to avoid SSRIs while on tamoxifen therapy are reasonable.

SOMATIC VARIANTS AS PREDICTORS OF DRUG RESPONSE

Somatic variations are acquired alterations in DNA that occur in cells other than the germ cells and are not inherited. Some of these mutations, detected in tumor DNA, predict response to cancer chemotherapy. The elucidation of the signal transduction networks that drive neoplastic transformation has led to rationally designed cancer therapeutics that target specific molecular events.[62] These targeted therapeutics, unlike traditional cancer chemotherapeutics, do not have narrow therapeutic indices. Many of the currently known drugs in this class are protein kinase inhibitors. Genes that encode protein kinases are often dysregulated and constitutively activated in cancer. Kinase inhibitors therefore reduce the activity of the activated protein

TABLE 13-2 Examples of somatic mutations in target genes reported to modulate response to kinase inhibitors.

Gene Product	Variants	Drugs	Treatment Outcome
BCR-ABL	T315I and others	Imatinib, dasatinib, nilotinib	Decreased efficacy, resistance
ERBB2	p95	Trastuzumab	Decreased efficacy, resistance
EGFR	G719A, G719C, L858R, L861Q, exon 19 intragenic deletion	Gefitinib	Increased efficacy

BCR-ABL, breakpoint cluster region-ABL; *ERBB2*, v-erb-b2 erythroblastic leukemia viral oncogene homolog 2, neuroblastoma/glioblastoma-derived oncogene homolog (avian); *EGFR*, epidermal growth factor receptor.

kinases, reducing the cellular oncogenic drive and inducing tumor regression. Three classic examples of somatic mutations of tumor DNA that predict response to kinase inhibitors are highlighted in Table 13–2.

BCR-ABL, KIT, PDGFRA Kinase Inhibitors

The BCR-ABL protein tyrosine kinase is the fusion of the BCR and non-receptor protein tyrosine kinase ABL that results from the reciprocal chromosomal translocation t(9;22) producing a shortened chromosome 22, called the Philadelphia (Ph) chromosome. This resultant chromosome has constitutive tyrosine kinase activity.[63] The BCR-ABL protein is associated predominantly with CML but also with ALL.[63] Imatinib was the first small molecule kinase inhibitor approved as treatment for CML that targets BCR-ABL. It binds to an inactive conformation of the BCR-ABL protein kinase.[64,65] Imatinib also has specificity for the platelet-derived growth factor receptor alpha (PDGFRA) and stem cell growth factor receptor (KIT) protein kinases, and is used in treatment of malignancies associated with dysregulated forms of those proteins.[64]

Treatment of CML patients with imatinib leads to complete cytogenetic and hematological remission; however, imatinib fails to deplete leukemic stem cells that harbor the BCR-ABL fusion protein.[66] Therefore, some patients develop resistance to imatinib, particularly in the advanced phases of CML and Ph-positive ALL.[67] Mechanisms of imatinib resistance involve BCR-ABL amplification and overexpression of mRNA and protein.[68,69] However, the most common mechanism of resistance is the acquisition of point mutations in the kinase domain of the *ABL* gene.[70]

Point mutations in the *ABL* gene are listed in Table 13–3. The first identified point mutation associated with imatinib resistance was T315I.[70] Crystal structures of an analogue of imatinib bound to the ABL kinase domain revealed that the T315 residue was crucial for the interaction between imatinib and ABL.[71] It was also found that a different mutation at the T315 residue (T315V) conferred constitutive kinase activity to ABL and was less sensitive to imatinib compared with wild-type ABL.[72] The T315I point mutation impairs imatinib binding, thereby reducing tyrosine kinase inhibition of ABL. More than 50 different point mutations in *ABL* associated with imatinib resistance have been reported.[67] Most are rare, and six amino acid residues (G250, Y253, E255, T315, M351, and F359) thus far account for 60–70% of imatinib-resistant mutations.[67]

Two of the more frequently detected *ABL* mutants, Y253F and E255K, have been shown to have high in vitro transforming potential. The in vitro finding is consistent with clinical findings that show P-loop mutations such as Y253F and E255K are associated with a greater likelihood of progression to blast crisis and

TABLE 13-3 Activity of BCR-ABL inhibitors against a selection of *BCR-ABL1* mutants found in patients with CML.

	Imatinib (nM)	Nilotinib (nM)	Dasatinib (nM)
P-loop			
Native BCR-ABL1	260	13	0.8
M244V	2,000	38	1.3
G250E	1,350	48	1.8
Q252H	1,325	70	3.4
Y253H	>6,400	450	1.3
Y253F	3,475	125	1.4
E255K	5,200	200	5.6
E255V	>6,400	430	11
V299L	540	NA	18
ATP binding site			
F311L	480	23	1.3
T315I	>6,400	>2,000	>200
T315A	971	61	125
F317L	1,050	50	7.4
F317V	350	NA	53
Catalytic domain			
M351T	880	15	1.1
E355G	2,300	NA	1.8
F359V	1,825	175	2.2
A-loop			
V379I	1,630	51	0.8
L387M	1,000	49	2
H396R	1,750	41	1.3
H396P	850	41	0.6

High sensitivity	Intermediate sensitivity	High insensitivity

All concentrations (nM) represent IC_{50} values. Reprinted with permission.[75]

decreased overall survival in imatinib-treated patients.[73] Similarly the T315I mutation, generally found in patients with advanced CML, has a worse overall survival compared with other *ABL* mutations in patients on imatinib therapy.[74] This is likely due to the fact that no FDA-approved tyrosine kinase inhibitors are effective against the T315I mutation. Current standard of care for patients with the T315I mutation is to enroll them in a clinical trial or refer them for stem cell transplant.

Drug-resistant BCR-ABL point mutations are found in imatinib-naïve CML or are acquired during imatinib treatment. Acquired imatinib resistance involves the re-emergence of BCR-ABL tyrosine kinase activity. This suggests that the mutant BCR-ABL protein is still a viable target for inhibition by small molecule inhibitors.[76,77] To this end, alternative therapies have been designed to overcome resistance to imatinib. One of these drugs, nilotinib, is approximately 30-fold more potent than imatinib as an ABL inhibitor.[67] A significant clinical response to nilotinib is demonstrated in patients with imatinib-resistant CML in all phases of disease and in patients with Ph-positive ALL.[78] Nilotinib also inhibits KIT and PDGFRB protein kinases.[79]

Another drug designed to overcome imatinib resistance is dasatinib. Dasatinib is a potent inhibitor of BCR-ABL, Src-family kinases, KIT, and PDGFR.[80,81] In contrast to imatinib and nilotinib, dasatinib binds to the active conformation of the ABL kinase.[82] Based on data from phase I and II trials in patients with imatinib-resistant CML and Ph-positive ALL patients, dasatinib is approved in the United States for the treatment of adults in all phases of CML with imatinib resistance or intolerance and in patients with Ph-positive ALL with imatinib resistance or intolerance.[83,84] The sensitivity of the point mutations in BCR-ABL to imatinib, nilotinib, and dasatinib is provided in Table 13–3. Clinically, the assessment of these point mutations is only done if a patient is not responding to therapy.

Most gastrointestinal stromal tumors (GISTs) harbor oncogenic *KIT* or *PDGFRA* receptor tyrosine kinase mutations.[85] The *KIT* or *PDGFRA* gain-of-function mutations are early events in GIST oncogenesis.[86] Imatinib, a potent inhibitor of KIT signaling, has recently become first-line treatment of metastatic GIST following in vitro studies suggesting a therapeutic potential for imatinib in a human GIST cell line.[87] Prior to imatinib, surgical resection of primary localized GIST was the only chance for cure.[88] GISTs are refractory to standard chemotherapy and radiation, with a predicted 5-year survival of 30%.[89] Prospective trials of imatinib in metastatic GIST have shown that approximately 80% of patients respond to imatinib or have stable disease.[90,91] In addition, 70% of metastatic GIST patients will have at least a 2-year disease-free survival and 50% will be free of disease progression.[92]

KIT mutations occur in up to 90% of GISTs and clinical response to imatinib is dependent on the presence of specific *KIT* mutations.[93] Exon 11 *KIT* mutations are found in 75% of GISTs and result in the abrogation of the juxtamembrane auto-inhibition of KIT kinase.[94] Patients with exon 11 *KIT* mutations have a higher response rate to imatinib treatment and longer time to treatment failure compared with patients with other *KIT* or *PDGFRA* mutations.[95] In addition, patients with the rare exon 13 *KIT* mutation or exon 17 *PDGFRA* mutation may respond to imatinib.[95] Patients without any detectable *KIT* or *PDGFRA* mutations respond less frequently to imatinib treatment compared with patients with exon 11 *KIT* mutations.[93] However, only up to 39% of those patients without *KIT* or *PDGFRA* mutations do respond to imatinib.[96] These data suggest that imatinib treatment ought to be considered for all GIST patients, regardless of *KIT* or *PDGFRA* mutation status.[95] The only exception may be patients with a primary imatinib-resistant mutation of *PDGFRA* (D842V).

The majority of metastatic GIST patients will develop resistance to imatinib. The most common resistance mechanisms involve the acquisition of secondary exon 13, 14, or 17 *KIT* mutations that prohibit imatinib binding.[95] Some of these secondary mutations, such as the frequently occurring V654A substitution, are intrinsically imatinib-resistant.[97] However, other mutations such as those involving the N822 residue are intrinsically imatinib-sensitive but are associated with clinical imatinib resistance when coincident with an exon 11 *KIT* mutation.[97]

Sunitinib, an inhibitor of KIT, PDGFRA, FLT3, and VEGFR2, has recently been approved for the treatment of imatinib-resistant GIST and in patients unable to tolerate imatinib therapy.[98] In a randomized phase III trial of sunitinib in patients who had progressed on imatinib therapy, sunitinib was found to prolong median time to tumor progression.[99] Sunitinib provides a temporary benefit for imatinib-resistant GIST patients. Therefore, additional therapeutic modalities are needed. Preclinical studies in GIST cell lines have shown that treatment with heat shock protein 90 (HSP90) inhibitors results in degradation of the KIT oncoprotein and may be of benefit in imatinib-resistant GIST.[100]

ERBB2 Kinase Inhibitors

ERBB2/HER2 gene amplification and protein overexpression occurs in approximately 30% of metastatic breast cancer[101] and also shows clinical correlation with earlier relapse and decreased overall survival.[102] Trastuzumab is a monoclonal antibody approved for the treatment of amplified or overexpressed ERBB2 in metastatic breast cancer.[103] It is active as a single agent and in combination with chemotherapy in ERBB2-overexpressing breast cancer. However, the response rates to trastuzumab monotherapy range from 12% to 34%.[104] Primary resistance to trastuzumab monotherapy occurs in approximately 66–88% of ERBB2-overexpressing metastatic breast tumors.[105,106] Trastuzumab with adjuvant chemotherapy (paclitaxel or docetaxel) significantly improves disease-free and overall survival in patients with early stage ERBB2-overexpressing breast cancers compared with trastuzumab monotherapy.[107–109]

ERBB2 is also overexpressed, to a lesser degree, in lung cancers, specifically adenocarcinomas and large-cell carcinomas, and is predictive of worse outcomes.[110–112] Intragenic mutations have also been found in the conserved kinase domain of the *ERBB2* gene in some lung cancers.[113,114] The *ERBB2* mutations seem to occur exclusively in non-small cell lung cancer (NSCLC) of an adenocarcinoma histology and are more common in female patients and non-smokers.[113] So far, benefit of trastuzumab monotherapy or as part of combination chemotherapy has not been demonstrated for the treatment of NSCLC with overexpressed ERBB2.[115–118]

Invariably, the majority of patients who achieve an initial response to trastuzumab-based regimens develop resistance within 1 year.[104] The mechanisms of resistance (primary or acquired) have not been fully elucidated. Elucidating the molecular mechanisms underlying primary or acquired trastuzumab resistance is critical to improving the survival of breast cancer patients whose tumors overexpress ERBB2.[119] Resistance to trastuzumab has been associated with increased expression of the membrane-associated glycoprotein MUC4.[120] MUC4 binds and sterically hinders ERBB2 from binding to trastuzumab.[120] In a trastuzumab-resistant cell line with ERBB2 amplification demonstrating primary resistance to trastuzumab, protein levels of MUC4 were inversely correlated with trastuzumab binding capacity.[121] Knockdown of MUC4 RNA increased the sensitivity of the resistant line to trastuzumab.[121]

Compensatory signaling from other EGFR family members can disrupt the inhibitory effect of trastuzumab. Trastuzumab binds the domain IV of ERBB2 and domain II is involved in heterodimerization with EGFR and ERBB3.[122] Additionally, increased signaling from other receptor types such as insulin growth factor-1 receptor (IGF-1R) has been shown to reduce trastuzumab-mediated growth arrest.[123] IGF-1R interacts with ERBB2 in trastuzumab-resistant cells but not in trastuzumab-sensitive cells.[124] Inhibition of IGF-1R by antibody blockade or tyrosine kinase inhibition increased trastuzumab sensitivity in vitro.[124]

Altered downstream signaling from ERBB2 has been shown to confer primary resistance to trastuzumab. ERBB2 signaling activates the PI3K signaling pathway. Constitutive PI3K/AKT activity has been shown to inhibit trastuzumab-mediated cell cycle arrest and apoptosis.[125] An ERBB2-overexpressing breast cancer cell line, BT474, resistant to trastuzumab had elevated levels of phosphorylated AKT compared with the parent line.[126] The resistant cells were sensitive to a small molecule inhibitor of PI3K.[126] Patients with phosphatase and tensin homolog (PTEN)–deficient, ERBB2-overexpressing breast tumors have a poorer response to trastuzumab-based therapy.[127] Subsequently, it was shown that in PTEN-deficient cells, PI3K inhibitors rescued trastuzumab resistance in vitro and in vivo.[127] Therefore, PTEN loss may serve as a predictor of trastuzumab resistance and PI3K inhibitors may be potential therapies in PTEN-deficient trastuzumab-resistant tumors.[104]

Novel therapeutic strategies are being employed to overcome resistance to trastuzumab. Pertuzumab is a monoclonal ERBB2 antibody that represents a new class of drugs called dimerization inhibitors.[104] It can block signaling by other EGFR family receptors, as well as inhibit signaling in cells expressing normal ERBB2 levels. Pertuzumab sterically blocks dimerization of ERBB2 with EGFR and ERBB3, inhibiting signaling from ERBB2/EGFR and ERBB2/ERBB3 heterodimers.[128] It is also able to disrupt

the interaction between ERBB2 and IGF-1R in trastuzumab-resistant cells.[124] Trastuzumab and pertuzumab bind to different epitopes in the extracellular domain of ERBB2.[129,130] The combination of trastuzumab and pertuzumab produced synergistic apoptosis in ERBB2-overexpressing trastuzumab-naïve breast cancer cells,[131] without any significant effect on the viability of trastuzumab-resistant breast cancer cells.[124]

Another alternative therapeutic agent against trastuzumab-resistant tumors is lapatinib, a dual tyrosine kinase inhibitor targeted against both EGFR and ERBB2. Binding of lapatinib to EGFR and ERBB2 is reversible but its dissociation is much slower. This allows for a prolonged downregulation of receptor tyrosine phosphorylation.[104] ERBB2 status, but not EGFR status, is a determinant of lapatinib activity.[104] It has been shown that combination of lapatinib with trastuzumab enhanced apoptosis of ERBB2-overexpressing breast cancer cells.[132] Resistance to lapatinib seems to be mediated by increased signaling from the estrogen receptor in estrogen receptor–positive ERBB2-overexpressing breast cancers.[133] This suggests that targeting of both the estrogen receptor and ERBB2 may be beneficial in a subset of cancer patients.[133] A recent phase III trial of trastuzumab-resistant ERBB2-overexpressing breast cancer patients demonstrated that the combination of lapatinib and capecitabine resulted in longer median progression-free survival compared with capecitabine alone.[134]

Trastuzumab resistance can also be seen in tumors that express a truncated form of HER2 (p95) with no extracellular domain containing trastuzumab binding site. In a study of 46 patients with metastatic breast cancer, only 1 of 9 patients expressing p95HER2 responded to trastuzumab, compared with 19 of 37 with full-length HER2 expression.[135] In another study, high levels of p95 predicted worse outcome in patients.[136] It is suggested that lapatinib may be a more effective treatment choice and this is being investigated in clinical trials. A combination strategy with trastuzumab and lapatinib has shown potential in breast cancer patients with ERBB2 overexpression.[137] Additional clinical trials are necessary to confirm these results.

EGFR Kinase Inhibitors

EGFR protein tyrosine kinase overexpression has been implicated in numerous cancer types.[138] Gefitinib and erlotinib are EGFR tyrosine kinase inhibitors marketed as single drug therapy for chemotherapy-refractory advanced NSCLC.[139,140] The mechanism of increased sensitivity of EGFR mutants to erlotinib and gefitinib is still unknown. However, it has been shown that somatic mutations in the conserved kinase domain of EGFR gene (exon 19 in-frame deletions and exon 21 L858R missense amino acid substitution) confer ligand-independent activation and prolonged kinase activity after ligand stimulation,[141,142] and are associated with sensitivity to gefitinib[141,142] and erlotinib.[143]

Somatic mutations of EGFR kinase domain are most common in NSCLC. EGFR mutations are rare in head and neck cancers, cholangiosarcomas, colon cancers, ovarian cancers, esophageal cancers, and pancreatic cancers.[144–149] In lung cancers,

EGFR kinase domain mutations are more common in adenocarcinomas, East Asians, women, and non-smokers.[150] Mutations outside of the kinase domain are rare in NSCLC.[141-143] However, mutations of the extracellular domain of *EGFR* are common in gliobastomas[151] and squamous cell lung cancers.[152]

In NSCLC, *EGFR* mutations are commonly associated with amplification.[153] Patients with EGFR amplification were more likely to respond to gefitinib or erlotinib and had longer median time to disease progression and overall survival compared with patients with normal *EGFR* copy number.[154] Conversely, it remains to be established whether amplification of wild-type *EGFR* contributes to lung cancer development and response to gefitinib or erlotinib.[154] Several mutations of *EGFR* have been reported. Thus far, there are five mutations known to confer sensitivity to EGFR tyrosine kinase inhibitors. The drug-sensitive mutations are point mutations in exon 18 (G719A or G719C), point mutations in exon 21 (L858R and L861Q), and in-frame deletions of exon 19 that eliminate four amino acids (LREA).[155] The most common of these drug-sensitive mutations are the exon 19 in-frame deletion and exon 21 missense amino acid substitution (L858R) accounting for up to 90% of *EGFR* mutations in NSCLC.[155]

In retrospective studies, the association between the presence of *EGFR* mutation and sensitivity to gefitinib and erlotinib is quite consistent showing 75% response rate for patients with *EGFR* mutations compared with 10% response rate for patients with wild-type *EGFR*.[156-160] Additional, prospective trials have confirmed these findings, whereby 78% of patients with a somatic exon 19 deletion or exon 21 L858R mutation had radiographic responses to gefitinib and erlotinib.[161-163]

Large phase III retrospective trials have been conducted where NSCLC patients were randomized to receive either standard cytotoxic chemotherapy alone or standard chemotherapy in combination with gefitinib or erlotinib.[156,164] These studies have reported that patients with *EGFR* mutations have prolonged survival compared with patients with wild-type *EGFR* treated with gefitinib or erlotinib. Interestingly, these studies have also found that the prolonged survival may occur in the absence of treatment with gefitinib, erlotinib, surgery, or standard cancer chemotherapy.[154] In the standard cytotoxic chemotherapy alone treatment arm, patients with *EGFR* mutation had prolonged progression-free and overall survival compared with patients with wild-type *EGFR*.[156,164] A prospective study was done in Japan of 230 patients with metastatic NSCLC with EGFR mutations who had not previously received chemotherapy. Subjects were randomized to receive gefitinib or standard of care chemotherapy with carboplatin–paclitaxel.[165] In the planned interim analysis progression-free survival was significantly longer in the gefitinib group than in the standard-chemotherapy group (hazard ratio for death or disease progression with gefitinib, 0.36; *P* <.001), resulting in early termination of the study. The gefitinib group had a significantly longer median progression-free survival (10.8 months vs. 5.4 months in the chemotherapy group; *P* <.001), as well as a higher response rate (73.7% vs. 30.7%; *P* <.001). The median overall survival was 30.5 months in the gefitinib group and 23.6 months in the chemotherapy group (*P* = .31).[165]

There are conflicting data regarding the clinical course between patients with exon 19 in-frame deletions and patients with exon 21 L858R missense substitution. One study reported that NSCLC patients with the L858R mutation treated with surgery alone have an increase in overall survival compared with NSCLC patients with exon 19 deletions.[150] In contrast, after treatment with gefitinib or erlotinib, NSCLC patients with *EGFR* exon 19 deletions have an increase in overall survival.[155]

Despite a dramatic initial response to gefitinib and erlotinib, NSCLC patients with *EGFR* mutations rarely achieve a complete response, and treatment resistance is inevitable. There are thus far three *EGFR* kinase domain mutations associated with drug resistance: an exon 19 point mutation (D761Y), an exon 20 point mutation (T790M), and an exon 20 insertion (D770_N771insNPG).[154] The most common of these drug-resistant mutations is the T790M reported to occur in about 50% of tumors after disease progression.[166,167] The T790M mutation has been predicted to block the binding of gefitinib or erlotinib to the kinase ATP binding pocket. This mutation is analogous to the acquired drug resistance to imatinib seen in GIST and CML.[154] Interestingly, the T790M mutation has been seen in the germline and tumor DNA of family members with hereditary bronchioloalveolar carcinoma.[168] In vitro data have suggested that irreversible EGFR inhibitors may have activity in patients with acquired resistance to gefitinib or erlotinib.[169,170] A phase II trial of HKI-272, an irreversible EGFR kinase inhibitor, is ongoing to determine the efficacy in patients who have progressed after initial treatment with gefitinib or erlotinib.[154]

Other molecular parameters involved in the EGFR signaling cascade are associated with gefitinib or erlotinib activity. In cDNA microarray analysis, increased expression of tumor growth factor alpha (TGF-α), a ligand for EGFR, is associated with poor response to gefitinib.[171] Increased expression of heregulin, a ligand for ERBB3, is also associated with insensitivity to gefitinib.[172] It has been reported that increased copy number of *ERBB2* in the presence of *EGFR* mutation is associated with response to gefitinib.[173] However, NSCLC patients with *ERBB2* mutations do not respond to gefitinib or erlotinib.[174]

Downstream of EGFR, it has been observed that NSCLC patients with *KRAS* mutations are resistant to gefitinib or erlotinib.[175] AKT is phosphorylated on EGFR activation transmitting signals for cell survival.[176] It has been reported that increased phosphorylation of AKT is predictive of response to gefitinib or erlotinib.[143,177] A novel drug-resistant gefitinib mutation has recently been reported that does not involve mutation of *EGFR*. It was reported that gefitinib-resistant clones from an *EGFR* mutant lung cancer cell line displayed amplification of hepatocyte growth factor receptor (*MET*) oncogene and maintained activation of epidermal growth factor receptor 3/phosphatidylinositol 3-kinase/v-akt murine thymoma viral oncogene homolog 1 (ERBB3/PI3K/AKT) signaling in the presence of gefitinib.[178] Following the initial observation in cell lines, a panel of 18 gefitinib- or erlotinib-resistant primary lung tumors was assessed for *MET* amplification. *MET* amplification was found to occur in 22% of those tumors.[178]

PHARMACOGENOMICS IN ONCOLOGY CLINICAL TRIALS

Potential benefits of incorporating pharmacogenomics in drug discovery and development include improved response rates, reduced sample size or shorter trial length, improved survival, and favorable economic impact. At first, reducing the target population by selectively enrolling patients may seem imperceptive to global drug development programs geared toward multi-billion dollar drugs. However, patient stratification using pharmacogenomic markers can prove advantageous especially for anti-cancer drugs with a low overall efficacy. In markets with multiple equally efficacious treatment options, a drug accompanied by companion diagnostics that can identify a subset of patients as responders would increase the market share of the drug.

Molecular Profiling for Oncology Pharmacogenomic Studies

Molecular profiling can be done at the level of DNA, RNA, and proteins. Gene expression profiling has been the most utilized technology due to its comprehensiveness and cost-effectiveness. A routine screen consisting of over 30,000 genes in the human genome can be performed in a single experiment using DNA chips or cDNA arrays. In addition, Reverse Phase Protein Array (RPPA), a high-throughput proteomics technology, has been successful in screening over 200 proteins (inactive and active states); however, it is currently not possible to screen the entire proteome in a single experiment. Even though the limitation of gene expression profiling is that the mRNA levels may not correlate with the levels of cognate proteins,[179,180] cluster analysis has been a common approach for pattern recognition,[181] which can be followed by more in-depth analysis of selected proteins. There are two common cluster analysis approaches: (1) unsupervised clustering can be used to discover unknown genes in one or more pathways to identify a subclass of tumor with a distinct clinical outcome, and (2) supervised clustering is used to validate a predictive signature or a gene panel correlated with favorable or unfavorable treatment outcome.[182]

Since transcriptional profiling is the most advanced profiling technique, it is used as a standard platform for analysis of tumor samples. Rapidly evolving proteomic technology will eventually facilitate global protein and metabolite profiling that can be used in conjunction with transcription profiling to provide a systematic approach to utilize pharmacogenomics. Finally, high-density SNP genotyping may also provide a valuable tool to understand responses of novel therapies to improve cancer treatment.

Retrospective Analyses and Genome-Wide Association Studies (GWAS)

Since the application of pharmacogenomics in oncology is relatively a modern field of research, the majority of studies are conducted first to generate and second to validate a hypothesis.

To prove a preliminary pharmacogenomic hypothesis in cancer patients, retrospective analyses using samples from already conducted studies are often performed. These include NCI-sponsored clinical trials, cooperative group or intergroup trials, NCI-sponsored Specialized Programs of Research Excellence, cancer centers-initiated or an individual investigator-initiated research project, and pharmaceutical company-sponsored studies. One of the successful outcomes of these types of analyses is the identification of activating somatic mutations of *KRAS* gene that is associated with lack of efficacy of EGFR-targeted therapy with cetuximab and panitumumab.[183,184] This important finding has led to establishment of guidelines by the American Society of Clinical Oncology (ASCO) to incorporate the analysis of *KRAS* mutations to improve the clinical outcome with these agents.[185] Furthermore, this result has also prompted the FDA and the European Medicines Agency (EMEA) to include these data in the prescribing information for cetuximab and panitumumab.

Alternatively, the "hypothesis-generating" exploratory analyses that employ GWAS techniques using previously collected biological specimens from existing and ongoing clinical trials have also been successful to identify important and novel genetic mutations that can be rapidly translated into clinical practice. A recent GWAS from the Postmenopausal Breast Cancer Adjuvant Trial MA.27 found four SNPs related to T-cell leukemia/lymphoma protein 1A (*TCL1A*) that were associated with musculoskeletal events in women receiving aromatase inhibitors as adjuvant therapy for early-stage breast cancer.[186] This novel finding may lead to identification of targets for prevention of musculoskeletal events with aromatase inhibitor therapy. Similarly, a better understanding of target mutation status and biological consequences will benefit development and clinical utility of existing and novel anti-cancer drugs. The application of pharmacogenomics in developing novel targeted therapeutics will largely depend on the discovery of novel surrogate biomarkers and identification of disease- and therapeutics-relevant polymorphisms, which again highlights importance of GWAS.

Findings from both retrospective analyses and exploratory studies typically need to be confirmed in a prospective study to provide evidence to support utilization of a routine pharmacogenomic test in making clinical decisions. However, this is often not feasible primarily due to the increasing cost of conducting clinical studies and challenges in patient recruitment. A reliable alternative is to include the pharmacogenomic analysis as a correlative part of large randomized prospective studies or to retrospectively evaluate the data from patients entered into large prospective clinical trials. A recent example of this is *CYP2D6* genotyping in predicting response to tamoxifen treatment. Retrospective analysis from two large clinical trials, ATAC[61] and BIG 1-98,[60] did not find an association between the *CYP2D6* genotype and the effectiveness of tamoxifen in preventing breast cancer recurrence. The findings from these analyses have been sufficient for not recommending *CYP2D6* testing in patients being considered for tamoxifen therapy.

Study Design and Conduct in Prospective Oncology Pharmacogenomic Studies

Incorporation of Pharmacogenomics in Preclinical Studies

Since drug discovery and development take a considerable amount of time and money, it is prudent to initiate exploration of markers of drug response before the first human efficacy studies. In drug discovery, preclinical models such as cell lines and xenografts can provide pharmacogenomic hypothesis to be tested prospectively in the human efficacy studies. One approach to the discovery of drug response markers involves testing of the compounds in cell lines or xenografts that express common polymorphisms in a target protein/pathway or a metabolizing enzyme for the class of compounds.[187,188] In vivo efficacy studies using primary xenografts with detailed tumor profiling may also help identification of pharmacogenomic markers. Another approach is transcriptional profiling of well-characterized panels of cell lines, marker profile of which matches well to panels of untreated tumor samples and ranking of optimal markers by various statistical approaches.[189] If the half-maximal inhibitory concentration (IC_{50}) values, determined for every cell line, are suggestive of a subset of tumors with better response to the compound in question, pharmacogenomics of these markers can be tested prospectively.

Implementing Pharmacogenomics in Clinical Trials

Among various phases of clinical trials, the phase II studies are likely the best place to initiate exploration of clinical pharmacogenomics in influencing treatment response and toxicity. In development of oncology drugs, the assessment of pharmacogenomic markers is not typically useful in phase 0/I studies since they consist of heterogeneous patients (various tumor types, different treatment history), most of whom are not exposed to effective doses of the drug. However, these phase 0/I studies may provide a good strategy to screen for genetic variations in drug transporters and drug-metabolizing enzymes to help evaluate pharmacokinetic differences and to identify differential host response to the drug early in clinical development. Samples can be collected in the phase I studies for future analysis in case of unanticipated pharmacokinetic differences.[190] Occasionally, strong preclinical evidence can also be investigated in patients in the Phase I studies.

In phase II studies, a sufficient number of patients are administered a dose to validate pharmacogenomic hypotheses from preclinical investigations as well as to identify new markers of treatment outcome. Here, pharmacokinetic as well as pharmacodynamic (tumor) markers can be studied in detail to explore various pharmacogenomic hypotheses. Pharmacogenomic markers identified in phase II studies should be confirmed in phase III studies. The need for pharmacogenomic analysis earlier in the clinical development is highlighted by the example that identification of activating *EGFR* mutations in nearly all responders of gefitinib treatment for NSCLC was made by post-marketing sequence analyses.[141,142] The transcription profiling in phase I–III clinical trials, if conducted to address pharmacogenomics of

EGFR-targeted therapy, could also have been able to determine this association and facilitated optimal patient selection much earlier on.

Biological Material for Oncology Pharmacogenomic Studies

Detection of soluble markers in the blood or markers in blood cells that can provide useful information about the efficacy of a drug is the most common way to assess biomarkers of treatment outcome. For pharmacogenomic studies, common SNPs in metabolizing enzymes, efflux pump, or other clearance pathways can be easily assessed using any genetic material collected at baseline. However, tumor biopsy before and/or during treatment to evaluate expression or activity of the target protein and pathway and its correlation to response is often critical in effective development of a new drug. For example, detection of *ERBB2* amplification or HER2 overexpression in breast cancer biopsies before starting the treatment has proven essential as an eligibility criterion.[109] In addition, mutations in the *BCR-ABL* gene responsible for resistance to imatinib may need to be assessed during treatment in CML patients who progress while being treated.[67,70] Even though detection of markers in tumor biopsy, which is invasive and expensive, is often essential, an alternate procedure for exploratory analysis of the markers is the use of surrogate tissues such as peripheral blood mononuclear cells (PBMCs).[191] The differential exposure of the drug to the tumor cells versus PBMCs as well as differences in expression and activity of target protein and pathways may however hinder effective interpretation of the data and may need to be confirmed using tumor biopsy.[192] PBMCs are also commonly used for the transcription profiling or proteomic profiling to explore potential pharmacogenomic markers of treatment outcome,[193–195] which have proven to supplement standard clinical and pathological subtyping of tumors in prediction of response.[196–199]

Patient Selection for Oncology Pharmacogenomic Studies

Patient selection is an important aspect of designing a pharmacogenomic study. In this aspect, various factors need to be considered. First, tumor-specific factors such as mutations in target protein or its signaling pathways may lead to altered efficacy. Previous studies conducted using EGFR-targeted therapies have emphasized the importance of mutations not only in the target receptor but also in the downstream signaling components (e.g., KRAS in the case of EGFR-targeted therapies).[175,183,184] When a drug targets multiple pathways, all the signaling components need to be evaluated for their importance in overall efficacy with the drugs. Although pharmacogenomic studies have mainly focused on tumor-specific genetic changes, germline changes are also of significant importance. Second, host-specific factors such as functional genotypic variants of metabolizing enzymes and clearance pathways may impact drug exposure for a given patient. For example, differences in allelic distribution of genes may significantly predict and validate ethnic differences in anti-neoplastic drug disposition in population-related pharmacogenomic studies.[200,201] The existence of ethnic differences, in particular, need to be considered for individual anti-cancer drugs as well as a therapeutic regimen proposed for the study to improve efficacy and minimize toxicity. Third, expression or mutation of some proteins and overactivity of certain pathways may confer resistance to a therapy. A significant amount of work needs to be done in this area since the response rate varies considerably among patients for any given anti-cancer drug or regimen.

Operational Issues in Oncology Pharmacogenomic Studies

The common and critical challenges of the oncology pharmacogenomic studies are adequate sample size and patient compliance. The issue of sample size can be addressed by adequate training of staff, close supervision of enrollment, and effective communication with clinical trial participants. The informed consent process in pharmacogenomic studies is quite complex due to inherent complexity of genomic technology and the terminology used to describe pharmacogenomics, which may hinder patient enrollment.[202] If the profiling is limited to transcriptional analysis requiring RNA samples, the investigator should distinguish it from genomic technologies, where DNA samples are being collected. In addition, explanation of the type of testing planned may increase the understanding of study participants and answer some of the ethical and privacy concerns and facilitate patient recruitment. The patients are more likely to enroll as research subjects if they are encouraged to ask questions with the knowledge that the participation in the study is completely voluntary and they have the right to withdraw their participation from the pharmacogenomic portion of the study without any reprimand.

On the other hand, patient compliance in voluntary pharmacogenomic sampling can be significantly improved by minimizing the burden on patients. Specifically, careful consideration should be given to the objectives and end points of a pharmacogenomic study including sample type (blood, normal tissue, tumor, etc.), sample collection time points, and alignment with other pharmacodynamic and clinical end points. It is critical to identify the least invasive source of tissue for the analysis of markers to increase enrollment and prevent dropouts. It is also recommended that pharmacogenomic sampling be coordinated with other scheduled clinical laboratory test for patient convenience. In almost all cases, a single baseline sample should be collected prior to the initiation of experimental therapy for transcriptional profiling for either prognostic or predictive markers of response. Acquisition of both pre-treatment and post-treatment samples provides a unique opportunity to evaluate transcriptional changes in response to the study drug and to identify profiles of acquired drug resistance and provides novel targets to effectively overcome this resistance.

SUMMARY

Pharmacogenomic strategies have been postulated to be most relevant for oncology drugs with (1) narrow therapeutic indices, (2) a high degree of variability in inter-individual response,

(3) little or no available method to monitor safety or efficacy, and (4) few alternative treatment options.[203] In general, pharmacogenomic strategies to optimize drug therapies are becoming more essential since focus in oncology drug development has shifted from broad-spectrum cytotoxic therapies to more specific targeted therapies. In addition to the monoclonal antibodies targeting a specific pathway, small molecule inhibitors that target one or multiple proteins and pathways also provide an example of drugs for which pharmacogenomic characterization is beneficial.

Pharmacogenomics has become intensely focused on the search for genomic biomarkers for use as classifiers to select patients in randomized controlled trials. The predictive utility of a genomic classifier has tremendous clinical appeal. Additionally, the use of a companion diagnostic will need to be considered and may become an integral part in the utilization of drugs in clinical practice. The credible mechanism to test the clinical utility of a genomic classifier is to employ the study results from a well-designed prospective trial. Such investigations will allow analysis of all relevant performance factors in the drug and diagnostic combinations including their sensitivity, specificity, and positive or negative predictive values.

REFERENCES

1. Brower V. New initiatives aim to test more cancer drugs for children. *J Natl Cancer Inst.* 2004;96(24):1808–1810.
2. Arrondeau J, Gan HK, Razak AR, Paoletti X, Le Tourneau C. Development of anti-cancer drugs. *Discov Med.* 2010;10(53):355–362.
3. Goldberger NE, Hunter KW. A systems biology approach to defining metastatic biomarkers and signaling pathways. *Wiley Interdiscip Rev Syst Biol Med.* 2009;1(1):89–96.
4. Renan MJ. How many mutations are required for tumorigenesis? Implications from human cancer data. *Mol Carcinog.* 1993;7(3):139–146.
5. Armitage P, Doll R. The age distribution of cancer and a multi-stage theory of carcinogenesis. *Br J Cancer.* 1954;8(1):1–12.
6. Nowell PC. The clonal evolution of tumor cell populations. *Science.* 1976;194(4260):23–28.
7. Fearon ER, Vogelstein B. A genetic model for colorectal tumorigenesis. *Cell.* 1990;61(5):759–767.
8. Vogelstein B, Kinzler KW. Cancer genes and the pathways they control. *Nat Med.* 2004;10(8):789–799.
9. Futreal PA, Coin L, Marshall M, et al. A census of human cancer genes. *Nat Rev Cancer.* 2004;4(3):177–183.
10. Weinberg RA. *The Biology of Cancer.* New York: Garland Science; 2007.
11. El-Deiry WS. *Tumor Suppressor Genes.* Totowa, NJ: Humana Press; 2003.
12. Knudson AG Jr. Hereditary cancer, oncogenes, and antioncogenes. *Cancer Res.* 1985;45(4):1437–1443.
13. Baylin SB. DNA methylation and gene silencing in cancer. *Nat Clin Pract Oncol.* 2005;2(suppl 1):S4–S11.
14. Knudson AG. Cancer genetics. *Am J Med Genet.* 2002;111(1):96–102.
15. Sherr CJ. Principles of tumor suppression. *Cell.* 2004;116(2):235–246.
16. Weinshilboum RM, Sladek SL. Mercaptopurine pharmacogenetics: monogenic inheritance of erythrocyte thiopurine methyltransferase activity. *Am J Hum Genet.* 1980;32(5):651–662.
17. McLeod HL, Relling MV, Liu Q, Pui CH, Evans WE. Polymorphic thiopurine methyltransferase in erythrocytes is indicative of activity in leukemic blasts from children with acute lymphoblastic leukemia. *Blood.* 1995;85(7):1897–1902.
18. Lennard L, Van Loon JA, Lilleyman JS, Weinshilboum RM. Thiopurine pharmacogenetics in leukemia: correlation of erythrocyte thiopurine

methyltransferase activity and 6-thioguanine nucleotide concentrations. *Clin Pharmacol Ther.* 1987;41(1):18–25.

19. Lennard L, Van Loon JA, Weinshilboum RM. Pharmacogenetics of acute azathioprine toxicity: relationship to thiopurine methyltransferase genetic polymorphism. *Clin Pharmacol Ther.* 1989;46(2):149–154.

20. Elion GB. The purine path to chemotherapy. *Science.* 1989;244(4900): 41–47.

21. Parks DA, Granger DN. Xanthine oxidase: biochemistry, distribution and physiology. *Acta Physiol Scand Suppl.* 1986;548:87–99.

22. Lennard L, Gibson BE, Nicole T, Lilleyman JS. Congenital thiopurine methyltransferase deficiency and 6-mercaptopurine toxicity during treatment for acute lymphoblastic leukaemia. *Arch Dis Child.* 1993;69(5): 577–579.

23. Evans WE, Horner M, Chu YQ, Kalwinsky D, Roberts WM. Altered mercaptopurine metabolism, toxic effects, and dosage requirement in a thiopurine methyltransferase-deficient child with acute lymphocytic leukemia. *J Pediatr.* 1991;119(6):985–989.

24. Schaeffeler E, Fischer C, Brockmeier D, et al. Comprehensive analysis of thiopurine *S*-methyltransferase phenotype–genotype correlation in a large population of German-Caucasians and identification of novel TPMT variants. *Pharmacogenetics.* 2004;14(7):407–417.

25. Yates CR, Krynetski EY, Loennechen T, et al. Molecular diagnosis of thiopurine *S*-methyltransferase deficiency: genetic basis for azathioprine and mercaptopurine intolerance. *Ann Intern Med.* 1997;126(8):608–614.

26. Evans WE, Hon YY, Bomgaars L, et al. Preponderance of thiopurine *S*-methyltransferase deficiency and heterozygosity among patients intolerant to mercaptopurine or azathioprine. *J Clin Oncol.* 2001;19(8): 2293–2301.

27. Goetz MP, Ames MM, Weinshilboum RM. Primer on medical genomics. Part XII: pharmacogenomics—general principles with cancer as a model. *Mayo Clin Proc.* 2004;79(3):376–384.

28. Donnan JR, Ungar WJ, Mathews M, Hancock-Howard RL, Rahman P. A cost effectiveness analysis of thiopurine methyltransferase testing for guiding 6-mercaptopurine dosing in children with acute lymphoblastic leukemia. *Pediatr Blood Cancer.* 2011;57(2):231–239.

29. Pinedo HM, Peters GF. Fluorouracil: biochemistry and pharmacology. *J Clin Oncol.* 1988;6(10):1653–1664.

30. Etienne MC, Lagrange JL, Dassonville O, et al. Population study of dihydropyrimidine dehydrogenase in cancer patients. *J Clin Oncol.* 1994;12(11):2248–2253.

31. Fleming RA, Milano G, Thyss A, et al. Correlation between dihydropyrimidine dehydrogenase activity in peripheral mononuclear cells and systemic clearance of fluorouracil in cancer patients. *Cancer Res.* 1992;52(10):2899–2902.

32. Harris BE, Song R, Soong SJ, Diasio RB. Relationship between dihydropyrimidine dehydrogenase activity and plasma 5-fluorouracil levels with evidence for circadian variation of enzyme activity and plasma drug levels in cancer patients receiving 5-fluorouracil by protracted continuous infusion. *Cancer Res.* 1990;50(1):197–201.

33. Lu Z, Zhang R, Diasio RB. Dihydropyrimidine dehydrogenase activity in human peripheral blood mononuclear cells and liver: population characteristics, newly identified deficient patients, and clinical implication in 5-fluorouracil chemotherapy. *Cancer Res.* 1993;53(22):5433–5438.

34. van Kuilenburg AB, Haasjes J, Richel DJ, et al. Clinical implications of dihydropyrimidine dehydrogenase (DPD) deficiency in patients with severe 5-fluorouracil-associated toxicity: identification of new mutations in the DPD gene. *Clin Cancer Res.* 2000;6(12):4705–4712.

35. Diasio RB, Beavers TL, Carpenter JT. Familial deficiency of dihydropyrimidine dehydrogenase. Biochemical basis for familial pyrimidinemia and severe 5-fluorouracil-induced toxicity. *J Clin Invest.* 1988;81(1):47–51.

36. Collie-Duguid ES, Etienne MC, Milano G, McLeod HL. Known variant DPYD alleles do not explain DPD deficiency in cancer patients. *Pharmacogenetics.* 2000;10(3):217–223.

37. Ezzeldin H, Diasio R. Dihydropyrimidine dehydrogenase deficiency, a pharmacogenetic syndrome associated with potentially life-threatening toxicity following 5-fluorouracil administration. *Clin Colorectal Cancer.* 2004;4(3):181–189.

38. Mattison LK, Fourie J, Desmond RA, Modak A, Saif MW, Diasio RB. Increased prevalence of dihydropyrimidine dehydrogenase deficiency in

African-Americans compared with Caucasians. *Clin Cancer Res.* 2006;12(18): 5491–5495.

39. Morel A, Boisdron-Celle M, Fey L, et al. Clinical relevance of different dihydropyrimidine dehydrogenase gene single nucleotide polymorphisms on 5-fluorouracil tolerance. *Mol Cancer Ther.* 2006;5(11):2895–2904.

40. Schwab M, Zanger UM, Marx C, et al. Role of genetic and nongenetic factors for fluorouracil treatment-related severe toxicity: a prospective clinical trial by the German 5-FU Toxicity Study Group. *J Clin Oncol.* 2008;26(13):2131–2138.

41. Ezzeldin HH, Lee AM, Mattison LK, Diasio RB. Methylation of the DPYD promoter: an alternative mechanism for dihydropyrimidine dehydrogenase deficiency in cancer patients. *Clin Cancer Res.* 2005;11(24 pt 1): 8699–8705.

42. Mathijssen RH, Marsh S, Karlsson MO, et al. Irinotecan pathway genotype analysis to predict pharmacokinetics. *Clin Cancer Res.* 2003;9(9): 3246–3253.

43. Kaneda N, Nagata H, Furuta T, Yokokura T. Metabolism and pharmacokinetics of the camptothecin analogue CPT-11 in the mouse. *Cancer Res.* 1990;50(6):1715–1720.

44. Iyer L, King CD, Whitington PF, et al. Genetic predisposition to the metabolism of irinotecan (CPT-11). Role of uridine diphosphate glucuronosyltransferase isoform 1A1 in the glucuronidation of its active metabolite (SN-38) in human liver microsomes. *J Clin Invest.* 1998;101(4):847–854.

45. Ando Y, Saka H, Ando M, et al. Polymorphisms of UDP-glucuronosyltransferase gene and irinotecan toxicity: a pharmacogenetic analysis. *Cancer Res.* 2000;60(24):6921–6926.

46. Innocenti F, Undevia SD, Iyer L, et al. Genetic variants in the UDP-glucuronosyltransferase 1A1 gene predict the risk of severe neutropenia of irinotecan. *J Clin Oncol.* 2004;22(8):1382–1388.

47. Marcuello E, Altes A, Menoyo A, Del Rio E, Gomez-Pardo M, Baiget M. UGT1A1 gene variations and irinotecan treatment in patients with metastatic colorectal cancer. *Br J Cancer.* 2004;91(4):678–682.

48. Rouits E, Boisdron-Celle M, Dumont A, Guerin O, Morel A, Gamelin E. Relevance of different UGT1A1 polymorphisms in irinotecan-induced toxicity: a molecular and clinical study of 75 patients. *Clin Cancer Res.* 2004;10(15):5151–5159.

49. Hu ZY, Yu Q, Pei Q, Guo C. Dose-dependent association between UGT1A1*28 genotype and irinotecan-induced neutropenia: low doses also increase risk. *Clin Cancer Res.* 2010;16(15):3832–3842.

50. Hu ZY, Yu Q, Zhao YS. Dose-dependent association between UGT1A1*28 polymorphism and irinotecan-induced diarrhoea: a meta-analysis. *Eur J Cancer.* 2010;46(10):1856–1865.

51. Palomaki GE, Bradley LA, Douglas MP, Kolor K, Dotson WD. Can UGT1A1 genotyping reduce morbidity and mortality in patients with metastatic colorectal cancer treated with irinotecan? An evidence-based review. *Genet Med.* 2009;11(1):21–34.

52. Obradovic M, Mrhar A, Kos M. Cost-effectiveness of UGT1A1 genotyping in second-line, high-dose, once every 3 weeks irinotecan monotherapy treatment of colorectal cancer. *Pharmacogenomics.* 2008;9(5):539–549.

53. Goetz MP, Knox SK, Suman VJ, et al. The impact of cytochrome P450 2D6 metabolism in women receiving adjuvant tamoxifen. *Breast Cancer Res Treat.* 2007;101(1):113–121.

54. Thurlimann B, Keshaviah A, Coates AS, et al. A comparison of letrozole and tamoxifen in postmenopausal women with early breast cancer. *N Engl J Med.* 2005;353(26):2747–2757.

55. Ingle JN, Suman VJ, Johnson PA, et al. Evaluation of tamoxifen plus letrozole with assessment of pharmacokinetic interaction in postmenopausal women with metastatic breast cancer. *Clin Cancer Res.* 1999;5(7): 1642–1649.

56. Lonning PE, Lien EA, Lundgren S, Kvinnsland S. Clinical pharmacokinetics of endocrine agents used in advanced breast cancer. *Clin Pharmacokinet.* 1992;22(5):327–358.

57. Jin Y, Desta Z, Stearns V, et al. CYP2D6 genotype, antidepressant use, and tamoxifen metabolism during adjuvant breast cancer treatment. *J Natl Cancer Inst.* 2005;97(1):30–39.

58. Stearns V, Johnson MD, Rae JM, et al. Active tamoxifen metabolite plasma concentrations after coadministration of tamoxifen and the selective serotonin reuptake inhibitor paroxetine. *J Natl Cancer Inst.* 2003;95(23):1758–1764.

59. Goetz MP, Rae JM, Suman VJ, et al. Pharmacogenetics of tamoxifen biotransformation is associated with clinical outcomes of efficacy and hot flashes. *J Clin Oncol.* 2005;23(36):9312–9318.

60. Leyland-Jones B, Regan MM, Bouzyk M, et al. Outcome according to CYP2D6 genotype among postmenopausal women with endocrine-responsive early invasive breast cancer randomized in the BIG 1-98 Trial. *Cancer Res.* 2010;70(24 suppl):Abstract number S1–S8.

61. Rae JM, Drury S, Hayes DF, et al. Lack of correlation between gene variants in tamoxifen metabolizing enzymes with primary endpoints in the ATAC Trial. *Cancer Res.* 2010;70(24 suppl):Abstract number S1–S7.

62. Sebolt-Leopold JS, English JM. Mechanisms of drug inhibition of signalling molecules. *Nature.* 2006;441(7092):457–462.

63. Manley PW, Cowan-Jacob SW, Buchdunger E, et al. Imatinib: a selective tyrosine kinase inhibitor. *Eur J Cancer.* 2002;38(suppl 5):S19–S27.

64. Capdeville R, Buchdunger E, Zimmermann J, Matter A. Glivec (STI571, imatinib), a rationally developed, targeted anticancer drug. *Nat Rev Drug Discov.* 2002;1(7):493–502.

65. Roskoski R Jr. STI-571: an anticancer protein-tyrosine kinase inhibitor. *Biochem Biophys Res Commun.* 2003;309(4):709–717.

66. Michor F, Hughes TP, Iwasa Y, et al. Dynamics of chronic myeloid leukaemia. *Nature.* 2005;435(7046):1267–1270.

67. Weisberg E, Manley PW, Cowan-Jacob SW, Hochhaus A, Griffin JD. Second generation inhibitors of BCR-ABL for the treatment of imatinib-resistant chronic myeloid leukaemia. *Nat Rev Cancer.* 2007;7(5):345–356.

68. le Coutre P, Tassi E, Varella-Garcia M, et al. Induction of resistance to the Abelson inhibitor STI571 in human leukemic cells through gene amplification. *Blood.* 2000;95(5):1758–1766.

69. Weisberg E, Griffin JD. Mechanism of resistance to the ABL tyrosine kinase inhibitor STI571 in BCR/ABL-transformed hematopoietic cell lines. *Blood.* 2000;95(11):3498–3505.

70. Gorre ME, Mohammed M, Ellwood K, et al. Clinical resistance to STI-571 cancer therapy caused by BCR-ABL gene mutation or amplification. *Science.* 2001;293(5531):876–880.

71. Schindler T, Bornmann W, Pellicena P, Miller WT, Clarkson B, Kuriyan J. Structural mechanism for STI-571 inhibition of Abelson tyrosine kinase. *Science.* 2000;289(5486):1938–1942.

72. Corbin AS, Buchdunger E, Pascal F, Druker BJ. Analysis of the structural basis of specificity of inhibition of the Abl kinase by STI571. *J Biol Chem.* 2002;277(35):32214–32219.

73. Soverini S, Martinelli G, Rosti G, et al. ABL mutations in late chronic phase chronic myeloid leukemia patients with up-front cytogenetic resistance to imatinib are associated with a greater likelihood of progression to blast crisis and shorter survival: a study by the GIMEMA Working Party on Chronic Myeloid Leukemia. *J Clin Oncol.* 2005;23(18):4100–4109.

74. Nicolini FE, Corm S, Le QH, et al. Mutation status and clinical outcome of 89 imatinib mesylate-resistant chronic myelogenous leukemia patients: a retrospective analysis from the French intergroup of CML (Fi(phi)-LMC GROUP). *Leukemia.* 2006;20(6):1061–1066.

75. Quintas-Cardama A, Cortes J. Molecular biology of bcr-abl1-positive chronic myeloid leukemia. *Blood.* 2009;113(8):1619–1630.

76. Barthe C, Gharbi MJ, Lagarde V, et al. Mutation in the ATP-binding site of BCR-ABL in a patient with chronic myeloid leukaemia with increasing resistance to STI571. *Br J Haematol.* 2002;119(1):109–111.

77. Branford S, Rudzki Z, Walsh S, et al. High frequency of point mutations clustered within the adenosine triphosphate-binding region of BCR/ABL in patients with chronic myeloid leukemia or Ph-positive acute lymphoblastic leukemia who develop imatinib (STI571) resistance. *Blood.* 2002;99(9):3472–3475.

78. Kantarjian H, Giles F, Wunderle L, et al. Nilotinib in imatinib-resistant CML and Philadelphia chromosome-positive ALL. *N Engl J Med.* 2006;354(24):2542–2551.

79. Manley PW, Cowan-Jacob SW, Mestan J. Advances in the structural biology, design and clinical development of Bcr-Abl kinase inhibitors for the treatment of chronic myeloid leukaemia. *Biochim Biophys Acta.* 2005;1754(1–2):3–13.

80. Das J, Chen P, Norris D, et al. 2-Aminothiazole as a novel kinase inhibitor template. Structure–activity relationship studies toward the discovery of N-(2-chloro-6-methylphenyl)-2-[[6-[4-(2-hydroxyethyl)-1-piperazinyl]-

81. Melnick JS, Janes J, Kim S, et al. An efficient rapid system for profiling the cellular activities of molecular libraries. *Proc Natl Acad Sci U S A.* 2006;103(9):3153–3158.

82. Tokarski JS, Newitt JA, Chang CY, et al. The structure of dasatinib (BMS-354825) bound to activated ABL kinase domain elucidates its inhibitory activity against imatinib-resistant ABL mutants. *Cancer Res.* 2006;66(11):5790–5797.

83. Cortes J, Rousselot P, Kim DW, et al. Dasatinib induces complete hematologic and cytogenetic responses in patients with imatinib-resistant or -intolerant chronic myeloid leukemia in blast crisis. *Blood.* 2007;109(8):3207–3213.

84. Talpaz M, Shah NP, Kantarjian H, et al. Dasatinib in imatinib-resistant Philadelphia chromosome-positive leukemias. *N Engl J Med.* 2006;354(24):2531–2541.

85. Fletcher JA, Rubin BP. KIT mutations in GIST. *Curr Opin Genet Dev.* 2007;17(1):3–7.

86. Corless CL, McGreevey L, Haley A, Town A, Heinrich MC. KIT mutations are common in incidental gastrointestinal stromal tumors one centimeter or less in size. *Am J Pathol.* 2002;160(5):1567–1572.

87. Tuveson DA, Willis NA, Jacks T, et al. STI571 inactivation of the gastrointestinal stromal tumor c-KIT oncoprotein: biological and clinical implications. *Oncogene.* 2001;20(36):5054–5058.

88. Gold JS, Dematteo RP. Combined surgical and molecular therapy: the gastrointestinal stromal tumor model. *Ann Surg.* 2006;244(2):176–184.

89. DeMatteo RP, Lewis JJ, Leung D, Mudan SS, Woodruff JM, Brennan MF. Two hundred gastrointestinal stromal tumors: recurrence patterns and prognostic factors for survival. *Ann Surg.* 2000;231(1):51–58.

90. Demetri GD. Identification and treatment of chemoresistant inoperable or metastatic GIST: experience with the selective tyrosine kinase inhibitor imatinib mesylate (STI571). *Eur J Cancer.* 2002;38(suppl 5):S52–S59.

91. Verweij J, van Oosterom A, Blay JY, et al. Imatinib mesylate (STI-571 Glivec, Gleevec) is an active agent for gastrointestinal stromal tumours, but does not yield responses in other soft-tissue sarcomas that are unselected for a molecular target. Results from an EORTC Soft Tissue and Bone Sarcoma Group phase II study. *Eur J Cancer.* 2003;39(14):2006–2011.

92. Verweij J, Casali PG, Zalcberg J, et al. Progression-free survival in gastrointestinal stromal tumours with high-dose imatinib: randomised trial. *Lancet.* 2004;364(9440):1127–1134.

93. Heinrich MC, Corless CL, Demetri GD, et al. Kinase mutations and imatinib response in patients with metastatic gastrointestinal stromal tumor. *J Clin Oncol.* 2003;21(23):4342–4349.

94. Tarn C, Merkel E, Canutescu AA, et al. Analysis of KIT mutations in sporadic and familial gastrointestinal stromal tumors: therapeutic implications through protein modeling. *Clin Cancer Res.* 2005;11(10):3668–3677.

95. Joensuu H. Gastrointestinal stromal tumor (GIST). *Ann Oncol.* 2006;17(suppl 10):x280–x286.

96. Heinrich MC, Corless CL. Gastric GI stromal tumors (GISTs): the role of surgery in the era of targeted therapy. *J Surg Oncol.* 2005;90(3):195–207 [discussion 207].

97. Heinrich MC, Corless CL, Blanke CD, et al. Molecular correlates of imatinib resistance in gastrointestinal stromal tumors. *J Clin Oncol.* 2006;24(29):4764–4774.

98. Joensuu H. Sunitinib for imatinib-resistant GIST. *Lancet.* 2006;368(9544):1303–1304.

99. Demetri GD, van Oosterom AT, Garrett CR, et al. Efficacy and safety of sunitinib in patients with advanced gastrointestinal stromal tumour after failure of imatinib: a randomised controlled trial. *Lancet.* 2006;368(9544):1329–1338.

100. Bauer S, Yu LK, Demetri GD, Fletcher JA. Heat shock protein 90 inhibition in imatinib-resistant gastrointestinal stromal tumor. *Cancer Res.* 2006;66(18):9153–9161.

101. Slamon DJ, Godolphin W, Jones LA, et al. Studies of the HER-2/neu proto-oncogene in human breast and ovarian cancer. *Science.* 1989;244(4905):707–712.

102. Perren TJ. c-erbB-2 oncogene as a prognostic marker in breast cancer. *Br J Cancer.* 1991;63(3):328–332.

103. Roskoski R Jr. The ErbB/HER receptor protein-tyrosine kinases and cancer. *Biochem Biophys Res Commun.* 2004;319(1):1–11.

104. Nahta R, Esteva FJ. Herceptin: mechanisms of action and resistance. *Cancer Lett.* 2006;232(2):123–138.

105. Baselga J, Tripathy D, Mendelsohn J, et al. Phase II study of weekly intravenous trastuzumab (Herceptin) in patients with HER2/neu-overexpressing metastatic breast cancer. *Semin Oncol.* 1999;26(4 suppl 12):78–83.

106. Vogel CL, Cobleigh MA, Tripathy D, et al. Efficacy and safety of trastuzumab as a single agent in first-line treatment of HER2-overexpressing metastatic breast cancer. *J Clin Oncol.* 2002;20(3):719–726.

107. Esteva FJ, Valero V, Booser D, et al. Phase II study of weekly docetaxel and trastuzumab for patients with HER-2-overexpressing metastatic breast cancer. *J Clin Oncol.* 2002;20(7):1800–1808.

108. Seidman AD, Fornier MN, Esteva FJ, et al. Weekly trastuzumab and paclitaxel therapy for metastatic breast cancer with analysis of efficacy by HER2 immunophenotype and gene amplification. *J Clin Oncol.* 2001;19(10):2587–2595.

109. Slamon DJ, Leyland-Jones B, Shak S, et al. Use of chemotherapy plus a monoclonal antibody against HER2 for metastatic breast cancer that overexpresses HER2. *N Engl J Med.* 2001;344(11):783–792.

110. Azzoli CG, Krug LM, Miller VA, Kris MG, Mass R. Trastuzumab in the treatment of non-small cell lung cancer. *Semin Oncol.* 2002;29(1 suppl 4):59–65.

111. Brabender J, Danenberg KD, Metzger R, et al. Epidermal growth factor receptor and HER2-neu mRNA expression in non-small cell lung cancer is correlated with survival. *Clin Cancer Res.* 2001;7(7):1850–1855.

112. Shi D, He G, Cao S, et al. Overexpression of the c-erbB-2/neu-encoded p185 protein in primary lung cancer. *Mol Carcinog.* 1992;5(3):213–218.

113. Shigematsu H, Takahashi T, Nomura M, et al. Somatic mutations of the HER2 kinase domain in lung adenocarcinomas. *Cancer Res.* 2005;65(5):1642–1646.

114. Stephens P, Hunter C, Bignell G, et al. Lung cancer: intragenic ERBB2 kinase mutations in tumours. *Nature.* 2004;431(7008):525–526.

115. Clamon G, Herndon J, Kern J, et al. Lack of trastuzumab activity in non-small cell lung carcinoma with overexpression of erb-B2: 39810: a phase II trial of Cancer and Leukemia Group B. *Cancer.* 2005;103(8):1670–1675.

116. Gatzemeier U, Groth G, Butts C, et al. Randomized phase II trial of gemcitabine–cisplatin with or without trastuzumab in HER2-positive non-small-cell lung cancer. *Ann Oncol.* 2004;15(1):19–27.

117. Langer CJ, Stephenson P, Thor A, Vangel M, Johnson DH. Trastuzumab in the treatment of advanced non-small-cell lung cancer: is there a role? Focus on Eastern Cooperative Oncology Group study 2598. *J Clin Oncol.* 2004;22(7):1180–1187.

118. Zinner RG, Glisson BS, Fossella FV, et al. Trastuzumab in combination with cisplatin and gemcitabine in patients with Her2-overexpressing, untreated, advanced non-small cell lung cancer: report of a phase II trial and findings regarding optimal identification of patients with Her2-overexpressing disease. *Lung Cancer.* 2004;44(1):99–110.

119. Nahta R, Yu D, Hung MC, Hortobagyi GN, Esteva FJ. Mechanisms of disease: understanding resistance to HER2-targeted therapy in human breast cancer. *Nat Clin Pract Oncol.* 2006;3(5):269–280.

120. Price-Schiavi SA, Jepson S, Li P, et al. Rat Muc4 (sialomucin complex) reduces binding of anti-ErbB2 antibodies to tumor cell surfaces, a potential mechanism for Herceptin resistance. *Int J Cancer.* 2002;99(6):783–791.

121. Nagy P, Friedlander E, Tanner M, et al. Decreased accessibility and lack of activation of ErbB2 in JIMT-1, a Herceptin-resistant, MUC4-expressing breast cancer cell line. *Cancer Res.* 2005;65(2):473–482.

122. Motoyama AB, Hynes NE, Lane HA. The efficacy of ErbB receptor-targeted anticancer therapeutics is influenced by the availability of epidermal growth factor-related peptides. *Cancer Res.* 2002;62(11):3151–3158.

123. Lu Y, Zi X, Zhao Y, Mascarenhas D, Pollak M. Insulin-like growth factor-I receptor signaling and resistance to trastuzumab (Herceptin). *J Natl Cancer Inst.* 2001;93(24):1852–1857.

124. Nahta R, Yuan LX, Zhang B, Kobayashi R, Esteva FJ. Insulin-like growth factor-I receptor/human epidermal growth factor receptor 2 heterodimerization contributes to trastuzumab resistance of breast cancer cells. *Cancer Res.* 2005;65(23):11118–11128.

125. Yakes FM, Chinratanalab W, Ritter CA, King W, Seelig S, Arteaga CL. Herceptin-induced inhibition of phosphatidylinositol-3 kinase and Akt Is required for antibody-mediated effects on p27, cyclin D1, and antitumor action. *Cancer Res.* 2002;62(14):4132–4141.

126. Chan CT, Metz MZ, Kane SE. Differential sensitivities of trastuzumab (Herceptin)-resistant human breast cancer cells to phosphoinositide-3 kinase (PI-3K) and epidermal growth factor receptor (EGFR) kinase inhibitors. *Breast Cancer Res Treat.* 2005;91(2):187–201.

127. Nagata Y, Lan KH, Zhou X, et al. PTEN activation contributes to tumor inhibition by trastuzumab, and loss of PTEN predicts trastuzumab resistance in patients. *Cancer Cell.* 2004;6(2):117–127.

128. Agus DB, Akita RW, Fox WD, et al. Targeting ligand-activated ErbB2 signaling inhibits breast and prostate tumor growth. *Cancer Cell.* 2002;2(2):127–137.

129. Cho HS, Mason K, Ramyar KX, et al. Structure of the extracellular region of HER2 alone and in complex with the Herceptin Fab. *Nature.* 2003;421(6924):756–760.

130. Franklin MC, Carey KD, Vajdos FF, Leahy DJ, de Vos AM, Sliwkowski MX. Insights into ErbB signaling from the structure of the ErbB2–pertuzumab complex. *Cancer Cell.* 2004;5(4):317–328.

131. Nahta R, Hung MC, Esteva FJ. The HER-2-targeting antibodies trastuzumab and pertuzumab synergistically inhibit the survival of breast cancer cells. *Cancer Res.* 2004;64(7):2343–2346.

132. Xia W, Gerard CM, Liu L, Baudson NM, Ory TL, Spector NL. Combining lapatinib (GW572016), a small molecule inhibitor of ErbB1 and ErbB2 tyrosine kinases, with therapeutic anti-ErbB2 antibodies enhances apoptosis of ErbB2-overexpressing breast cancer cells. *Oncogene.* 2005;24(41):6213–6221.

133. Xia W, Bacus S, Hegde P, et al. A model of acquired autoresistance to a potent ErbB2 tyrosine kinase inhibitor and a therapeutic strategy to prevent its onset in breast cancer. *Proc Natl Acad Sci U S A.* 2006;103(20):7795–7800.

134. Geyer CE, Forster J, Lindquist D, et al. Lapatinib plus capecitabine for HER2-positive advanced breast cancer. *N Engl J Med.* 2006;355(26):2733–2743.

135. Scaltriti M, Rojo F, Ocaña A, et al. Expression of p95HER2, a truncated form of the HER2 receptor, and response to anti-HER2 therapies in breast cancer. *J Natl Cancer Inst.* 2007;99(8):628–638.

136. Sáez R, Molina MA, Ramsey EE, et al. p95Her-2 predicts worse outcome in patients with Her-2-positive breast cancer. *Clin Cancer Res.* 2006;12(2):424–431.

137. Chang JCN, Mayer IA, Forero-Torres A, et al. TBCRC 006: a multicenter phase II study of neoadjuvant lapatinib and trastuzumab in patients with HER2-overexpressing breast cancer. *J Clin Oncol.* 2011;29(suppl):Abstract number 505.

138. Sridhar SS, Seymour L, Shepherd FA. Inhibitors of epidermal-growth-factor receptors: a review of clinical research with a focus on non-small-cell lung cancer. *Lancet Oncol.* 2003;4(7):397–406.

139. Fukuoka M, Yano S, Giaccone G, et al. Multi-institutional randomized phase II trial of gefitinib for previously treated patients with advanced non-small-cell lung cancer (the IDEAL 1 Trial) [corrected]. *J Clin Oncol.* 2003;21(12):2237–2246.

140. Kris MG, Natale RB, Herbst RS, et al. Efficacy of gefitinib, an inhibitor of the epidermal growth factor receptor tyrosine kinase, in symptomatic patients with non-small cell lung cancer: a randomized trial. *JAMA.* 2003;290(16):2149–2158.

141. Lynch TJ, Bell DW, Sordella R, et al. Activating mutations in the epidermal growth factor receptor underlying responsiveness of non-small-cell lung cancer to gefitinib. *N Engl J Med.* 2004;350(21):2129–2139.

142. Paez JG, Janne PA, Lee JC, et al. EGFR mutations in lung cancer: correlation with clinical response to gefitinib therapy. *Science.* 2004;304(5676):1497–1500.

143. Pao W, Miller VA, Venkatraman E, Kris MG. Predicting sensitivity of non-small-cell lung cancer to gefitinib: is there a role for P-Akt? *J Natl Cancer Inst.* 2004;96(15):1117–1119.

144. Guo M, Liu S, Lu F. Gefitinib-sensitizing mutations in esophageal carcinoma. *N Engl J Med.* 2006;354(20):2193–2194.

145. Gwak GY, Yoon JH, Shin CM, et al. Detection of response-predicting mutations in the kinase domain of the epidermal growth factor receptor gene in cholangiocarcinomas. *J Cancer Res Clin Oncol.* 2005;131(10):649–652.

146. Kwak EL, Jankowski J, Thayer SP, et al. Epidermal growth factor receptor kinase domain mutations in esophageal and pancreatic adenocarcinomas. *Clin Cancer Res.* 2006;12(14 pt 1):4283–4287.

147. Lee JW, Soung YH, Kim SY, et al. Somatic mutations of EGFR gene in squamous cell carcinoma of the head and neck. *Clin Cancer Res.* 2005;11(8):2879–2882.

148. Nagahara H, Mimori K, Ohta M, et al. Somatic mutations of epidermal growth factor receptor in colorectal carcinoma. *Clin Cancer Res.* 2005;11(4):1368–1371.

149. Schilder RJ, Sill MW, Chen X, et al. Phase II study of gefitinib in patients with relapsed or persistent ovarian or primary peritoneal carcinoma and evaluation of epidermal growth factor receptor mutations and immunohistochemical expression: a Gynecologic Oncology Group Study. *Clin Cancer Res.* 2005;11(15):5539–5548.

150. Shigematsu H, Lin L, Takahashi T, et al. Clinical and biological features associated with epidermal growth factor receptor gene mutations in lung cancers. *J Natl Cancer Inst.* 2005;97(5):339–346.

151. Mellinghoff IK, Wang MY, Vivanco I, et al. Molecular determinants of the response of glioblastomas to EGFR kinase inhibitors. *N Engl J Med.* 2005;353(19):2012–2024.

152. Ji H, Zhao X, Yuza Y, et al. Epidermal growth factor receptor variant III mutations in lung tumorigenesis and sensitivity to tyrosine kinase inhibitors. *Proc Natl Acad Sci U S A.* 2006;103(20):7817–7822.

153. Kaye FJ. A curious link between epidermal growth factor receptor amplification and survival: effect of "allele dilution" on gefitinib sensitivity? *J Natl Cancer Inst.* 2005;97(9):621–623.

154. Riely GJ, Politi KA, Miller VA, Pao W. Update on epidermal growth factor receptor mutations in non-small cell lung cancer. *Clin Cancer Res.* 2006;12(24):7232–7241.

155. Riely GJ, Pao W, Pham D, et al. Clinical course of patients with non-small cell lung cancer and epidermal growth factor receptor exon 19 and exon 21 mutations treated with gefitinib or erlotinib. *Clin Cancer Res.* 2006;12(3 pt 1):839–844.

156. Bell DW, Lynch TJ, Haserlat SM, et al. Epidermal growth factor receptor mutations and gene amplification in non-small-cell lung cancer: molecular analysis of the IDEAL/INTACT gefitinib trials. *J Clin Oncol.* 2005;23(31):8081–8092.

157. Han SW, Kim TY, Hwang PG, et al. Predictive and prognostic impact of epidermal growth factor receptor mutation in non-small-cell lung cancer patients treated with gefitinib. *J Clin Oncol.* 2005;23(11):2493–2501.

158. Mitsudomi T, Kosaka T, Endoh H, et al. Mutations of the epidermal growth factor receptor gene predict prolonged survival after gefitinib treatment in patients with non-small-cell lung cancer with postoperative recurrence. *J Clin Oncol.* 2005;23(11):2513–2520.

159. Tsao MS, Sakurada A, Cutz JC, et al. Erlotinib in lung cancer—molecular and clinical predictors of outcome. *N Engl J Med.* 2005;353(2):133–144.

160. Uramoto H, Sugio K, Oyama T, et al. Epidermal growth factor receptor mutations are associated with gefitinib sensitivity in non-small cell lung cancer in Japanese. *Lung Cancer.* 2006;51(1):71–77.

161. Inoue A, Suzuki T, Fukuhara T, et al. Prospective phase II study of gefitinib for chemotherapy-naive patients with advanced non-small-cell lung cancer with epidermal growth factor receptor gene mutations. *J Clin Oncol.* 2006;24(21):3340–3346.

162. Sunaga N, Tomizawa Y, Yanagitani N, et al. Phase II prospective study of the efficacy of gefitinib for the treatment of stage III/IV non-small cell lung cancer with EGFR mutations, irrespective of previous chemotherapy. *Lung Cancer.* 2007;56(3):383–389.

163. Sutani A, Nagai Y, Udagawa K, et al. Gefitinib for non-small-cell lung cancer patients with epidermal growth factor receptor gene mutations screened by peptide nucleic acid-locked nucleic acid PCR clamp. *Br J Cancer.* 2006;95(11):1483–1489.

164. Eberhard DA, Johnson BE, Amler LC, et al. Mutations in the epidermal growth factor receptor and in KRAS are predictive and prognostic indicators in patients with non-small-cell lung cancer treated with chemotherapy alone and in combination with erlotinib. *J Clin Oncol.* 2005;23(25):5900–5909.

165. Maemondo M, Inoue A, Kobayashi K, et al. Gefitinib or chemotherapy for non-small-cell lung cancer with mutated EGFR. *N Engl J Med.* 2010;362(25):2380–2388.

166. Kobayashi S, Boggon TJ, Dayaram T, et al. EGFR mutation and resistance of non-small-cell lung cancer to gefitinib. *N Engl J Med.* 2005;352(8):786–792.

167. Pao W, Miller VA, Politi KA, et al. Acquired resistance of lung adenocarcinomas to gefitinib or erlotinib is associated with a second mutation in the EGFR kinase domain. *PLoS Med.* 2005;2(3):e73.

168. Bell DW, Gore I, Okimoto RA, et al. Inherited susceptibility to lung cancer may be associated with the T790M drug resistance mutation in EGFR. *Nat Genet.* 2005;37(12):1315–1316.

169. Kobayashi S, Ji H, Yuza Y, et al. An alternative inhibitor overcomes resistance caused by a mutation of the epidermal growth factor receptor. *Cancer Res.* 2005;65(16):7096–7101.

170. Kwak EL, Sordella R, Bell DW, et al. Irreversible inhibitors of the EGF receptor may circumvent acquired resistance to gefitinib. *Proc Natl Acad Sci U S A.* 2005;102(21):7665–7670.

171. Kakiuchi S, Daigo Y, Ishikawa N, et al. Prediction of sensitivity of advanced non-small cell lung cancers to gefitinib (Iressa, ZD1839). *Hum Mol Genet.* 2004;13(24):3029–3043.

172. Zhou BB, Peyton M, He B, et al. Targeting ADAM-mediated ligand cleavage to inhibit HER3 and EGFR pathways in non-small cell lung cancer. *Cancer Cell.* 2006;10(1):39–50.

173. Cappuzzo F, Varella-Garcia M, Shigematsu H, et al. Increased HER2 gene copy number is associated with response to gefitinib therapy in epidermal growth factor receptor-positive non-small-cell lung cancer patients. *J Clin Oncol.* 2005;23(22):5007–5018.

174. Wang SE, Narasanna A, Perez-Torres M, et al. HER2 kinase domain mutation results in constitutive phosphorylation and activation of HER2 and EGFR and resistance to EGFR tyrosine kinase inhibitors. *Cancer Cell.* 2006;10(1):25–38.

175. Pao W, Wang TY, Riely GJ, et al. KRAS mutations and primary resistance of lung adenocarcinomas to gefitinib or erlotinib. *PLoS Med.* 2005;2(1):e17.

176. Sordella R, Bell DW, Haber DA, Settleman J. Gefitinib-sensitizing EGFR mutations in lung cancer activate anti-apoptotic pathways. *Science.* 2004;305(5687):1163–1167.

177. Cappuzzo F, Magrini E, Ceresoli GL, et al. Akt phosphorylation and gefitinib efficacy in patients with advanced non-small-cell lung cancer. *J Natl Cancer Inst.* 2004;96(15):1133–1141.

178. Engelman JA, Zejnullahu K, Mitsudomi T, et al. MET amplification leads to gefitinib resistance in lung cancer by activating ERBB3 signaling. *Science.* 2007;316(5827):1039–1043.

179. Chen G, Gharib TG, Huang CC, et al. Discordant protein and mRNA expression in lung adenocarcinomas. *Mol Cell Proteomics.* 2002;1(4):304–313.

180. Griffin TJ, Gygi SP, Ideker T, et al. Complementary profiling of gene expression at the transcriptome and proteome levels in *Saccharomyces cerevisiae. Mol Cell Proteomics.* 2002;1(4):323–333.

181. Ramaswamy S, Tamayo P, Rifkin R, et al. Multiclass cancer diagnosis using tumor gene expression signatures. *Proc Natl Acad Sci U S A.* 2001;98(26):15149–15154.

182. Frades I, Matthiesen R. Overview on techniques in cluster analysis. *Methods Mol Biol.* 2010;593:81–107.

183. Benvenuti S, Sartore-Bianchi A, Di Nicolantonio F, et al. Oncogenic activation of the RAS/RAF signaling pathway impairs the response of metastatic colorectal cancers to anti-epidermal growth factor receptor antibody therapies. *Cancer Res.* 2007;67(6):2643–2648.

184. Lievre A, Bachet JB, Le Corre D, et al. KRAS mutation status is predictive of response to cetuximab therapy in colorectal cancer. *Cancer Res.* 2006;66(8):3992–3995.

185. Allegra CJ, Jessup JM, Somerfield MR, et al. American Society of Clinical Oncology provisional clinical opinion: testing for KRAS gene mutations in patients with metastatic colorectal carcinoma to predict response to anti-epidermal growth factor receptor monoclonal antibody therapy. *J Clin Oncol.* 2009;27(12):2091–2096.

186. Ingle JN. Genome-wide case–control study of musculoskeletal adverse events and functional genomics in women receiving aromatase inhibitors: going beyond associations. *Breast Cancer Res.* 2010;12(suppl 4):S17.

187. Walsh AC, Feulner JA, Reilly A. Evidence for functionally significant polymorphism of human glutamate cysteine ligase catalytic subunit: association with glutathione levels and drug resistance in the National Cancer Institute tumor cell line panel. *Toxicol Sci.* 2001;61(2):218–223.

188. Charasson V, Hillaire-Buys D, Solassol I, et al. Involvement of gene poly-morphisms of the folate pathway enzymes in gene expression and anti-cancer drug sensitivity using the NCI-60 panel as a model. *Eur J Cancer.* 2009;45(13):2391–2401.

189. Eisen MB, Spellman PT, Brown PO, Botstein D. Cluster analysis and display of genome-wide expression patterns. *Proc Natl Acad Sci U S A.* 1998;95(25):14863–14868.

190. Baird RD, Kitzen J, Clarke PA, et al. Phase I safety, pharmacokinetic, and pharmacogenomic trial of ES-285, a novel marine cytotoxic agent, admin-istered to adult patients with advanced solid tumors. *Mol Cancer Ther.* 2009;8(6):1430–1437.

191. Rockett JC, Burczynski ME, Fornace AJ, Herrmann PC, Krawetz SA, Dix DJ. Surrogate tissue analysis: monitoring toxicant exposure and health sta-tus of inaccessible tissues through the analysis of accessible tissues and cells. *Toxicol Appl Pharmacol.* 2004;194(2):189–199.

192. Sims P, Coffman RL, Hessel EM. Biomarkers measuring the activity of Toll-like receptor ligands in clinical development programs. *Methods Mol Biol.* 2009;517:415–440.

193. DePrimo SE, Wong LM, Khatry DB, et al. Expression profiling of blood samples from an SU5416 phase III metastatic colorectal cancer clinical trial: a novel strategy for biomarker identification. *BMC Cancer.* 2003;3:3.

194. Panelli MC, Wang E, Phan G, et al. Gene-expression profiling of the response of peripheral blood mononuclear cells and melanoma metastases to systemic IL-2 administration. *Genome Biol.* 2002;3(7):RESEARCH0035.

195. Twine NC, Stover JA, Marshall B, et al. Disease-associated expression pro-files in peripheral blood mononuclear cells from patients with advanced renal cell carcinoma. *Cancer Res.* 2003;63(18):6069–6075.

196. Ayers M, Symmans WF, Stec J, et al. Gene expression profiles predict complete pathologic response to neoadjuvant paclitaxel and fluorouracil, doxorubicin, and cyclophosphamide chemotherapy in breast cancer. *J Clin Oncol.* 2004;22(12):2284–2293.

197. Lossos IS, Czerwinski DK, Alizadeh AA, et al. Prediction of survival in diffuse large-B-cell lymphoma based on the expression of six genes. *N Engl J Med.* 2004;350(18):1828–1837.

198. Rosenwald A, Wright G, Chan WC, et al. The use of molecular profiling to predict survival after chemotherapy for diffuse large-B-cell lymphoma. *N Engl J Med.* 2002;346(25):1937–1947.

199. van de Vijver MJ, He YD, van't Veer LJ, et al. A gene-expression signature as a predictor of survival in breast cancer. *N Engl J Med.* 2002;347(25):1999–2009.

200. Gandara DR, Kawaguchi T, Crowley J, Moon J, Furuse K, Kawahara M, Teramukai S, Ohe Y, Kubota K, Williamson SK, Gautschi O, Lenz HJ, McLeod HL, Lara PN Jr, Coltman CA Jr, Fukuoka M, Saijo N, Fukushima M, Mack PC. Japanese-US common-arm analysis of pacli-taxel plus carboplatin in advanced non-small-cell lung cancer: a model for assessing population-related pharmacogenomics. *J Clin Oncol.* 2009;27(21):3540–3546.

201. de Jong FA, Marsh S, Mathijssen RH, King C, Verweij J, Sparreboom A, McLeod HL. ABCG2 pharmacogenetics: ethnic differences in allele fre-quency and assessment of influence on irinotecan disposition. *Clin Cancer Res.* 2004;10(17):5889–5894.

202. Anderson DC, Gomez-Mancilla B, Spear BB, et al. Elements of informed consent for pharmacogenetic research; perspective of the pharmacogenetics working group. *Pharmacogenomics J.* 2002;2(5):284–292.

203. Flowers CR, Veenstra D. The role of cost-effectiveness analysis in the era of pharmacogenomics. *Pharmacoeconomics.* 2004;22(8):481–493.

14

Psychiatry and Addiction Medicine

David A. Mrazek, MD, FRCPsych

LEARNING OBJECTIVES

- Discuss pharmacogenomic implications as it relates to psychiatric illness.

- Outline how pharmacogenomics relates to response to a variety of drugs used in the treatment of various psychiatric diseases.

- Review the use of pharmacogenomic testing as it relates to the treatment of various psychiatric diseases.

It is now possible to use genetic testing to minimize adverse responses to psychiatric medications and to increase the probability of identifying medications that will be more likely to provide a therapeutic response for an individual patient.[1] It has been known for many years that variations in drug-metabolizing enzyme genes (DME genes), such as the cytochrome P450 2D6 gene (CYP2D6), are associated with differential pharmacokinetic profiles for psychotropic medications.[2] While individual clinical laboratories began testing for drug-metabolizing genes before 2004, the FDA approval of the AmpliChip developed by Roche Diagnostics was a landmark event that facilitated the utilization of clinical genotyping in a greatly expanded number of clinical settings.[3]

DRUG-METABOLIZING ENZYME GENES RELEVANT FOR GUIDING TREATMENT WHEN USING PSYCHOTROPIC MEDICATIONS

Variations in the DME genes have been shown to alter the responses of patients to psychotropic medications. Specifically, the cytochrome P450 family of genes has been studied extensively. Five of the many cytochrome P450 genes that are particularly relevant for the management of psychotropic medications will be reviewed.

The Cytochrome P450 2D6 Gene

The CYP2D6 was the first DME gene that was widely tested to identify poor metabolizers. Additionally, the identification of ultrarapid metabolizers of 2D6 substrate medications has proven to be clinically useful. There are more than 70 medications that are currently metabolized by the 2D6 enzyme. Many of these drugs are widely used psychotropic medications.

CYP2D6 is located on the 22nd chromosome and codes for the CYP2D6 enzyme. It is highly variable and there are currently more than 100 formally recognized variants. These CYP2D6 allelic variants have been classified as being upregulated, normal, deficient, or completely inactive. A variety of methodologies for predicting 2D6 phenotypes based on CYP2D6 genotypes have been suggested. However, the most widely used methodologies for phenotype specification are designed to identify patients as having one of four metabolic capacities. These categories are usually labeled as poor, intermediate, extensive (i.e., normal), and ultrarapid.

There is considerable variability in the allele frequency of 2D6 gene variants based on the ancestral origin of a population. For example, the completely inactive *3 allele is essentially found only in European populations. Similarly, the deficient *17 allele is primarily found in sub-Saharan Africa populations. Yet another example is the *10 allele, which is the most common allele found in Japanese populations.[4]

The results of pharmacogenomic testing provide an estimate of a metabolic capacity phenotype. However, a more active genotype can produce a CYP2D6 enzyme that is subsequently inhibited as a consequence of a drug interaction. Strong inhibition of patients who have one or even two normal CYP2D6 alleles can result in decreased metabolic capacity. However, poor metabolizers who have two inactive copies of the 2D6 gene have no 2D6 metabolic capacity. Consequently, the metabolism of these individuals cannot be further inhibited.

While many antidepressant medications are metabolized to some degree by the 2D6 enzyme, there are five antidepressants that are primarily metabolized by 2D6. These include two selective serotonin reuptake inhibitors, fluoxetine and paroxetine, the selective norepinephrine reuptake inhibitor venlafaxine, and two tricyclic antidepressants, desipramine and nortriptyline.

Similarly, many antipsychotic medications have some 2D6 enzyme involvement in their metabolism. However, there are five antipsychotic medications that are predominantly metabolized by 2D6. These include four typical antipsychotic medications, chlorpromazine, thioridazine, haloperidol, and perphenazine, as well as the atypical antipsychotic medication, risperidone.

Atomoxetine is a medication that is used for the treatment of attention deficit hyperactivity disorder. The primary mode of metabolism of atomoxetine is also by the 2D6 enzyme. Caution in using atomoxetine is advised in patients who are poor CYP2D6 metabolizers, given that they may achieve a 10-fold higher AUC and a 5-fold higher peak concentration to a given dose. Consequently, poor metabolizers are at a higher rate for the adverse effects when prescribed standard doses of atomoxetine.[5]

Some analgesics such as codeine and tramadol are prodrugs. A prodrug is an inactive compound and must be transformed to an active metabolite in order to have a therapeutic effect. In the case of codeine, its active metabolite is morphine. A patient must have some CYP2D6 metabolic capacity for this transformation from codeine to morphine to take place.

A primary consideration in treatment of patients with 2D6 substrate medications is that those patients who have diminished metabolic capacity must be treated with lower than traditional doses. Conversely, patients who have ultrarapid CYP2D6 metabolic capacity are unlikely to respond to treatment with 2D6 substrate medications at traditional doses.

The Cytochrome P450 2C19 Gene

The cytochrome P450 2C19 gene (CYP2C19) is a large gene that codes for an enzyme containing 490 amino acids. CYP2C19 is somewhat less variable than 2D6. However, there are CYP2C19 alleles that are upregulated, normal, have decreased metabolic activity, or are completely inactive. Like CYP2D6, CYP2C19 has dramatic variation in allelic distributions based on geographical ancestry. For example, patients who are of Asian ancestry are more likely to have intermediate or poor metabolic 2C19 phenotypes than patients of European ancestry.

Both citalopram and escitalopram are primarily metabolized by the 2C19 enzyme as are imipramine and amitriptyline. In contrast to the 2D6 enzyme, the 2C19 enzyme usually plays a relatively minor role in the metabolism of antipsychotic medications.

The Cytochrome P450 1A2 Gene

The cytochrome P450 1A2 gene (CYP1A2) is the only commonly genotyped cytochrome P450 enzyme drug-metabolizing gene that is easily inducible. CYP1A2 is located on chromosome 15 and codes for the 1A2 enzyme composed of 516 amino acids. Allele frequency of the inducible CYP1A2 allele (i.e.,*1F) has been reported to be approximately 33% in populations of European ancestry. The most common inducer of 1A2 activity is tobacco smoke.

Fluvoxamine is an antidepressant that is primarily metabolized by the 1A2 enzyme. However, the CYP1A2 enzyme also plays a role in the metabolism of duloxetine, clomipramine, and imipramine. The 1A2 enzyme plays an important role in the metabolism of both clozapine and olanzapine. Given that alleles of this gene are inducible when patients are exposed to tobacco smoke, induction can result in clinical complications of acutely psychotic patients who have an enhanced 1A2 metabolic capacity.

The Cytochrome P450 2B6 Gene

The cytochrome P450 2B6 gene (CYP2B6) is located on chromosome 19 and consists of 27,098 nucleotides. CYP2B6 codes for the 2B6 enzyme composed of 491 amino acids. It is the primary enzyme for the metabolism of bupropion, which is used both as an antidepressant and to decrease craving for nicotine.[6]

A specific polymorphism of CYP2B6 has been demonstrated to result in a coding change that decreases the functionality of the enzyme. Patients with the T allele of this polymorphism are less likely to respond to bupropion treatment.[7] CYP2B6 also may influence nicotine replacement therapy as it can metabolize nicotine.

The Cytochrome P450 2A6 Gene

The cytochrome P450 2A6 gene (CYP2A6) is located on chromosome 19 and consists of 6,909 nucleotides. CYP2A6 codes for the 2A6 enzyme that is composed of 494 amino acids. It plays a major role in the metabolism of nicotine and consequently slow CYP2A6 metabolizers are able to achieve higher levels of plasma nicotine when taking standard nicotine replacement therapy.

PHARMACOGENOMIC TARGET GENES RELEVANT FOR GUIDING TREATMENT WHEN USING PSYCHOTROPIC MEDICATIONS

The term "target gene" refers to those genes that code for proteins that play a role in the pharmacodynamic response of patients to medications. A pharmacodynamic response requires that the patient have an adequate exposure to the medication. The most common target genes of interest for psychiatric pharmacogenomic testing are neurotransmitter transporter genes and neurotransmitter receptor genes. The effectiveness of a transporter molecule to facilitate the "reuptake" of a neurotransmitter to the interior of the neuron has implications for psychotropic medications that influence the reuptake process. For example, the serotonin transporter protein is the primary target of selective serotonin reuptake inhibitors. As a consequence of this inhibition, the concentration of serotonin in the neural cleft is increased with the objective of achieving a decrease in the severity of depressive symptoms. Neurotransmitter receptors, similarly, are variable and this variation can result in differences in their sensitivity to medications. Genetic variance has been associated with variation in sensitivity.

Serotonin Transporter Gene

The serotonin transporter gene (SLC6A4) is the most widely studied pharmacogenomically relevant target gene that has been demonstrated to predict the probability of psychotropic medication response. SLC6A4 is located on chromosome 17 and codes for the serotonin transporter protein that plays a primary role in the reuptake of serotonin in the neural synapse.

The most widely studied variant of SLC6A4 is the indel promoter polymorphism, which is frequently referred to as 5HTTLPR. This indel consists of a variant that is either 43 or 44 base pairs (bp) in size. There are actually many variations of both the long allele and the short allele. Furthermore, there has been some evidence that there is an interaction between a single nucleotide polymorphism (SNP) (i.e., rs25531) located immediately upstream of the indel polymorphism and the activity level of the long allele of the transporter protein.

Yet another significant variant of SLC6A4 is a variable number tandem repeat (VNTR) located in intron 2. This variant is sometimes referred to as the STin2 VNTR. Four variants of this VNTR have been reported. The most common alleles are the 10- and 12-repeat.

Variations in SLC6A4 allele frequencies occur across ancestral populations. For example, the long allele of the indel polymorphism occurs with an allele frequency of approximately 82% in African American populations. In contrast, the frequency of the long allele is only 20% in Japanese populations.

The most extensive work related to pharmacogenomic variability of SLC6A4 focused on the antidepressant medication response to selective serotonin reuptake inhibitor medications. Early studies of European populations reported that patients with the long form of the indel promoter polymorphism were more likely to respond to medications such as fluvoxamine.[8] This finding of a better response in patients who are homozygous for the long allele has not been demonstrated in every study. In some Asian populations, the more common short allele has been associated with better response. However, a large study of citalopram in patients of European ancestry reported an association between indel promoter polymorphism and the second intron VNTR and medication response.[9] A meta-analysis of 15 studies concluded that patients who are homozygous for the long allele and are of European ancestry have a more consistent therapeutic response to SSRI treatment.[10]

The Serotonin 2A Receptor Gene

The serotonin 2A receptor gene (HTR2A) has a number of common variants that have been associated with psychotropic medication response. HTR2A is located on the 13th chromosome and codes for the serotonin 2A receptor.

Two widely studied HTR2A variants are rs6311 (i.e., −1438G/A) and rs6313 (i.e., 102T/C). These two variants are believed to be in almost complete linkage disequilibrium. As a consequence of this linkage disequilibrium, the guanine allele of rs6311 is linked to the cytosine allele of rs6313. Conversely, the adenine allele rs6311 is paired with the thymine allele of rs6313.

Yet another important variant of HTR2A is rs7997012. This variant is a SNP in the second intron but has been associated with medication response. Specifically, patients with this second intron variant who have the adenine allele have been reported to have a better response to citalopram than patients without this allele.[11] It has also been reported that variance in rs6313 is associated with greater intolerance to paroxetine.[12]

Variants of HTR2A have been associated with extrapyramidal symptoms.[13] Specifically, the cytosine allele of rs6313 has been shown to be associated with dyskinesia in schizophrenic patients.

The Serotonin 2C Receptor Gene

The serotonin 2C receptor gene (HTR2C) has a number of common variants that have been associated with psychotropic medication response. HTR2C is located on the 13th chromosome and codes for the serotonin 2C receptor. The cytosine allele of rs3813929 (i.e.,−759C/T) has been consistently associated with weight gain in patients taking antipsychotic medications. A meta-analysis of the association between the −759C/T variance and weight gain concluded that the thymine allele was associated with less weight gain.[14] As a result, the prescription of atypical antipsychotic medications that have been demonstrated to stimulate weight gain should be minimized in patients who do not have a copy of the protective thymine allele.

GENES ASSOCIATED WITH ANTICRAVING MEDICATION RESPONSE

The Mu-Opioid Receptor Gene

The mu-opioid receptor gene (OPRM1) is located on chromosome 6 and consists of 236,366 nucleotides. ORPM1 codes for the mu-opioid receptor that is composed of 493 amino acids. Patients who have alcohol dependence and have either one or two copies of the G allele have been reported to be more likely to have a positive response to treatment with naltrexone.[15]

The Period Homolog 2 Clock Gene

The period homolog 2 clock gene (PER2) is located on chromosome 2 and consists of 44,529 nucleotides. PER2 codes for the clock gene PER2 protein that is composed of 1,255 amino acids. There has been some evidence to suggest that variation in

PER2 may be related to a differential response to acamprosate, but further research is needed before this finding can be used to predict response to acamprosate.[16]

The Dopamine 4 Receptor Gene

The dopamine 4 receptor gene (DRD4) is located on chromosome 11 and consists of 3,399 nucleotides. DRD4 codes for the dopamine 4 receptor that is composed of 419 amino acids. Patients with one or two copies of the seven-repeat allele of DRD4 have been reported to have more positive reactions to alcohol. However, the seven-repeat allele has also been shown to be associated with a greater decrease in the consumption of alcohol when patients are treated with olanzapine. The mechanism of action of olanzapine is believed to involve both the D2 receptor and the DRD4 receptor.[17]

A GENE ASSOCIATED WITH DRUG SAFETY

The major histocompatibility complex gene (HLA-B) is located on chromosome 6 and consists of 3,341 nucleotides. HLA-B codes for a major histocompatibility complex protein that is composed of 362 amino acids. Patients with the HLA-B*1502 allele are at increased risk of developing Stevens–Johnson syndrome when prescribed carbamazepine.[18]

CLINICAL UTILITY OF PHARMACOGENOMIC TESTING

Although psychiatric pharmacogenomic testing has been conducted for nearly a decade, no large-scale prospective randomized controlled trials have been initiated. The primary reason for not conducting such trials has been that this traditional methodology of demonstrating clinical benefit in the general population is not an efficient methodology for defining the implications of relatively rare variants that influence medication response. An important paper in 2004 focused on hundreds of small studies that demonstrated some effect related to specific variations.[19] Subsequently, it has become clear that a more efficient approach to demonstrate clinical utility is to study patients who have atypical genotypes. Furthermore, to improve the usefulness of pharmacogenomic testing, multiple gene interactions must be considered. Given the complexity of interpreting the impact of multiple pharmacogenomically relevant genes, it is quite interesting, and somewhat surprising, that a single gene variant such as the long alleles of SLC6A4 has an effect that is independent of the influence of other genes.

ETHICAL CONSIDERATIONS

The ethical considerations for the clinical utilization of pharmacogenomic testing are similar to the considerations related to the use of any laboratory evaluation that has the potential to demonstrate adverse outcomes or increased risk. Therefore, it is essential to consider the utilization of pharmacogenomic testing within the context of other strategies that are used to minimize the risk that patients may experience. A number of principles should be considered.

First, pharmacogenomic testing must be preceded by appropriate consent. Second, this consent must include specific clarification that clinical testing is a voluntary procedure. Third, confidentiality of the results of the testing must be maintained. Finally, the reliability of the testing must be well established.

CLINICAL IMPLICATIONS

The Case of a Very Poor Metabolizer

The most obvious indication for using pharmacogenomic testing is to identify poor metabolizers. Metabolic capacity can be evaluated on a continuum of the ability of a patient to metabolize a medication. Consequently, there is variability in the metabolic activity of patients who have been classified using the traditional metabolic categories. Specifically, "poor" metabolizers of each of the relevant cytochrome P450 enzymes represent a spectrum of metabolic capacities that extends from very decreased to completely absent. There have been many examples of extremely adverse events that have occurred in patients who are poor metabolizers.[20,21] Clarifying whether a patient has adequate metabolic capacity provides a clinician with a straightforward strategy to minimize side effects. Essentially, there are two options that are available to manage a patient who has reduced metabolic capacity. The first is to choose a medication that is metabolized by an alternative enzyme. The second is to use a substrate medication despite limited metabolic capacity, but modify the dosing strategy by beginning at a low dose and slowly titrating the dose upward.

Managing the Risk of Relapse of Psychosis

Patients who are treated for psychotic symptoms on an inpatient unit with either clozapine or olanzapine may have problems related to the inducibility of some forms of CYP1A2. Given that smoking is restricted in most psychiatric inpatient units, administration of appropriate antipsychotic medication and titration of dosage is often conducted while patients have minimal exposure to tobacco smoke. Nearly 50% of the patients of European ancestry have either one or two copies of an inducible allele of CYP1A2. This presents a practical problem if a patient with one or two of these alleles begins to smoke on discharge. As the induction of the CYP1A2 takes place, the serum concentration of a 1A2 substrate medication such as olanzapine or clozapine will begin to drop. Without pharmacogenomic testing, many of these patients who relapse are accused of nonadherence when in fact they are taking their medications appropriately.

Increasing the Odds of Success

The selection of an appropriate antidepressant for an individual patient who presents with moderate to severe depression and who has no history of previous treatment can be a challenge.

Prior to the introduction of pharmacogenomic testing, standard practice was to select a serotonin reuptake inhibitor based on the family history of the patient or the side effect profile of the medication. If the first antidepressant did not work, other antidepressants were prescribed until the patient finally responded. It is now possible to improve the likelihood of identifying a drug that will be effective. For example, there is now reasonable evidence to suggest that choosing an antidepressant that is not a selective serotonin reuptake inhibitor is a prudent alternative strategy for patients of European ancestry who are homozygous for the short form of the serotonin transporter indel allele.

FACTORS AFFECTING THE IMPLEMENTATION OF PSYCHIATRIC PHARMACOGENOMICS

Initially, cost was the primary barrier preventing the use of pharmacogenomic testing. However, as genotyping technologies have become less expensive, comprehensive genotypic profiles can be obtained for far less than the cost of a single day of psychiatric hospitalization. Given the increasing amount of information linking variability in either pharmacokinetically or pharmacodynamically relevant genes with side effects, identification of vulnerabilities prior to the onset of treatment is now a cost-effective strategy. This is particularly true if generic medications can be selected based on a prediction that they are likely to tolerate the generic medication and have a relatively low risk of side effects when compared with other medication choices.

Currently, it is primarily the lack of understanding of the implications of pharmacogenomic testing that limits its use.[22] Difficulty in grasping the implications of pharmacogenomic testing is an issue for both clinicians and their patients. However, with increasing evidence of the clinical benefit of testing a number of genes, awareness of the benefits of testing has become more widespread. What will continue to be the problem is the complexity of determining the implications of multiple variants. Realistically, this is a multivariant problem of considerable complexity that will increasingly require the use of computerized algorithms to assess the influence of multiple variations. Such systems have been developed and increasingly sophisticated enhancements will further improve their accuracy and usefulness.

THE USE OF PSYCHIATRIC PHARMACOGENOMIC TESTING IN THE FUTURE

With the decreased cost of testing and the increased awareness of the clinical implications of minimizing adverse events, it is quite probable that in the relatively near future, pharmacogenomic testing will be a standard component of both inpatient and outpatient psychiatric care when it involves the use of psychotropic medications. With consideration of more comprehensive sets of relevant genes, it is reasonable to expect that the prognosis of patients with the full range of psychiatric diagnoses will improve. Additionally, it is certain that the number of adverse events related to psychotropic medication exposure will be decreased.

Case 1: Unemployed House Painter

Mr JS is a 47-year-old unemployed house painter who has been hospitalized on the inpatient psychiatric service for the past 7 days. He has a history of chronic schizophrenia with multiple hospitalizations over the past 10 years. His medication history includes unsuccessful treatment trials of haloperidol, perphenazine, olanzapine, and aripiprazole. He has recently begun taking clozapine and has been titrated as an outpatient to a daily dose 600 mg. At admission, he was taking clozapine, quetiapine 50 mg at bedtime, one capsule of vitamin E daily, and multivitamins. A family member related a recent history of bizarre behavior including ritualistic shuffling before entering doorways, getting out of bed multiple times during the night to check that the house was locked, and repeatedly checking that light bulbs throughout the house were screwed in tightly. Further history includes consumption of two to four cans of beer per day and smoking one pack of cigarettes daily. The patient was continued on his admission medications with the exception of quetiapine being discontinued and the addition of fluvoxamine 100 mg daily. After 3 days of hospitalization, the patient displayed less obsessive-compulsive behavior but became increasingly agitated when asked to participate in group functions. One week after admission, the patient was found on the floor of his room experiencing a generalized seizure.

Question: What pharmacogenetic issues could be important in understanding this patient's hospital course?

Answer: Clozapine is a highly effective antipsychotic drug for patients who are resistant to other drugs in this class. A few patients will experience obsessive-compulsive symptoms after therapy begins that may require treatment. Clozapine is metabolized by CYP1A2 and cigarette smoking is a major cause of CYP1A2 induction. As many inpatient units forbid patients to smoke, the reversal of CYP1A2 induction can change the clearance of drugs such as clozapine. It is likely that the reduced clearance resulted in a sufficient increase in clozapine plasma concentration to precipitate a drug-induced seizure, a known adverse event associated with high doses of clozapine. Fluvoxamine, which is also metabolized by CYP1A2, would be subject to the same effects on metabolic clearance as clozapine from cigarette smoking. While fluvoxamine is labeled for the treatment of obsessive-compulsive symptoms, its use for depression has been associated with better response in patients possessing the long form of the insertion/deletion polymorphism in the serotonin transporter promoter region (SLC6A4 allele).

Case 2: Elementary School Pupil with Excessive Weight Gain

KR is a 7-year-old boy who was diagnosed with autistic disorder 3 years ago. He has been undergoing an intensive behavioral management program to minimize his irritability and temper outbursts. This effort has only been partly successful and his special education teacher has complained to his parents that he disrupts the classroom and prevents the other children from receiving proper instruction. His pediatrician started him on 0.5 mg of risperidone a day 3 months ago. Improvement in behavior has been noticeable by both the teacher and parents but both feel his behavior needs further control. In addition, the patient has an insatiable appetite at dinner and throws food and objects from the table if his demands for more food are not met. His mother now complains to the pediatrician that his clothes no longer fit. The pediatrician is considering a switch in medication to aripiprazole or possibly an increase in risperidone dosage but wants to run some genetic tests before making this decision.

Question: What genetic tests might be informative to the pediatrician in making a choice of pharmacotherapy for a child with autistic disorder?

Answer: Both risperidone and aripiprazole are FDA approved for the treatment of irritability associated with autistic disorder in children as young as age 7. Risperidone is metabolized extensively by CYP2D6 to its pharmacologically active metabolite, 9-hydroxy-risperidone. If the metabolite were not active, then a genotype of being an ultrarapid metabolizer would suggest either an increase in dosage that might be useful or a change to another medication. However, there are no data that address differences in pharmacodynamic effects by genotype in the use of risperidone in autistic disorder. Aripiprazole is metabolized by CYP3A4 and is unlikely to be as influenced by CYP genotype as risperidone. In adults, aripiprazole is associated with less weight gain than risperidone but is considerably more expensive. The serotonin 2C receptor gene can be expressed as a variant with a cytosine or thymine allele (rs3813929, −759C/T). The cytosine allele has been consistently associated with weight gain in patients taking antipsychotic drugs. If this patient's genotype includes the cytosine allele, then a switch to aripiprazole may be indicated in spite of its increased cost.

REFERENCES

1. Mrazek DA. *Psychiatric Pharmacogenomics*. New York, NY: Oxford University Press; 2010.
2. Dalen P, Dahl ML, Ruiz ML, Nordin J, Bertilsson L. 10-Hydroxylation of nortriptyline in white persons with 0, 1, 2, 3, and 13 functional CYP2D6 genes. *Clin Pharmacol Ther*. 1998;63(4):444–452.
3. Mrazek DA. New tool: genotyping makes prescribing safer, more effective. *Curr Psychiatry*. 2004;3(9):11–12, 15–18, 23.
4. Ingelman-Sundberg M. Genetic polymorphisms of cytochrome P450 2D6 (CYP2D6): clinical consequences, evolutionary aspects and functional diversity. *Pharmacogenomics J*. 2005;5(1):6–13.
5. O'Hare A, ed. *Physicians' Desk Reference*. 65th ed. Montvale, NJ: PDR Network; 2011.
6. Hesse LM, Venkatakrishnan K, Court MH, et al. CYP2B6 mediates the in vitro hydroxylation of bupropion: potential drug interactions with other antidepressants. *Drug Metab Dispos*. 2000;28(10):1176–1183.
7. Lerman C, Shields P, Wileyto E, et al. Pharmacogenetic investigation of smoking cessation treatment. *Pharmacogenetics*. 2002;12:627–634.
8. Smeraldi E, Zanardi R, Benedetti F, Bella D, Perez J, Catalano M. Polymorphism within the promoter of the serotonin transporter gene and antidepressant efficacy of fluvoxamine. *Mol Psychiatry*. 1998;3:508–511.
9. Mrazek DA, Rush AJ, Biernacka JM, et al. SLC6A4 variation and citalopram response [research article]. *Am J Med Genet B Neuropsychiatr Genet*. 2009;150B(3):341–351.
10. Serretti A, Kato M, De Ronchi D, Kinoshita T. Meta-analysis of serotonin transporter gene promoter polymorphism (5-HTTLPR) association with selective serotonin reuptake inhibitor efficacy in depressed patients [original article]. *Mol Psychiatry*. 2007;12(3):247–257.
11. McMahon FJ, Buervenich S, Charney D, et al. Variation in the gene encoding the serotonin 2A receptor is associated with outcome of antidepressant treatment. *Am J Hum Genet*. 2006;78:804–814.
12. Murphy GM, Kremer C, Rodrigues HE, Schatzberg AF. Pharmacogenetics of antidepressant medication intolerance. *Am J Psychiatry*. 2003;160: 1830–1835.
13. Segman RH, Heresco-Levy U, Finkel B, et al. Association between the serotonin 2A receptor gene and tardive dyskinesia in chronic schizophrenia. *Mol Psychiatry*. 2001;6(2):225–229.
14. De Luca V, Mueller DJ, de Bartolomeis A, Kennedy J. Association of the HTR2C gene and antipsychotic induced weight gain: a meta-analysis [review article]. *Int J Neuropsychopharmacol*. 2007;10:697–704.
15. Anton RF, Oroszi G, O'Malley S, et al. An evaluation of mu-opioid receptor (OPRM1) as a predictor of naltrexone response in the treatment of alcohol dependence: results from the Combined Pharmacotherapies and Behavioral Interventions for Alcohol Dependence (COMBINE) study. *Arch Gen Psychiatry*. 2008;65(2):135–144.
16. Spanagel R, Pendyala G, Abarca C, et al. The clock gene Per2 influences the glutamatergic system and modulates alcohol consumption. *Nat Med*. 2005;11(1):35–42.
17. Hutchison KE, Ray L, Sandman E, et al. The effect of olanzapine on craving and alcohol consumption. *Neuropsychopharmacology*. 2006;31(6): 1310–1317.
18. Chen P, Lin JJ, Lu CS, et al. Carbamazepine-induced toxic effects and HLA-B*1502 screening in Taiwan. *N Engl J Med*. 2011;364(12):1126–1133.
19. Kirchheiner J, Nickchen K, Bauer M, et al. Pharmacogenetics of antidepressants and antipsychotics: the contribution of allelic variations to the phenotype of drug response. *Mol Psychiatry*. 2004;9:442–473.
20. Koski A, Ojanpera I, Sistonen J, Vuori E, Sajantila A. A fatal doxepin poisoning associated with a defective CYP2D6 genotype. *Am J Forensic Med Pathol*. 2007;28(3):259–261.
21. Sallee FR, DeVane CL, Ferrell RE. Fluoxetine-related death in a child with cytochrome P-450 2D6 genetic deficiency. *J Child Adolesc Psychopharmacol*. 2000;10(1):27–34.
22. Mrazek DA, Lerman C. Facilitating clinical implementation of pharmacogenomics. *JAMA*. 2011;306(3):304–305.

15

Immunology, Transplantation, and Vaccines

Mary S. Hayney, PharmD, MPH, FCCP, BCPS

LEARNING OBJECTIVES

- Hypothesize how genetic polymorphisms within the immune system may lead to variability in responses to infection, transplantation, or immunization

- Consider the outcome advantages of human leukocyte antigen matching in solid organ transplantation
- Describe how genetic diversity may influence response to vaccines

IMMUNOLOGY

The human body has a great capacity to resist the many organisms and toxins with which it comes in contact. This defensive mechanism is called immunity and involves an intricate system consisting of both innate and acquired immunity. Innate immunity consists of general processes that are present at birth. These processes are considered the first line of defense against an infectious organism and include skin, gastric acid, mucus, neutrophils, and complement. It is different from acquired immunity in that it is nonspecific, has a fast response, and does not have a memory in response to previous infections.

Active immunity involves humoral and cellular compartments. Although each compartment in the immune system is unique with its own specialized cells, the system works in concert to protect the body from infectious organisms. Active immunity occurs following an initial invasion by a foreign organism or toxin. Each toxin and organism has a unique makeup of proteins or large polysaccharides that differentiates it from other compounds. These proteins and polysaccharides are called antigens.

The fact that not all those exposed to a particular pathogen will develop infection is an important point in infectious disease.

The processes involved in the development of infection are likely the virulence of the pathogen and the host susceptibility. In this section we will focus on the components of the immune system that are known to be polymorphic in humans and may contribute to host susceptibility.

Antigen Recognition

B and T cells must have the capacity to recognize and virtually an infinite number of antigens. Both types of lymphocytes have specially adapted receptors for that purpose. The B cell receptor has the same antigen specificity as the antibody it secretes. The T cell receptor is specific and critical for antigen presentation. The genes for these receptors possess unique capacity to undergo deletion, rearrangement, and somatic mutation. The genes for antigen recognition portion of antibodies and T cell receptors are organized in regions. Several copies of the same gene are located within each region. Each copy of the gene is different from the others. These gene cassettes can be rearranged or deleted during the antigen recognition process. In addition, the genes can undergo limited somatic mutation in an effort to create an antibody or T cell receptor that has high affinity for the antigen of interest. These processes allow for the possibility that nearly an infinite number of receptors for antigen recognition can be generated.

Human Leukocyte Antigen

Human leukocyte antigen (HLA) displays an unequaled degree of genetic polymorphism among functional human genes.[1] Each individual has HLA genes for class I, HLA-A, HLA-B, and HLA-C, and for class II, HLA-DRB, HLA-DQA, HLA-DQB, HLA-DPA, and HLA-DPB. The HLA genes are located on chromosome 6, and each individual has two alleles for each gene—one set from each parent. The function of HLA is to present peptides from pathogens to T cell receptors to initiate an immune response. HLA is part of the coordinated interaction between antigen-presenting cells and T cells whereby the immune system recognizes self from nonself allowing it to discriminately mount responses to nonself that it recognizes as antigens. The array of possible HLA glycoproteins makes it very unlikely that any pathogen will evade an immune response by all humans. It is also very unlikely that two unrelated humans would have identical HLA genotypes.

HLA class I glycoproteins are ubiquitous and are expressed on the surfaces of every nucleated human cell. They present endogenous peptides derived from the cell itself to cytotoxic T cells. HLA class I glycoproteins play an important role in viral infections. Since viruses use their host cells' machinery for replication, these cells present viral proteins on their surfaces using HLA class I glycoproteins. The presentation of viral peptides elicits a cell-mediated immune response that destroys the virally infected cell.

HLA class II glycoproteins expressed on an antigen-presenting cell display antigenic peptides derived from the pathogen. A pathogen undergoes phagocytosis by an antigen-presenting cell. The pathogen is digested in a lysosome and digested peptides associated with HLA class II glycoprotein can be presented on the cell surface. A T cell recognizes the antigenic peptide as foreign and initiates an immune response to the antigen.

The antigenic peptide must fit into the peptide binding cleft of either HLA class I or class II glycoprotein. Both size and the composition of the peptide determine the fit. For HLA class I glycoproteins, the length of the peptide is typically between 9 and 14 amino acids. For HLA class II, the fit of the antigenic peptide is relatively forgiving as the ends of the peptide binding cleft are open so that the peptide can hang off the ends of the HLA.

The sequence of the antigenic peptide is determined by the pathogen. However, the bulk and charge of the amino acids determine if it will fit in the peptide binding cleft. The polymorphisms within both HLA class I and class II are found almost exclusively in the part of the glycoprotein that makes up the peptide binding cleft (Figure 15–1). Based on the particular surface of the peptide binding cleft, some antigenic peptides may be preferentially presented while others may not be presented at all. The resulting diversity of the HLA peptide binding clefts is advantageous for the survival of the species. The diversity of the peptide binding clefts across the population translates into the

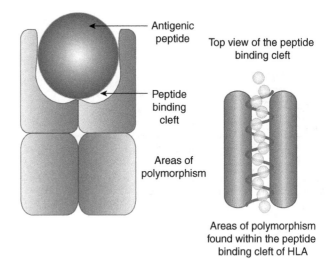

FIGURE 15–1 HLA class II glycoprotein. Two glycoproteins encoded in the HLA region on chromosome 6 form an HLA class 2 glycoprotein. The pocket at the top of the protein is called the peptide binding cleft. The polymorphisms are found in the peptide binding cleft. The top view shows an antigenic peptide in the peptide binding cleft. HLA class II glycoproteins are permissive in their binding as the peptide can hang off the ends of the peptide binding cleft. The polymorphisms found in the peptide binding cleft can change the amino acids that can affect the charge and bulk of the antigenic peptide that can be bound.

ability to recognize and generate an immune response to virtually any pathogen. The type of antigenic peptide that is displayed in the peptide binding cleft is an important factor in the immune response that is generated.

HLA and Drug Reaction and Disease Associations

Because of its biology and polymorphisms, a number of disease associations have been made with HLA types. Associations between HLA types and development and progression of autoimmune diseases are well established.[2] HLA polymorphisms may contribute to susceptibility to infection.[3]

Recently, two HLA types have been identified for risk of carbamazepine hypersensitivity reactions. HLA-A*3101 in Europeans and HLA-B*1502 in Asians have been shown to dramatically increase the risk of mild macropapular rash to severe toxic epidermal necrolysis or Stevens–Johnson syndrome.[4,5] The risk is important enough that some experts are recommending HLA typing before initiating carbamazepine therapy.[4,5]

Importantly, the prevalence and frequency of HLA types vary with populations and ethnicities. Clinicians must be cautious when using the literature to evaluate the risk of disease or response due to HLA polymorphisms. The patient under consideration may have to be from a similar ethnic or racial group as the one in which the study was done in order for the association to be applicable.[6]

Rheumatoid arthritis serves as an example of an autoimmune disease with a well-established connection to HLA polymorphisms. Environmental and other genetic factors contribute to the development of rheumatoid arthritis. Rheumatoid arthritis presents in a wide array of clinical severity. Antibodies to self-proteins are characteristically found in many autoimmune diseases. Anticitrullinated protein antibodies are just one type of autoantibodies that are commonly found in patients with rheumatoid arthritis. Patients with anticitrullinated protein are likely to have rheumatoid arthritis that is more rapidly progressive and severe. HLA-DRB alleles in several ethnic groups have been associated with rheumatoid arthritis. A string of amino acids common to several HLA-DRB alleles confers susceptibility to rheumatoid arthritis with anticitrullinated protein antibodies. The shared epitope contains QKRAA, QRRAA, or RRRAA in the glycoprotein.[7] Currently, any HLA-DRB allele that has this shared epitope is believed to increase the risk of rheumatoid arthritis. About one third of the risk for rheumatoid arthritis can be attributed to HLA-DRB gene polymorphisms.[8]

TRANSPLANTATION

Pharmacogenomics in the field of transplantation is extraordinarily complicated. The genetic basis of tissue antigenicity, immune response, drug metabolism, risk of adverse reactions, and susceptibility to infectious diseases can all be considered. Other chapters cover drug metabolism, adverse events, and infectious diseases in detail.

Tissue typing makes transplantation possible. Blood group is the most basic tissue typing done. ABO blood group antigens are present on most tissues and can be targets of immune response in the recipient. Across-blood-group transplantation is done only in rare circumstances because it is riskier and may involve more intense immunosuppression.

Human Leukocyte Antigen Polymorphisms

HLA matching has been demonstrated to improve outcome in transplantation. Less acute rejection and longer survival is associated with closely matched HLA between recipient and graft. Clinically, matching donor and recipient for HLA-A, HLA-B, and HLA-DR is practical. HLA-C, HLA-DQ, and HLA-DP are antigenic, but it would be impossible to find appropriate matches for these many HLA types. Given the possible combinations, even matching on just HLA-A, HLA-B, and HLA-DR rarely is a six-antigen match made even with the thousands of individuals on the kidney transplant waiting list. However, priority is given to a recipient with a complete match for a kidney. HLA matching for liver transplantation does not improve outcomes.[9] A priori HLA matching is not done for lung or heart transplantation. Size matching and severity of illness also factor into the allocation of donor organs. In addition, hearts and lungs do not function as well when subjected to a prolonged ischemia

time so the transplant must occur quickly, and the organ cannot be shipped across the country.

Some transplant candidates have preformed antibody responses to HLA. These responses can be initiated by exposure to blood products and are often found in multiparous women. Sometimes, no known risk factor is identified. These anti-HLA antibodies are called panel reactive antibodies (PRA). Traditionally, PRA was measured using a panel of lymphocytes from donors chosen to represent a wide array of HLA types. The PRA was measured by the percentage of lymphocytes from the panel that were killed when mixed with the recipient's serum. Newer methods take advantage of bead technology and fluorescent labeling. Beads coated with HLA glycoproteins are incubated with the patient's serum and then with fluorescently labeled antibodies to human antibodies. The degree of coating can be measured by flow cytometry. Individual and clusters of HLA types to which the patient has preformed antibodies can be identified. These preformed antibodies are associated with more rapid graft rejection.

Cytokine Polymorphisms

Production of a number of cytokines known to be important in solid organ transplant rejection is under polymorphic control. Single nucleotide polymorphisms (SNPs) in the gene promoter regions of interferon γ (IFNγ), tumor necrosis factor α (TNFα), interleukin-10 (IL-10), and transforming growth factor β_1 (TGF-β_1) affect cytokine production. Results of studies linking cytokine gene polymorphisms to transplant graft outcomes have drawn inconsistent conclusions. However, reasonable evidence of an association between high TNFα production and acute rejection of kidney and liver transplants exists.[10] This association is biologically plausible because TNFα activates inflammatory cells, increases adhesion molecule expression on vascular endothelium that increases the ability of immune cells to infiltrate the graft, and upregulates the expression of HLA. Some evidence exists that this association is more important when HLA mismatches between recipient and donor are present.[11]

Chemokine, Costimulation, Growth Factor, and Adhesion Molecule Polymorphisms

Several investigations of associations between transplant outcomes and vascular endothelial growth factor (VEGF), CTLA-4, regulated on activation of normal T cell expressed and secreted (RANTES), adhesion molecules, and chemokine receptors have been conducted. The results are mixed, and often the studies are underpowered with follow-up time that is too short to detect a difference in transplant outcome.[10,12]

Progress toward understanding an association between heart transplant outcome and Fas has been made. Activated T cells and macrophages express Fas and FasL on their surfaces. These transmembrane proteins initiate apoptosis. Apoptosis may be part of the vascular injury that occurs with acute rejection and leads to chronic rejection that manifests as obliteration of cardiac blood vessels known as cardiac allograft vasculopathy. Cardiac allograft vasculopathy is a form of chronic rejection of heart transplants. Genetically determined high production of Fas has been associated with heart transplant rejection. This risk appears to be more apparent in pediatric heart transplantation and adds to the risk of age at transplant and race.[12]

Renin–Angiotensin System

The renin–angiotensin system (RAS) possesses a number of pharmacologic targets.[13] Angiotensin-converting enzyme (ACE) inhibitors and angiotensin receptor blockers are used extensively in transplant patients for their antihypertensive effects. However, components of RAS have immunomodulatory effects. Angiotensin II increases vascular permeability and recruits cells during the inflammatory process. RAS components are expressed on dendritic cells, natural killer cells, and T cells. In the presence of a stimulator, angiotensin II promotes proliferation of natural killer cells and T cells. ACE polymorphisms are presented in more detail in Chapter 17B. In kidney transplant patients, the DD variant of ACE contributes to higher angiotensin II production and more renal transplant dysfunction. Genetically determined high producers of angiotensin II are at higher risk for renal transplant dysfunction. Pediatric heart transplant patients who are high angiotensin II producers have been shown to be at higher risk of rejection with hemodynamic compromise.[12] The RAS polymorphism association with renal and heart transplant outcome has only recently been recognized. More and larger studies are needed to determine the importance of RAS polymorphisms and transplantation.

Ultimately, the discovery of a combination of gene polymorphisms that includes the genetically polymorphic immune responsiveness of the graft as well as the recipient may be useful to choose aggressive immunosuppression regimens for those at higher risk of acute rejection and graft loss. Low-risk patients may be spared some of the toxicities of immunosuppression and benefit from less surveillance for acute rejection. Given the complexity of the immune response to a transplanted organ, a combination of genotypes is more likely to explain risks of immune responsiveness and graft outcomes. Based on results thus far, a combination of a high cytokine producer with a low immune regulatory genotype may be predisposed to acute rejection.[12,14]

Polymorphic Metabolism of Immunosuppressants

The immunosuppressant medications in clinical use have narrow therapeutic windows and high interindividual pharmacokinetic variability. Identifying pharmacogenomic targets for dosing of and predicting adverse events would be extremely valuable.

Mycophenolic Acid

Mycophenolic acid is metabolized primarily by glucuronidation. UDP-glucuronosyltransferase (UGT) 1A9 is the isoform catalyzing 55%, 75%, and 50% of the mycophenolic acid phenyl glucuronide production in the liver, kidney, and intestinal mucosa, respectively.[15] Polymorphisms in the promoter region of the UGT1A9 gene result in 17-fold variability in enzyme expression. Individuals with high UGT genotypes have significantly lower mycophenolic acid exposure.[16] Lower exposure to mycophenolic acid increases the risk of acute rejection. Routine UGT genotyping has not replaced trough or area-under-the-curve blood concentration monitoring in the clinic.[16]

Diarrhea is a common and dose-limiting adverse event with mycophenolic acid use. Additionally, the use of mycophenolic acid in combination with tacrolimus increases the risk of diarrhea compared with the combination of mycophenolic acid and cyclosporine. The decreased incidence of diarrhea with cyclosporine use is likely because cyclosporine inhibits biliary excretion of mycophenolic acid metabolites. Several studies have been done to identify the exact mechanism and genetic associations for mycophenolic acid–induced diarrhea.[17] UGT1A8, which is expressed in the intestinal mucosa, has been identified as a target gene. Two main allelic variants of the UGT1A8 gene exist. UGT1A8*2 is associated with a lower capacity for producing acyl mycophenolic acid phenyl glucuronide but similar ability to produce mycophenolic acid phenyl glucuronide compared with UGT1A8*1. Therefore, the UGT1A8*2 offers a protective effect from mycophenolic acid–associated diarrhea. The effect is more pronounced in individuals using cyclosporine.[18]

Calcineurin Inhibitors

Both cyclosporine and tacrolimus undergo extensive metabolism by CYP3A4 and CYP3A5. Both are also P-glycoprotein substrates. CYP3A5 is variably expressed in humans and has significant influence on the pharmacokinetics of calcineurin inhibitors, but the consequences of this are not particularly important for cyclosporine dosing.[17] However, studies have shown that genotyping for CYP3A5 variants may help guard against underdosing of tacrolimus in CYP3A5 expressers. Because tacrolimus blood concentration monitoring is the standard of care, the clinical impact of routine CYP3A5 genotyping may be small.[17]

GENETIC PREDICTORS OF RESPONSE TO VACCINES

Pharmacogenomics distinguishes itself by focusing on genetic influences on drug response. Variability of vaccine responsiveness is high, and some of the variability may be explained through single or complex multiple gene effects. An interesting aspect to the pharmacogenomics of vaccines is the opportunity to consider the genomes of both the host and the pathogen. Both genomes are important in determining the optimal immune response.

Vaccination relies on immunological memory to induce a response that is protective against disease on subsequent exposures. The immune response to the vaccine should resemble that induced by the natural infection to ideally produce protective immunity.[19–23] Vaccines could be used as probes of the immune system for identifying disease susceptibility genes.

The identification of disease susceptibility genes improves diagnostics. This information should aid in understanding the pathogenesis of infectious diseases and may lead to new therapeutic strategies. Public health initiatives to prevent disease may be targeted to individuals and populations most susceptible to infection.

The complete genome sequencing of a number of pathogens has presented scientists with a tremendous opportunity and challenge. The array of information that can be obtained from these sequences is phenomenal. The value of the whole genome sequence will result in antigenic determinants for vaccine development. However, the translation of this information into prophylactic and therapeutic interventions is still in its infancy.

Pathogen Genome for Antigen Identification

Serogroup B *Neisseria meningitides* sequence represents a good example of the use of the pathogen's genome to explore vaccine development.[24] Although serogroup B causes approximately one third of all cases of invasive *N. meningitides* infections, the meningococcal conjugate vaccine in clinical use covers only for serogroups A, C, Y, and W135. The serogroup B polysaccharide antigen resembles the human carbohydrate, polysialic acid, and, therefore, is poorly immunogenic or may even induce autoantibodies.[25] To overcome these obstacles, the entire serogroup B *N. meningitides* genome was sequenced to identify vaccine candidates. Three hundred and fifty antigens were expressed in *Escherichia coli* and used to immunize mice. Those antigens that induce a bactericidal antibody response were chosen for further study with the goal of developing a vaccine to protect against serogroup B *N. meningitides* infection, other serogroups, and possibly other pathogenic strains of *Neisseria*.[26]

Another strategy for translating the pathogen genome to a potential vaccine is to identify immunologically important peptides for cytotoxic T lymphocytes called CTL epitopes. Cytotoxic T lymphocyte responses are often critical for an immune response to a viral infection. The role of cytotoxic T lymphocytes is to seek out virally infected cells by the recognizing peptides presented by HLA glycoproteins on the cell surface and killing the infected cells. The viral peptide presented by the HLA complex that is recognized by a cytotoxic T cell is the CTL epitope.

Identification of these peptides has been greatly facilitated by the knowledge of the entire genome of the pathogen. Since each of the potentially antigenic peptides is about 10 amino acids in length, simple translation of the genome into protein sequences yields some information. The amino acid sequence is divided into peptides 10 amino acids in length, each overlapping the previous peptide by 9 amino acids. All possible peptides of 10 amino acids are represented in the dataset (Figure 15–2). For example, the West Nile virus genome translates to 3,433 amino acids. There are 3,424 peptides that are 10 amino acids in length.

Many researchers have spent years synthesizing peptides and measuring cytotoxic T lymphocyte responses to them. Bioinformatics is speeding up the process of selecting CTL epitopes.[26] A computer-based algorithm that matches the antigenic peptide with HLA glycoproteins based on likelihood of binding is being developed and tested.[27] From our West Nile virus example, 20 peptides were selected for testing based on their likelihood of binding. The algorithm eliminated more than 99% of the peptides that needed to be screened based on low probability of binding to the HLA. Indeed, the relatively few peptides screened yielded peptides that vigorously stimulated cytotoxic T lymphocyte responses when tested in biological systems. This approach dramatically decreased the time needed and cost of identification of CTL epitopes. These CTL epitopes may lead to the development of a subunit vaccine. (Hepatitis B vaccine is an example of a subunit vaccine.)

Vaccine antigens may also be produced by genetic engineering technology. These products are sometimes referred to as recombinant vaccines. Four genetically engineered vaccines are currently available in the United States. Hepatitis B and human papillomavirus (HPV) vaccines are produced by insertion of a segment of the respective viral gene into the gene of a yeast cell. The modified yeast cell produces pure hepatitis B surface antigen or HPV capsid protein when it grows. Live typhoid vaccine (Ty21a) is *Salmonella* Typhi bacteria that have been genetically modified to not cause illness. Live attenuated influenza vaccine has been engineered to replicate effectively in the mucosa of the nasopharynx but not in the lungs.

Measles Vaccine

Pharmacogenomics can also be used to predict which individuals may be likely to have a vigorous or poor response to a vaccine. Some apparently healthy individuals fail to mount an immune response to a particular vaccine. Measles vaccine response is well studied and will be used as an example.

Measles is a highly contagious viral infection characterized by high fever and rash. A live attenuated vaccine is used for prevention of this infection. A study of antibody response to measles vaccine was conducted among healthy school children. Ten percent of the population was seronegative, and seronegative individuals were clustered in families.[28] This observation is certainly suggestive of a genetic effect. The investigators pursued identification of a genetic effect with HLA genes as the candidate genes.

Both HLA class I and class II alleles were associated with measles vaccine responses. Class I HLA-B8, HLA-B13, and HLA-B44

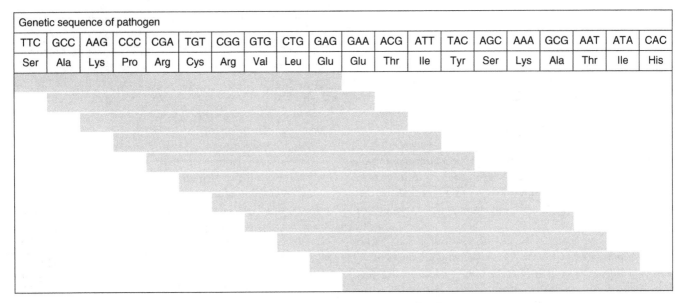

Genetic sequence of pathogen																			
TTC	GCC	AAG	CCC	CGA	TGT	CGG	GTG	CTG	GAG	GAA	ACG	ATT	TAC	AGC	AAA	GCG	AAT	ATA	CAC
Ser	Ala	Lys	Pro	Arg	Cys	Arg	Val	Leu	Glu	Glu	Thr	Ile	Tyr	Ser	Lys	Ala	Thr	Ile	His

FIGURE 15–2 Identification of potential cytotoxic T cell (CTL) epitopes from the genetic sequence of the pathogen. This protein from a hypothetical pathogen is translated from mRNA (step not shown) that was transcribed from the DNA sequence. The sequence of the protein made depends on the sequence of the genomic DNA. CTL epitopes are generated from the translated protein. Each peptide can be tested for its ability to elicit a vigorous immune response individually or after selection using computer modeling. With a sequence of only 20 amino acids, 10 peptides were generated. Computer algorithms increase the capacity to identify CTL epitopes that are immunogenic.

alleles and class II HLA-DRB1*03 and HLA-DQA1*0201 are associated with low measles antibody responses.[29,30] Interestingly, HLA homozygosity increases the risk of measles vaccine nonresponse.[31] Homozygosity within the HLA has also been associated with poor response to hepatitis B vaccines.[32–34] It is hypothesized that lack of diversity in antigen presentation may explain decreased vaccine response.

The pathogen interaction with the host can be another source of genetically determined variability. Both signaling lymphocyte activation molecule (SLAM) and CD46, a membrane protein that is part of the regulation of the complement system, are cellular targets for measles virus binding and entry into the host cell. SLAM and CD46 polymorphisms have been associated with measles vaccine antibody concentrations.[35] Presumably, SLAM polymorphisms in the receptors change the conformation and make binding of the live measles vaccine virus less favorable. The proposed mechanism for CD46 SNP to influence measles vaccine antibody concentrations is less clear. The important SNP is in an intron that may affect gene transcription.

Influenza Vaccine

Influenza infections cause significant seasonal morbidity and mortality. This RNA virus undergoes frequent mutation so that it is able to escape immune recognition and continue to circulate in the human population. Annual influenza immunization

is necessary. Variability in immune responses to currently used influenza vaccines has been noted.[36] Antibody responses to influenza A/H1N1 have been associated with HLA-A gene polymorphisms. HLA-A*1101 and HLA-1*6801 are associated with higher H1N1 influenza antibody production. Both H1 and H3 antibody responses were correlated with IL-1 receptor, IL-2 receptor, IL-6, IL-10 receptor, and IL-12B polymorphisms.[37] HLA class II polymorphisms have also been associated with influenza vaccine response with HLA-DRB1*0701 being found more frequently among responders and fewer HLA-DQB1*0603-9/14 among nonresponders.[38] The genetic polymorphisms associated with influenza vaccine at this time should be considered very preliminary. Influenza viruses and presumably the nature of the immune response change seasonally. No studies have been done over multiple influenza seasons. However, given the importance of influenza as a public health burden, these studies should be high priority to improve protection conferred by influenza immunization.

Pharmacogenomics has the potential to revolutionize prevention, diagnosis, and treatment of immunological diseases. Both the genome of the antigen and the human genome present potential targets for intervention and will likely yield multiple targets for drug development. Nevertheless, the interplay between the host and the antigen adds a layer of complexity. Innovative diagnostic, susceptibility, and therapeutic interventions are being developed. However, the pharmacogenomics of immunological diseases is in its infancy.

HLA Matching Case

Jill has renal failure secondary to hypertension and diabetic nephropathy. She has two siblings who are potential donors. Which sibling is a better HLA match for her?

HLA typing results

Jill	
A1	A2
B8	B27
DR1	DR4

Dan	
A2	A2
B6	B8
DR1	DR3

Jenny	
A1	A2
B8	B44
DR1	DR1

Match and mismatch are terms used to describe similarity at the HLA loci. When an individual is homozygous at a locus, mismatch is a better description of the immunological risk. Dan is homozygous at HLA-A, and Jenny is homozygous at HLA-DR.

Dan is a two-antigen mismatch with Jill. He carries HLA-B6 and DR3 that Jill's immune system will see as foreign or not-self. Jenny is a one-antigen mismatch with Jill with only B44 being mismatched. Jenny is the better matched donor in this case.

How does the Situation Change if Dan is the Kidney Recipient?

Jill is a two-antigen mismatch with Dan. Dan will see B27 and DR4 as mismatched antigens. Jenny is also a two-antigen mismatch with Dan. She carries A1 and B44 that Dan does not. However, DR mismatches are higher risk mismatches than class I. Therefore, Jenny is the preferred donor for Dan.

Vaccine Case

Dr Horn has noticed that several members of the three families have fallen ill with a hypothetical infectious virus during the current outbreak. All members of the family were immunized according to the currently recommended schedule. She doubts that the vaccine was compromised due to improper storage or poor vaccine administration technique because the members of these families were immunized over the course of several years. She hypothesizes that the vaccine failures may have a genetic link. What are likely hypotheses that she could consider as her laboratory investigates this outbreak?

Several techniques are available to investigate a possible genetic link for vaccine failure. A genome-wide association study could be done. HLA typing may be a narrow focus and is reasonable as response to other vaccines has HLA associations. Cytokine, growth factors, adhesion molecules, or their receptors could be considered. Also, the cellular receptor for the virus attachment or mechanism of cell entry may be polymorphic and render some individuals more susceptible to infection or to vaccine failure.

REFERENCES

1. Charron D. HLA, immunogenetics, pharmacogenetics and personalized medicine. *Vox Sang.* 2011;100(1):163–166.
2. Mackay IR. Clustering and commonalities among autoimmune diseases. *J Autoimmun.* 2009;33(3–4):170–177.
3. Marquet S, Schurr E. Genetics of susceptibility to infectious diseases: tuberculosis and leprosy as examples. *Drug Metab Dispos.* 2001;29:479–483.
4. McCormack M, Alfirevic A, Bourgeois S, et al. HLA-A*3101 and carbamazepine-induced hypersensitivity reactions in Europeans. *N Engl J Med.* 2011;364(12):1134–1143.
5. Chen P, Lin J-J, Lu C-S, et al. Carbamazepine-induced toxic effects and HLA-B*1502 screening in Taiwan. *N Engl J Med.* 2011;364(12):1126–1133.
6. McCarthy MI, Abecasis GR, Cardon LR, et al. Genome-wide association studies for complex traits: consensus, uncertainty and challenges. *Nat Rev Genet.* 2008;9(5):356–369.
7. Bax M, van Heemst J, Huizinga T, Toes R. Genetics of rheumatoid arthritis: what have we learned? *Immunogenetics.* 2011;63(8):459–466.
8. Perricone C, Ceccarelli F, Valesini G. An overview on the genetic of rheumatoid arthritis: a never-ending story. *Autoimmun Rev.* 2011;10(10):599–608.
9. Moroso V, van der Meer A, Tilanus HW, et al. Donor and recipient HLA/KIR genotypes do not predict liver transplantation outcome. *Transpl Int.* 2011;24(9):932–942.
10. Nickerson P. The impact of immune gene polymorphisms in kidney and liver transplantation. *Clin Lab Med.* 2008;28(3):455–468.
11. Sankaran D, Asderakis A, Ashraf S, et al. Cytokine gene polymorphisms predict acute graft rejection following renal transplantation. *Kidney Int.* 1999;56(1):281–288.
12. Girnita DM, Ohmann EL, Brooks MM, et al. Gene polymorphisms impact the risk of rejection with hemodynamic compromise: a multicenter study. *Transplantation.* 2011;91:1326–1332.
13. Geara AS, Azzi J, Jurewicz M, Abdi R. The renin–angiotensin system: an old, newly discovered player in immunoregulation. *Transplant Rev.* 2009;23(3):151–158.
14. Girnita DM, Webber SA, Zeevi A. Clinical impact of cytokine and growth factor genetic polymorphisms in thoracic organ transplantation. *Clin Lab Med.* 2008;28(3):423–440.
15. Picard N, Ratanasavanh D, Premaud A, Le Meur Y, Marquet P. Identification of the UDP-glucuronosyl transferase isoforms involved in mycophenolic acid phase II metabolism. *Drug Metab Dispos.* 2005;33(1):139–146.
16. Cantarovich M, Brown NW, Ensom MHH, et al. Mycophenolate monitoring in liver, thoracic, pancreas, and small bowel transplantation: a consensus report. *Transplant Rev.* 2011;25(2):65–77.
17. Picard N, Marquet P. The influence of pharmacogenetics and cofactors on clinical outcomes in kidney transplantation. *Expert Opin Drug Metab Toxicol.* 2011;7(6):731–743.
18. Woillard J-B, Rerolle J-P, Picard N, et al. Risk of diarrhoea in a long-term cohort of renal transplant patients given mycophenolate mofetil: the significant role of the UGT1A8*2 variant allele. *Br J Clin Pharmacol.* 2010;69(6):675–683.
19. Gazzinelli RT, Hakim FT, Hieny S, Shearer GM, Sher A. Synergistic role of CD4+ and CD8+ T lymphocytes in IFN-gamma production and protective immunity induced by an attenuated *Toxoplasma gondii* vaccine. *J Immunol.* 1991;146(1):286–292.
20. Romani L, Mocci S, Bietta C, Lanfaloni L, Puccetti P, Bistoni F. Th1 and Th2 cytokine secretion patterns in murine candidiasis: association of Th1 responses with acquired resistance. *Infect Immun.* 1991;59(12):4647–4654.
21. Sher A, Coffman RL, Hieny S, Cheever AW. Ablation of eosinophil and IgE responses with anti-IL-5 or anti-IL-4 antibodies fails to affect immunity against *Schistosoma mansoni* in the mouse. *J Immunol.* 1990;145(11):3911–3916.
22. Tang YW, Graham BS. Anti-IL-4 treatment at immunization modulates cytokine expression, reduces illness, and increases cytotoxic T lymphocyte activity in mice challenged with respiratory syncytial virus. *J Clin Invest.* 1994;94(5):1953–1958.
23. Paul WE, Seder RA. Lymphocyte responses and cytokines. *Cell.* 1994;76(2):241–251.

24. Pizza M, Scarlato V, Masignani V, et al. Identification of vaccine candidates against serogroup B meningococcus by whole-genome sequencing. *Science.* 2000;287:1816–1820.

25. Hayrinen J, Jennings H, Raff HV, et al. Antibodies to polysialic acid and its *N*-propyl derivative: binding properties and interaction with human embryonal brain glycopeptides. *J Infect Dis.* 1995;171: 1480–1490.

26. Moriel DG, Scarselli M, Serino L, Mora M, Rappuoli R, Masignani V. Genome-based vaccine development: a short cut for the future. *Hum Vaccines.* 2008;4(3):184–188.

27. De Groot AS, Saint-Aubin C, Bosma A, Sbai H, Rayner J, Martin W. Rapid determination of HLA B*07 ligands from the West Nile virus NY99 genome. *Emerg Infect Dis.* 2001;7(4):706–713.

28. Poland GA. Immunogenetic mechanisms of antibody response to measles vaccine: the role of HLA genes. *Vaccine.* 1999;17:1719–1725.

29. Ovsyannikova IG, Jacobson RM, Vierkant RA, Shane Pankratz V, Jacobsen SJ, Poland GA. Associations between human leukocyte antigen (HLA) alleles and very high levels of measles antibody following vaccination. *Vaccine.* 2004;22(15–16):1914–1920.

30. Poland GA, Ovsyannikova IG, Jacobson RM, et al. Identification of an association between HLA class II alleles and low antibody levels after measles immunization. *Vaccine.* 2001;20(3–4):430–438.

31. Sauver JLS, Ovsyannikova IG, Jacobson RM, et al. Associations between human leukocyte antigen homozygosity and antibody levels to measles vaccine. *J Infect Dis.* 2002;185(11):1545–1549.

32. Craven DE, Awdeh ZL, Kunches LM, et al. Nonresponsiveness to hepatitis B vaccine in health care workers. Results of revaccination and genetic typings. *Ann Intern Med.* 1986;105(3):356–360.

33. Hayney MS, Welter DL, Reynolds AM, Francois M, Love RB. High dose hepatitis B vaccine in patients waiting for lung transplantation. *Pharmacotherapy.* 2003;23(5):555–560.

34. Kruskall MS, Alper CA, Awdeh Z, Yunis EJ, Marcus-Bagley D. The immune response to hepatitis B vaccine in humans: inheritance patterns in families. *J Exp Med.* 1992;175(2):495–502.

35. Dhiman N, Poland GA, Cunningham J, et al. Variations in measles vaccine-specific humoral immunity by polymorphisms in SLAM and CD46 measles virus receptors. *J Allergy Clin Immunol.* 2007;120:666–672.

36. Lambkin R, Novelli P, Gelder CM. Human genetics and responses to influenza vaccination. Clinical implications. *Am J Pharmacogenomics.* 2004;4(5):293–298.

37. Poland GA, Ovsyannikov IG, Jacobson RM. Immunogenetics of seasonal influenza vaccine response. *Vaccine.* 2008;26(suppl 4):D35–D40.

38. Gelder CM, Lambkin R, Hart KW, et al. Associations between human leukocyte antigens and nonresponsiveness to influenza vaccine. *J Infect Dis.* 2002;185(1):114–117.

Pharmacogenomics in Neurology

Francis M. Gengo, PharmD, FCP, &
Michelle M. Rainka, PharmD

LEARNING OBJECTIVES

- Review specific neurological disease states and the pharmacogenomics of these.
- Discuss how pharmacogenomics affects response to drug therapy and its implications.

- Outline how pharmacogenomics and pharmacogenomic testing will have an impact on diagnosis and treatment of neurological disease states.

INTRODUCTION

Knowledge of pharmacogenomics is becoming increasingly important in neurology, as in many fields of medicine, for practicing pharmacotherapeutics. The effectiveness and toxicities of medications used in secondary stroke prophylaxis, dementia, seizure disorders, multiple sclerosis (MS), and Parkinson disease (PD) are all influenced by genetic polymorphisms. These include but go beyond variability in metabolism by Phase I/II enzymes. Genetic variability plays a role in how prodrugs work by controlling metabolism to their active form, as in the case of clopidogrel; how drugs bind to receptors, as in the case of MS; or how drugs are eliminated or inactivated as in the case of anticonvulsants and agents for Alzheimer's disease (AD).[1] In recent AD clinical trials, for example, it has been found that a certain apolipoprotein E (APOE) allele can affect whether patients respond positively to a drug treatment. Susceptibility to life-threatening hypersensitivity reactions is also related to specific polymorphisms. Future research may provide genetic explanations for multiple drug resistance in epileptic patients.

ANTIPLATELET AGENTS FOR STROKE PROPHYLAXIS

Antiplatelet therapy is the standard of care for prevention and treatment of atherothrombotic events, including myocardial infarction and stroke prophylaxis.[2] Variability in antiplatelet response to all classes of these drugs has been well documented and lack of response to antiplatelet therapy has been established as a risk factor for developing secondary atherothrombotic events. While pharmacokinetics and disease severity play a role in the variability in response to antiplatelet agents, genetic polymorphisms contribute to variability in response to aspirin, the thienopyridines, and the GPIIb/IIIa inhibitors. Patients with certain genotypes may benefit from individualized therapy to reduce their risk of secondary thrombotic events.

Thienopyridines

Clopidogrel is commonly used and indicated for acute myocardial infarction, myocardial infarction prophylaxis, stroke prophylaxis, and percutaneous coronary intervention.[3] It is administered as an inactive drug that requires activation, largely by CYP2C19, CYP3A4 and CYPA12, to an active metabolite for a therapeutic effect to be produced (Figure 16–1). Antiplatelet effect is produced by the active metabolite of clopidogrel irreversibly inhibiting adenosine diphosphate (ADP)–induced platelet aggregation by preventing ADP binding to its $P2Y_{12}$ platelet receptor. It is estimated that up to 40% of patients do not achieve an optimal antiplatelet effect with clopidogrel, which puts these patients at higher risk of developing an atherothrombotic event.[4]

Mega et al. tested the association between genetic variants in CYP genes and antiplatelet response in 162 healthy patients taking clopidogrel.[5] They additionally examined the association

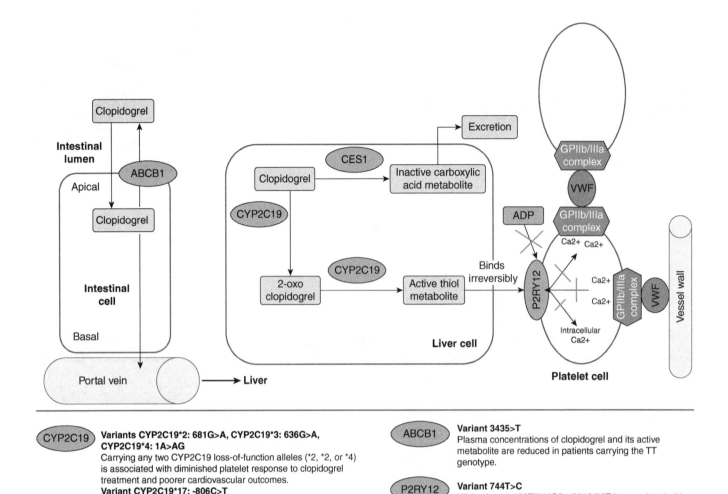

CYP2C19 — Variants CYP2C19*2: 681G>A, CYP2C19*3: 636G>A, CYP2C19*4: 1A>AG
Carrying any two CYP2C19 loss-of-function alleles (*2, *2, or *4) is associated with diminished platelet response to clopidogrel treatment and poorer cardiovascular outcomes.
Variant CYP2C19*17: -806C>T
The CYP2C19*17 carrier status significantly associated with enhanced response to clopidogrel and an increased risk of bleeding.

ABCB1 — Variant 3435>T
Plasma concentrations of clopidogrel and its active metabolite are reduced in patients carrying the TT genotype.

P2RY12 — Variant 744T>C
H2 haplotype 139T/744C/ins801A/52T is associated with enhanced platelet reactivity, coronary artery disease, and poor response to clopidrogel.

FIGURE 16–1 Genetic polymorphisms associated with clopidogrel.[127] (With permission from Vance JM., Tekin D. Genomic medicine and neurology. Continuum: lifelong learning in neurology. *Neurogenetics*. 2011;17(2):249–267. Copyright © 2011, American Academy of Neurology).

between these genetic variants and cardiovascular outcomes in a cohort of 1,477 subjects. Patients with a reduced function allele for CYP2C19 had a relative reduction of 32.4% of the active metabolite exposure compared with patients without a reduced function allele (*P* <.001). The ex vivo antiplatelet effect measured in these patients was 25% less than that in patients without the reduced function allele. Patients with the ultrarapid metabolizer (UM) genotypes had the highest concentration of active metabolite and the greatest platelet inhibition, and subjects with poor metabolizer (PM) genotypes had the lowest concentration of active metabolite and the lowest platelet inhibition. A similar trend was observed for patients with a reduced function allele for CYP2B6. There was no association of reduced function alleles for CYP2C9, 3A5, and 1A2 and production of the active metabolite of clopidogrel or in antiplatelet response. Patients with at least one reduced function CYP2C19 allele were at a significantly higher risk for death due to cardiovascular causes, myocardial infarctions, or stroke compared with patients with a normal functioning CYP2C19. The most common reduced function allele was CYP2C19*2. There was no an association between the primary efficacy outcome and any of the other CYP genotypes.

Patients with CYP2C19*2 had significantly lower concentrations of active metabolite of clopidogrel, decreased platelet inhibition, and a higher rate of major cardiovascular events. These findings have been confirmed in numerous other studies.[6–8]

Other reports have investigated the response variability to clopidogrel in patients with genetic polymorphisms CYP2C19*2, *3, and *17, CYP3A4*1B, and CYP3A5*3.[9] Previous results show that CYP2C19*2 allele carriers had significantly increased platelet aggregation. There were no other associations between the other genotypes and platelet aggregation. This has been replicated in other studies[8,10] by Mega et al.[5] and Simon et al.[8]

Some individuals may have an increased response to clopidogrel, which would increase their risk of bleeding complications. Data from a retrospective study of 598 patients after the administration of 600 mg of clopidogrel demonstrated that the CYP2C19*17 genotype was associated with extensive metabolism of clopidogrel and better platelet response to clopidogrel, while the *4, *5, and *6 alleles did not produce significant effects. The *17 allele was associated with an increased risk of bleeding.[10] Prospective studies by Geisler et al.[9] and Mega et al.[5] failed to find an association between patients with the

*17 allele and an altered response to clopidogrel, but Frere et al.[10] and Sibbing et al.[16] found that patients with this allele may have a better antiplatelet response to clopidogrel. Further, findings from Sibbing et al. showed that these patients were at an increased risk of bleeding. Considering the implications of putting patients at a higher risk of bleeding, genetic testing may be appropriate to determine which patients have this gain-of-function allele, specifically for patients already at high risk for bleeding. More clinical studies are needed to clarify the effects of having a *CYP2C19*17* allele when taking clopidogrel.

Although Figure 16–1 does not include the CYP1A2 enzyme, it has been shown to influence the production of the active metabolite of clopidogrel. Medications that induce the CYP1A2 enzyme have been shown to enhance the antiplatelet effects of clopidogrel. These would include insulins, modafinil, some beta-lactam antibiotics, and tobacco. There have been several reanalyses of large studies including CAPRIE, CURE, CREDO, and CLARITY TIMI. Endpoints for CAPRIE included stroke but the endpoints for the others were death or coronary events. The reanalysis stratified patients as active smokers vs nonsmokers or former smokers. Each of these analyses demonstrated that clopidogrel was much more efficacious in smokers compared with nonsmokers, and attributes this finding to the induction of the CYP1A2 enzyme in smokers.[11]

It is clear that genomic polymorphisms are associated with variability in response to clopidogrel. This is more relevant when clopidogrel is used in the setting of acute stroke than in the setting of acute coronary syndrome. In acute coronary syndrome a loading dose of 300–600 mg is often used that would at least temporally avoid the problem of inadequate production of the active thiol metabolite. However, because of the risk of hemorrhagic transformation of a cerebral infarction, loading doses are not commonly used following an acute stroke. The polymorphisms associated with reduced clopidogrel metabolism can and do significantly limit its effectiveness particularly in the days following an acute stroke when the risk of reinfarction is the highest.

Aspirin

Aspirin has remained the gold standard for secondary stroke prophylaxis.[12] Acetylsalicylic acid acetylates a serine moiety on the COX-1 enzyme rendering it incapable of metabolizing arachidonic acid to thromboxane, a potent agonist for platelet aggregation. Because platelets are without a nucleus and incapable of protein synthesis, the COX-1 enzyme cannot be regenerated, and the platelets' ability to aggregate is permanently disrupted. The effects of a single dose of aspirin reverse only as the population of platelets is turned over and replaced by new platelets. Acetylsalicylic acid is the only salicylate that affects platelet aggregation, and it is deacetylated rapidly, largely in the portal circulation. Many studies have reported "aspirin resistance." Our own series reports an inadequate antiplatelet response to aspirin in 20% of patients being treated for secondary stroke prophylaxis.

Patients resistant to 81 mg do respond to higher aspirin doses. However, there are a substantial number of patients who do not achieve an antiplatelet effect at any aspirin dose. There are some data to suggest that genomic polymorphisms may contribute to this lack of responsiveness to aspirin. Halushka et al. studied 38 healthy volunteers to assess if genetic variation of COX-1 influenced response to aspirin.[13] They performed genomic sequencing of the patients' cDNA of COX-1 and measured platelet aggregation as well as production of thromboxane B_2 and prostaglandin $F_{2\infty}$. After genomic sequencing, nine different polymorphisms of COX-1 were identified. Four of these polymorphisms were common, with heterozygosity greater than 10%, and included A-842G, C50T, C644A, and C22T. Two of these polymorphisms, A-842G and C50T, were found to be in complete linkage disequilibrium. These polymorphisms were further evaluated for association with activity of COX-1. There were no significant differences in thromboxane B_2 production found between homozygotes for the common alleles and heterozygotes for any of these polymorphisms. Response to aspirin as measured by formation of prostaglandin $F_{2\infty}$ was decreased in heterozygous patients for A-842G and C50T versus the common allele homozygous patients indicating that patients with this genetic variant in COX-1 may have an increased sensitivity to aspirin. There were no significant differences found in the response to aspirin for patients with the C644A or C22T polymorphisms. Platelet aggregation following aspirin showed a reduced response in patients homozygous for the common allele of A-842G and C50T, compared with that in heterozygous patients. These data represent a starting point for future in vivo studies to build upon to determine the significance of the A-842G and C50T genetic variant and aspirin response.

These results, however, conflict with subsequent work of others who report that the COX-1 haplotypes were associated with different antiplatelet response. There was an association between haplotype GCGCC, including A-842G, and increased platelet aggregation and thromboxane production (i.e., decreased sensitivity to aspirin).[14]

It has also been postulated that a polymorphism in glycoprotein IIIa may influence aspirin response variability. Szczeklik et al. investigated the effect of the polymorphism T1565C (Leu33Pro, P1A1/A2) of glycoprotein IIIa on response to aspirin in healthy men.[15] Bleeding time was shorter before aspirin ingestion in patients with the P1A2 allele and aspirin prolonged bleeding time in both groups. In 7 out of 26 patients with the P1A2 allele aspirin shortened bleeding time by 30 seconds, compared with 1 out of 54 patients with the common allele. While bleeding time is not a precise measure of the effects of aspirin, there does seem to be an association between P1A2 allele and the reduced response to aspirin. The P1[A1/A2] and P1[A2/A2] polymorphisms have been studied by others.[16] Patients with P1A2 were significantly more sensitive to the platelet inhibition by acetylsalicylic acid than P1A1 patients, contradicting Szczeklik's[17] results that indicated patients with the P1A2 allele were more resistant to platelet inhibition by acetylsalicylic acid.

These conflicting results may have been due to technical differences in the way that response to aspirin was measured or because platelets were incubated with aspirin rather than administering aspirin to the subject. Mechanisms to explain "aspirin resistance" are varied including pharmacokinetic, disease, and environmental influence and now the beginnings of data to suggest genetic factors.

GPIIb/IIIa Inhibitors

GPIIb/IIIa inhibitors are a class of antiplatelet drugs that are largely used for percutaneous coronary intervention and myocardial infarction prophylaxis and include abciximab, tirofiban, and eptifibatide.[17] They act by inhibiting glycoprotein IIb/IIIa and preventing the attachment of adhesive ligands to the glycoprotein IIb/IIIa receptor on activated platelets. These drugs also have a documented response variability, which may put patients at risk for cardiovascular events.

It has been suggested that patients with a P1A2 polymorphism may have an altered response to GPIIb/IIIa inhibitors, such as abciximab.[18] Differences were found in inhibition of platelet aggregation among different genotypes, with heterozygotes having a lower IC_{50} than homozygotes for P1A2. The IC_{50} for heterozygote patients was 1.9 ± 0.21 µg/mL, compared with 2.27 ± 0.19 µg/mL for patients homozygous for A1 and 2.13 ± 0.14 µg/mL for patients homozygous for A2. It appears that patients heterozygous for P1A2 were more sensitive to the inhibition of platelet aggregation by abciximab.

Conclusions

Based on the studies reviewed, it was shown that clopidogrel, aspirin, and GPIIb/IIIa inhibitors all have genetic variability that could influence antiplatelet response. There are the most data for clopidogrel, and these studies largely support the claim that individuals with particular polymorphisms will have an altered response to the antiplatelet effect of clopidogrel. The genotype with the most supporting data is for individuals expressing a CYP2C19*2 allele, which is a loss-of-function allele. Numerous trials have shown that individuals carrying this allele have a reduced amount of the active metabolite of clopidogrel, lower platelet inhibition, and an increased risk for cardiovascular events.[5-8] Considering these significant results, genetic testing may play an important role in determining patient selection for clopidogrel. In fact, in May 2009 the FDA added a warning to the Plavix package insert stating that PM of CYP2C19 are at a higher risk of developing cardiovascular events and that genetic testing is available to determine patients who are PM.[3] Additionally, they recommended that alternative treatment be used in these patients. The evidence for an altered response to clopidogrel in patients with a *CYP2C19*17* allele, a gain-of-function allele, is not as clear and more clinical studies are warranted, particularly considering the implications of increased bleeding.

There are also conflicting data on the role of genetic polymorphisms in controlling aspirin response variability. The most common polymorphisms studied have been polymorphisms of COX-1, specifically A-842G/C50T which are in linkage disequilibrium. Halushka et al. found that patients with an A-842G/C50T polymorphism may have an increased sensitivity to aspirin, as patients with this polymorphism had an increased inhibition of formation of prostaglandin H_2 by acetylsalicylic acid compared with patients with the common allele.[13] Maree et al., conversely, showed that patients with an A-842G/C50T allele actually had a decreased sensitivity to aspirin.[14] Together, these studies show that more pharmacogenomic research is required to clarify the effects of this polymorphism on aspirin response.

A polymorphism in glycoprotein IIIa, P1A1A2, has also been linked to variations in aspirin response as well as GPIIb/IIIa inhibitors response. Two trials in healthy volunteers studied the effect of this polymorphism on bleeding time and platelet aggregation after treatment with aspirin.[15,18] They produced conflicting results, with Szczeklik et al.[15] showing that patients with this polymorphism had a decreased sensitivity to aspirin due to shortened bleeding time and Andrioli et al.[18] finding that patients with this polymorphism had an increased sensitivity to platelet inhibition by aspirin. Additionally, conflicting results were also produced when patients with this polymorphism were treated with GPIIb/IIIa inhibitors. An in vitro study by Michelson et al.[19] found these patients to have an increased sensitivity to abciximab, whereas Weber et al.[20] could not show any significant difference. Therefore, it cannot be concluded that patients with the P1A1A2 polymorphism have an altered response to either aspirin or GPIIb/IIIa inhibitors, although this may be the case. Future studies should focus on this polymorphism to determine if any association can be made with response variability. At this time, scientific evidence does not support a recommendation for genetic screening to identify individuals with this polymorphism before receiving aspirin prophylaxis.

ANTICOAGUALANTS IN STROKE PROPHYLAXSIS

Atrial fibrillation is a common disorder that increases the risk of ischemic stroke. The incidence of atrial fibrillation in 2007 was more than 5% of individuals over the age of 65 in the western world.[21] Warfarin, a vitamin K antagonist, has been the mainstay therapy to prevent such related thromboembolism. It has long been thought of as a difficult drug to manage as a result of its narrow therapeutic index in that toxic doses are not significantly higher than effective doses. However, warfarin is also difficult to dose due to genetic variants in the CYP2C9 and VKORC1 genes (Figure 16–2). Patient responses to warfarin's anticoagualant effects are highly variable. Warfarin is a racemic mixture of *R*- and *S*-warfarin, with *S*-warfarin being the more potent of the two isomers. *S*-Warfarin is predominantly metabolized by the CYP2C9 enzyme. The major variants of CYP2C9 are the *2 and *3 alleles, and they are associated with reduced enzyme function and thus slower clearance resulting in higher drug concentrations. Patients with the CYP2C9*2 and CYP2C9*3 variants, when compared with patients with wild genotype CYP2C9*1/*1, took a longer time to reach therapeutic international normalized ratio (INR), had an increased rate of above range INR and increased risk of bleeding, and required a lower maintenance dose of warfarin.[22] VKORC1 is the target enzyme of warfarin, and VKORC1 haplotypes A and B account for 25% of warfarin dose variance.[23] Patients with haplotype A require a lower warfarin dose, whereas those with haplotype B require a higher warfarin dose. The FDA has provided specific dosing recommendations for those with CYP2C9 and VKORC1 variants as of January 2010. The recommended ranges for maintenance

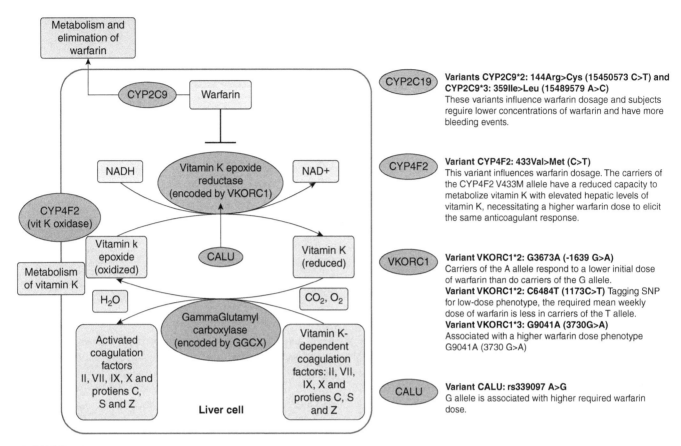

FIGURE 16–2 Genetic polymorphisms associated with warfarin.[127] (With permission from Vance JM., Tekin D. Genomic medicine and neurology. Continuum: lifelong learning in neurology. *Neurogenetics.* 2011;17(2):249–267. Copyright © 2011, American Academy of Neurology).

doses for genetic variants are included in the Coumadin package insert, and should be considered on dose initiation.[24]

Schwarz et al. conducted a prospective study to evaluate the CYP2C9 and VKORC1 contributions to initial (the first 4 weeks of therapy) variability in INR response. CYP2C9 and VKORC1 genotyping was performed, and major variants, such as CYP2C9*2 and CYP2C9*3 genotypes and VKORC1 A and non-A haplotypes, were identified.[25] The allelic frequencies of CYP2C9*2, CYP2C9*3, and VKORC1 haplotype A in the patients were 12.0%, 4.8%, and 32.6%, respectively. Clearly patients who were VKORC1 A/A homozygotes had a 2.4 times faster rate of achieving therapeutic INR than VKORC1 non-A/ non-A homozygotes ($P < .001$). The A/A homozygotes also had a 2.5 times higher rate of achieving an INR greater than 4.0 than non-A/non-A homozygotes ($P < .009$). Patients who were A/non-A heterozygotes were at higher risk as well. A/A homozygotes were above therapeutic INR for a longer period of time. Overall, they required a lower average dose of warfarin. CYP2C9 variants did not significantly affect the time to first therapeutic INR and time above an INR >4.0. However, patients with CYP2C9 variants had a shorter time to a first INR >4.0 ($P = .03$). In the initial stages of warfarin therapy, INR variations are contributed to VKORC1 haplotype A.

The International Warfarin Pharmacogenetics Consortium developed a pharmacogenetic dose algorithm for warfarin and to compare it with clinical dose and fixed-dose algorithms.[26] Clinical and genetic data for 5,700 patients were obtained from 21 different research groups. Of particular interest were the patients' demographics, concurrent medications, primary indication for warfarin, maintenance dose of warfarin, target INR, and CYP2C9 and VKORC1 genotypes. Combining clinical and genetic data, a pharmacogenetic dose algorithm was developed (available at www.warfarindosing.org). The results of the study show that the pharmacogenetic dose algorithm was more accurate in estimating doses than either clinical or fixed-dose algorithms (Figure 16–3). For patients who required low-dose warfarin (defined as <21 mg of warfarin per week), 35% of the dose estimations fell within 20% of the actual dose using the pharmacogenetic algorithm as compared with 24% using the clinical algorithm ($P < .001$) and 0% using the fixed-dose algorithm ($P < .001$). The pharmacogenetic algorithm also provided significantly less overestimations than the clinical and fixed-dose algorithms. For patients who required high-dose warfarin (defined as >49 mg of warfarin per week), 32.8% of the dose estimations fell within 20% of the actual dose using the pharmacogenetic algorithm as compared with 13.3% using the clinical algorithm ($P < .001$) and 0% using the fixed-dose algorithm ($P < .001$). The pharmacogenetic algorithm also provided significantly less underestimations than the clinical and fixed-dose algorithms. For patients who required intermediate-dose

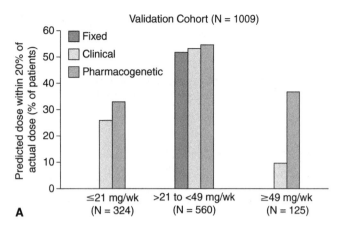

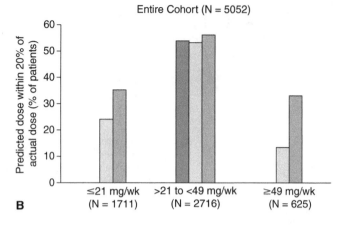

FIGURE 16–3 Warfarin pharmacogenetic dose algorithm.[26]

warfarin (defined as >21 and <49 mg of warfarin per week), there was no significant difference among the three approaches in estimating ideal warfarin doses. The study concluded that the pharmacogenetic dose algorithm that was developed provided better dose estimates than the clinical and fixed-dose algorithms for patients who required low or high doses of warfarin.

Another approved oral anticoagulant for nonvalvular atrial fibrillation is dabigatran etexilate, which is a prodrug that is rapidly hydrolyzed by plasma and hepatic esterases to dabigatran. Dabigatran further undergoes hepatic glucuronidation to active acylglucuronide isomers. The dosing for dabigatran etexilate is fixed at 150 mg BID except for individuals with reduced renal function (i.e., CrCl 15–30 mL/min), in whom the dosing is 75 mg BID. Dabigatran is a direct thrombin inhibitor and, unlike warfarin, is not metabolized by CYP enzymes.[27]

The RELY trial compared two doses of dabigatran (110 mg BID and 150 mg BID) with adjusted-dose warfarin in the prevention of stroke in patients with atrial fibrillation.[28] Results indicate that dabigatran 110 mg was noninferior to adjusted-dose warfarin in the prevention of thromboembolism and had less risks of bleeding (P<.001 and <.003, respectively). Dabigatran 150 mg was superior to adjusted-dose warfarin in the prevention of thromboembolism and had similar risks of bleeding (P<.001 and = 0.31, respectively).

Response to warfarin therapy is highly dependent on the CYP2C9 and VKORC1 genes. The CYP2C9 *2 and *3 variants are associated with decreased enzyme activity and decreased time to first therapeutic INR, increased rate of above 4.0 INRs, increased risk of bleeding, and lower maintenance doses. VKORC1 haplotype A is associated with faster time to therapeutic INR, faster time to an INR >4.0, and increased time over an INR >4.0, especially in the initial stages of therapy. The CYP2C9 and VKORC1 variants described require a lower dose of warfarin. This is especially important in the earlier stages of therapy, when a maintenance dose of warfarin has not yet been established. The risk of overanticoagulation is high. A patient's response to warfarin may vary drastically depending on his or her genetic makeup.

ALZHEIMER'S DISEASE

AD is an age-related, progressive neurodegenerative disorder that develops over a period of years. The neurodegeneration is thought to begin 10–20 years before patients initially present with symptoms. The brain disorder begins with loss of memory and confusion and can later progress into behavior and personality changes, a decline in cognitive skills, and inability to make decisions and carry out activities of daily living (ADL). Age is the greatest risk factor for development of AD, but as more evidence emerges, genetics seem to play an increasingly important role. Currently, the disease affects one of eight patients over the age of 65, but 50% of patients over the age of 85.[29] Other risk factors that are still under investigation for placing one at increased risk include female sex, lower levels of education, and history of head trauma. The hallmark signs of AD are amyloid plaques, neurofibrillary tangles (NFT), and loss of neurons responsible for memory and learning in the cortical areas and medial temporal lobe structures of the brain, which begin principally in the hippocampus and eventually affect all areas of the brain as neurodegeneration progresses.[30]

Two forms of AD exist: early onset Alzheimer's disease (EOAD) and late-onset Alzheimer's disease (LOAD). Individuals who develop symptoms before age 60–65 are considered to have EOAD that accounts for only 1–5% with dominantly inherited gene alterations on chromosomes 1, 14, and 21. LOAD has an onset after age 60–65 and is the predominant form of AD. Autosomal dominant AD occurs in at least three individuals over the span of two or more generations with two of the individuals as first-degree relatives. It represents less than 5% of cases and almost exclusively occurs in EOAD.[31] Familial AD occurs in more than one individual; at least two of the affected individuals are third degree or closer. These are seen in LOAD (15–25%) but can also be seen in about 47% of EOAD. Sporadic AD occurs as an isolated case or cases are separated by more than three generations in a family, and it accounts for 7% of cases.[31] Sporadic AD is usually LOAD, although there have been cases of EOAD (40%). LOAD is the predominant form of AD accounting for 95% of cases.

Amyloid Precursor Protein and Amyloid Plaques

Three deterministic autosomal dominant gene mutations have been implicated in the progression of amyloid plaques and EOAD: amyloid precursor protein (APP), presenilin 1 (PSEN1), and presenilin 2 (PSEN2). These mutations only account for 1–5% of EOAD cases and likely other genes are involved in EOAD.[31,32] APP and PSEN1 demonstrate complete penetrance, whereas PSEN2 demonstrates 95% penetrance.[31] Conversely APOE is a susceptibility gene for AD, with three isoforms ε2, ε3, and ε4. ε4 is associated with increased risk of AD, usually in LOAD, but also in EOAD. On the other hand, ε2 is thought to be protective.[31] Most of the disease-associated genes differ by a single point mutation making them potential targets for gene silencing trials.[32] Also because clinical trials are now focusing on manipulating the pathophysiology of the disease, genes affecting the development of amyloid plaques, NFT, and neurodegeneration will likely play a larger role in future treatments than in currently approved treatments.

APP is an integral membrane protein concentrated in synapses of neurons. Although its exact function is not known, it takes part in synapse formation, neural plasticity, and iron export.[33] In normal conditions amyloid-beta is degraded by neprilysin, an insulin-degrading peptidase, and by endothelin-converting enzyme. It is then cleared from the brain by a balanced process mediated by low-density lipoprotein receptor-related protein and the receptor for advanced glycation end products. In AD, an imbalance between the production and clearance of amyloid-beta in the brain initiates the accumulation, ultimately leading to neuronal degeneration and dementia.[30]

Alterations in the protein or any component in the pathway can cause the buildup of A-beta 42 and lead to these senile plaques. Imbalances in the process begin with a mutation on chromosome 21 creating an abnormal APP.[30] When there is a mutation on the APP protein, an abnormal A-beta is excised by the beta and gamma secretases, rather than being preferentially cleaved by alpha secretase. This form of A-beta cannot be cleared and catabolized because it does not complex with the exporter and is therefore built up over time into senile plaques. Thirty-two mutations have been identified as causing an amino acid substitution and cause conformational changes in the APP protein.[34] Those affected by trisomy of chromosome 21 are more so affected because of an extra APP gene and tend to develop plaques earlier in life.[35]

A-beta is excised by two enzymes from APP labeled as beta-secretase and gamma secretase. Gamma secretase is an intramembranous protease complex consisting of four components: PSEN1, nicastrin, PSEN2, and APH-1. The PSEN proteins are thought to stabilize the gamma secretase.[36] Beta-secretase activity comes from an integral membrane aspartyle protease called beta-site APP-cleaving enzyme (BACE-1).[37] Mutations on both chromosomes 14 and 1 involve the formation of abnormal presenilin. When the components on the gamma secretase are mutated, the enzyme misprocesses APP, leading to an altered ratio between A-beta 42 and A-beta 40 and further deposition of A-beta 42 into plaques. With so many different mutations that are possible for PSEN1, the likelihood of developing AD in later stages of life is very high.[38] It has been suggested that the gamma secretase may have substrates other than APP and the altered processing of these other substrates may also be involved in the pathophysiology of AD.[39] Recent studies have shown that silencing the PSEN1 mutant gene is able to decrease the expression of the mutant PSEN1 protein and therefore a decrease in the accumulation of the toxic A-beta 42.[32]

APOE gene found on chromosome 19 may be involved in increasing risk. This gene codes for a protein that helps carry cholesterol in the bloodstream. APOE ε2 is the rarest form and may actually protect an individual against the disease. It may either protect a person or prolong the onset of the disease if present. APOE ε3 is the most common form and neither helps nor hurts the risk of developing Alzheimer. At least one of the APOE ε4 alleles occurs in 50–70% of the AD population. The risk increases in a dose-dependent manner where those with familial risk factors and more than one allele of the APOE e4 type will increase risk.[31]

Neurofibrillary Tangles

As AD progresses, NFT begin to spread throughout the brain starting in the neocortex. NFT are formed when tau, a microtubule-associated protein, becomes hyperphosphoyrlated. The tau-encoding gene, microtubule-associated protein tau (MAPT), consists of 16 exons.[34] Tau assists in the formation and stabilization of microtubules.[40] When tau is unable to bind to the microtubules, they become unstable and disintegrate. The aggregation of unbounded tau into an insoluble form results in pretangles that accumulate further into NFTs interfering with numerous cellular functions.[30] A novel agent T-817MA, 1-(3-[2-(1-benzothiophen-5-yl)ethoxy]propyl)azeti-din-3-ol maleate, was studied in mice with the mutated tau gene and it seems to be a neuroprotective agent that can aid in inhibiting neuronal degeneration, thus improving motor and cognitive impairments.[41]

Fyn kinase is also thought to be involved in phosphorylating tau and exacerbating A-beta-mediated synaptic dysfunction. Fyn also increases the nonpathological cleavage of APP, suggesting that this opposes the progression of AD. In a study of transgenic mice, ultimately, loss of Fyn at early stages of the disease was found to increase soluble A-beta accumulation and worsens spatial learning in the absence of changes in tau phosphorylation.[42]

Other Genes

Researchers have begun using genome-wide associated studies (GWAS) to speed up the discovery process of risk factor genes. SORL1 gene on chromosome 11 was discovered as being another susceptibility gene involved in late-onset AD. It is involved in transporting APP within cells and when SORL1 was underexpressed, the beta amyloid levels increased and likewise when a similar gene, SORCS1, was underexpressed, gamma secretase activity and levels of amyloid increased.[43]

Another gene on chromosome 6, MTHFD1L, encodes methyltetrahydrofolate reductase (MTHFR) that converts folic acid to its active form, l-methylfolate, and is associated with risk of late-onset Alzheimer's disease. Individuals possessing mutations may be twice as likely to develop the disease and may also possess elevated homocysteine levels in the body, which plays a role in AD.[44] Therefore, in individuals with MTHFD1L mutations, therapy may focus on replacing the active form of folic acid, l-methylfolate theoretically (Deplin), but clinical trials need to be conducted to determine if this will be efficacious.

Current Treatments: Acetylcholinesterase Inhibitors and NMDA Antagonists

Current treatments for AD involve acetylcholinesterase inhibitors (AChEI) (donepezil, galantamine, rivastigmine) and moderate-affinity N-methyl-d-aspartate (NMDA) antagonist, memantine. In AD, there is a reduction in the activity of cholinergic neurons and AChEIs are employed to reduce the rate at which acetylcholine (ACh) is broken down, thereby increasing the concentration of ACh in the brain and decreasing the loss of ACh caused by the death of cholinergic neurons.[45,46] Memantine, on the other hand, is believed to protect neurons from excitotoxicity.[34] Both of these approved pharmacological treatment options and most others in the pipeline only slow the apparent progression of AD; they do not improve cognitive decline, and they also do not modulate the genetic mutations. Once there are damages to the neurons and synapses, they cannot be reversed.

Response to AChEI can be altered by genetics. Donepezil and galantamine are metabolized by cytochrome P450 2D6, 3A4, and 1A2.[47] CYP 2D6 genotypes consist of extensive metabolizers (EM), intermediate metabolizers (IM), PM, and UM and it is plausible that metabolizer status could affect efficacy or toxicity of cholinesterase inhibitors.[48] Fifteen percent of Alzheimer patients may metabolize AChEI abnormally whereby about half would be UM, requiring higher doses. On the other hand, approximately half would be PM, increasing the likelihood of toxicity or adverse events.[47] Patients with PM and UM phenotypes as well as ε4 genes tend to have worse treatment responses, whereas those with EM or IM phenotypes tend to respond more favorably.[47] In addition, the gene encoding choline transferase (ChAT) that encodes the major catalytic enzyme of the cholinergic pathway is associated with response to AChEIs.[49] ChAT is reduced in AD and is also correlated with the severity of dementia.[49] Single nucleotide polymorphism (SNP) rs733722 in the promoter region of ChAT accounts for 6% of the variance in response to AChEIs.[49] Another gene, SLC18A3, encodes for a vesicular ACh transporter that incorporates ChAT into synaptic vesicles and has also been implicated in disease susceptibility. rs733722 is present in approximately 33% of the population.[49]

Recent clinical trials have been aimed at interfering with A-beta deposition, vaccination with A-beta, selective A-beta 42–lowering agents, gamma secretase inhibition, and modulation of tau deposition. Unfortunately, many of the pitfalls of some of these trials have been significantly detrimental side effects or lack of significant improvement over placebo over extended periods of time.[34] Although the currently approved treatments are only modestly

affected by genetics, pharmacogenomics will continue to play an increasing role in Alzheimer's treatments as newer treatments target the pathophysiology that is more tightly tied to genetics.

EPILEPSY

The estimated prevalence of epilepsy is 1%, resulting in over 50 million treated patients worldwide. Obtaining good seizure control without intolerable adverse effects can generally be achieved in 70–75% of patients; however, identifying the dose to achieve this is generally empiric. Unfortunately the introduction of several drugs newer than phenytoin (PHT), phenobarbital, and valproic acid has done little to improve seizure control in patients with refractory seizures. The understanding of genetic polymorphism in anticonvulsant metabolism enables less variability in dose concentration relationships. Pharmacogenomic factors are also useful in identifying patients with a higher susceptibility to adverse events unrelated to drug concentrations. Finally, pharmacogenomic factors have been studied to determine if anticonvulsant resistance leading to intractable seizures is due to overexpression of genes controlling energy-dependent efflux pumps leading to reduced exposure of the brain to that anticonvulsant.

Polymorphism in Anticonvulsant Metabolism

Of the current AEDs, old and new, the only drugs affected by cytochrome P450 polymorphisms are PHT and phenobarbital.[50] While other AEDs are partly, or even extensively, metabolized by CYP enzymes, no evidence has been shown to correlate any CYP polymorphism with clinical response, serum drug concentrations, or other measurable outcomes.[51] While both PHT and phenobarbital are metabolized by CYP2C9 and CYP2C19, more evidence exists that clinical outcomes rely on CYP polymorphisms with PHT than with phenobarbital. It has been shown that PHT metabolism varies based on various CYP2C9 alleles.[52] This study demonstrated that the mean PHT dose required to achieve steady-state concentrations between 10 and 20 μg/mL in patients with one or two mutant alleles (CYP2C9*2 and CYP2C9*3) was 37% lower than that in patients homozygous for the wild type. In the same study, the PHT doses required to achieve therapeutic steady state were not significantly different between carriers of the CYP2C19 mutant allele. Case studies have also reported unexpected PHT toxicity in patients with at least one mutant CYP2C9*3 allele. One such case study reported a 41-year-old woman who on admission to the hospital for seizures was given 15 mg/kg over 30 minutes and became nonresponsive with low respiratory rate.[53] Subsequent serum PHT concentration was 79 μg/mL and genotyping revealed she carried one wild-type and one mutant CYP2C9*3 allele.

A study of Japanese epileptics using phenobarbital showed a correlation to genotype and clearance of phenobarbital.[54] This study measured serum concentrations and calculated clearance rates for 79 patients treated with phenobarbital and genotyped them for both CYP2C9 and CYP2C19. The authors found that patients with a mutant CYP2C9 allele had significantly reduced clearance of phenobarbital compared with wild-type homozygotes. They found no correlation between CYP2C19 genotype and phenobarbital clearance.

This suggests that there may be utility in genotyping for CYP2C9 to determine patients who may have reduced metabolism of PHT or phenobarbital before initiating therapy with these agents. These results also suggest that although both drugs are apparent substrates of CYP2C19, the genotype of the patient has not been shown to correlate to clinical outcomes such as maintenance dose or clearance.

Genomic Predictors of Higher Susceptibility to Adverse Events Unrelated To Drug Concentrations

Drug hypersensitivity reactions that commonly involve skin and mucosa can, in severe cases, result in aplastic anemia, renal failure, hepatitis, and death. Carbamazepine, an older but effective anticonvulsant, is also used widely for mood stabilization in bipolar disorder, for neuropathic pain syndromes, and an adjunct in chronic pain syndromes. In rare cases it can cause the life-threatening hypersensitivity reactions of Stevens–Johnson syndrome (SJS) and toxic epidermal necrolysis (TEN). While both are rare, they are clearly associated with AEDs but more commonly seen with carbamazepine.[55] Recent research has shown that the human leukocyte antigen (HLA) HLA-B*1502 shows a strong association with carbamazepine-induced SJS in Han Chinese.[56] Although this association was not found in any Caucasian populations, the finding prompted the FDA to change the labeling information of carbamazepine to include information about HLA-B*1502, and the FDA now recommends genotyping individuals of Asian ancestry for the allele prior to using the drug.[57] After the FDA recommendations were published, another study suggested a strong association between the allele and both carbamazepine- and PHT-induced SJS in a Thai population, providing evidence that the correlation may not be limited to Han Chinese.[58] Considering the structural similarities between carbamazepine and other AEDs, a study was conducted by Hung et al. to test whether a similar association existed between the HLA-B*1502 allele and drug-induced SJS/ TEN during therapy with other commonly used AEDs, specifically PHT, lamotrigine (LTG), and oxcarbazepine (OXC).[59]

This was a case–control association study by identifying cases of SJS and TEN induced from PHT, LTG, or OXC from various hospital systems in Taiwan from 2002 to 2008. The authors enrolled 26 PHT-induced cases, 6 LTG-induced cases, and 3 OXC-induced cases. In all enrolled cases, the drug was considered the cause of the SJS/TEN if onset was within 2 months of starting the drug. For control cases, 113 patients using PHT and 67 using LTG for over 3 months without any adverse drug reactions were enrolled. To control for OXC, a Taiwanese population study was used and 93 healthy subjects were randomly selected. All enrolled individuals were Han Chinese living in Taiwan. Individuals were then HLA genotyped to determine A,

B, C, and DRB1 alleles. The authors found HLA-B*1502 present in 30.8% of PHT-related SJS/TEN, 33% of LTG-related SJS, and 100% of OXC-related SJS with odds ratios of 5.1 (95% CI: 1.8–15.1; $P = .0041$), 5.1 (95% CI: 0.8–33.8; $P = .1266$), and 80.7 (95% CI: 3.8–1,714.4; $P = 8.4 \times 10^{-4}$), respectively. HLA-B*1502 is a common risk allele for multiple aromatic antiepileptic drugs.

Considering the potential for SJS or TEN, the FDA recommends genotyping patients of Asian ancestry prior to treatment with carbamazepine. Combined with evidence that other AEDs may have the same increased risk with the HLA-B*1502 allele, genetic testing for Asian patients may prove extremely useful for reducing the risk of this adverse reaction. The association between the allele and carbamazepine has not been demonstrated in non-Asian populations.[60] This is likely because SJS/ TEN and the frequency of the allele in non-Asians are so rare that the sample sizes are not large enough to detect it.

Pharmacogenomic Factors and Anticonvulsant Resistance

It has been hypothesized that patients with uncontrolled seizures despite treatment with multiple anticonvulsants may have a genetic overexpression of energy-dependent drug efflux transporters at the blood brain barrier (BBB) rendering them anticonvulsant resistant. Several studies have investigated whether polymorphisms in *ABCB1*—the gene that encodes the efflux transporter ABCB1 (also known as P-glycoprotein [P-gp] and MDR1)—are correlated with the nonresponse to antiepileptic drugs, with conflicting results.

In a report by Siddiqui et al., 115 drug-responsive epileptics, 200 drug-resistant epileptics, and 200 control patients were genotyped at ABCB1 3435 for the C or T polymorphism.[61] There was a significantly higher likelihood for drug-resistant epileptics to have the CC genotype rather than the TT genotype compared with drug-responsive epileptics with an odds ratio of 2.66 and a 95% confidence interval of 1.32–5.38. Unfortunately these results could not be replicated by two subsequent and similar studies.[62,63]

While a genetic variation of the ABCB1 transporter is a reasonable potential cause of multiple drug resistance in epileptics, it does not seem that response or nonresponse can be predicted from the C3435T polymorphism. It would seem possible that either anticonvulsants are not dependent on P-gp for transport into the brain or anticonvulsants are not high-affinity substrates for P-gp. That P-gp is not involved in drug resistance to anticonvulsants can also be seen in animal data. Data shown in Figure 16–1 show that there is little, if any, significant change in brain/plasma ratio following a known P-gp inhibitor for several anticonvulsants.[50] Moreover, the relationship between plasma and CSF concentrations for older anticonvulsants is linear rather than nonlinear as would be expected if an energy-dependent transporter were involved. These results do not necessarily suggest that variation in the ABCB1 transporter plays no role in multiple drug resistance, but instead suggest that whatever role the transporter plays in resistance may not be clearly predicted by genotyping for the C3435T polymorphism. Conflicting results may be further explained by Kimchi-Sarfaty et al. These authors explain that a synonymous SNP found in the ABCB1 transporter gene results in an altered P-gp response, despite producing no changes in the amino acid that is produced. The authors hypothesize that, although the amino acid composition itself remains unchanged, this rare codon causes altered protein folding and therefore conformational changes at the P-gp receptor, and, thus, can change the substrate-receptor response.[64] Clearly, more research should be performed to determine if these changes translate into clinically meaningful effects on drug response.

In summary, genomic study is clearly useful in identifying populations of patients likely to need higher or lower doses of PHT and phenobarbital owing to differences in rate of metabolism. Genomic study is also useful in identifying populations of patients and individual patients more susceptible to hypersensitivity reactions. Unfortunately, existing data do not suggest that genomic study will be useful in explaining anticonvulsant resistance.

MULTIPLE SCLEROSIS

MS is a chronic autoimmune disease of the central nervous system involving pathological inflammation, demyelination, and neuron degeneration characterized by progressive physical and cognitive dysfunction.[65] The pathogenesis of MS is not fully understood, but appears to involve both environmental and genetic mechanisms. The clinical course of MS is extensively variable between individuals. An initial triggering event is thought to produce a subclinical presentation of neurodegenerative changes. This latent period is succeeded by an initial demyelinating event, called a clinically isolated syndrome (CIS). MS diagnosis is confirmed on a second isolated event and evidence of new inflammatory lesions on brain MRI. MS may remain subclinical in some individuals throughout an entire lifetime, while in others, an initial clinical isolated syndrome is followed by a mild course of disease. Eighty-five percent of patients develop a relapsing-remitting course (RRMS), which can progress into secondary progressive MS (SPMS) characterized by progressive neurological decline without periods of remission. In 10–15% of cases, disease is progressive from the initial event and is termed primary progressive (PPMS) that may also be relapsing in nature (PRMS).

The susceptibility of individuals to developing MS appears to be heterogeneous and involves complex non-Mendelian inheritance.[66,67] Risk factors for developing MS appear to include female sex, family history of MS, and Caucasian ethnicity.[67,68] Environmental factors have also been explored. Antibodies against the Epstein–Barr virus have been associated with gray matter atrophy in MS.[69,70] Smoking is associated with greater disability, lesions, and neurodegeneration in MS.[71,72] Additionally, vitamin D deficiency and polymorphisms in the vitamin D receptor have been associated with increased risk of developing MS and accelerated disease progression.[73] The improvement of genetic testing, particularly of genome-wide association studies (GWAS), has identified several genes that may confer susceptibility to developing MS. In particular, the polymorphisms in the HLA have consistently shown to confer 20–60% of the genetic susceptibility to MS. Polymorphisms in other immune system components, including IL2RA, IL7RA, CD58, CLEC16A, and CD226, may increase disease susceptibility.[66,74]

Given the extensive heterogeneity of susceptibility and clinical course of MS, treatment of MS is equally complex. Current strategies aim at symptomatic management and delaying disease progression, but do not offer a cure. Disease-modifying therapies downregulate various pathogenic immune processes and have shown to effectively reduce relapses, lessen brain MRI activity, and slow progression of disability.[75,76] Despite these advantages, studies indicate large differences in treatment response between individuals. While some patients appear to respond well, up to half of those treated are nonresponders to therapy, and some develop serious side effects.[77,78] Interestingly, treatment failure with one agent does not appear to correlate with ineffectiveness of a second agent. The ability to predict patient response would allow for individualized therapy that may reduce both the economic and disease burdens of MS. Pharmacogenomic research has attempted to identify genetic differences that may provide insight into this puzzle. The ability to predict patient response would allow for individualized therapy that may reduce both the economic and disease burdens of MS.

Interferon-β

Interferon therapy has been used as a first-line treatment for MS for many years. Interferon-beta is a naturally occurring immunoregulator in humans and has antiproliferative, proapoptotic, and antiviral properties.[79] The precise mechanism of action of IFN-β in MS is unknown; however, it may involve inhibition of production of proinflammatory cytokines, decreased brain penetration of T-cells, and promotion of remyelination.[80] There are currently three interferons approved for use in MS, including Avonex (IFN-β1a), Rebif (IFN-β1a), and Betaferon (IFN-β1b). All of these interferons bind to the same receptor, IFNAR, which consists of two subunits, IFNAR1 and IFNAR2. These receptors are coded by genes on chromosome 21q22.1, which are under study.[81] Side effects from interferon therapy include injection site reactions, flu-like symptoms, depression, bronchospasms, and hepatotoxicity. In responders, interferon therapy decreases relapse rate and severity and slows clinical progression; however, relapse rates occur in up to 50% of people treated with interferon.[82] IFN-β therapy has been shown to evoke antibody production in some individuals. These antibodies can lead to immunogenic responses and can neutralize IFN-β and directly decrease therapeutic efficacy. The development of binding antibodies (BABs), some of which are neutralizing (NABs), are thought to decrease the efficacy of interferons to varying degrees.[83] Given the incongruity in treatment response to interferon therapy, genomic studies have attempted to identify loci that may predict treatment response among MS patients. In particular, candidate gene studies were performed for HLA and interferon receptor polymorphisms, and one genome-wide analysis was performed. Studies varied greatly in response definition and genetic marker studies (Table 16–1).

TABLE 16–1 Pharmacogenomic studies of disease-modifying therapies in multiple sclerosis.

Therapy	Patient Population	Genetic Markers	Response Definition	Response Rate	Association
Sriram et al.[81] IFN-β	RRMS, ≥2 relapses in 2 years prior to therapy	8 SNPS in IFNAR1 and IFNAR2: • IFNAR1-SNP PROM 408 • IFNAR1-SNP 2627 • IFNAR1-SNP 16469 • IFNAR1-SNP 16725 • IFNAR1-SNP 18417 • IFNAR2-SNP 7126 • IFNAR2-SNP 11876 • IFNAR2-SNP 32499	0 relapses and no increase in EDSS in 2 years of follow-up	57 responders 48 nonresponders 42 undefined	*None*, trend in SNP16469 (A/T), third intron of IFNAR1 (modest association with relapse-free status, requires confirmation)
Leyva et al.[87] IFN-β	RRMS (*n* = 100) Secondary progressive (*n* = 47)	3 SNPS in IFNAR1 and IFNAR2: • IFNAR1-SNP PROM 408 • IFNAR1-SNP 18417 • IFNAR2-SNP 11876	Nonresponders: relapse within previous year or increase of 0.5 points in EDSS score after first year of treatment	104 responders 43 nonresponders	*None* to interferon response, but IFNAR1-SNP 18417, IFNAR2-SNP 11876 related to disease susceptibility
Byun et al.[88] IFN-β	RRMS ≥2 relapses in 2 years prior to treatment	35 SNPs selected as candidates from genome-wide analysis: • HAPLN1 SNP rs 2266137 • GPC5 SNP rs 10492503 • BMP8B TRIT1 SNP rs1493663 • LOC645097 LOC729006 SNP rs4698555 • LRRC49 SNP rs986393 • DIRAS2 SNP rs1172902 • PTGER3 SNP rs132764 • FLJ32978 SNP rs952084 • E2F7 NAV3 SNP rs10506738 • GPC5 SNP rs9301789 • COL25A1 SNP rs794143 • FAM5C RGS18 SNP rs230275 • DAB2 SNP rs10512706 • LOC574040 SNP rs1421784	0 relapses and no increase in EDSS in 2 years of follow-up	99 responders 107 nonresponders	18 SNPs associated with response: • HAPLN1 SNP rs 2266137 • GPC5 SNP rs 10492503 • LOC645097 LOC729006 SNP rs4698555 • LRRC49 SNP rs986393 • FLJ32978 SNP rs952084 • GPC5 SNP rs9301789 • COL25A1 SNP rs794143 • DAB2 SNP rs10512706 • LOC574040 SNP rs1421784 • LOC39118 SNP rs10494649 • LOC653214 SNP rs2212774 • POFUT2 SNP rs1999333 • MCTP2 LOC220311 SNP rs7169847

(Continued)

TABLE 16-1 Pharmacogenomic studies of disease-modifying therapies in multiple sclerosis. (*Continued*)

Therapy	Patient Population	Genetic Markers	Response Definition	Response Rate	Association
		· LOC39118 SNP rs10494649			· C80RF4 ZMAT4 SNP rs10504026
		· LOC653214 SNP rs2212774			· CAST SNP rs10510779
		· CCDC102B DOK6 SNP rs1573400			· LOC442331 SNP rs6944054
		· RASGEF1B COX5BL1 SNP rs538307			· TAFA1 SNP rs4855469
		· POFUT2 SNP rs1999333			· NPAS3 SNP rs4128599
		· DACH2 KLHL4 SNP rs1389357			
		· TTK SNP rs239586			
		· MCTP2 LOC220311 SNP rs7169847			
		· SEP15 HS2ST1 SNP rs479341			
		· C80RF4 ZMAT4 SNP rs10504026			
		· CAST SNP rs10510779			
		· DBIL2 SNP rs9294145			
		· LOC442331 SNP rs6944054			
		· DMD SNP rs10521996			
		· STK39 SNP rs9287889			
		· CDH13 SNP rs1109542			
		· LOC402059 SNP rs137219			
		· FBX038 SNP rs9325096			
		· SEP15 SNP rs581405			
		· TAFA1 SNP rs4855469			
		· NPAS3 SNP rs4128599			
Hoffmann et al.[83]	MS	HLA-I and HLA-II DRB1, DQB1	Antibody production	202 antibody (+) 296 antibody (−)	HLA-DRB1*0401 and *0408 related to antibodies to IFN-β, but are not necessarily related to whether they are NABS
Villoslada et al.[84]	RRMS ≥2 relapses in last 2 years	HLA-A, -B, -DRB1, -DQB1	0 relapses and no increase in EDSS in 2 years of follow-up	48 responders 57 nonresponders	*None* to interferon response, but DRB1*1501, DQB1*0602 related to disease susceptibility
Comabella et al.[85]	RRMS	HLA-A, -B, -C, -DRB1, -DQA1, and -DQB1	0 relapses and no increase in EDSS in 2 years of follow-up	74 responders 75 nonresponders	*None*

| Gross et al.[90] | IFN-β
Glatiramer acetate | HLA-DRB1*1501
IRF8 | RRMS (n = 723)
PRMS (n = 10)
CIS (n = 23) | First event described as:
(a) Clinical relapse or
(b) Change in T2 hyperintense lesion or new gadolinium-enhancing lesion on MRI
Or an (c) EDSS increase of 1 or more points over 6 months | 424 IFN-β:
(a) 155 events
(b) 115 events
(c) 35 events
332 GA:
(a) 39 events
(b) 34 events
(c) 8 events | Homozygous HLA-DRB1*1501 ↑ time to first event in GA more than IFN-β
Homozygous IRF8 ↑ time to first event in GA more than IFN-β and ↓ time to first event in IFN-β |
| Grossman et al.[91] | Glatiramer acetate | 61 candidate SNPs on:
TRB@
MBP
MOG
CTSS
MMP9
CD80
CD86
CTLA4
APOE
IFNG
IL1R1
IL1R2
IL@RA
IL2RB
IL2RB1
IL2RB2
SPP1
TGFB1
TGFB2
TGFB3
CCL3
CCL5
CCR3
CASP1
FAS
ESR1
ESR2 | RRMS (n = 174 consented to genomic testing) | No relapse over 9 months and no more than one T1-enhancing lesions
Or
No new gadolinium-enhanced lesion over first 6 months
Or
0 relapses and no increase in EDSS in 2 years of follow-up | 89 untreated
85 GA | TRB@ CTSS
Nominal significance for MBP, CD86, FAS, IL1R1, IL12RB2 |

Human Leukocyte Antigen

HLA are critical components of T-cell activation and differentiation, and HLA alleles have consistently shown to confer disease susceptibility in MS and may be involved in disease progression. They are located on major histocompatibility complex (MHC) on chromosome 6p21.3.[84] Therefore, HLA alleles have been studied extensively in relation to treatment response of disease-modifying therapies and association with antibody production against IFN-β. HLA-A, -B, -C, -DRB1*1501, and -DQB1*0602 have been studied. No association was found with HLA status and treatment outcome, but DRB1*1501 and DQB1*0602 were related to disease susceptibility.[85,86]

Hoffmann et al.[83] studied the association of HLA class II alleles and the development of and treatment response in MS patients in Germany. Patients carrying the HLA-DRB1*0401 and -DRB1*0408 carriers had increased risk of developing IFN-β antibodies. However, these alleles were not consistently associated with NAB production. Although allelic variation has been correlated with antibody production, it has not been directly correlated with treatment response.

Interferon Receptors

The primary mechanism of interferon action is thought to involve binding of interferon to the interferon type I receptor, a cell-surface receptor responsible for activation of the JAK-STAT pathway and subsequent stimulation of an immunological signaling cascade.[86] The interferon receptor is comprised of two subunits, IFNAR1 and IFNAR2, which have been tested for polymorphisms in association with treatment response. These receptors are coded for by genes on chromosome 21q22.1, which are under study.[81] Only SNP 16469 on the IFNAR1 gene showed a moderate association with relapse-free status.[81] However, IFNAR1 (SNP 18417) and IFNAR2 (SNP 11876) have shown a relationship to disease susceptibility.[87] Conversely, Byun et al. did not find a relationship between SNPs detected in or near IFNAR1 or IFNAR2, but the findings were limited as the authors analyzed only SNPS detected by their microarrays.[88]

Genome-Wide Analysis

Byun et al.[88] performed a genome-wide analysis to assess the role of various polymorphisms in interferon treatment response. Two hundred and six patients were recruited at four medical centers in the Mediterranean Basin. Patients needed to have RRMS, current treatment with beta-interferon, and a history of two or more relapses in 2 years prior to therapy initiation for inclusion. They were followed for 2 years with disease assessments by neurologists every 3 months. Clinical response was defined as zero relapses and no increase in EDSS throughout the entire 2-year follow-up period. Overall, 99 patients were considered responders while 107 were nonresponders. Genome-wide analysis of patient DNA was used to identify potential SNP candidates based on allelic frequencies and clustering. Thirty-five candidate SNPs were selected, 18 of which remained significant after analysis, including glypican, collagen type XXV α1, hyaluronan

proteoglycan link protein, calpastatin, TAFA1 (chemokine-like), LOC442331 (similar to dynein), and neuronal PAS dominant protein 3 which are located within genes. The remaining SNPS are in intergenic regions. Of note, SNPs related to ion channels and signal transduction pathways varied most frequently among responders and nonresponders. In particular, glypican 5 SNPs were common. Glypicans alter cytokine responsiveness and aid in axon regeneration and synapse formation, and are associated with MS plaques. Peripherally, they are also required for Schwann cell myelination. Interferon therapy may alter expression of glypicans and SNPs could potentially alter this effect. Polymorphisms in hyaluronan proteoglycans and collagen may affect the binding of matrix metalloproteases released by leukocytes to aid in their penetration through basement membranes. Interferon-beta has shown to inhibit these proteins. SNP variations in these proteins may prevent IFN-β's inhibitory effect. Interestingly, no association was found with interferon receptors, further corroborating reports of previous trials (Table 16–1). This study was limited in that it could only examine SNPs detected by the authors' microarray and that the authors did not control for NABs or BABs.[88]

Glatiramer Acetate (Copaxone)

Glatiramer acetate (GA) is a peptide similar in structure to myelin basic protein, which may modify the immune response of myelin antigens in MS patients and increase repair of neural tissue.[89] In clinical trials, Copaxone produced a 30% reduction in relapse rate, increased time between relapses and number of patients who were relapse-free, and did slow disease progression in MS patients. Injection site reactions are common and use of GA may produce transient chest pain, flushing, and palpitations. Two studies to date have looked at the role of genetic markers in conferring treatment response in patients receiving GA therapy. GA binds to MHC class II molecules, some of which are encoded by DRB1.

Gross et al.[90] performed a retrospective analysis on the association with the HLA-DRB1*1501 allele as well as interferon response factor 8 (IRF8) in time to first event in patients treated with either IFN-β or GA (Table 16–1). Time to first event was defined as clinical relapse, change in T2 hyperintense lesion or new gadolinium-enhancing lesion on MRI, or an EDSS increase of 1 or more points over 6 months. Overall, time to first event was not different between GA and IFN-β. The HLA-DRB1*1501 allele correlated with a better treatment response in GA-treated patients. Association of this allele was not found in the IFN-β subset. Although this association explained some of the hazard-free survival in GA-treated patients, the authors conclude that it likely only exerts a modest effect on treatment response with GA therapy. In addition, those homozygous for IRF8 had demonstrated longer times to first event in the GA population more than the IFN-β population and appeared to be associated with shorter time to first event in the IFN-β population.[90] However, this was not able to be replicated in IFN-β treated subjects with negative antibody status. IRF8 is associated with susceptibility to MS and upregulation of interferon response genes and patients with increased interferon response genes seem to be at an increased risk of relapse.[90]

Grossman et al. recruited patients from 2 previous clinical trials of GA versus placebo treatment, and assessed the relationship between treatment response and 63 SNPs.[91] One hundred and one patients from the European/Canadian MRI trial and 73 patients from the US pivotal trail were enrolled and genotypes were analyzed. Responders in the E/C trial were previously defined as having no clinical relapse in the 9 months of follow-up and no more than one T1-enhancing lesion, or no new T1-enhancing lesion appearance in the first 6 months of therapy, while US trial responders were identified as patients who remained relapse-free with no increase in EDSS score over the duration of the 2-year trial. Results indicated two genes were predictive of GA response, TRB@ and CTSS. TRB@ is a molecular complex thought to be associated with GA mechanism of action, and was associated with treatment response in both E/C and US responders (OR 6.85). CTSS may be involved in GA metabolism, and was associated with treatment response in the E/C trial. In addition, it plays a role in MHC II chain processing. Of note, the HLA-DRB1*1501 was not associated with drug response, but the study may have been underpowered to detect an association. Nominal significance was seen for MBP, CD86, FAS, IL1R1, and IL12RB2. MBP is thought to be the primary myelin autoantigen attacked by the immune system, which is inhibited by GA.

Natalizumab (Tysabri)

Natalizumab is a recombinant humanized monoclonal antibody that inhibits VLA-4 adhesion to VCAM expressed on activated endothelium.[92] Inhibition of VLA-4 results in impaired T-cell migration across the BBB and apoptosis. In patients with RRMS, natalizumab reduces the probability of disease progression, increases probability of remaining relapse-free, and reduces the appearance of new lesions on MRI. Despite treatment response in most patients, Tysabri is currently considered a second-line agent in the treatment of MS due to the risk of progressive multifocal leukoencephalopathy (PML).[93] PML is caused by JC polyomavirus (JCV), an opportunistic pathogen which infects oligodendrocytes and causes rapid neuronal demyelination and death. Although an estimated 50–60% of MS patients are infected with JCV, most individuals will remain asymptomatic unless immunocompromised. JCV exists in two distinct subtypes, a benign form and a pathogenic form capable of infecting nerve cells. This pathogenic form has been associated with multiple mutations of the noncoding control region (NCCR) involved in gene replication.

To identify how JCV genotype or specific mutations may confer susceptibility to developing PML, Reid et al.[93] conducted a genomic analysis of viral isolates collected from 17 PML patients treated with natalizumab. Isolates were obtained from plasma, urine, and CSF of selected patients and JCV genotype, NCCR variations, and VP1 capsid protein sequences were analyzed using PCR amplification. Results indicated multiple JCV genotypes between individuals, with each patient being infected with a single genotype. No association was found between JCV genotype and PML development. In blood and CSF, NCCR and VP1 mutations were found in 100% and 81% of isolates, respectively. In contrast, urine samples of JCV contained no mutations in these regions. These results indicate that after infection with the benign form of the virus, NCCR and VP1 mutations occur via an unknown mechanism that creates the pathogenic, infectious form of the virus responsible for PML. How natalizumab may act to facilitate this transformation is unknown, but warrants further study. Identification of susceptibility loci on the viral genome may help identify patients at risk for PML development and allow for more selective use of natalizumab.

Fingolimod (Gilenya)

Fingolimod is the first oral therapy available for MS and reduces frequency of relapses and delays disability.[94] It binds to sphingosine 1-phosphate receptor subtypes 1, 3, 4, and 5, which reduces lymphocyte levels in the blood by inhibiting release from lymph nodes. In a clinical trial comparing fingolimod with interferon-β, patients experienced lower annual relapse rates (17% vs. 30%) and reduced appearance of gadolium-enhanced lesions on MRI.[95] Side effects of fingolimod include macular edema, transient bradycardia on initial administration, and immunosuppression. At present, no pharmacogenomic studies have been performed on fingolimod, as heterogeneous treatment responses or side effect profiles are not yet apparent with this therapy.

Mitoxantrone (Novantrone)

Mitoxantrone (MX) is an antineoplastic agent indicated for SPMS and has shown to reduce relapse rates and decrease the rate of disability.[96] MX inhibits DNA and RNA synthesis and has many immunomodulatory effects that are thought to influence MS disease progression. Currently, the clinical utility of MX is limited due to an increased risk of hematological malignancy and dose-limiting cardiotoxicity.

Therapeutic efficacy of MX appears to be influenced by polymorphisms in the ATP-binding cassette transporter genes responsible for drug efflux. Cotte et al. studied the association between ABC polymorphisms and treatment response and side effect profile of MS patients treated with MX.[97] Genotypic data were analyzed retrospectively from 309 MX or MX-corticosteroid-treated patients for ABCB1 2677G>T, 3435C>T, ABCG2 V12M, and Q141K. Clinical response was analyzed between 9 and 12 months, and defined by EDSS stability or improvement, improvement in relapse rate, MSFC stability/improvement, MRI activity, and physician discretion. In patients receiving MX monotherapy, 78.1% were considered responders and 59.1% of MX/CS-treated patients were considered responders. Twenty-eight patients experienced severe cardiac effects and eight had hematological effects. When compared with healthy subjects, no difference was found in genotypic frequencies. An in vitro assay was performed to assess ABC-transporter-mediated MX efflux in CD56+ cells. Patients homozygous for common ABCB1/ABCB2 alleles had higher MX efflux and less CD56+ cell death than patients with at least one variant allele. When correlated with therapeutic response, patients with two variant alleles had higher response rates (83%) than patients with two common alleles (62.5). Heterozygous patients had an intermediate effect (79.6%). In MX/CS-treated patients, no association was found between variant ABC alleles and therapeutic response; however, this cohort was small. No correlation was found between ABC-transporter alleles and cardiotoxicity or hematotoxicity. It appears ABCB1 and ABCG2 alleles may be useful in identifying potential responders to MX treatment.

Conclusions

The current body of evidence indicates that pharmacogenomic analysis may play an important role in both the efficacy and toxicity of MS treatments. In patients treated with beta-interferons, polymorphisms in the interferon receptor or HLA do not correlate with treatment response, while HLA-DRB1*0401 and *0408 loci correlate with antibody production. Recently, genome-wide analysis revealed SNPs in glypticans and extracellular matrix proteins show a relationship to treatment response. Increased time to first event with GA therapy has been associated with HLA-DRB1*1501, and TRB@ and CTSS genes were associated with treatment response. PML found in natalizumab patients may be associated with specific viral polymorphisms of the JCV. MX responsiveness appears to be related to ABCB1/ABCB2 polymorphisms.

The aforementioned pharmacogenomic studies have been useful in identifying possible mechanisms conferring response or toxicity to treatment. The continued utilization of genome-wide screening will expectantly provide more information on the complex genetic and environmental interactions involved in MS susceptibility, disease course, and treatment. These findings will be crucial in improving the clinical course and outlook of MS.

PARKINSON DISEASE

PD is a degenerative neurological disorder that results in death of dopaminergic neurons in the substantia nigra. The exact etiology of PD is yet to be determined, but it has been hypothesized that both genetic and environmental factors may play a role. The loss of dopaminergic neurons of the nigrostriatal pathway results in inhibition of thalamic activity, which thereby reduces activity of the motor cortex. This decrease in motor function results in the hallmark features of PD including tremor at rest, bradykinesia, postural instability, and rigidity. Advanced stages of the disease may even precipitate behavioral and cognitive impairment.[98]

Although there is no cure for PD, several pharmacological treatments have proven to be efficacious in reducing motor symptoms and improving quality of life. Such classes of medications include dopamine precursors, monoamine oxidase type B (MAO-B) inhibitors, catechol-*O*-methyltransferase (COMT)

inhibitors, dopamine receptor agonists, and NMDA receptor antagonists. However, the interindividual variability with respect to both treatment response and tolerability is large.

In recent years, there has been growing interest in genetic variability as an explanation for the large interindividual variability in antiparkinson drug efficacy and toxicity. Numerous gene candidates have been identified including, but not limited to, genes encoding COMT (*COMT* gene), dopamine receptors (*DRD1, DRD2, DRD3* genes), dopamine beta-hydroxylase (*DBH* gene), dopamine transporter (*DAT* gene), monoamine oxidases (*MAOA, MAOB* genes), and cytochrome P450 enzymes.[99]

Dopamine Precursors

Levodopa (L-dopa) is the immediate metabolic precursor of dopamine and is the cornerstone treatment for PD. L-dopa is administered with carbidopa, a noncompetitive l-amino acid decarboxylase inhibitor that prevents the conversion of L-dopa to dopamine in the periphery and GI tract. Since carbidopa does not cross the BBB while L-dopa does, concomitant administration of these two drugs substantially increases the bioavailability of L-dopa in the central nervous system. Once past the BBB, L-dopa is converted to dopamine by aromatic l-amino acid decarboxylase (DOPA decarboxylase) in the substantia nigra where it is stored in presynaptic dopaminergic neurons. When stimulated for release, the decarboxylated L-dopa reserve binds to postsynaptic D_1 and D_2 receptors.

Dopamine and its precursors undergo immediate degradation by the enzymes COMT and MAO-B.[98] Genetic polymorphisms of COMT and MAO-B enzymes have been hypothesized to influence the effectiveness of L-dopa therapy. Perhaps the most studied genetic polymorphism of the COMT enzyme is the Val[158]Met polymorphism, which is an SNP caused by a valine to methionine substitution. This SNP results in a low-activity allele COMT L and may result in three possible genotypes with varying activity—low-activity COMT$^{L/L}$, intermediate-activity COMT$^{L/H}$, and high-activity COMT$^{H/H}$. The COMT$^{H/H}$ variant is up to four times more active in the degradation of dopamine versus the low-activity variant.

Reilly et al. were one of the first to correlate COMT activity with patient response to L-dopa therapy.[100] Their study in 14 patients found that those with higher erythrocyte COMT activity experienced less favorable clinical responses to L-dopa than patients with lower erythrocyte COMT activity. Their study set the stage for future research into the genetic polymorphisms that affect the activity level of the COMT enzyme. Bialecka et al. demonstrated a possible link between SNPs of the *COMT* gene and interpatient variability in therapeutic response as measured by the daily optimal L-dopa dose during the fifth year of treatment.[101] This case–control study of 679 patients of Caucasian origin observed that the mean L-dopa dose at year 5 of treatment increased with the activity of functional haplotypes. Significantly higher mean doses (604 mg per day vs. 512 mg per day, $P < .05$) were associated with high-activity COMT$^{H/H}$ haplotype carriers as compared with low-activity COMT$^{L/L}$ haplotype carriers. However, COMT genotype was not found to be associated with the development of L-dopa-induced dyskinesias. Yet, a smaller retrospective study conducted by Bialecka et al. failed to observe significant differences between COMT and MAO-B genotypes on effective L-dopa daily doses.[102]

In contrast, a prospective study of 104 PD patients of Italian descent conducted by Contin et al. investigated the effect of COMT Val[158]Met polymorphism on L-dopa response and rate of adverse events using pharmacokinetic (T_{max}) and pharmacodynamic (C_{max}) parameters.[103] Neither did they find statistically significant differences in pharmacokinetic and pharmacodynamic parameters in patients with varying COMT haplotypes nor were they able to correlate the COMT polymorphisms with oral bioavailability in their study population. Similar studies in Korean and Japanese patients also found no statistically significant differences between COMT genotypes and pharmacokinetic and pharmacodynamic responses to L-dopa therapy.[104,105]

Associations between genetic polymorphisms and L-dopa-induced side effects, particularly dyskinesias, have also been examined to some extent. Several investigators observed statistically significant correlations between L-dopa-induced peak-dose dyskinesias with the DRD2 CAn-STR gene polymorphism, which include four common alleles (13, 14, 15, or 16 CA repeats). Oliveri et al. found that patients with the at least 1 of the 13 or 14 alleles of the DRD2 CAn-STR gene had a risk reduction in development of dyskinesias when compared with those who carried none (OR = 0.28, 95% CI: 0.11–0.77).[106] Zappia et al. confirmed their result only in male subjects (OR = 0.34, 95% CI: 0.14–0.84).[107] Strong et al. observed that patients with the 14 allele or 14/15 genotype of the DRD2 CAn-STR gene actually had an increased risk of early dyskinesia (OR = 3.4, CI: 1.1–10.4; OR = 27.2, CI: 1.4–510).[108]

As evidenced by the mixed results in the studies just previously highlighted, the verdict is still out on the influence of COMT polymorphisms on L-dopa efficacy. Genetic variability of the COMT enzyme has demonstrated at least some influence on the dosing of L-dopa, which may be useful in designing individualized treatment regimens. Stronger pharmacogenetic associations have emerged as they pertain to L-dopa-induced adverse effects, but the body of evidence is still inadequate to make definitive assertions. What is obvious from these investigations is that the clinical implications of such genetic variability on L-dopa therapy remain inconclusive with respect to therapeutic response and limited with regard to drug toxicity.

Monoamine Oxidase Type B Inhibitors

MAO-B is the primary enzyme in the brain responsible for the breakdown of dopamine. MAO-B inhibitors are used concomitantly with L-dopa therapy to potentiate the effects of L-dopa. This combination therapy results in both beneficial dopaminergic effects on motor function and the potential for the dose reductions of L-dopa, which may help to decrease rates of significant adverse events. Currently, there are two FDA-approved

MAO-B inhibitors indicated for the treatment of PD—selegiline and rasagiline. Selegiline is a selective, noncompetitive antagonist of the MAO-B enzyme and is indicated as an adjuvant agent to L-dopa therapy. Rasagiline is a selective, irreversible inhibitor of MAO-B with 5–10 times greater potency than selegiline and is therefore indicated for monotherapy in early stages of PD.[109]

Genetic polymorphisms of the cytochrome P450 superfamily of enzymes have been postulated to play a role influencing treatment of PD with MAO-B inhibitors. Selegiline has been found to be associated with gene polymorphisms of the CYP450 superfamily of enzymes, most notably CYP2B6. CYP2B6 had long been regarded a minor contributor in drug metabolism. In recent years, however, it has been discovered that CYP2B6 makes up approximately 1–10% of hepatic CYP content and is the major metabolizing enzyme for numerous drugs, including selegiline.[110] Furthermore, it has been noted that there is up to a 250-fold interindividual variation in CYP2B6 expression due to genetic polymorphisms with 29 allelic variants identified to date (CYP2B6*1– *29).[111,112] There have been several important allelic variants that have been identified that alter the level of activity of CYP2B6, although most do not translate into changes in enzymatic function. In an in vitro study performed by Watanabe et al., several allelic variants were found to affect the metabolism of selegiline.[113] Two allelic variants—CYP2B6*10 and CYP2B6*14—appeared to have significantly lower enzymatic activity for selegiline N-demethylation compared with the wild-type allele.

It has been proposed that rasagiline may be associated with gene polymorphisms in CYP1A2, MAO-B, and the B-cell lymphoma 2 (Bcl-2).[114] Rasagiline is metabolized by CYP1A2 and thereby might be thought to be affected by genetic polymorphisms in this enzyme. To date, however, no allelic variants in CYP1A2 have been found to affect treatment with rasagiline, and genetic polymorphisms in BCL-2 and MAO-B have not been studied to any extent with relation to rasagiline therapy.

The knowledge regarding the effect of genetic variability on MAO-B inhibitors is still in its infancy and it is not yet known exactly how these genetic variations will affect treatment efficacy and toxicity. The available information regarding the effect of genetic polymorphisms on the metabolism of selegiline is limited, but the findings thus far warrant future studies to investigate the clinical implications. Considering the important role CYP2B6 plays in selegiline metabolism, genetic polymorphisms of this enzyme may prove to have some impact on drug exposure and clinical effectiveness in PD patients. More research is needed to evaluate the role of genetic polymorphism on rasagiline therapy, and this will most likely focus on variations of the CYP1A2, MAOB, and BCL2 genes.

Catechol-O-Methyltransferase Inhibitors

COMT is an enzyme that functions alongside DOPA decarboxylase to convert L-dopa to a less active metabolite, 3-O-methyldopa (3-OMD). COMT is found to its greatest extent in the liver and kidneys but is also present throughout other peripheral sites and centrally in neuronal tissues. COMT inhibitors—entacapone and tolcapone—are another class of medications used as an adjunct to L-dopa therapy in the treatment of PD. They are utilized to extend the half-life and duration of action of L-dopa, which also may allow the use of smaller L-dopa dose for therapeutic effect. Entacapone is reversible COMT inhibitor that acts only in the periphery and is more often used specifically for patients who experience "wearing off" symptoms associated with long-term L-dopa treatment. Tolcapone is a selective, reversible COMT inhibitor that acts at both peripheral and central sites and, thus, it is more potent and longer-acting than entacapone. However, tolcapone has been issued a black box warning for possible hepatotoxicity while entacapone has not, making the latter agent the preferred COMT inhibitor.[115,116]

Genetic polymorphisms of the genes that encode COMT and UDP-glucuronosyltransferase 1A9 (UGT1A9) have been studied with respect to the COMT inhibitors. The Val[158]Met polymorphism implicated in L-dopa therapy has also been thought to contribute to the efficacy of COMT inhibitors. Lee et al. investigated the effect of different COMT genotypes on the therapeutic efficacy of entacapone but concluded that COMT genotype was at best a minor factor contributing to clinical response.[117] Conversely, Corvol et al. found that COMT[H/H] and COMT[L/L] polymorphisms may in fact play a role in affecting the clinical response of L-dopa–entacapone therapy.[118] Their investigation was a randomized crossover clinical trial in 33 PD patients, each genotyped for COMT polymorphism, with the primary objective of assessing the gain in "on" time (i.e., period when symptoms are alleviated). The gain in "on" time in the COMT[H/H] group was significantly higher than that in the COMT[L/L] group (39 ± 10 minutes vs. 9 ± 9 minutes, $P = .04$). The authors also observed a significant interaction between COMT genotype and the response to entacapone on the pharmacokinetics of L-dopa ($P = .04$).

Both entacapone and tolcapone are eliminated by glucuronidation through UGT1A9. Genetic mutations associated with UGT1A9 have been shown to affect glucuronidation of other drugs.[119,120] Allelic variants of UGT1A9 have been less studied as it pertains to COMT inhibitors, but they may play a critical role in tolcapone-induced hepatotoxicity. There have been two case reports of female PD patients receiving tolcapone, both genotyped to be UGT1A9 PM, who developed severe hepatocellular injury.[121] These cases of hepatotoxicity prompted the FDA to issue a black box warning and require more stringent monitoring parameters for tolcapone.[122]

As seen with the boxed warning issued for tolcapone hepatotoxicity, genetic polymorphisms of UGT1A9 hold great potential to shape the way we approach PD treatment using COMT inhibitors. Conflicting results regarding COMT polymorphism, however, underlie the importance of more replicative or confirmatory investigations to establish a clinically relevant link to PD pharmacotherapy.

Dopamine Agonists

Dopamine agonists include bromocriptine, pramipexole, and ropinirole, all of which are approved for monotherapy or in combination with L-dopa. Use as monotherapy may extend the time before L-dopa therapy is required. Use as an adjuvant drug allows for reduction in the L-dopa dose.

Bromocriptine is an ergot derivative that acts as an agonist on dopamine D_2 receptors and an antagonist on dopamine D_1 receptors in the CNS. It has been shown to be a substrate for the efflux transporter P-gp at the BBB in mice, and efficacy of bromocriptine is thought to be associated with genetic polymorphisms in the *ABCB1* gene, which encodes P-gp.[114,123] It is suggested that changes in P-gp expression or efflux activity as a consequence of genetic polymorphisms would significantly alter bromocriptine disposition in the brain, hence affecting the efficacy and toxicity. Over 100 allelic variants have been identified thus far in the *ABCB1* gene and have been found to alter the activity levels of the efflux transporter.[124] However, there have been no studies to date specifically evaluating the influence of allelic variants of ABCB1 on bromocriptine efficacy and toxicity in PD.

Pramipexole is also an ergot derivative and has been found to have large interpatient variability in therapeutic response and rates of adverse reactions. This variation in efficacy is thought to be a result of SNPs in the dopamine receptor genes *DRD2* and *DRD3*, specifically the *DRD2* TaqIA and *DRD3* Ser9Gly variants. A prospective study by Liu et al. of 30 Chinese PD patients administered pramipexole investigated *DRD2* TaqIA gene polymorphisms (allelic variances A1 and A2) and *DRD3* Ser9Gly gene polymorphisms (allelic variances Ser/Ser, Ser/Gly, and Gly/Gly) on treatment response.[125] No significant associations were observed with the DRD2 genotypes, but patients homozygous for Ser/Ser were found to have a statistically significant higher response to pramipexole over patients with the Gly allele ($P = .024$).

Genetic variations in dopamine receptor D_3 may indeed explain variability in pramipexole treatment efficacy, and more studies are needed to determine whether this holds true. The hypothetical impact of different ABCB1 genotypes on bromocriptine efficacy and toxicity seems worthwhile to pursue, considering that many ABCB1 allelic variants have been shown to affect P-gp activity. Again, additional studies are necessary to evaluate whether genetic polymorphisms will affect decisions in the treatment of PD patients with dopamine agonists.

NMDA Receptor Antagonist

Amantadine is the only NMDA receptor antagonist approved for use as monotherapy and as an adjuvant agent for the treatment of PD. Its exact mechanism has not been fully elucidated, but it is thought to potentiate dopaminergic responses that in turn increases dopamine release and inhibits reuptake.[126] These actions are independent of its antiviral effects. Amantadine has been found to be associated with polymorphisms in the genes

Neurology Cases

Case 1: 39-year-old homemaker

Mrs CF is a 39-year-old Caucasian homemaker who was previously employed as a symphony violinist. She has no significant medical history except a past diagnosis of essential hypertension treated for the past 5 years with olmesartan (Benicar) 20 mg once daily and hydrochlorothiazide 25 mg daily. She consumes two glasses of red wine a day. She has never smoked and has not been hospitalized since the birth of her only daughter 6 years ago. She is seeking a medical evaluation for a complaint of difficulty in swallowing when eating dinner. Over the past 3 months, she has experienced an estimated six episodes of choking on solid food and she would sometimes gasp for air until the food passed into her stomach. These episodes were relieved by drinking fluids but the last experience also included the regurgitation of food before her airway was sufficiently open to take a full breath. Twice during the past 6 months she awoke during the night with severe heart burn and epigastric pain that was relieved by a liquid antacid. The patient also complains of occasional mild diarrhea. Further inquiry into her social history revealed that she lost her job as a violinist due to deteriorating performance. Her physical exam was nonremarkable and all vital signs were normal. An upper gastroscopy examination was ordered that revealed the presence of Barrett's esophagus. Gastrointestinal esophageal reflux disease, asymptomatic (GERD), was diagnosed and the patient begun on a regimen of esomeprazole (Nexum), 20 mg twice a day. A tentative diagnosis of MS was included in a plan of further diagnostic tests that included an MRI, a lumbar puncture for CSF examination, and genetic screening for MS.

Question: If a suspicion of MS is confirmed, what would be the pertinent pharmacogenetic considerations for this woman before she is begun on pharmacotherapy?

Answer: MS can be difficult to diagnosis since its signs and symptoms overlap those of other medical disorders. Mrs CF had erosive esophagitis that was caused by GERD to which she was essentially asymptomatic until the appearance of dysphagia. The difficulty in swallowing disappeared rapidly on appropriate treatment with a proton pump inhibitor. Esomeprazole is the S-isomer of omeprazole and is extensively metabolized by the polymorphic enzyme CYP 2C19. PM via 2C19 will have high area under the drug concentration versus time curve (AUC) of omeprazole compared with the administration of the same dose to EM. The genetic background of

patients with MS strongly implicates the HLA locus of the genome and two or more interleukin receptor genes, IL2RA and IL7RA, as being associated with the disease. Given the episodic nature of MS symptoms, patients are likely to receive multiple drugs and highly variable dosage regimens in an attempt to maintain symptom remission. The often-used medications include corticosteroids, interferon, glatiramer, natalizumab and fingolimod, and MS. These drugs are given by injection with the exception of fingolimod, the first oral drug specifically for MS. Specific dosage recommendations based on pharmacogenetic tests related to these drugs are equivocal at this time with the exception that ABCB1/ABCB2 mutant alleles may predict a better response to MS. A variety of genetic biomarkers related to immune response are being investigated to predict therapeutic benefit from all of the MS therapies. Even without specific guidelines, MS patients are likely to take a variety of medications that are metabolized by the P450 system. Knowledge of metabolic pathways and whether drugs are CYP inducers or inhibitors is generally useful in predicting drug interactions. For example, CYP3A4 inducers would be expected to increase the clearance of corticosteroids and decrease their effectiveness in the treatment of MS.

Case 2: 64-year-old college professor

BJ is a 64-year-old professor of engineering. Over the past semester, he has become increasingly forgetful of basic principles that he has taught in class for over 20 years. He was unable to finish a mathematical derivation on the blackboard in a freshman class and had to relinquish control of the class to a graduate student. The following day he was admitted to the hospital after being brought by his wife to the emergency room because his eyes and skin had developed a yellow color and he had become disoriented to a point that he did not recognize her when he awoke in the morning. Physical examination revealed a distended liver, a pulse of 94, blood pressure of 145/89, and normal respirations. Significant laboratory findings included an elevated bilirubin (2.0 mg/dL; normal 0.1–1.0), an ALT of 200 U/L (normal 8–20), and a GGT of 75 U/L (normal 0–65). A mental status exam was significant for a Mini-Mental State Exam (MMSE) score of 22 (mild AD typically 19–24). His wife relayed a history of taking a drug for the past 4 months for his memory prescribed by his internist, but she could not remember the name of the medication.

(Continued)

Neurology Cases (*Continued*)

Question: What is the most likely cause of this man's problem and the relationship to pharmacogenetics?

Answer: Early onset AD (younger than 60–65) is associated with specific genetic findings on chromosomes 1, 14, and 21. Mutations on chromosome 21 cause the formation of abnormal APP. One of the most significant findings in this field is the association of the APOE gene on chromosome 19 with late-onset AD. APOE4 is present in about 40% of the population with late-onset Alzheimer's. At the present time, the APOE gene profile is used to identify people who are at risk. The principal drugs used in treatment are the AChEI. A number of candidate genes, described in the chapter text, have been investigated as predictors of response. Tacrine, the first drug available for Alzheimer's dementia, has caused liver enzyme elevations, principally ALT, in up to 50% of patients during the first few months of therapy. Various genes are thought to be associated with tacrine hepatotoxicity with mutations in ABCB4 (coding for multidrug resistance protein 3) being highly suspected. Tacrine is extensively metabolized by CYP1A2, glucuronidation, and minor pathways including CYP2D6. Genetic testing has become increasingly popular to profile metabolic capability in designing dosage regimens for tacrine, but the improved efficacy and tolerability of the alternative drugs are displacing this drug.

that encode dopamine receptors D_1 and D_2, but no studies to date have been undertaken to correlate this with efficacy or tolerability of the drug.[114]

Conclusions

It is without question that genetic variability to some extent is involved in the interindividual variability seen with pharmacological PD treatments. Some progress has been made in establishing links between variability in genes encoding drug receptors and metabolizing enzymes with response and toxicity of antiparkinson drugs. As discussed, interesting associations have emanated between PD pharmacotherapeutics and genetic polymorphisms—L-dopa with COMT and dopamine receptors, COMT inhibitors with COMT and UGT1A9, selegiline with CYP2B6, bromocriptine with P-gp, and pramipexole with dopamine receptor D_3. Yet, the clinical relevance of such genetic variability has not been conclusively determined with respect to therapeutic response and tolerability to PD pharmacotherapy.

Genetic polymorphisms in the proteins involved in the pharmacology of antiparkinson therapeutics may have significant clinical implications for effective and safe treatment. At the present time, PD patients are not routinely genotyped, as most of the information to date has not yielded unequivocal results. The various PD pharmacogenetic studies completed thus far have included relatively small samples sizes and may be underpowered to detect statistical differences. Furthermore, many of these studies were conducted in homogenous patient groups, which limit generalization to a broader population. Additional investigations with larger sample sizes and more heterogeneous patient populations are necessary to discover whether genetic polymorphisms may be used to minimize interindividual variability and guide pharmacological treatment of PD. Advancements in the fields of pharmacogenetics and pharmacogenomics will most certainly spur future exploratory and confirmatory genetic research in PD, which in turn may result in more individualized treatment approaches based on genetic variations (Table 16–2).

FREQUENTLY USED TERMS

Abbreviation and Synonyms	Definition
HLA	Major histocompatibility complex
ABCB1, MDR1 (multidrug resistant)	ATP-binding cassette subfamily B member 1; encodes for P-glycoprotein (P-gp) efflux transport
ABCG2	ATP-binding cassette subfamily G member 2; breast cancer resistance protein
COMT	Catechol-*O*-methyltransferase
MAO-B	Monoamine oxidase B
DRD3	Dopamine receptor (D_3)
IGTB3, GPIIIa	Glycoprotein IIIa

ACKNOWLEDGMENTS

The authors would like to thank Pharm.D. candidates Elizabeth Badgley, Christina Behney, Megan Connaughton, Krystina Geiger, Christina Hew, Christina Manciocchi, Huy Van Nguyen, Katherine Nguyen, Scott Pickford, and Vanessa Schmouder for their contributions to this chapter.

TABLE 16–2 Anticoagulation and antiplatelet therapy: drug properties and pharmacogenetic variants.

	Genetic Variants of Interest	Metabolism	Efflux Pump Substrate	Receptor	Target Enzymes and Proteins	Other Genetic Variants: Enzymes or Proteins
Antiplatelet therapy						
Clopidogrel	CYP2C19, ABCB1, P2RY12	CYP2C19 (S)[1], CYP3A4[128]	ABCB1 (S)[1]	P2RY12 (S)[1]	—	—
Aspirin	COX-1, GPIIIa—P1A1/A2	Esterase, hepatic conjugation[128]	—	GPIIIa—P1A1/A2 polymorphism (C)[15,17]	COX-1 (C)[13,14]	—
GPIIb/IIIaInh						
Abciximab	GPIIb/IIIa—P1A1/A2	Proteolytic cleavage[128]	—	GPIIb/IIIa—P1A1/A2 polymorphism (S)[18]	—	—
Tirofiban	—	Minimally hepatic[128]	—	GPIIb/IIIa	—	—
Eptifibatide	—	—	—	GPIIb/IIIa	—	—
Anticoagulation therapy						
Warfarin	CYP2C9, VKORC1, CYP4F2, CALU	CYP2C9 (S),[25] minor pathways: CYP2C8, 2C18, 2C19, 1A2, 3A4[128]	—	—	VKORC1 (S)[23,25]	CYP4F2 (S)[127], CALU (S)[127]
						Other Genetic Variants: Disease Susceptibility Genes; Other Enzymes or Proteins
Alzheimer disease: drug properties and pharmacogenetic variants						
Alzheimer disease	APP, PSEN1, PSEN2, MAPT, APOE, SORL1, MTHFR, ChAT, SLC18A3	—	—	—	—	APP, PSEN1, PSEN2, MAPT, APOE, SORL1, MTHFR (S),[31,32,34] ChAT (SNP rs733722), SLC18A3 (S)[49]
AChEIs						
Donepezil	CYP2D6	CYP2D6,[47,48] CYP3A4, CYP1A2[128]	—	—	AChE	ApoE[128]
Galantamine	—	CYP2D6, CYP3A4[128]	—	—	AChE	ApoE[128]
Rivastigmine	—	Cholinesterase; minimal CYP[128]	—	—	AChE	ApoE[128]
NMDA antagonists						
Memantine	—	Partially hepatic, primarily independent of CYP[128]	—	NMDA[128]	—	—

(Continued)

TABLE 16–2 Anticoagulation and antiplatelet therapy: drug properties and pharmacogenetic variants. (Continued)

	Genetic Variants of Interest	Metabolism	Efflux Pump Substrate	Receptor	Target Enzymes and Proteins	Other Genetic Variants: Enzymes or Proteins
Other						
l-Methylfolate	MTHFR	—	—	—	—	MTHFR (S)[44]
Anticonvulsant therapy: drug properties and pharmacogenetic variants						
Drug						
Phenytoin	CYP2C9, HLA-B*1502	CYP2C9 (S),[50-53] CYP2C19 (I)[52]	ABCB1[128]	—	—	HLA-B*1502 (S)[59]
Phenobarbital	CYP2C9	CYP2C9 (S),[54] CYP2C19 (I)[53]	—	—	—	—
Carbamazepine	HLA-B*1502	CYP3A4[128]	ABCB1[128]	—	—	HLA-B*1502 (S)[56,57,59]
Oxcarbazepine	HLA-B*1502	Hepatic[128]	—	—	—	HLA-B*1502 (S)[59]
MS therapy: drug properties and pharmacogenetic variants						
Multiple sclerosis	IL2RA, IL7RA, CD58, CLEC16A, CD226, HLA class II alleles	—	—	—	—	IL2RA, IL7RA, CD58, CLEC16A, CD226 (S),[66,74] HLA-DRB1*1501 (S),[84,85] HLA-DRB1*0602 (S),[84,85] HLA-DRB1*0401 (S),[83] HLA-DRB1*0408 (S),[83] IFNAR1 (SNP 18417), IFNAR2 (SNP 11876) (S)[87]
Drug						
Interferon-β1a, interferon-β1b	IFNAR1, glypican, collagen type XXV α1, hyaluronan proteoglycan link protein, calpastatin, TAFA1, LOC442331, neuronal PAS dominant protein 3	—	—	IFNAR1 (SNP 16469) (S)[81]	—	Glypican, collagen type XXV α1, hyaluronan proteoglycan link protein, calpastatin, TAFA1, LOC442331, neuronal PAS dominant protein 3 (S),[88] IRF8 (S),[90] HLA-DRB1*1501 (I)[90]
Glatiramer acetate	IRF8, TRB@, CTSS, HLA-DRB1*1501	—	—	—	—	IRF8 (S),[90] TRB@ (S), CTSS (S),[91] HLA-DRB1*1501 (S),[90] MBP, FAS, CD86, IL1R1, IL12RB2 (I)[91]
Natalizumab	JCV genotype	—	—	—	α4 integrin	JCV genotype (S)[93]
Fingolimod	No studies available	—	—	Sphingosine 1-receptor subtypes 1, 3, 4, 5[95]	—	—
Mitoxantrone	ABCB1/ABCB2	—	ABCB1/ABCB2 (S)[97]	—	—	—

Parkinson disease therapy: drug properties and pharmacogenetic variants

Drug						
Levodopa	DRD2 Can-STR, COMT	Aromatic-l-amino-acid decarboxylase, COMT (C),[100,101,103-105] MAO-B[98]	—	D1, D2 receptors[128]	—	DRD2 Can-STR gene (S)[106]
Carbidopa	—	—	—	—	Decarboxylase[128]	—
MAO-B inhibitors						
Selegiline	CYP2B6	CYP2B6 (S)[113]	—	—	MAO-B	—
Rasagiline	—	CYP1A2 (I)[114]	—	—	MAO-B	Bcl-2 (I),[114] MAO-B (I)[114]
COMT inhibitors						
Entacapone	UGT1A9, COMT	UGT1A9 (S)[119]	—	—	COMT (C)[117,118]	
Tolcapone	UGT1A9, COMT	UGT1A9 (S)[122]	—	—	COMT (C)[117,118]	
Dopamine agonists						
Bromocriptine	—	CYP3A[128]	ABCB1[114,123]	D1, D2 receptors[128]		—
Pramipexole	DRD3 gene	Negligible[128]	—	D1, D2, D3, D4 receptors; DRD2 gene (I),[125] DRD3 gene (S)[125]		—
Ropinirole	—	CYP1A2[128]	'	D2, D3 receptors[128]		—
NMDA receptor antagonists						
Amantadine	—	—	—	NMDA, polymorphisms at D2 and D2 receptors (I)[114]		—

(S) Studies indicate significant genetic influence on drug response or disease course/susceptibility; (C) studies produced conflicting results to support genetic influence on drug response or disease course/susceptibility; (I) studies available do not support genetic influence on drug response or disease course/susceptibility.

REFERENCES

1. Vance JM, Tekin D. Genomic Medicine and Neurology. *Continuum Lifelong Learning Neurol.* 2011;17:249–267.

2. Zuern C, Schwab M, Gawaz M, Geisler T. Platelet pharmacogenomics. *J Thromb Haemost.* 2010;8(6):1147–1158.

3. Plavix (clopidogrel) [package insert]. Bridgewater, NJ: Bristol-Myers Squibb/Sanofi Pharmaceuticals Partnership; August 2010.

4. Xie HG, Chen SL, Hu ZY, Zhang JJ, Ye F, Zou JJ. Individual variability in the disposition of and response to clopidogrel: pharmacogenomics and beyond. *Pharmacol Ther.* 2011;129(3):267–289.

5. Mega JL, Close SL, Wiviott SD, et al. Cytochrome p-450 polymorphisms and response to clopidogrel. *N Engl J Med.* 2009;360(4):354–362.

6. Sibbing D, Stegherr J, Latz W, et al. Cytochrome P450 2C19 loss-of-function polymorphism and stent thrombosis following percutaneous coronary intervention. *Eur Heart J.* 2009;30(8):916.

7. Giusti B, Gori AM, Marcucci R, et al. Relation of cytochrome P450 2C19 loss-of-function polymorphism to occurrence of drug-eluting coronary stent thrombosis. *Am J Cardiol.* 2009;103(6):806–811.

8. Simon T, Verstuyft C, Mary-Krause M, et al. Genetic determinants of response to clopidogrel and cardiovascular events. *N Engl J Med.* 2009;360(4):363–375.

9. Geisler T, Schaeffeler E, Dippon J, et al. CYP2C19 and nongenetic factors predict poor responsiveness to clopidogrel loading dose after coronary stent implantation. *Pharmacogenomics.* 2008;9(9):1251–1259.

10. Frere C, Cuisset T, Gaborit B, Alessi MC, Hulot JS. The CYP2C19* 17 allele is associated with better platelet response to clopidogrel in patients admitted for non ST acute coronary syndrome. *J Thromb Haemost.* 2009;7(8):1409–1411.

11. Gurbel PA, Nolin TD, Tantry US. *JAMA.* 2012;237(23):2495.

12. Faraday N, Becker DM, Becker LC. Pharmacogenomics of platelet responsiveness to aspirin. *Pharmacogenomics.* 2007;8(10):1413–1425.

13. Halushka MK, Walker LP, Halushka PV. Genetic variation in cyclooxygenase 1: effects on response to aspirin. *Clin Pharmacol Ther.* 2003;73(1):122–130.

14. Maree A, Curtin R, Chubb A, et al. Cyclooxygenase 1 haplotype modulates platelet response to aspirin. *J Thromb Haemost.* 2005;3(10):2340–2345.

15. Szczeklik A, Undas A, Sanak M, et al. Relationship between bleeding time, aspirin and the P1A1/A2 polymorphism of platelet glycoprotein IIIa. *Br J Haematol.* 2000;110:965–967.

16. Sibbing D, Koch W, Gebhard D, et al. Cytochrome 2C19* 17 allelic variant, platelet aggregation, bleeding events, and stent thrombosis in clopidogrel-treated patients with coronary stent placement. *Circulation.* 2010;121(4):512–518.

17. Di Castelnuovo A, de Gaetano G, Donati MB, et al. Platelet glycoprotein IIb/IIIa polymorphism and coronary artery disease. *Am J Pharmacogenomics.* 2005;5(2):93–99.

18. Andrioli G, Minuz P, Solero P, et al. Defective platelet response to arachidonic acid and thromboxane A2 in subjects with PlA2 polymorphism of 3 subunit (glycoprotein IIIa). *Br J Haematol.* 2000;110(4):911–918.

19. Michelson AD, Furman MI, Goldschmidt-Clermont P, et al. Platelet GP IIIa P1A polymorphisms display different sensitivities to agonists. *Circulation.* 2000;101:1013–1018.

20. Weber AA, Jacobs C, Meila D, et al. No evidence for an influence of the human platelet antigen-1 polymorphism on the antiplatelet effects of glycoprotein IIb/IIIa inhibitors. *Pharmacogenet Genomics.* 2002;12(7):581.

21. Ravn LS, Benn M, Nordestgaard BG, et al. Angiotensinogen and ACE gene polymorphisms and risk of atrial fibrillation in the general population. *Pharmacogenet Genomics.* 2008;18(6):525.

22. Higashi MK, Veenstra DL, Kondo LM, et al. Association between CYP2C9 genetic variants and anticoagulation-related outcomes during warfarin therapy. *JAMA.* 2002;287(13):1690.

23. Rieder MJ, Reiner AP, Gage BF, et al. Effect of VKORC1 haplotypes on transcriptional regulation and warfarin dose. *N Engl J Med.* 2005;352(22):2285–2293.

24. Coumadin® (warfarin sodium) [package insert]. Princeton, NJ: Bristol-Myers Squibb Pharma Company; September 2011.

25. Schwarz UI, Ritchie MD, Bradford Y, et al. Genetic determinants of response to warfarin during initial anticoagulation. *N Engl J Med.* 2008;358(10):999–1008.

26. Lee M, Chen Y, Wen M, et al. Estimation of the warfarin dose with clinical and pharmacogenetic data. *N Engl J Med.* 2009;360(8):753–764.

27. Stangier J. Clinical pharmacokinetics and pharmacodynamics of the oral direct thrombin inhibitor dabigatran etexilate. *Clin Pharmacokinet.* 2008;47(5):285–295.

28. Connolly SJ, Ezekowitz MD, Yusuf S, et al. Dabigatran versus warfarin in patients with atrial fibrillation. *N Engl J Med.* 2009;361(12):1139–1151.

29. 2011 Alzheimer's disease facts and figures. Alzheimer's Association. Fact sheet; March 2011. Available at: http://www.alz.org/documents_custom/2011_Facts_Figures_Fact_Sheet.pdf.

30. Blennow K, de Leon MJ, Zetterberg H. Alzheimer's disease. *Lancet.* 2006;368(9533):387–403.

31. Goldman JS, Hahn SE, Catania JW, et al. Genetic counseling and testing for Alzheimer disease: joint practice guidelines of the American College of Medical Genetics and the National Society of Genetic Counselors. *Genet Med.* 2011;13(6):597–605.

32. Sierant M, Paduszynska A, Kazmierczak-Baranska J, et al. Specific silencing of L392V PSEN1 mutant allele by RNA interference. *Int J Alzheimers Dis.* 2011;2011:809218.

33. Guo Q, Wang Z, Li H, Wiese M, Zheng H. APP physiological and pathophysiological functions: insights from animal models. *Cell Res.* 2012;22(1):78–89.

34. Galimberti D, Scarpini E. Disease-modifying treatments for Alzheimer's disease. *Ther Adv Neurol Disord.* 2011;4(4):203.

35. Sleegers K, Brouwers N, Gijselinck I, et al. APP duplication is sufficient to cause early onset Alzheimer's dementia with cerebral amyloid angiopathy. *Brain.* 2006;129(11):2977.

36. Gandy S. The role of cerebral amyloid beta accumulation in common forms of Alzheimer disease. *J Clin Invest.* 2005;115(5):1121–1129.

37. Vassar R, Bennet BD, Babu-Khan S, et al. Beta-secretase cleavage of Alzheimer's amyloid precursor protein by the transmembrane aspartic protease BACE. *Science.* 1999;286:735–741.

38. Farkas E, Luiten PGM. Cerebral microvascular pathology in aging and Alzheimer's disease. *Prog Neurobiol.* 2001;64(6):575–611.

39. Hata S, Saito Y, Suzuki T. Alzheimer's disease as a membrane associated enzymopathy of amyloid precursor protein (APP) secretases. In: Jelinek R, ed. *Lipids and Cellular Membranes in Amyloid Diseases.* Weinheim, Germany: Wiley-VCH Verlag GmbH & Co KgaA; 2011:177–194.

40. Su B, Wang X, Lee H, et al. Chronic oxidative stress causes increased tau phosphorylation in M17 neuroblastoma cells. *Neurosci Lett.* 2010;468(3):267–271.

41. Fukushima T, Nakamura A, Iwakami N, et al. T-817MA, a neuroprotective agent, attenuates the motor and cognitive impairments associated with neuronal degeneration in P301L tau transgenic mice. *Biochem Biophys Res Commun.* 2011;407(4):730–734.

42. Minami SS, Clifford TG, Hoe HS, Matsuoka Y, Rebeck GW. Fyn knock-down increases A [beta], decreases phospho-tau, and worsens spatial learning in 3 Tg-AD mice. *Neurobiol Aging.* 2012;33(4):825.e15–825.e24.

43. Reitz C, Tokuhiro S, Clark LN, et al. SORCS1 alters amyloid precursor protein processing and variants may increase Alzheimer's disease risk. *Ann Neurol.* 2011;69(1):47–64.

44. Naj AC, Beecham GW, Martin ER, et al. Dementia revealed: novel chromosome 6 locus for late-onset Alzheimer disease provides genetic evidence for folate-pathway abnormalities. *PLoS Genet.* 2010;6(9):e1001130.

45. Geula C, Mesulam M. Cholinesterases and the pathology of Alzheimer disease. *Alzheimer Dis Assoc Disord.* 1995;9(suppl 2):23–28.

46. Stahl SM. The new cholinesterase inhibitors for Alzheimer's disease, Part 2: illustrating their mechanisms of action. *J Clin Psychiatry.* 2000;61(11):813–814.

47. Cacabelos R, Llovo R, Fraile C, Fernandez-Novoa L. Pharmacogenetic aspects of therapy with cholinesterase inhibitors: the role of CYP 2D6 in Alzheimer's disease pharmacogenetics. *Curr Alzheimer Res.* 2007;4(4):479–500.

48. Cacabelos R. Pharmacogenomics and therapeutic prospects in dementia. *Eur Arch Psychiatry Clin Neurosci.* 2008;258(suppl 1):2–47.

49. Harold D, MacGregor S, Patterson CE, et al. A single nucleotide polymorphism in CHAT influences response to acetylcholinesterase inhibitors in Alzheimer's disease. *Pharmacogenet Genomics*. 2006;16(2):75.

50. Anderson GD. Pharmacokinetic, pharmacodynamic, and pharmacogenetic targeted therapy of antiepileptic drugs. *Ther Drug Monit*. 2008;30(2):173.

51. Ferraro TN, Buono RJ. The relationship between the pharmacology of antiepileptic drugs and human gene variation: an overview. *Epilepsy Behav*. 2005;7(1):18–36.

52. van der Weide J, Steijns LSW, van Weelden MJM, de Haan K. The effect of genetic polymorphism of cytochrome P450 CYP2C9 on phenytoin dose requirement. *Pharmacogenet Genomics*. 2001;11(4):287.

53. Citerio G, Nobili A, Airoldi L, Pastorelli R, Patruno A. Severe intoxication after phenytoin infusion: a preventable pharmacogenetic adverse reaction. *Neurology*. 2003;60(8):1395.

54. Goto S, Seo T, Murata T, et al. Population estimation of the effects of cytochrome P450 2C9 and 2C19 polymorphisms on phenobarbital clearance in Japanese. *Ther Drug Monit*. 2007;29(1):118.

55. Roujeau JC, Kelly JP, Naldi L, et al. Medication use and the risk of Stevens–Johnson syndrome or toxic epidermal necrolysis. *N Engl J Med*. 1995;333(24):1600–1608.

56. Chung WH, Hung SI, Hong HS, et al. Medical genetics: a marker for Stevens–Johnson syndrome. *Nature*. 2004;428(6982):486.

57. Ferrell PB, McLeod HL. Carbamazepine, HLA-B* 1502 and risk of Stevens–Johnson syndrome and toxic epidermal necrolysis: US FDA recommendations. *Pharmacogenomics*. 2008;9(10):1543–1546.

58. Locharernkul C, Loplumlert J, Limotai C, et al. Carbamazepine and phenytoin induced Stevens Johnson syndrome is associated with HLA B* 1502 allele in Thai population. *Epilepsia*. 2008;49(12):2087–2091.

59. Hung SI, Chung WH, Liu ZS, et al. Common risk allele in aromatic antiepileptic-drug induced Stevens–Johnson syndrome and toxic epidermal necrolysis in Han Chinese. *Pharmacogenomics*. 2010;11(3):349–356.

60. Alfirevic A, Jorgensen AL, Williamson PR, Chadwick DW, Park BK, Pirmohamed M. HLA-B locus in Caucasian patients with carbamazepine hypersensitivity. *Pharmacogenomics*. 2006;7(6):813–818.

61. Siddiqui A, Kerb R, Weale ME, et al. Association of multidrug resistance in epilepsy with a polymorphism in the drug-transporter gene ABCB1. *N Engl J Med*. 2003;348(15):1442–1448.

62. Sills GJ, Mohanraj R, Butler E, et al. Lack of association between the C3435T polymorphism in the human multidrug resistance (MDR1) gene and response to antiepileptic drug treatment. *Epilepsia*. 2005;46(5):643–647.

63. Tan N, Heron S, Scheffer IE, et al. Failure to confirm association of a polymorphism in ABCB1 with multidrug-resistant epilepsy. *Neurology*. 2004;63(6):1090.

64. Kimchi-Sarfaty C, Oh JM, Kim IW, et al. A "silent" polymorphism in the MDR1 gene changes substrate specificity. *Science*. 2007;315:525–528.

65. Compston A, Coles A. Multiple sclerosis. *Lancet*. 2008;372(9648):1502–1517.

66. Ebers GC, Sadovnick AD. The role of genetic factors in multiple sclerosis susceptibility. *J Neuroimmunol*. 1994;54(1–2):1–17.

67. Sawcer S, Goodfellow PN. Inheritance of susceptibility to multiple sclerosis. *Curr Opin Immunol*. 1998;10(6):697–703.

68. Siva A. The spectrum of multiple sclerosis and treatment decisions. *Clin Neurol Neurosurg*. 2006;108(3):333–338.

69. Lindsey JW, Hatfield LM. Epstein–Barr virus and multiple sclerosis: cellular immune response and cross-reactivity. *J Neuroimmunol*. 2010;229(1–2):238–242.

70. Vaughan JH, Riise T, Rhodes GH, Nguyen MD, Barrett-Connor E, Nyland H. An Epstein Barr virus-related cross reactive autoimmune response in multiple sclerosis in Norway. *J Neuroimmunol*. 1996;69(1–2):95–102.

71. Pittas F, Ponsonby A-L, van der Mei I, et al. Smoking is associated with progressive disease course and increased progression in clinical disability in a prospective cohort of people with multiple sclerosis. *J Neurol*. 2009;256(4):577–585.

72. Kakalacheva K, Lünemann JD. Environmental triggers of multiple sclerosis. *FEBS Lett*. In press.

73. Greer JM, McCombe PA. Role of gender in multiple sclerosis: clinical effects and potential molecular mechanisms. *J Neuroimmunol*. 2011;234(1–2):7–18.

74. Dutta R, Trapp BD. Gene expression profiling in multiple sclerosis brain. *Neurobiol Dis*. In press.

75. Miller A, Avidan N, Tzunz-Henig N, et al. Translation towards personalized medicine in multiple sclerosis. *J Neurol Sci*. 2008;274(1–2):68–75.

76. Graber JJ, McGraw CA, Kimbrough D, Dhib-Jalbut S. Overlapping and distinct mechanisms of action of multiple sclerosis therapies. *Clin Neurol Neurosurg*. 2010;112(7):583–591.

77. Khan OA, Tselis AC, Kamholz JA, Garbern JY, Lewis RA, Lisak RP. A prospective, open-label treatment trial to compare the effect of IFN beta-1a (Avonex), IFNbeta-1b (Betaseron), and glatiramer acetate (Copaxone) on the relapse rate in relapsing-remitting multiple sclerosis. *Eur J Neurol*. 2001;8(2):141–148.

78. Flechter S, Vardi J, Pollak L, Rabey JM. Comparison of glatiramer acetate (Copaxone) and interferon beta-1b (Betaferon) in multiple sclerosis patients: an open-label 2-year follow-up. *J Neurol Sci*. 2002;197(1–2):51–55.

79. Zhang J, Hutton G, Zang Y. A comparison of the mechanisms of action of interferon beta and glatiramer acetate in the treatment of multiple sclerosis. *Clin Ther*. 2002;24(12):1998–2021.

80. Heine S, Ebnet J, Maysami S, Stangel M. Effects of interferon-beta on oligodendroglial cells. *J Neuroimmunol*. 2006;177(1–2):173–180.

81. Sriram U, Barcellos LF, Villoslada P, et al. Pharmacogenomic analysis of interferon receptor polymorphisms in multiple sclerosis. *Genes Immun*. 2003;4(2):147–152.

82. Revel M. Interferon-[beta] in the treatment of relapsing-remitting multiple sclerosis. *Pharmacol Ther*. 2003;100(1):49–62.

83. Hoffmann S, Cepok S, Grummel V, et al. HLA-DRB1*0401 and HLA-DRB1*0408 are strongly associated with the development of antibodies against interferon-beta therapy in multiple sclerosis. *Am J Hum Genet*. 2008;83(2):219–227.

84. Villoslada P, Barcellos LF, Rio J, et al. The HLA locus and multiple sclerosis in Spain. Role in disease susceptibility, clinical course and response to interferon-[beta]. *J Neuroimmunol*. 2002;130(1–2):194–201.

85. Comabella M, Fernández-Arquero M, Río J, et al. HLA class I and II alleles and response to treatment with interferon-beta in relapsing-remitting multiple sclerosis. *J Neuroimmunol*. 2009;210(1–2):116–119.

86. Domanski P, Colamonici OR. The type-I interferon receptor. The long and short of it. *Cytokine Growth Factor Rev*. 1996;7(2):143–151.

87. Leyva L, Fernández O, Fedetz M, et al. IFNAR1 and IFNAR2 polymorphisms confer susceptibility to multiple sclerosis but not to interferon-beta treatment response. *J Neuroimmunol*. 2005;163(1–2):165–171.

88. Byun E, Caillier SJ, Montalban X, et al. Genome-wide pharmacogenomic analysis of the response to interferon beta therapy in multiple sclerosis. *Arch Neurol*. 2008;65(3):337–344.

89. Johnson KP, Brooks BR, Cohen JA, et al. Copolymer 1 reduces relapse rate and improves disability in relapsing-remitting multiple sclerosis: results of a phase III multicenter, double-blind placebo-controlled trial. The Copolymer 1 Multiple Sclerosis Study Group. *Neurology*. 1995;45(7):1268–1276.

90. Gross R, Healy BC, Cepok S, et al. Population structure and HLA DRB1*1501 in the response of subjects with multiple sclerosis to first-line treatments. *J Neuroimmunol*. 2011;233(1–2):168–174.

91. Grossman I, Avidan N, Singer C, et al. Pharmacogenetics of glatiramer acetate therapy for multiple sclerosis reveals drug-response markers. *Pharmacogenet Genomics*. 2007;17(8):657–666.

92. Polman CH, O'Connor PW, Havrdova E, et al. A randomized, placebo-controlled trial of natalizumab for relapsing multiple sclerosis. *N Engl J Med*. 2006;354(9):899–910.

93. Reid CE, Li H, Sur G, et al. Sequencing and analysis of JC virus DNA from natalizumab-treated PML patients. *J Infect Dis*. 2011;204(2):237–244.

94. Ingwersen J, Aktas O, Kuery P, Kieseier B, Boyko A, Hartung H-P. Fingolimod in multiple sclerosis: mechanisms of action and clinical efficacy. *Clin Immunol*. In press.

95. Khatri B, Barkhof F, Comi G, et al. Comparison of fingolimod with interferon beta-1a in relapsing-remitting multiple sclerosis: a randomised extension of the TRANSFORMS study. *Lancet Neurol*. 2011;10(6):520–529.

96. Wundes A, Kraft GH, Bowen JD, Gooley TA, Nash RA. Mitoxantrone for worsening multiple sclerosis: tolerability, toxicity, adherence and efficacy in the clinical setting. *Clin Neurol Neurosurg*. 2010;112(10):876–882.

97. Cotte S, von Ahsen N, Kruse N, et al. ABC-transporter gene-polymorphisms are potential pharmacogenetic markers for mitoxantrone response in multiple sclerosis. *Brain*. 2009;132(pt 9):2517–2530.

98. Joseph DP, Talbert R, Yee G, Matzke G, Wells B, Posey L. *Pharmacotherapy: A Pathophysiologic Approach*. The McGraw-Hill Companies; 2008.

99. Gilgun-Sherki Y, Djaldetti R, Melamed E, Offen D. Polymorphism in candidate genes: implications for the risk and treatment of idiopathic Parkinson's disease. *Pharmacogenomics J*. 2004;4(5):291–306.

100. Reilly DK, Rivera-Calimlim L, Van Dyke D. Catechol-O-methyltransferase activity: a determinant of levodopa response. *Clin Pharmacol Ther*. 1980;28(2):278–286.

101. Bialecka M, Kurzawski M, Klodowska-Duda G, Opala G, Tan EK, Drozdzik M. The association of functional catechol-O-methyltransferase haplotypes with risk of Parkinson's disease, levodopa treatment response, and complications. *Pharmacogenet Genomics*. 2008;18(9):815.

102. Bialecka M, Drozdzik M, Klodowska-Duda G, et al. The effect of monoamine oxidase B (MAOB) and catechol-O-methyltransferase (COMT) polymorphisms on levodopa therapy in patients with sporadic Parkinson's disease. *Acta Neurol Scand*. 2004;110(4):260–266.

103. Contin M, Martinelli P, Mochi M, Riva R, Albani F, Baruzzi A. Genetic polymorphism of catechol O methyltransferase and levodopa pharmacokinetic–pharmacodynamic pattern in patients with Parkinson's disease. *Mov Disord*. 2005;20(6):734–739.

104. Lee MS, Lyoo CH, Ulmanen I, Syvänen AC. Genotypes of catechol-O-methyltransferase and response to levodopa treatment in patients with Parkinson's disease. *Neurosci Lett*. 2001;298(2):131–134.

105. Watanabe M, Harada S, Nakamura T, et al. Association between catechol-O-methyltransferase gene polymorphisms and wearing-off and dyskinesia in Parkinson's disease. *Neuropsychobiology*. 2000;48(4):190–193.

106. Oliveri R, Annesi G, Zappia M, et al. Dopamine D2 receptor gene polymorphism and the risk of levodopa-induced dyskinesias in PD. *Neurology*. 1999;53(7):1425.

107. Zappia M, Annesi G, Nicoletti G, et al. Sex differences in clinical and genetic determinants of levodopa peak-dose dyskinesias in Parkinson disease: an exploratory study. *Arch Neurol*. 2005;62(4):601.

108. Strong JA, Dalvi A, Revilla FJ, et al. Genotype and smoking history affect risk of levodopa induced dyskinesias in Parkinson's disease. *Mov Disord*. 2006;21(5):654–659.

109. Chen JJ, Swope DM. Clinical pharmacology of rasagiline: a novel, second-generation propargylamine for the treatment of Parkinson disease. *J Clin Pharmacol*. 2005;45(8):878.

110. Turpeinen M, Raunio H, Pelkonen O. The functional role of CYP2B6 in human drug metabolism: substrates and inhibitors in vitro, in vivo and in silico. *Curr Drug Metab*. 2006;7(7):705–714.

111. Benetton SA, Fang C, Yang Y, et al. P450 phenotyping of the metabolism of selegiline to desmethylselegiline and methamphetamine. *Drug Metab Pharmacokinet*. 2007;22(2):78–87.

112. Wang H, Tompkins LM. CYP2B6: new insights into a historically overlooked cytochrome P450 isozyme. *Curr Drug Metab*. 2008;9(7):598.

113. Watanabe T, Sakuyama K, Sasaki T, et al. Functional characterization of 26 CYP2B6 allelic variants (CYP2B6.2–CYP2B6.28, except CYP2B6.22). *Pharmacogenet Genomics*. 2010;20(7):459.

114. PharmKGB. National Institute of Health; 2011. Available at: http://pharmgkb.com/index.jsp. Accessed 07/12/11.

115. Tasmar (tolcapone) [package insert]. Nutley, NJ: Roche Laboratories Inc; February 2006.

116. Comtan (entacapone) [package insert]. East Hanover, NJ: Novartis Pharmaceuticals Corporation; September 2010.

117. Lee M, Kim H, Cho E, Lim J, Rinne J. COMT genotype and effectiveness of entacapone in patients with fluctuating Parkinson's disease. *Neurology*. 2002;58(4):564.

118. Corvol JC, Bonnet C, Charbonnier Beaupel F, et al. The COMT Val158Met polymorphism affects the response to entacapone in Parkinson's disease: a randomized crossover clinical trial. *Ann Neurol*. 2011;69(1):111–118.

119. Paoluzzi L, Singh AS, Price DK, et al. Influence of genetic variants in UGT1A1 and UGT1A9 on the in vivo glucuronidation of SN-38. *J Clin Pharmacol*. 2004;44(8):854.

120. Villeneuve L, Girard H, Fortier LC, Gagné JF, Guillemette C. Novel functional polymorphisms in the UGT1A7 and UGT1A9 glucuronidating enzymes in Caucasian and African-American subjects and their impact on the metabolism of 7-ethyl-10-hydroxycamptothecin and flavopiridol anticancer drugs. *J Pharmacol Exp Ther*. 2003;307(1):117.

121. Martignoni E, Cosentino M, Ferrari M, et al. Two patients with COMT inhibitor–induced hepatic dysfunction and UGT1A9 genetic polymorphism. *Neurology*. 2005;65(11):1820.

122. Olanow CW. Tolcapone and hepatotoxic effects. *Arch Neurol*. 2000;57(2):263.

123. Vautier S, Lacomblez L, Chacun H, et al. Interactions between the dopamine agonist, bromocriptine and the efflux protein, P-glycoprotein at the blood–brain barrier in the mouse. *Eur J Pharm Sci*. 2006;27(2–3):167–174.

124. Vautier S, Milane A, Fernandez C, Buyse M, Chacun H, Farinotti R. Interactions between antiparkinsonian drugs and ABCB1/P-glycoprotein at the blood–brain barrier in a rat brain endothelial cell model. *Neurosci Lett*. 2008;442(1):19–23.

125. Liu YZ, Tang BS, Yan XX, et al. Association of the DRD2 and DRD3 polymorphisms with response to pramipexole in Parkinson's disease patients. *Eur J Clin Pharmacol*. 2009;65(7):679–683.

126. Symmetrel® (amantadine) [package insert]. Chadds Ford, PA: Endo Pharmaceuticals; February 2007.

127. Vance JM, Tekin D. Continuum: lifelong learning in neurology. *Neurogenetics*. 2011;17(2):249–267.

128. Lexi-Comp Online. Lexi-Comp Inc; 2011.

Pharmacogenomics of Gastrointestinal Drugs: Focus on Proton Pump Inhibitors

Takahisa Furuta, MD, PhD, Mitsushige Sugimoto, MD, PhD, & Naohito Shirai, MD, PhD

LEARNING OBJECTIVES

- Discuss pharmacogenomics as it relates to gastroenterology with the focus on *H. pylori* infection.
- Outline the effects of genetic polymorphism on proton pump inhibitors and their efficacy in *H. pylori*.
- Illustrate how pharmacogenomics can be used to tailor therapy with proton pump inhibitors.

INTRODUCTION

Proton pump inhibitors (PPIs), such as omeprazole, lansoprazole, rabeprazole, esomeprazole, and pantoprazole, are now clinically used as the potent gastric acid inhibitors. They are derivatives of benzimidazole. They are absorbed in the small intestine and reach, via systemic circulation, the gastric parietal cells, where they bind to the proton pump (H^+/K^+-ATPase) irreversibly and disturb the function of proton pump, thereby resulting in a potent acid inhibition.[1] The major indications of PPIs are acid-related diseases, such as peptic ulcer, gastroesophageal reflux diseases (GERD), and Zollinger–Ellison syndrome.[2–6] PPIs are also used for the eradication of *H. pylori* with antimicrobial agents.[7–9]

PPIs undergo the hepatic metabolism by the cytochrome P450 (CYP) system. The principal enzyme involved in the metabolism of PPIs is CYP2C19. CYP3A4 is also involved in PPI metabolism.[10–14] For example, omeprazole, a representative and first clinically available PPI, is mainly metabolized by CYP2C19 to 5-hydroxyomeprazole, which is metabolized by CYP3A4 to 5-hydroxyomeprazole sulfone. Omeprazole is partially first metabolized by CYP3A4 to omeprazole sulfone, which is metabolized by CYP2C19 to 5-hydroxyomeprazole sulfone (Figure 17A–1). There are interindividual differences in the activity of CYP2C19. Recent reports have revealed that pharmacokinetics and pharmacodynamics of PPIs are affected by the CYP2C19 polymorphism.

EFFECTS OF CYP2C19 POLYMORPHISM ON THE PHARMACOKINETICS AND PHARMACODYNAMICS OF PPIs

Polymorphism of Cytochrome P450 Enzymes

There are more than 20 kinds of CYP enzymes in the liver. These enzymes hydrolyze a variety of drugs. Among CYP enzymes, CYP1A2, 2C8, 2C9, 2C19, 2D6, and 3A4 are important in the metabolism of drugs in humans.[15] Most of CYP450 enzymes show a genetic polymorphism associated with their enzyme activities

FIGURE 17A–1 Metabolism of omeprazole (OME) in relation to cytochrome P450 (CYP) isoenzymes. Weight of arrows indicates the relative contribution of different enzyme pathways. OME is mainly metabolized by CYP2C19 to 5-hydroxyomeprazole (5-OH-OME), which is then metabolized to 5-hydroxyomeprazole sulfone (5-OH-OME-SFN). OME is also metabolized by CYP3A4 to omeprazole sulfone (OME-SFN), which is then metabolized by CYP2C19 to 5-OH-OME-SFN.

(http://www.imm.ki.se/CYPalleles/default.htm). Plasma concentrations and effects of drugs metabolized by these enzymes differ among different individuals with their different enzyme activities genetically determined.

Genetic Differences in the Main PPI-Metabolizing Enzyme, CYP2C19

PPIs are mainly metabolized by CYP2C19 (Figure 17A–1). There are interindividual differences in the activity of this enzyme, which was first characterized by the racemic antiepileptic agent, mephenytoin, of which the *S*-enantiomer undergoes hydroxylation through CYP2C19.[10,15,16] The polymorphism of this enzyme is classified into the three genotype groups: rapid metabolizer (RM) (=homozygous extensive metabolizer [homEM]), intermediate metabolizer (IM) (=heterozygous extensive metabolizer [hetEM]), and poor metabolizer (PM). In RMs, both of the alleles have no inactivating mutations and the enzyme can be generated from both of the nonmutated alleles. In IMs, the one allele has the mutation in the coding region of CYP2C19 (see Chapter 6). However, the other allele has no mutation and normal enzyme can be generated from this allele. In PMs, both of the alleles have mutations in the CYP2C19 genes, and, therefore, normal enzyme cannot be generated from any of the two mutated alleles, resulting in the deficiency of the enzyme activity.

There are interethnic differences in the frequencies of PMs of this enzyme: 2.5% in the white Americans, 2.0% in the African Americans, 3.5% in the white Europeans, 4.8% in Shona Zimbabweans, 19.8% in the Chinese-Han population, 13.4% in the Chinese-Bai population, 12.6% in the Korean population, and 18.0–22.5% in the Japanese population.[17–24]

Various genetic mutations involved in the CYP2C19 polymorphism have been discovered from ethnically different populations (http://www.imm.ki.se/CYPalleles/cyp2c19.htm).

However, the PM-related CYP2C19 polymorphism of Japanese and Caucasian people essentially can be explained by two point mutations generating inactive alleles, that is, *CYP2C19*2* (exon 5 mutation) and *CYP2C19*3* (exon 4).[22,25,26]

Effect of CYP2C19 Genotypic Differences on the Pharmacokinetics and Pharmacodynamics of PPIs

When 20 mg of omeprazole (the active drug) is given as a single dose, plasma omeprazole concentrations differ among the three different CYP2C19 genotype (RM, IM, and PM) groups (Figure 17A–2A).[27] Plasma omeprazole concentrations in the PM group are sustained for a long time after dosing. On the other hand, plasma concentrations of 5-hydroxyomeprazole, which is formed from omeprazole via CYP2C19, in the PM group are lower than those in the RM and IM groups. Hydroxylation of omeprazole in PMs is mediated by CYP3A4.[28] In PMs, the sulfoxidation of omeprazole is the main metabolic pathway and omeprazole sulfone cannot be metabolized to 5-hydroxyomeprazole sulfone by CYP2C19 in the PM group, because PMs lack CYP2C19. Therefore, plasma omeprazole sulfone concentrations are sustained for a long time after dosing in the PM group (Figure 17A–2C). The mean value for the area under the plasma concentration–time curves (AUC) of omeprazole in the PM group is about 13 times as high as that of the RM group (Figure 17A–3A). There are also significant differences in the two omeprazole metabolite, 5-hydroxyomeprazole and omeprazole sulfone, concentrations among the three different CYP2C19 genotype groups (Figures 17A–3B and C).

The intragastric pH profile also differs among the three different genotype groups (Figure 17A–4A). The mean 24-hour intragastric pH level in the RM group is the lowest, that of the IM group comes next, and that in the PM group is highest (Figure 17A–4B). The acid inhibition achieved by omeprazole in

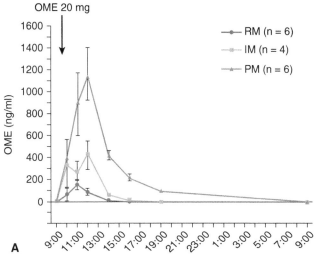

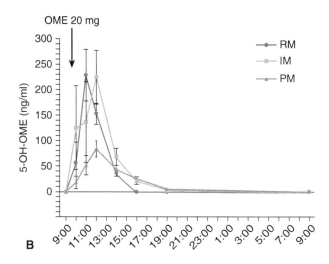

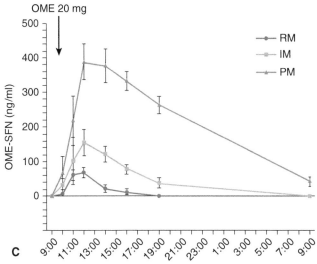

FIGURE 17A–2   Mean (±SE) plasma concentrations of omeprazole (OME) (**A**), 5-hydroxyomeprazole (5-OH-OME) (**B**), and omeprazole sulfone (OME-SFN) (**C**) as a function of CYP2C19 genotype. (**A**) Plasma concentration of OME was highest in the PM group, intermediate in the IM group, and lowest in the RM group. (**B**) The peak concentration (C_{max}) of 5-OH-OME was observed first in the RM group. Plasma concentration of OH-OME was lowest in the PM group. (**C**) Plasma concentration of OME-SFN was highest in the PM group, intermediate in the IM group, and lowest in the RM group. *Abbreviations*: RM, rapid metabolizer; IM, intermediate metabolizer; PM, poor metabolizer.

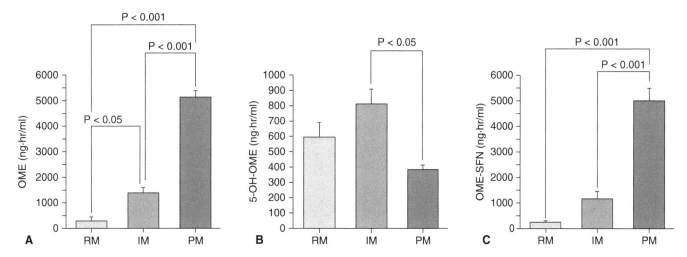

FIGURE 17A–3   Means (±SE) of the areas under the plasma concentration–time curves (AUC) for omeprazole (OME) (**A**), 5-hydroxyomeprazole (5-OH-OME) (**B**), and omeprazole sulfone (OME-SFN) (**C**) as a function of CYP2C19 genotype when 20 mg of omeprazole is once dosed. (**A**) The mean AUC for OME was highest in the PM group, intermediate in the IM group, and lowest in the RM group. (**B**) The mean AUC for 5-OH-OME in the PM group was lowest of the three groups. (**C**) The mean AUC for OME-SFN was highest in the PM group, intermediate in the IM group, and lowest in the RM group. See abbreviations in the legend of Figure 17A–2.

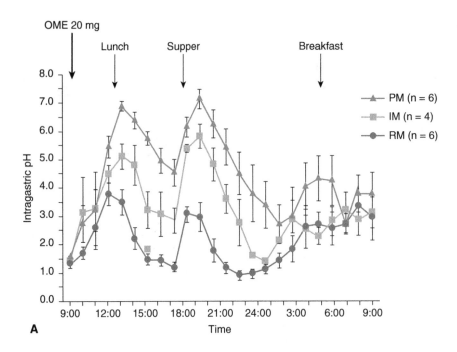

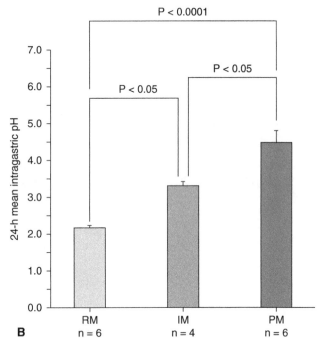

FIGURE 17A–4   Profiles of intragastric pH values (**A**) and the 24-hour mean intragastric pHs (**B**) as a function of CYP2C19 genotype status for 20 mg of omeprazole (OME) dosing. The mean intragastric pH values differed significantly ($P = .0001$) among the three groups when 20 mg of OME was once dosed.

the RM group seems insufficient under the so-called standardized dosing scheme,[27,29] as discussed below.

Plasma concentration–time curves after oral dosing of 20 mg of omeprazole, 30 mg of lansoprazole, and 20 mg of rabeprazole for 8 days as a function of CYP2C19 genotype status are also affected by CYP2C19 genotype status (Figure 17A–5A). The mean values for the AUCs of omeprazole, lansoprazole, and rabeprazole in subjects with RM, IM, or PM genotype of CYP2C19 are summarized in Figure 17A–5B. Intragastric pH profiles after repeated dosing of 20 mg of omeprazole, 30 mg of lansoprazole, or 20 mg of rabeprazole for 8 days are also affected by CYP2C19

genotype status (Figure 17A–6A),[30–32] although the difference in acid inhibitory effect of a PPI among different CYP2C19 genotype statuses becomes smaller by the repeated dosing of a PPI (compare the pH data in Figure 17A–6A with those in Figure 17A–4A). The differences in acid inhibition by a PPI among the different CYP2C19 genotype groups are considered to come from different plasma concentrations among the different genotype groups: profound acid inhibition in PMs is considered to be derived from higher plasma PPI concentrations for a longer period in PMs and low acid inhibition in RMs is supposed to be ascribable to low plasma PPI concentrations in them.

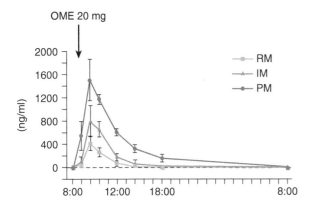

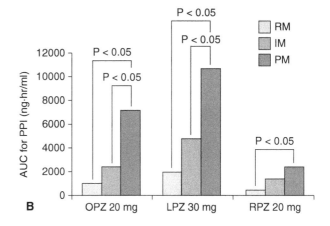

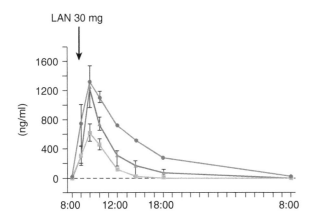

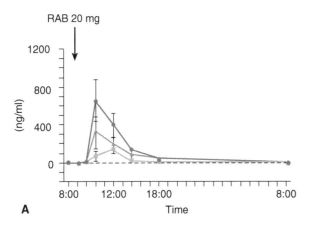

A

FIGURE 17A–5 (**A**) Mean (±SE) plasma levels of 20 mg of omeprazole (OME), 30 mg of lansoprazole (LAN), and 20 mg of rabeprazole (RAB) as a function of CYP2C19 genotype for 8 days. Plasma concentrations of OME, LAN, and RAB were highest in the PM group, intermediate in the IM group, and lowest in the RM group. (**B**) Area under the plasma concentration–time curves for omeprazole (OME), lansoprazole (LAN), and rabeprazole (RAB) as a function of CYP2C19 phenotype. AUC values of OME, LAN, and RAB were highest in the PM group, intermediate in the IM group, and lowest in the RM group.

However, when 30 mg of lansoprazole is dosed four times daily in order to sustain the plasma lansoprazole concentrations all day long (Figure 17A–7), a complete acid inhibition can be achieved even in RMs (Figure 17A–8). Because of the irreversible blockade of the proton pump and the involvement of metabolites in the effects of PPIs, the time course and extent of acid suppression is not directly linked to plasma concentrations. Interestingly, the peak plasma concentration (C_{max}) of lansoprazole in RMs when 30 mg of lansoprazole is dosed four times daily is not increased in comparison with the case of once-daily dosing of 30 mg of lansoprazole (Figure 17A–7) and

is not as high as that observed in PMs, although sufficient acid inhibition is achieved in RMs when lansoprazole was dosed four times daily. This indicates that the faster elimination of lansoprazole rather than its lower C_{max} is the primary reason for the insufficient acid inhibition in RMs. In other words, the acid inhibitory effect of PPIs depends more on the plasma elimination half-life time ($t_{1/2}$) than on C_{max}. Therefore, the dosing scheme of a PPI is a key point to attain an appropriate intragastric pH level and should be determined on the basis of the individual CYP2C19 genotype status for a sufficient acid inhibition.

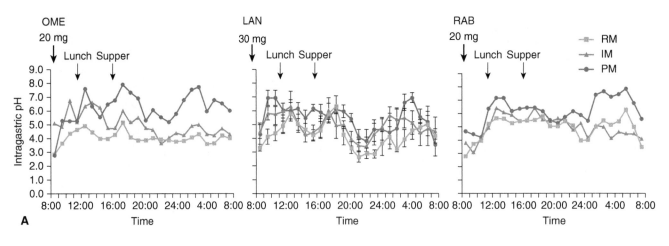

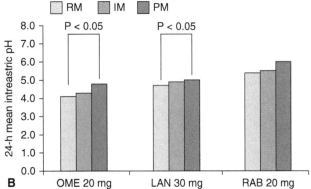

FIGURE 17A–6 (**A**) Mean (±SE) intragastric pH values as a function of CYP2C19 genotype status for 20 mg of omeprazole (OME), 30 mg of lansoprazole (LAN), or 20 mg of rabeprazole (RAB) dosing for 8 days. (**B**) Median of the 24 hour-mean intragastric pH values as a function of CYP2C19 phenotype status for 20 mg of omeprazole (OME), 30 mg of lansoprazole (LAN), or 20 mg of rabeprazole (RAB) dosing. The 24-hour mean intragastric pH value was highest in the PM group, intermediate in the IM group, and lowest in the RM group. Statistical significant difference was observed between the RM group and the PM group when 20 mg of OME or 30 mg of LAN was dosed. See the legend of Figure 17A–2 for the abbreviations.

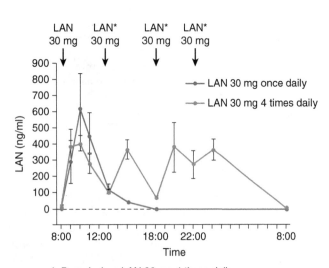

*: Dosed when LAN 30 mg 4 times daily

FIGURE 17A–7 Mean (±SE) plasma concentration–time curves for lansoprazole (LAN) after the final dosings of 30 mg of LAN once daily and 30 mg of lansoprazole four times daily for 8 days in the five RMs. By four times daily dosing of 30 mg of LAN, plasma levels of LAN are sustained during each of the dosing intervals in the five RMs.

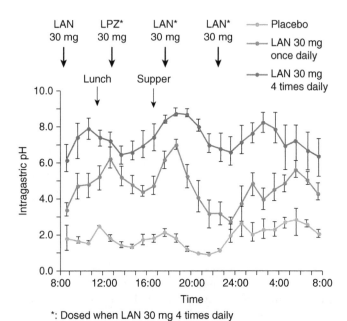

*: Dosed when LAN 30 mg 4 times daily

FIGURE 17A–8 Mean (±SE) intragastric pH values versus time course after the last dosings when placebo, 30 mg of LAN once daily, and 30 mg of LAN four times daily were dosed. Although the pH values were decreased to the levels less than 4.0 for several hours during nocturnal time when LAN 30 mg was dosed once daily for 8 days, no such decrease in the pH levels was observed when LAN 30 mg was dosed four times daily for 8 days. Complete acid inhibition (i.e., intragastric pH around 7.0) can be achieved by LAN 30 mg four times daily dosing for 8 days.

EFFECT OF CYP2C19 POLYMORPHISM ON GERD TREATMENT BY A PPI

GERD is a common disorder, which represents a major indication for PPIs. The cure rates of GERD attained by PPIs are around 90%, while there are some patients who do not respond to the usual standard dose of a PPI (e.g., 20 mg of omeprazole or 30 mg of lansoprazole).[33–35] Recently, one of the reasons for GERD refractory to the PPI treatment has been shown to be associated with the metabolism of a PPI as discussed below.

When 30 mg of lansoprazole was dosed in GERD patients positive for mucosal breaks (grades A–D in Los Angeles classification) for 8 weeks, cure rates of mucosal breaks significantly depended on CYP2C19 genotype status.[36] The cure rate of mucosal breaks in the RM group was lowest, that in the IM group came next, and that in the PM group was highest (Figure 17A–9), with the observation that the cure rate of grade C or D of GERD in patients with the RM genotype of CYP2C19 was dramatically low (1/6 = 16.7%, CI: 0.4–64.1%).[36] Plasma lansoprazole concentrations at 3 hours after the last dose depended on the CYP2C19 genotype status (Figure 17A–10A) and were associated with cure rates of mucosal breaks of GERD. The mean plasma lansoprazole concentration in the successfully treated group was significantly higher than that in the unsuccessfully treated group (Figure 17A–10B). Similarly,

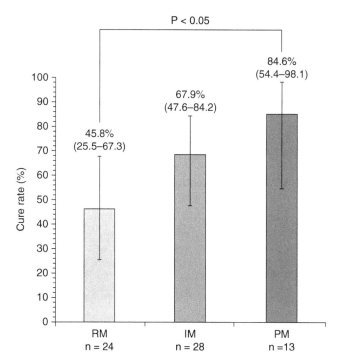

FIGURE 17A–9 Cure rates of GERD with a daily dose of 30 mg of lansoprazole for 8 weeks in the different CYP2C19 genotype groups. Bars indicate 95% confidence intervals (95% CI). There was a significant difference in the cure rates among the three different CYP2C19 genotype groups. The cure rate in the RM group was lowest, that in the IM group came next, and that in the PM group was the highest. *P*-Value was derived from Fisher's exact test.

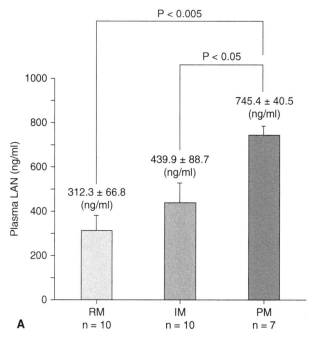

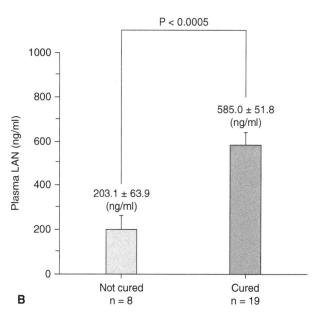

FIGURE 17A–10 The mean ± SE concentrations of plasma lansoprazole (LAN) at 3 hours after the final 30-mg dose of LAN in the different CYP2C19 genotype groups (**A**) and in the unsuccessfully or successfully treated groups (**B**). *P*-Values were derived from Scheffe's multiple comparison test (**A**) and Student's *t*-test (**B**). Significant differences in the mean plasma LAN concentrations among different CYP2C19 genotype groups were observed. The mean plasma LAN concentration in the RM group was lowest, that in the IM group came next, and that in the PM group was highest of the three genotype groups (**A**). The mean plasma LAN concentration in the group without cure of GERD was significantly lower than that in the successfully treated group (**B**).

Kawamura et al.[37] also reported that the cure rate of mucosal breaks treated with lansoprazole 30 mg daily for 8 weeks in the RM patients was lowest of the three different CYP2C19 genotype groups. Recurrence of GERD symptoms during the maintenance therapy with a PPI after cure of mucosal breaks is also affected by CYP2C19 genotype status.[38] Acid inhibition achieved by a daily dose of 30 mg of lansoprazole in the PM genotype group appears to be clinically sufficient for GERD treatment, and those in IMs and RMs might be insufficient in several cases.

Nocturnal acid breakthrough (NAB), which is defined as an intragastric pH lower than 4 lasting for more than 1 hour during the overnight period, is now considered as one of the factors associated with the success or failure of treatment of GERD with PPIs.[39–42] Interestingly, the frequency of NAB depends on the CYP2C19 genotype status and NAB is most frequently seen in subjects with the RM genotype pattern of CYP2C19,[31,32] resulting in the lowest cure rate of GERD of the RM patients among the three different genotype groups.[36,37]

On the basis of the above discussion, an increased dose of a PPI is recommended for the RM GERD patients who are refractory to the treatment with a usual standard dose of a PPI. In fact, a usual dose of a PPI, such as 20 mg of omeprazole daily, was reported to be therapeutically insufficient for some patients in western countries, whereas an increased dose of omeprazole, up to 80 mg daily, successfully treated such patients,[43] although the majority of westerners have the RM genotype of CYP2C19.[44] A more frequent daily dosing of lansoprazole (e.g., 30 mg four times a day) can achieve sufficient acid suppression (i.e., intragastric pH around 7) in the RM genotype group as noted above.[32] Therefore, an increased dose of PPIs might be one of the therapeutic strategies for the treatment of GERD refractory to the usual dose of a PPI in patients with the RM genotype of CYP2C19.

It has been reported that the acid inhibitory effect of histamine 2 (H2) receptor antagonists, such as famotidine, is not affected by the CYP2C19 genotype status and superior to that of lansoprazole in the RM patients during the nighttime.[31] Adding an evening dose of an H2 receptor antagonist to a morning dose of a PPI has also been reported to be effective for the control of NAB in individuals who are resistant to a usual PPI treatment.[45–47] Therefore, concomitant treatment with a PPI plus an H2 receptor antagonist appears to be another therapeutic strategy for RM patients with GERD refractory to treatment with a usual constant dose of a PPI alone.

Accordingly, CYP2C19 genotype status is considered as one of the predictable determinants for the results of a PPI-based GERD therapy. If CYP2C19 genotype status is determined before treatment, an optimal dose of a PPI can be prescribed, based on this predetermined pharmacogenomic status. Therefore, the individualized therapeutic strategy based on the individual CYP2C19 genotype status should be conducted in such a therapeutic manner as performed with an increased dose of a PPI or adding an H2 receptor antagonist, particularly in the patients with the RM genotype of CYP2C19 and severe GERD

(i.e., grade C or D). This predetermined therapeutic strategy should be expected to increase the cure rates achieved by the initial treatment for GERD.

THE EFFECTS OF CYP2C19 POLYMORPHISM ON PPI-BASED ERADICATION THERAPY OF *H. PYLORI*

H. pylori is clearly associated with the pathogenesis of a variety of upper gastrointestinal disorders, such as peptic ulcer, mucosa-associated lymphoid tissue lymphoma, and gastric cancer.[48–51] Eradication of this pathogen is now an important treatment strategy for the cure of these diseases. Current regimens for the eradication of *H. pylori* consist of a PPI plus one or two antibacterial agents, such as amoxicillin, clarithromycin, and metronidazole.

The roles of PPIs in an *H. pylori* eradication therapy are as follows. First, PPIs make antibiotics more stable and bio-available in the stomach by raising intragastric pH to neutral levels.[52] Second, neutralization of intragastric pH levels allows *H. pylori* to shift into the growth phase and thus they become more sensitive to antibiotics, such as amoxicillin.[53–55] Third, suppression of acid secretion by a PPI increases the concentration of an antibiotic, such as amoxicillin, in the stomach.[56] Fourth, PPIs per se have an anti–*H. pylori* effect.[57] It is assumed that the weaker the effect of a PPI is, the lower the eradication rate is, and that the more potent the effect of a PPI is, the higher the eradication rate is. As a matter of fact, the cure rates achieved by treatment with two antibacterial agents (amoxicillin plus clarithromycin or clarithromycin plus metronidazole) without a PPI were significantly lower than those achieved by the treatment with the same two antibacterial agents plus omeprazole, a representative PPI.[58] Therefore, coadministration of a PPI with an antibiotic or antibiotics is essential for the treatment of *H. pylori* infection.

DUAL PPI/AMOXICILLIN ERADICATION THERAPY FOR *H. PYLORI* INFECTION IN RELATION TO CYP2C19 POLYMORPHISM

Dual Omeprazole/Amoxicillin Therapy

The eradication rates for *H. pylori* by dual omeprazole/amoxicillin (omeprazole 20 mg once daily plus amoxicillin 500 mg four times daily for 2 weeks) are approximately 30% in the RMs, 60% in the IMs, and 100% in the PMs (Figure 17A–11).[59] Differences in plasma omeprazole concentrations among the different CYP2C19 genotype groups are assumed to reflect the different eradication rates among the correspondent genotype groups. Aoyama et al.[60] reported that eradication rates by dual omeprazole/amoxicillin therapy (omeprazole 40 mg plus amoxicillin 2,000 mg daily for 1 week) were 33%

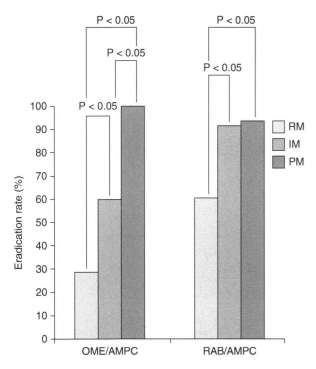

FIGURE 17A–11 Cure rates for *H. pylori* infection by dual therapy with 20 mg of omeprazole plus 2,000 mg of amoxicillin for 2 weeks (OME/AMPC) and the dual therapy with 20 mg of rabeprazole plus 1,500 mg of amoxicillin for 2 weeks (RAB/AMPC) as a function of CYP2C19 genotype groups. Statistical significances in cure rates among the three different genotype groups were assessed by Fisher's exact test. There were significant differences in cure rates among the three different genotype groups in the case of OME/AMPC therapy, whereas significant differences in cure rates were observed between the RM and IM groups and between the RM and PM groups in the case of RAB/AMPC therapy and no statistically significant difference in the cure rates was seen between the IM and PM groups. See the legend of Figure 17A–2 for the abbreviations.

in the RMs, 30% in the IMs, and 100% in the PMs. These two reports[59,60] indicate that eradication rates are higher in the PMs in comparison with those in the RMs and IMs when the same dual dosing scheme is conducted for patients with different CYP2C19 genotypes, suggesting that the longer sustained plasma omeprazole concentrations attained in the PM patients contribute to much higher eradication rates in dual omeprazole/amoxicillin therapy. Moreover, if the sufficient acid suppression observed in CYP2C19 PMs by omeprazole 20 mg is attained, *H. pylori* can be eradicated with amoxicillin 500 mg four times daily.

Dual Rabeprazole/Amoxicillin Therapy

Although the metabolism of rabeprazole was previously reported to be less affected by genetic polymorphism of CYP2C19,[61,62] recent reports have revealed that

pharmacokinetics of rabeprazole is significantly affected by genetic difference in CYP2C19.[30,63,64] However, the acid inhibitory effect of rabeprazole is so potent[65] that a sufficient acid inhibition can be achieved by rabeprazole at the usual standard dose in RMs,[30,66] and, therefore, high cure rates for *H. pylori* infection are expected to be achieved by dual rabeprazole/amoxicillin therapy. Kawai et al.[67] reported that a dual therapy with 20 mg of rabeprazole plus 2,000 mg of amoxicillin achieved a cure rate >80%, which was almost the same as that achieved by the triple PPI/amoxicillin/clarithromycin therapy in their study. In another study, the total average cure rate achieved by a dual therapy with 10 mg of rabeprazole twice daily plus 500 mg of amoxicillin three times daily for 2 weeks was around 80%.[68] However, the cure rates were affected by the different CYP2C19 genotype status (Figure 17A–11).[68] Significant differences in plasma rabeprazole concentrations among the different CYP2C19 genotype groups[30,63,64] might account for the different cure rates among the different CYP2C19 genotype groups, because rabeprazole per se has an anti–*H. pylori* effect.[69,70] Moreover, thioether rabeprazole, which is a metabolite formed via nonenzymatic reduction from the parent drug and is a potent inhibitor of *H. pylori* growth,[69,70] is metabolized by CYP2C19 to demethylated thioether rabeprazole. Therefore, significant differences in plasma thioether rabeprazole levels might have existed among the different CYP2C19 genotype groups, thereby resulting in the different cure rates among the three different CYP2C19 genotype groups.

Interestingly, the cure rate achieved by the dual rabeprazole/amoxicillin therapy in the IM plus PM groups (92.2%)[68] was very high as that achieved by current PPI-based triple therapies.[7,58,71–73] However, current triple therapies have problems of bacterial resistance to clarithromycin or metronidazole.[74–76] Metronidazole has also been reported to exhibit a risk of later development of lung cancer; however, the clinical significance of this is unclear.[77] Because 65–70% of Asians and 20–25% of Caucasian individuals are IM or PM genotypes or phenotypes of CYP2C19[44,78–80] and there are quite few amoxicillin-resistant strains of *H. pylori*,[81] the dual rabeprazole/amoxicillin therapy would yield, on a theoretical basis, a better than 90% success rate in curing *H. pylori* infection in 65–70% of Asians and 20–25% of Caucasian patients, without the second antibacterial agent, such as clarithromycin or metronidazole. Moreover, a dual high-dose rabeprazole (10 mg, four times daily) plus amoxicillin (500 mg, four times daily) therapy used as a second-line therapy is sufficiently effective even for RM patients.[82–84] Therefore, if patients' CYP2C19 genotype status is determined before the treatment, an individualized optimal treatment schedule (e.g., rabeprazole 10 mg qid plus amoxicillin 500 mg qid for RMs, and rabeprazole 10 mg bid plus amoxicillin 500 mg tid or qid for IMs and PMs) can be performed and the cure rate achieved by the initial treatment is expected to become higher. Therefore, the genotyping test of CYP2C19 is assumed to be a clinically useful tool for an optimal treatment selection of a PPI-based *H. pylori* eradication therapy.

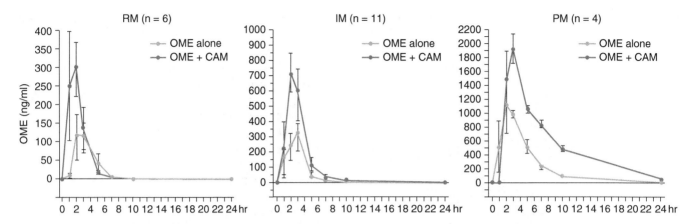

FIGURE 17A–12 Mean (±SE) plasma levels of omeprazole (OME) in the RM, IM, and PM groups with and without clarithromycin (CAM). Plasma concentrations of omeprazole were increased by CAM in the three different CYP2C19 genotype groups. See the legend of Figure 17A–2 for the abbreviations.

TRIPLE PPI/AMOXICILLIN/ CLARITHROMYCIN THERAPY FOR *H. PYLORI* INFECTION IN RELATION TO CYP2C19 POLYMORPHISM

Interaction Between PPI and Clarithromycin

One of the current regimens for eradication of *H. pylori* is the triple PPI/amoxicillin/clarithromycin therapy.[8] In addition, the possible drug–drug interaction between PPIs and clarithromycin must be considered. Clarithromycin is not only metabolized by CYP3A4 but also a potent inhibitor of CYP3A4. CYP3A4 is involved in the sulfoxidation of PPIs.[85] It also affects the activity of CYP2C19.[86] Therefore, when a PPI and clarithromycin are coadministered, a drug–drug interaction between the PPI and clarithromycin can occur.

Figure 17A–12 shows the effects of clarithromycin on plasma omeprazole concentrations as a function of CYP2C19 genotype status. Plasma omeprazole concentrations increase by coadministration with clarithromycin in each of the different CYP2C19 genotype groups. Particularly plasma omeprazole concentrations in PMs are extremely high, because PMs lacks CYP2C19, and, therefore, CYP3A4, which is an important PPI-metabolizing enzyme in PMs,[28] is inhibited by clarithromycin. Another study demonstrates that clarithromycin increases plasma lansoprazole concentrations by inhibiting the CYP3A4 activity in patients who undergo treatment with the triple lansoprazole/amoxicillin/clarithromycin therapy.[87] These results indicate that the drug–drug interaction between clarithromycin and a PPI may underlie the high cure rate for the eradication of *H. pylori* obtained by a triple PPI/amoxicillin/clarithromycin therapy. Plasma clarithromycin concentrations also differ among the different CYP2C19 genotype groups (Figure 17A–13),[28] which is assumed to be related to different eradication rates among the different CYP2C19 genotype groups.

Impact of CYP2C19 Polymorphism on Triple PPI/Amoxicillin/Clarithromycin Therapy for *H. Pylori* Infection at the Usual Dose

Differences in plasma clarithromycin and PPI concentrations among the different CYP2C19 genotype groups are assumed to be reflected by different cure rates for *H. pylori* infection as noted above. It was reported that eradication rates for *H. pylori* infection by a triple therapy with daily doses of omeprazole 40 mg or lansoprazole 60 mg, amoxicillin 1,500 mg, and clarithromycin 600 mg for 1 week were 72.7% in RMs, 92.1% in IMs, and 97.8% in PMs (Figure 17A–14).[88] The incidence of the RM genotype was higher in the group without eradication or with

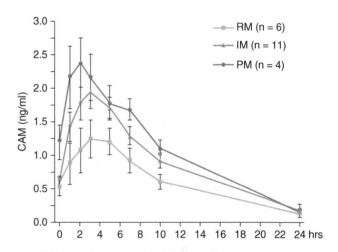

FIGURE 17A–13 Mean (±SE) plasma concentration–time curves of clarithromycin (CAM) in the three different genotype groups. Significant differences in plasma clarithromycin concentrations were observed among the three different CYP2C19 genotype groups. See the legend of Figure 17A–2 for the abbreviations.

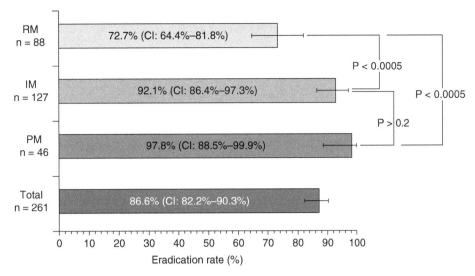

FIGURE 17A–14 *H. pylori* eradication rates achieved by the triple PPI/amoxicillin/clarithromycin therapy in total and for different CYP2C19 genotype groups. Bars indicate 95% confidence intervals (95% CI). There was a significant difference in eradication rate among the three different CYP2C19 genotype groups. See the legend of Figure 17A–2 for the abbreviations.

therapeutic failure, while the incidence of the PM genotype in patients without eradication was very low (Figure 17A–15A). Aoyama et al.[60] reported that cure rates by triple omeprazole/amoxicillin/clarithromycin therapy were 81% in RMs, 94.5% in IMs, and 100% in PMs. Tanigawara et al.[89] also reported the similar results. Dojo et al.[90] reported that cure rates by triple omeprazole/amoxicillin/clarithromycin therapy were 73.3% in RMs, 86.1% in IMs, and 85.0% in PMs (not statistically significant). Taken together, these reports suggest that one of the reasons for the eradication failure of *H. pylori* by triple PPI/amoxicillin/clarithromycin therapies is considered to be the insufficient dose of a PPI (omeprazole or lansoprazole) in RMs. Therefore, the RM genotype of CYP2C19 is one of the possible causes for the eradication failure of *H. pylori* infection by a triple PPI/amoxicillin/clarithromycin therapy as well as by a dual PPI/amoxicillin therapy.

Another important factor associated with success or failure of *H. pylori* eradication by a triple PPI/amoxicillin/clarithromycin therapy is bacterial resistance to clarithromycin. More than half of patients without eradication were infected with the clarithromycin-resistant strain of *H. pylori* (Figure 17A–15B). Bacterial resistance to clarithromycin is caused by mutation in 23S rRNA gene, which can be detected by molecular analyses.[91–94] It was reported that eradication rates in RM, IM, and PM patients infected with clarithromycin-sensitive strain of *H. pylori* were relatively high, whereas the eradication rate in RM patients infected with clarithromycin-resistant strain of *H. pylori* was dramatically low (7.1%) (Figure 17A–16).[88] Therefore, it can be concluded that the major factors associated with success or failure of the eradication of *H. pylori* by a triple PPI/amoxicillin/clarithromycin therapy are not only CYP2C19 genotype status of patients but also bacterial resistance to clarithromycin of *H. pylori* strains.

Retreatment Strategy for Eradication Failure by PPI/Amoxicillin/Clarithromycin Therapy at the Usual Dose

The majority of patients who fail in the eradication of *H. pylori* infection by PPI/amoxicillin/clarithromycin therapy at the usual doses have the RM genotype of CYP2C19 or are infected with a clarithromycin-resistant strain of *H. pylori*. However, the amoxicillin-resistant strain of *H. pylori* is quite rare,[81] and, therefore, treatment with an increased dose of PPI and amoxicillin is expected to succeed in the eradication of *H. pylori* in patients who have had therapeutic failure by the initial treatment with the triple therapy with a PPI, amoxicillin, and clarithromycin at the usual dose. Bayerdorffer et al.[95] reported that around 90% of the eradication rate could be achieved by the dual therapy with 120 mg of omeprazole plus 2.25 g of amoxicillin daily for 2 weeks, indicating that sufficient cure rates for *H. pylori* infection can be obtained by the dual therapy with a PPI and amoxicillin at a high dose. The dual therapy with high doses of PPI plus amoxicillin for the retreatment strategy is performed as the rescue therapy, where lansoprazole 30 mg or rabeprazole 10 mg plus 500 mg of amoxicillin is dosed four times daily for 2 weeks and sufficient cure rates higher than 90% have been obtained,[82,84,88] because four times daily dosing of a PPI can yield a sufficient acid inhibition (intragastric pH is kept at around 7 throughout the 24 hours of the day). In addition, amoxicillin is more bioavailable under a higher intragastric pH (i.e., around 7.0) attained by the CYP2C19-related PPI dosing scheme and the bactericidal effect of amoxicillin is expected to be fully enhanced. Miehlke et al.[96] also reported

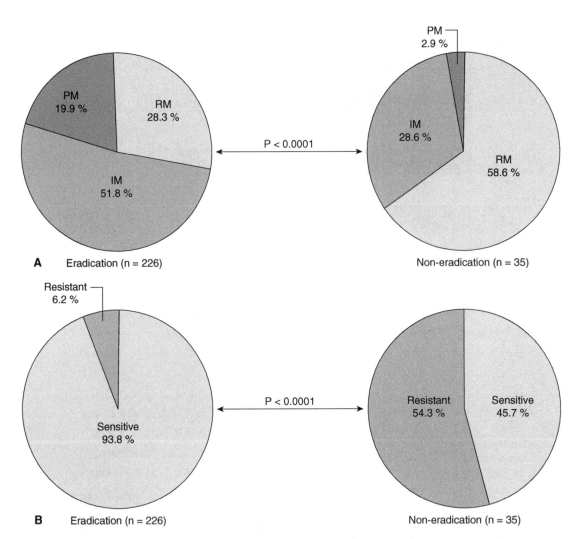

FIGURE 17A–15 (**A**) Frequencies of CYP2C19 genotypes in patients with eradication and noneradication of *H. pylori* infection by triple PPI/ amoxicillin/clarithromycin therapy. Note that most (>97%) patients with noneradication of *H. pylori* had EM genotypes of CYP2C19 (RM or IM), while only one PM patient belonged to the noneradication group. (**B**) Frequencies of clarithromycin-sensitive and -resistant strains of *H. pylori* in patients with and without eradication of *H. pylori* infection achieved with triple PPI/amoxicillin/clarithromycin therapy. Note that more than half (54.3%) of patients without eradication of *H. pylori* were infected with a clarithromycin-resistant strain of *H. pylori*, while only 6.2% of patients with eradication of *H. pylori* were infected with a clarithromycin-resistant strain of *H. pylori*. See the legend of Figure 17A–2 for the abbreviations.

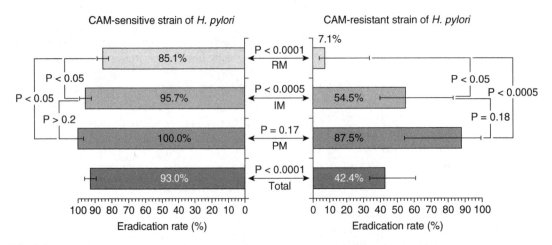

FIGURE 17A–16 *H. pylori* eradication rates achieved with triple PPI/amoxicillin/clarithromycin (CAM) therapy for CAM-sensitive and -resistant strains of *H. pylori* in total and for different CYP2C19 genotype groups. Bars indicate 95% confidence intervals (95% CI). There was a significant difference in eradication rate among the three genotype groups, for both CAM-resistant and -sensitive strains of *H. pylori*. See the legend of Figure 17A–2 for the abbreviations.

TABLE 17A–1 Cure rates of *H. pylori* infection by treatment with high doses of a PPI plus amoxicillin.

Regimen	Cure Rates (% PP)	Reference
OME 40 mg three times daily + AMP 750 mg three times daily	91	[95]
LAN 30 mg four times daily + AMPC 500 mg four times daily	96.7	[88]
RAB 10 mg four times daily + AMPC 500 mg four times daily	93.8	[84]
RAB 10 mg four times daily + AMPC 500 mg four times daily	100.0	[83]

PP, per protocol analysis; OME, omeprazole; LAN, lansoprazole; RAB, rabeprazole; AMPC, amoxicillin.

that the dual therapy with very high doses of omeprazole and amoxicillin was as effective as a quadruple therapy for the second-line regimen. The reported cure rates of *H. pylori* infection by treatment with high doses of a PPI plus amoxicillin are summarized in Table 17A–1.

Tailored Strategy for *H. Pylori* Infection Based on Pharmacogenomics

Pharmacogenomics-based tailored strategy for *H. pylori* infection was reported.[97] As the tailored strategy for *H. pylori* infection, patients infected with a clarithromycin-sensitive strain of *H. pylori* were treated with 200 mg of clarithromycin tid, 500 mg of amoxicillin tid, and personalized doses of

lansoprazole (i.e., 30 mg tid in RMs, 15 mg tid in IMs, and 15 mg bid in PMs) for 1 week, while patients infected with a clarithromycin-resistant strain of *H. pylori* were treated with 500 mg of amoxicillin qid and personalized dose of lansoprazole (i.e., 30 mg qid in RMs, 15 mg qid in IMs, and 15 mg bid in PMs) for 2 weeks (Figure 17A–17). This tailored strategy yielded nearly complete eradication rates (i.e., 96.6% PP analysis). Interestingly, the cost for genotyping test can be offset by the higher eradication rates obtained with the tailored strategy when compared with the standard regimen in Japan.[97] In the personalized treatment group, CYP2C19 genotype-dependent differences in cure rates are not observed (Figure 17A–18). Especially, the low cure rate in the CYP2C19 RM patients infected with clarithromycin-resistant strains of *H. pylori* is

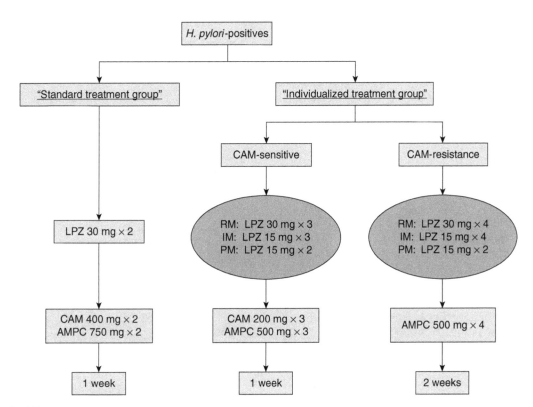

FIGURE 17A–17 Flow of standard versus tailored strategy of eradication of *H. pylori* based on genotypes of CYP2C19 and *H. pylori* 23S rRNA.

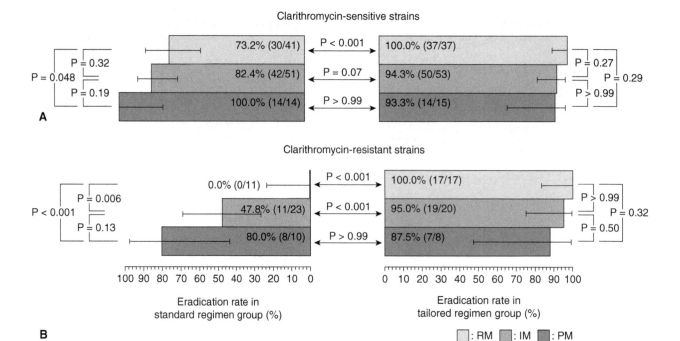

FIGURE 17A–18 *H. pylori* eradication rates (ITT) with standard and tailored regimens as a function of CYP2C19 genotype status in the first-line therapy, illustrating eradication rates of both clarithromycin-sensitive (**A**) and clarithromycin-resistant (**B**) strains of *H. pylori*.[97] Bars indicate the 95% confidence intervals of eradication rates. *Abbreviations*: CI = AMPC, amoxicillin; LPZ, lansoprazole; CAM-S, clarithromycin-sensitive strain of *H. pylori*; CAM-R, clarithromycin-resistant strain of *H. pylori*; RM, rapid metabolizer of CYP2C19; IM, intermediate metabolizer of CYP2C19; PM, poor metabolizer of CYP2C19.

dramatically improved in the tailored strategy group (Figure 17A–18B). Therefore, pharmacogenomics-based personalized eradication therapy is a useful strategy.

It should however also be mentioned that PPIs have a quite large therapeutic range and thus another option would be to increase standard doses without taking CYP2C19 genotype into account, achieving appropriate action in RMs without causing a relevant risk for PMs despite high concentrations. Cost-effectiveness needs to be compared between this option and genotype-adjusted therapy for a definite conclusion.

Key Points in the Eradication of *H. Pylori*

The basic strategy for *H. pylori* eradication from the viewpoint of clinical pharmacology is summarized as follows: first, to select the antibacterial agent to which *H. pylori* is sensitive and to dose it in an appropriate dosing manner (i.e., four times daily for amoxicillin, twice daily for clarithromycin); second, to make the environmental condition in the stomach more optimal under which the selected antibacterial agent becomes more stable and bioavailable, by coadministering the sufficient dose of a PPI chosen in relation to the individual CYP2C19 genotype status. The treatment plan individualized on the basis of above-mentioned items is expected to increase the eradication rate by the initial therapy. In general, therapy with any PPI can be used initially.

DRUG–DRUG INTERACTIONS BETWEEN PPI AND OTHER DRUGS IN RELATION TO CYP2C19 POLYMORPHISMS

Effects of PPIS on the Activity of P450

PPIs are often coadministered with other drugs including substrates of P450. The drug–drug interaction of PPIs with other drugs is of clinically important study subjects. Stedman and Barclay[98] summarized the drug–drug interaction of different PPIs via CYP and reported that there was some variation in their potential for drug interactions due to differences in enzyme inhibition. Kodaira et al.[99] reported the effect of different PPIs on the activity of P450 assessed by the [13C]-aminopyrine breath test in relation to CYP2C19 polymorphisms. They reported that different PPIs inhibited CYP activity to different extents.

Interaction Between PPIS and Clopidogrel

In 2008, the consensus and guidelines of the American College of Cardiology Foundation (ACCF), the American College of Gastroenterology (ACG), and American Heart Association (AHA) on antiplatelet therapy were published,[100–102] and stated that patients with a risk of peptic ulcer and/or treated with two or more antiplatelet agents are recommended to be treated

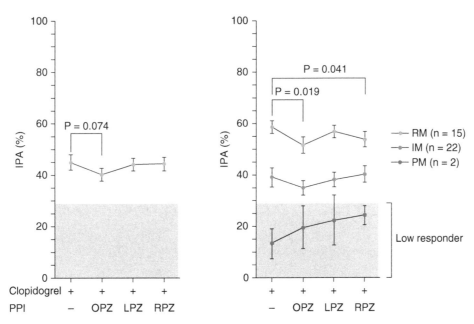

FIGURE 17A–19 The changes in the inhibition of platelet aggregation (IPA) by clopidogrel with different PPIs as a whole (**A**) and in different CYP2C19 genotype groups (**B**). The antiplatelet function of clopidogrel appeared influenced by any of the three PPIs, omeprazole (OPZ), lansoprazole (LPZ), and rabeprazole (RPZ), to the different degrees, but not statistically significantly, as a whole (**A**). When separately analyzed according to the CYP2C19 genotype groups, statistically significant difference in the inhibition of platelet aggregation by clopidogrel was found (**B**). This difference was maintained during the concomitant dosing with different PPIs. Omeprazole (OPZ) and rabeprazole (RPZ) significantly attenuated the inhibition of platelet aggregation by clopidogrel in rapid metabolizers (RMs) of CYP2C19 (**B**).

with a PPI. Therefore, patients treated with clopidogrel have a greater chance to be treated with a PPI. However, clopidogrel is activated by CYP2C19. Therefore, the plasma concentration of the active metabolite of clopidogrel depends on the activity of CYP2C19. The inhibitory effect of clopidogrel on platelet aggregation depends on CYP2C19 genotype status[103] and is also associated the clinical events.[104] Moreover, concomitant use of clopidogrel and a PPI induces a drug–drug interaction via CYP2C19, resulting in decreased activation of clopidogrel. Juurlink et al.[105] reported that concomitant therapy with a PPI was associated with an increased risk of reinfarction. Ho et al.[106] reported that concomitant use of clopidogrel and a PPI was associated with an increased risk of adverse outcomes compared with the use of clopidogrel without a PPI and they suggested that the use of a PPI might be associated with attenuation of benefits of clopidogrel. Together, there are merits (i.e., gastric protection) and demerits (i.e., attenuation of clopidogrel efficacy) in the concomitant use of a PPI in patients undergoing antiplatelet therapy including clopidogrel. This is the therapeutic dilemma of prophylaxis use of PPI in antiplatelet therapy.

Furuta et al.[107] studied the effects of omeprazole, lansoprazole, and rabeprazole on the antiplatelet functions of clopidogrel in relation to CYP2C19 genotype status and found that three PPIs attenuated the antiplatelet functions of clopidogrel in different degrees (Figure 17A–19A) and that the levels of attenuation of clopidogrel by PPIs depended on CYP2C19 genotype status (Figure 17A–19B). Although the efficacy of clopidogrel was decreased by a PPI in RMs of CYP2C19, the levels of

antiplatelet function of clopidogrel after attenuation by a PPI in this group were not mostly problematic (i.e., rarely decreased to the levels of "low responder [IPA <30%]"). On the other hand, in patients with the IM genotype of CYP2C19, conversion from responder to a lower chance of responding easily occurs. The subjects with the PM genotype of CYP2C19 were low responders irrespective of PPI use.

CONCLUSION AND SUMMARY POINTS

Not only pharmacokinetics and pharmacodynamics but also clinical outcomes by PPI-based therapy are affected by CYP2C19 genotype or pharmacogenomics. PPIs are now the first choice for acid inhibition. Moreover, a PPI is dosed for a long time for GERD patients. Clinical effects of PPIs depend on the CYP2C19 genotype status of patient. Therefore, this genotyping test is a useful clinical tool for the optimal PPI treatment. The cost-effectiveness of this genotyping test needs to be tested in a future study.

REFERENCES

1. Sachs G, Shin JM, Briving C, Wallmark B, Hersey S. The pharmacology of the gastric acid pump: the H+,K+ ATPase. *Annu Rev Pharmacol Toxicol.* 1995;35:277–305.
2. Blum RA. Lansoprazole and omeprazole in the treatment of acid peptic disorders. *Am J Health Syst Pharm.* 1996;53(12):1401–1415.
3. Lockhart SP. Clinical review of lansoprazole. *Br J Clin Pract Suppl.* 1994;75:48–55 [discussion 56–57].

4. Langtry HD, Wilde MI. Lansoprazole. An update of its pharmacological properties and clinical efficacy in the management of acid-related disorders. *Drugs.* 1997;54(3):473–500.

5. Inatomi N, Nagaya H, Takami K, Shino A, Satoh H. Effects of a proton pump inhibitor, AG-1749 (lansoprazole), on reflux esophagitis and experimental ulcers in rats. *Jpn J Pharmacol.* 1991;55(4):437–451.

6. Carswell CI, Goa KL. Rabeprazole: an update of its use in acid-related disorders. *Drugs.* 2001;61(15):2327–2356.

7. Unge P. Review of *Helicobacter pylori* eradication regimens. *Scand J Gastroenterol Suppl.* 1996;215:74–81.

8. Asaka M, Sugiyama T, Kato M, et al. A multicenter, double-blind study on triple therapy with lansoprazole, amoxicillin and clarithromycin for eradication of *Helicobacter pylori* in Japanese peptic ulcer patients. *Helicobacter.* 2001;6(3):254–261.

9. Furuta T, Futami H, Arai H, Hanai H, Kaneko E. Effects of lansoprazole with or without amoxicillin on ulcer healing: relation to eradication of *Helicobacter pylori. J Clin Gastroenterol.* 1995;20(suppl 2):S107–S111.

10. Andersson T, Regardh CG, Dahl-Puustinen ML, Bertilsson L. Slow omeprazole metabolizers are also poor *S*-mephenytoin hydroxylators. *Ther Drug Monit.* 1990;12(4):415–416.

11. Andersson T, Regardh CG, Lou YC, Zhang Y, Dahl ML, Bertilsson L. Polymorphic hydroxylation of *S*-mephenytoin and omeprazole metabolism in Caucasian and Chinese subjects. *Pharmacogenetics.* 1992;2(1):25–31.

12. Sohn DR, Kobayashi K, Chiba K, Lee KH, Shin SG, Ishizaki T. Disposition kinetics and metabolism of omeprazole in extensive and poor metabolizers of *S*-mephenytoin 4'-hydroxylation recruited from an Oriental population. *J Pharmacol Exp Ther.* 1992;262(3):1195–1202.

13. Pearce RE, Rodrigues AD, Goldstein JA, Parkinson A. Identification of the human P450 enzymes involved in lansoprazole metabolism. *J Pharmacol Exp Ther.* 1996;277(2):805–816.

14. Yamazaki H, Inoue K, Shaw PM, Checovich WJ, Guengerich FP, Shimada T. Different contributions of cytochrome P450 2C19 and 3A4 in the oxidation of omeprazole by human liver microsomes: effects of contents of these two forms in individual human samples. *J Pharmacol Exp Ther.* 1997;283(2):434–442.

15. Ishizaki T, Horai Y. Review article: cytochrome P450 and the metabolism of proton pump inhibitors—emphasis on rabeprazole. *Aliment Pharmacol Ther.* 1999;13(suppl 3):27–36.

16. Kupfer A, Preisig R. Pharmacogenetics of mephenytoin: a new drug hydroxylation polymorphism in man. *Eur J Clin Pharmacol.* 1984;26(6):753–759.

17. Ishizaki T, Sohn DR, Kobayashi K, et al. Interethnic differences in omeprazole metabolism in the two *S*-mephenytoin hydroxylation phenotypes studied in Caucasians and Orientals. *Ther Drug Monit.* 1994;16(2):214–215.

18. Xiao ZS, Goldstein JA, Xie HG, et al. Differences in the incidence of the CYP2C19 polymorphism affecting the *S*-mephenytoin phenotype in Chinese Han and Bai populations and identification of a new rare CYP2C19 mutant allele. *J Pharmacol Exp Ther.* 1997;281(1):604–609.

19. Xie HG, Kim RB, Stein CM, Wilkinson GR, Wood AJ. Genetic polymorphism of (*S*)-mephenytoin 4'-hydroxylation in populations of African descent. *Br J Clin Pharmacol.* 1999;48(3):402–408.

20. Marinac JS, Balian JD, Foxworth JW, et al. Determination of CYP2C19 phenotype in black Americans with omeprazole: correlation with genotype. *Clin Pharmacol Ther.* 1996;60(2):138–144.

21. Masimirembwa C, Bertilsson L, Johansson I, Hasler JA, Ingelman-Sundberg M. Phenotyping and genotyping of *S*-mephenytoin hydroxylase (cytochrome P450 2C19) in a Shona population of Zimbabwe. *Clin Pharmacol Ther.* 1995;57(6):656–661.

22. de Morais SM, Goldstein JA, Xie HG, et al. Genetic analysis of the *S*-mephenytoin polymorphism in a Chinese population. *Clin Pharmacol Ther.* 1995;58(4):404–411.

23. Kubota T, Chiba K, Ishizaki T. Genotyping of *S*-mephenytoin 4'-hydroxylation in an extended Japanese population. *Clin Pharmacol Ther.* 1996;60(6):661–666.

24. Roh HK, Dahl ML, Tybring G, Yamada H, Cha YN, Bertilsson L. CYP2C19 genotype and phenotype determined by omeprazole in a Korean population. *Pharmacogenetics.* 1996;6(6):547–551.

25. De Morais SM, Wilkinson GR, Blaisdell J, Meyer UA, Nakamura K, Goldstein JA. Identification of a new genetic defect responsible for the polymorphism of (*S*)-mephenytoin metabolism in Japanese. *Mol Pharmacol.* 1994;46(4):594–598.

26. de Morais SM, Wilkinson GR, Blaisdell J, Nakamura K, Meyer UA, Goldstein JA. The major genetic defect responsible for the polymorphism of *S*-mephenytoin metabolism in humans. *J Biol Chem.* 1994;269(22):15419–15422.

27. Furuta T, Ohashi K, Kosuge K, et al. CYP2C19 genotype status and effect of omeprazole on intragastric pH in humans. *Clin Pharmacol Ther.* 1999;65(5):552–561.

28. Furuta T, Ohashi K, Kobayashi K, et al. Effects of clarithromycin on the metabolism of omeprazole in relation to CYP2C19 genotype status in humans. *Clin Pharmacol Ther.* 1999;66(3):265–274.

29. Saitoh T, Fukushima Y, Otsuka H, et al. Effects of rabeprazole, lansoprazole and omeprazole on intragastric pH in CYP2C19 extensive metabolizers. *Aliment Pharmacol Ther.* 2002;16(10):1811–1817.

30. Shirai N, Furuta T, Moriyama Y, et al. Effects of CYP2C19 genotypic differences in the metabolism of omeprazole and rabeprazole on intragastric pH. *Aliment Pharmacol Ther.* 2001;15(12):1929–1937.

31. Shirai N, Furuta T, Xiao F, et al. Comparison of lansoprazole and famotidine for gastric acid inhibition during the daytime and nighttime in different CYP2C19 genotype groups. *Aliment Pharmacol Ther.* 2002;16(4):837–846.

32. Furuta T, Shirai N, Xiao F, Ohashi K, Ishizaki T. Effect of high-dose lansoprazole on intragastic pH in subjects who are homozygous extensive metabolizers of cytochrome P4502C19. *Clin Pharmacol Ther.* 2001;70(5):484–492.

33. Bardhan KD, Hawkey CJ, Long RG, et al. Lansoprazole versus ranitidine for the treatment of reflux oesophagitis. UK Lansoprazole Clinical Research Group. *Aliment Pharmacol Ther.* 1995;9(2):145–151.

34. Bardhan KD. The role of proton pump inhibitors in the treatment of gastro-oesophageal reflux disease. *Aliment Pharmacol Ther.* 1995; 9(suppl 1):15–25.

35. Kirchgatterer A, Aschl G, Hinterreiter M, Stadler B, Knoflach P. Current concepts in therapy of reflux disease. *Wien Med Wochenschr.* 2001;151(11–12):266–269.

36. Furuta T, Shirai N, Watanabe F, et al. Effect of cytochrome P4502C19 genotypic differences on cure rates for gastroesophageal reflux disease by lansoprazole. *Clin Pharmacol Ther.* 2002;72(4):453–460.

37. Kawamura M, Ohara S, Koike T, et al. The effects of lansoprazole on erosive reflux oesophagitis are influenced by CYP2C19 polymorphism. *Aliment Pharmacol Ther.* 2003;17(7):965–973.

38. Furuta T, Sugimoto M, Kodaira C, et al. CYP2C19 genotype is associated with symptomatic recurrence of GERD during maintenance therapy with low-dose lansoprazole. *Eur J Clin Pharmacol.* 2009;65(7):693–698.

39. Peghini PL, Katz PO, Bracy NA, Castell DO. Nocturnal recovery of gastric acid secretion with twice-daily dosing of proton pump inhibitors. *Am J Gastroenterol.* 1998;93(5):763–767.

40. Adachi K, Fujishiro H, Katsube T, et al. Predominant nocturnal acid reflux in patients with Los Angeles grade C and D reflux esophagitis. *J Gastroenterol Hepatol.* 2001;16(11):1191–1196.

41. Klinkenberg-Knol EC, Meuwissen SG. Combined gastric and oesophageal 24-hour pH monitoring and oesophageal manometry in patients with reflux disease, resistant to treatment with omeprazole. *Aliment Pharmacol Ther.* 1990;4(5):485–495.

42. Ours TM, Fackler WK, Richter JE, Vaezi MF. Nocturnal acid breakthrough: clinical significance and correlation with esophageal acid exposure. *Am J Gastroenterol.* 2003;98(3):545–550.

43. Leite LP, Johnston BT, Just RJ, Castell DO. Persistent acid secretion during omeprazole therapy: a study of gastric acid profiles in patients demonstrating failure of omeprazole therapy. *Am J Gastroenterol.* 1996;91(8):1527–1531.

44. Xie HG, Stein CM, Kim RB, Wilkinson GR, Flockhart DA, Wood AJ. Allelic, genotypic and phenotypic distributions of *S*-mephenytoin 4'-hydroxylase (CYP2C19) in healthy Caucasian populations of European descent throughout the world. *Pharmacogenetics.* 1999;9(5):539–549.

45. Xue S, Katz PO, Banerjee P, Tutuian R, Castell DO. Bedtime H2 blockers improve nocturnal gastric acid control in GERD patients on proton pump inhibitors. *Aliment Pharmacol Ther.* 2001;15(9):1351–1356.

46. Peghini PL, Katz PO, Castell DO. Ranitidine controls nocturnal gastric acid breakthrough on omeprazole: a controlled study in normal subjects. *Gastroenterology.* 1998;115(6):1335–1339.

47. Kinoshita Y, Adachi K, Fujishiro H. Therapeutic approaches to reflux disease, focusing on acid secretion. *J Gastroenterol*. 2003;38(suppl 15):13–19.

48. Blaser MJ. Hypotheses on the pathogenesis and natural history of *Helicobacter pylori*-induced inflammation. *Gastroenterology*. 1992;102(2):720–727.

49. Parsonnet J, Blaser MJ, Perez-Perez GI, Hargrett-Bean N, Tauxe RV. Symptoms and risk factors of *Helicobacter pylori* infection in a cohort of epidemiologists. *Gastroenterology*. 1992;102(1):41–46.

50. Wotherspoon AC. *Helicobacter pylori* infection and gastric lymphoma. *Br Med Bull*. 1998;54(1):79–85.

51. Uemura N, Okamoto S, Yamamoto S, et al. *Helicobacter pylori* infection and the development of gastric cancer. *N Engl J Med*. 2001;345(11):784–789.

52. Grayson ML, Eliopoulos GM, Ferraro MJ, Moellering RC Jr. Effect of varying pH on the susceptibility of *Campylobacter pylori* to antimicrobial agents. *Eur J Clin Microbiol Infect Dis*. 1989;8(10):888–889.

53. Scott D, Weeks D, Melchers K, Sachs G. The life and death of *Helicobacter pylori*. *Gut*. 1998;43(suppl 1):S56–S60.

54. Scott DR, Weeks D, Hong C, Postius S, Melchers K, Sachs G. The role of internal urease in acid resistance of *Helicobacter pylori*. *Gastroenterology*. 1998;114(1):58–70.

55. Graham DY, Fischbach L. *Helicobacter pylori* treatment in the era of increasing antibiotic resistance. *Gut*. 2010;59(8):1143–1153.

56. Goddard AF, Jessa MJ, Barrett DA, et al. Effect of omeprazole on the distribution of metronidazole, amoxicillin, and clarithromycin in human gastric juice. *Gastroenterology*. 1996;111(2):358–367.

57. Midolo PD, Turnidge JD, Lambert JR, Bell JM. Oxygen concentration influences proton pump inhibitor activity against *Helicobacter pylori* in vitro. *Antimicrob Agents Chemother*. 1996;40(6):1531–1533.

58. Lind T, Megraud F, Unge P, et al. The MACH2 study: role of omeprazole in eradication of *Helicobacter pylori* with 1-week triple therapies. *Gastroenterology*. 1999;116(2):248–253.

59. Furuta T, Ohashi K, Kamata T, et al. Effect of genetic differences in omeprazole metabolism on cure rates for *Helicobacter pylori* infection and peptic ulcer. *Ann Intern Med*. 1998;129(12):1027–1030.

60. Aoyama N, Tanigawara Y, Kita T, et al. Sufficient effect of 1-week omeprazole and amoxicillin dual treatment for *Helicobacter pylori* eradication in cytochrome P450 2C19 poor metabolizers. *J Gastroenterol*. 1999;34(suppl 11):80–83.

61. Yasuda S, Horai Y, Tomono Y, et al. Comparison of the kinetic disposition and metabolism of E3810, a new proton pump inhibitor, and omeprazole in relation to S-mephenytoin 4'-hydroxylation status. *Clin Pharmacol Ther*. 1995;58(2):143–154.

62. Sakai T, Aoyama N, Kita T, et al. CYP2C19 genotype and pharmacokinetics of three proton pump inhibitors in healthy subjects. *Pharm Res*. 2001;18(6):721–727.

63. Ieiri I, Kishimoto Y, Okochi H, et al. Comparison of the kinetic disposition of and serum gastrin change by lansoprazole versus rabeprazole during an 8-day dosing scheme in relation to CYP2C19 polymorphism. *Eur J Clin Pharmacol*. 2001;57(6–7):485–492.

64. Horai Y, Kimura M, Furuie H, et al. Pharmacodynamic effects and kinetic disposition of rabeprazole in relation to CYP2C19 genotypes. *Aliment Pharmacol Ther*. 2001;15(6):793–803.

65. Williams MP, Sercombe J, Hamilton MI, Pounder RE. A placebo-controlled trial to assess the effects of 8 days of dosing with rabeprazole versus omeprazole on 24-h intragastric acidity and plasma gastrin concentrations in young healthy male subjects. *Aliment Pharmacol Ther*. 1998;12(11):1079–1089.

66. Adachi K, Katsube T, Kawamura A, et al. CYP2C19 genotype status and intragastric pH during dosing with lansoprazole or rabeprazole. *Aliment Pharmacol Ther*. 2000;14(10):1259–1266.

67. Kawai T, Oguma K, Kudou T. Comparison of dual therapy of rabeprazole plus amoxicillin and triple therapy for cure of *Helicobacter pylori*. *Gastroenterology*. 2001;120(suppl 1):A584.

68. Furuta T, Shirai N, Takashima M, et al. Effects of genotypic differences in CYP2C19 status on cure rates for *Helicobacter pylori* infection by dual therapy with rabeprazole plus amoxicillin. *Pharmacogenetics*. 2001;11(4):341–348.

69. Kawakami Y, Akahane T, Yamaguchi M, et al. In vitro activities of rabeprazole, a novel proton pump inhibitor, and its thioether derivative alone and

in combination with other antimicrobials against recent clinical isolates of *Helicobacter pylori*. *Antimicrob Agents Chemother*. 2000;44(2):458–461.

70. Tsuchiya M, Imamura L, Park JB, Kobashi K. *Helicobacter pylori* urease inhibition by rabeprazole, a proton pump inhibitor. *Biol Pharm Bull*. 1995;18(8):1053–1056.

71. Bell GD, Powell KU, Burridge SM, et al. Rapid eradication of *Helicobacter pylori* infection. *Aliment Pharmacol Ther*. 1995;9(1):41–46.

72. Lind T, Veldhuyzen van Zanten S, Unge P, et al. Eradication of *Helicobacter pylori* using one-week triple therapies combining omeprazole with two antimicrobials: the MACH I Study. *Helicobacter*. 1996;1(3):138–144.

73. Walsh JH, Peterson WL. The treatment of *Helicobacter pylori* infection in the management of peptic ulcer disease. *N Engl J Med*. 1995;333(15):984–991.

74. Cederbrant G, Kahlmeter G, Ljungh A. Proposed mechanism for metronidazole resistance in *Helicobacter pylori*. *J Antimicrob Chemother*. 1992;29(2):115–120.

75. Results of a multicentre European survey in 1991 of metronidazole resistance in *Helicobacter pylori*. European Study Group on Antibiotic Susceptibility of *Helicobacter pylori*. *Eur J Clin Microbiol Infect Dis*. 1992;11(9):777–781.

76. Peterson WL, Graham DY, Marshall B, et al. Clarithromycin as monotherapy for eradication of *Helicobacter pylori*: a randomized, double-blind trial. *Am J Gastroenterol*. 1993;88(11):1860–1864.

77. Beard CM, Noller KL, O'Fallon WM, Kurland LT, Dahlin DC. Cancer after exposure to metronidazole. *Mayo Clin Proc*. 1988;63(2):147–153.

78. Alvan G, Bechtel P, Iselius L, Gundert-Remy U. Hydroxylation polymorphisms of debrisoquine and mephenytoin in European populations. *Eur J Clin Pharmacol*. 1990;39(6):533–537.

79. Ferguson RJ, De Morais SM, Benhamou S, et al. A new genetic defect in human CYP2C19: mutation of the initiation codon is responsible for poor metabolism of S-mephenytoin. *J Pharmacol Exp Ther*. 1998;284(1):356–361.

80. Nakamura K, Goto F, Ray WA, et al. Interethnic differences in genetic polymorphism of debrisoquin and mephenytoin hydroxylation between Japanese and Caucasian populations. *Clin Pharmacol Ther*. 1985;38(4):402–408.

81. Adamek RJ, Suerbaum S, Pfaffenbach B, Opferkuch W. Primary and acquired *Helicobacter pylori* resistance to clarithromycin, metronidazole, and amoxicillin—influence on treatment outcome. *Am J Gastroenterol*. 1998;93(3):386–389.

82. Furuta T, Shirai N, Xiao F, et al. High-dose rabeprazole/amoxicillin therapy as the second-line regimen after failure to eradicate H. pylori by triple therapy with the usual doses of a proton pump inhibitor, clarithromycin and amoxicillin. *Hepatogastroenterology*. 2003;50(54):2274–2278.

83. Furuta T, Sugimoto M, Kodaira C, et al. The dual therapy with 4 times daily dosing of rabeprazole and amoxicillin as the 3rd rescue regimen for eradication of H. pylori. *Hepatogastroenterology*. 2010;57:1314–1319.

84. Shirai N, Sugimoto M, Kodaira C, et al. Dual therapy with high doses of rabeprazole and amoxicillin versus triple therapy with rabeprazole, amoxicillin, and metronidazole as a rescue regimen for *Helicobacter pylori* infection after the standard triple therapy. *Eur J Clin Pharmacol*. 2007;63(8):743–749.

85. Andersson T, Miners JO, Veronese ME, Birkett DJ. Identification of human liver cytochrome P450 isoforms mediating secondary omeprazole metabolism. *Br J Clin Pharmacol*. 1994;37(6):597–604.

86. Rodrigues AD, Roberts EM, Mulford DJ, Yao Y, Ouellet D. Oxidative metabolism of clarithromycin in the presence of human liver microsomes. Major role for the cytochrome P4503A (CYP3A) subfamily. *Drug Metab Dispos*. 1997;25(5):623–630.

87. Ushiama H, Echizen H, Nachi S, Ohnishi A. Dose-dependent inhibition of CYP3A activity by clarithromycin during *Helicobacter pylori* eradication therapy assessed by changes in plasma lansoprazole levels and partial cortisol clearance to 6beta-hydroxycortisol. *Clin Pharmacol Ther*. 2002;72(1):33–43.

88. Furuta T, Shirai N, Takashima M, et al. Effect of genotypic differences in CYP2C19 on cure rates for *Helicobacter pylori* infection by triple therapy with a proton pump inhibitor, amoxicillin, and clarithromycin. *Clin Pharmacol Ther*. 2001;69(3):158–168.

89. Tanigawara Y, Aoyama N, Kita T, et al. CYP2C19 genotype-related efficacy of omeprazole for the treatment of infection caused by *Helicobacter pylori*. *Clin Pharmacol Ther*. 1999;66(5):528–534.

90. Dojo M, Azuma T, Saito T, Ohtani M, Muramatsu A, Kuriyama M. Effects of CYP2C19 gene polymorphism on cure rates for *Helicobacter pylori* infection by triple therapy with proton pump inhibitor (omeprazole or rabeprazole), amoxycillin and clarithromycin in Japan. *Dig Liver Dis*. 2001;33(8):671–675.

91. Versalovic J, Osato MS, Spakovsky K, et al. Point mutations in the 23S rRNA gene of *Helicobacter pylori* associated with different levels of clarithromycin resistance. *J Antimicrob Chemother*. 1997;40(2):283–286.

92. Stone GG, Shortridge D, Versalovic J, et al. A PCR-oligonucleotide ligation assay to determine the prevalence of 23S rRNA gene mutations in clarithromycin-resistant *Helicobacter pylori*. *Antimicrob Agents Chemother*. 1997;41(3):712–714.

93. Menard A, Santos A, Megraud F, Oleastro M. PCR-restriction fragment length polymorphism can also detect point mutation A2142C in the 23S rRNA gene, associated with *Helicobacter pylori* resistance to clarithromycin. *Antimicrob Agents Chemother*. 2002;46(4):1156–1157.

94. Furuta T, Sagehashi Y, Shirai N, et al. Influence of CYP2C19 polymorphism and *Helicobacter pylori* genotype determined from gastric tissue samples on response to triple therapy for *H. pylori* infection. *Clin Gastroenterol Hepatol*. 2005;3(6):564–573.

95. Bayerdorffer E, Miehlke S, Mannes GA, et al. Double-blind trial of omeprazole and amoxicillin to cure *Helicobacter pylori* infection in patients with duodenal ulcers. *Gastroenterology*. 1995;108(5):1412–1417.

96. Miehlke S, Kirsch C, Ochsenkuehan T. High-dose omeprazole/amoxicillin therapy versus quadruple therapy for treatment of *Helicobacter pylori* resistant against both metronidazole and clarithromycin: a prospective, randomised cross-over study. *Gastroenterology*. 2001;120(suppl):A120.

97. Furuta T, Shirai N, Kodaira M, et al. Pharmacogenomics-based tailored versus standard therapeutic regimen for eradication of *H. pylori*. *Clin Pharmacol Ther*. 2007;81(4):521–528.

98. Stedman CA, Barclay ML. Review article: comparison of the pharmacokinetics, acid suppression and efficacy of proton pump inhibitors. *Aliment Pharmacol Ther*. 2000;14(8):963–978.

99. Kodaira C, Uchida S, Yamade M, et al. Influence of different proton pump inhibitors on activity of cytochrome P450 assessed by [13C]-aminopyrine breath test. *J Clin Pharmacol*. 2012;52(3):432–439.

100. Bhatt DL, Scheiman J, Abraham NS, et al. ACCF/ACG/AHA 2008 expert consensus document on reducing the gastrointestinal risks of antiplatelet therapy and NSAID use: a report of the American College of Cardiology Foundation Task Force on Clinical Expert Consensus Documents. *J Am Coll Cardiol*. 2008;52(18):1502–1517.

101. Bhatt DL, Scheiman J, Abraham NS, et al. ACCF/ACG/AHA 2008 expert consensus document on reducing the gastrointestinal risks of antiplatelet therapy and NSAID use. *Am J Gastroenterol*. 2008;103(11):2890–2907.

102. Bhatt DL, Scheiman J, Abraham NS, et al. ACCF/ACG/AHA 2008 expert consensus document on reducing the gastrointestinal risks of antiplatelet therapy and NSAID use: a report of the American College of Cardiology Foundation Task Force on Clinical Expert Consensus Documents. *Circulation*. 2008;118(18):1894–1909.

103. Umemura K, Furuta T, Kondo K. The common gene variants of CYP2C19 affect pharmacokinetics and pharmacodynamics in an active metabolite of clopidogrel in healthy subjects. *J Thromb Haemost*. 2008;6(8):1439–1441.

104. Collet JP, Hulot JS, Pena A, et al. Cytochrome P450 2C19 polymorphism in young patients treated with clopidogrel after myocardial infarction: a cohort study. *Lancet*. 2009;373(9660):309–317.

105. Juurlink DN, Gomes T, Ko DT, et al. A population-based study of the drug interaction between proton pump inhibitors and clopidogrel. *CMAJ*. 2009;180(7):713–718.

106. Ho PM, Maddox TM, Wang L, et al. Risk of adverse outcomes associated with concomitant use of clopidogrel and proton pump inhibitors following acute coronary syndrome. *JAMA*. 2009;301(9):937–944.

107. Furuta T, Iwaki T, Umemura K. Influences of different proton pump inhibitors on the anti-platelet function of clopidogrel in relation to CYP2C19 genotypes. *Br J Clin Pharmacol*. 2010;70(3):383–392.

Genomics and the Kidney

Melanie S. Joy, PharmD, PhD

LEARNING OBJECTIVES

- To inform clinicians about the role of genetic variants as risk factors for kidney diseases.
- To assist clinicians in understanding how genomics can influence kidney disease progression.
- To inform clinicians about the contribution of pharmacogenomics toward patient care for kidney disorders.

- To provide clinicians with an understanding of how polymorphisms in drug metabolism and disposition genes can influence risks for drug-induced nephrotoxicity.

INTRODUCTION

Chronic kidney disease (CKD) afflicts at least 21 million persons in the United States.[1] The majority of CKD is due to long-standing and uncontrolled diabetes mellitus and hypertension. In addition to treatments aimed at reducing blood sugar and blood pressure, other common approaches for preserving kidney function include angiotensin-converting enzyme inhibitors (ACEIs) and angiotensin receptor blockers (ARBs) for reducing proteinuria, immunosuppressants and cytotoxic compounds for glomerulonephritis, and immunosuppressants for kidney transplantation. There has been a large expansion of studies within the nephrology research community to identify genetic variants that pose a risk for a particular form of CKD or serve as a risk factor for its progression (Table 17B–1). The role of genetic polymorphisms on drug metabolism and disposition (DMD) in patients with CKD has more recently gathered interest. This aspect is important as CKD, independent of genetic variants, is known to influence both the renal and non-renal clearance of drugs. Together, genomic and nongenomic factors could considerably influence the pharmacokinetics of drugs and overall responses to treatments in the CKD population. This chapter undergoes an extensive review of genomics

in order that a comprehensive understanding of its role in nephrology is provided to clinicians and researchers (Figure 17B–1). This information will be necessary for clinicians as the field evolves to treatments targeted toward genes or aberrant proteins. Additionally, clinicians will need to understand how to provide adequate therapy regimens in the face of physiological and genetic alterations that are present in CKD patients.

DRUG-INDUCED NEPHROTOXICITY

Data are emerging that implicate a role for genetic polymorphisms in drug-induced nephrotoxicity. This is important since nephrotoxicity due to drugs contributes to between 8% and 60% of acute kidney injury (AKI) cases.[2] In adult and pediatric intensive care units, prescriptions for nephrotoxic drugs account for ~25% of all drug orders.[3] Kidney biopsies are not standard of care to diagnose suspected AKI due to drugs. However, the diagnosis of nephrotoxicity is usually classified according to the kidney location or process affected by the toxicity, for example, hemodynamic, glomerular, tubular, tubulointerstitial, and obstructive. Clinically, nephrotoxicity is manifest as a

TABLE 17B-1 Chronic kidney diseases with associated genetic polymorphisms.

Disease	Gene	Variant	Kidney Location
Nephrotoxicity	CYP3A4	*1b, A-392G	PT+
	CYP3A5	*3, A6986G	PT+
	ABCB1	G2677T	PT+
		C3435T	
		C1236T	
	SLC22A2	G808T	PT+
Albuminuria	CUBN	I2984V	G
	MYH9	T36695247G	G
		T36695428C	
		T36695942C	
		C36710183T	
	ACE	I/D	G+
	AGT	M235T	G
	AGTR1	A1166C	G
	AGRT2	A1818T	G
	CYP11B2	C-344T	G
	CYP2C9	*2, Arg144Cys	G+
		*3, Ile359Leu	G+
	PLA$_2$R	C1110G	G
	NPHS2	Arg229Glu	G
	FCRγIIIa	Val158Phe	G+
	FCRγIIIb	NA1	G
		NA2	
	FCRγIIa	Arg131His	G
	NRF2	G-653A	G+
	CYP2B6	Arg487Cys	G+
	CYP2C19	Iso331Val	G+
	UGT1A7	T622C	G+
	UGT2B7	C802T	G+
	GLUT1	C21793T	G
		C23063A	
	SLC22A2	Arg270Ser	G+
	PPARγ	Pro12Ala	G+

Key: "+" denotes that the gene has influence on drugs prescribed in patients with kidney disease.

rise in serum creatinine and blood urea nitrogen several days after exposure to drugs that cause the initial insult to the kidney. Newer, sensitive markers such as kidney injury molecule 1 (Kim-1), neutrophil gelatinase–associated lipocalin (NGAL), N-acetyl-β-glucosaminidase (NAG), clusterin, cystatin C, and β2 microglobulin can detect nephrotoxicity earlier in its clinical course, with suggestions that these improvements could enable damage to be detected within several hours after an initial insult. This is advantageous to the patient, as offending drugs can be discontinued early and/or strategies, such as appropriate hydration, and/or dosage modification can be implemented in an expeditious manner.

Clinicians are seeking early detection and improved prediction tools that may be useful in eliminating or reducing the impact of drug-induced nephrotoxicity. Pharmacogenomics and toxicogenomics are emerging areas that have gained interest in nephrotoxicity due to drugs and chemicals. The possibility of preemptively screening patients for polymorphisms

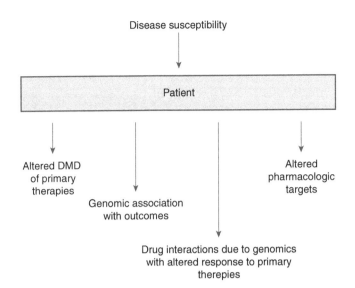

FIGURE 17B-1 Implications for genomics and kidney diseases. DMD, drug metabolism and disposition.

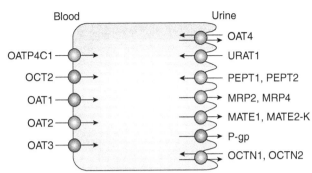

FIGURE 17B-2 Proximal tubule and transporters: kidney locations for pharmacogenomic effects. MATE, multidrug and toxin extrusion transporter; MRP2, multidrug resistance-associated protein transporter; OAT, organic anion transporter; OATP, organic anion transporting polypeptide; OCT, organic cation transporter; OCTN, carnitine/organic cation transporter; PEPT, peptide transporter; P-gp, multidrug resistance transporter; URAT, urate transporter.

that may enhance the risks of nephrotoxicity on exposure to a particular drug, prior to therapy initiation, is appealing. While this area of research is currently evolving, there are several publications that support a role for genetic polymorphisms in drug metabolism and/or drug transport pathways as risk factors for nephrotoxicity. The kidney itself is a high-risk candidate for toxicities and drug interactions secondary to genetic polymorphisms due to the presence of numerous transporters

and metabolizing enzymes in this eliminating organ (Figures 17B–2 and 17B–3). In general, for transport proteins localized to the nephron, polymorphisms that increase the activity of efflux transporters and decrease the activity of uptake transporters are protective for nephrotoxicity. The nephrotoxicity risk of enhanced-activity versus reduced-activity polymorphisms in drug metabolism genes is dependent on whether the parent or a metabolite is implicated as the main nephrotoxic

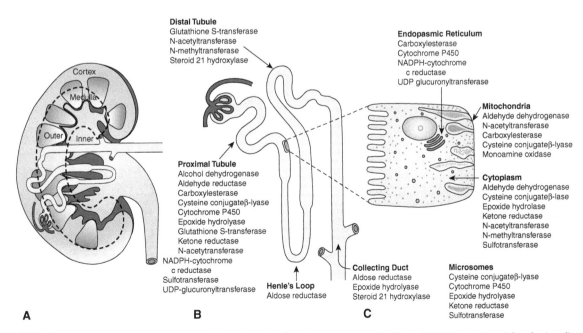

FIGURE 17B-3 (**A–C**) Drug metabolism in the kidney: locations for pharmacogenomic effects. NADPH, nicotinamide adenine dinucleotide phosphate; UDP, uridine diphosphate.

component. Other genes, in addition to those regulating drug metabolism and transport, have also been suggested to contribute to nephrotoxicity. This section will describe the available information concerning the role of genomics in nephrotoxicity due to immunosuppressants of the calcineurin inhibitor class, for example, cyclosporine and tacrolimus, and the chemotherapy agent cisplatin.

Calcineurin Inhibitors

Calcineurin inhibitors are used therapeutically in transplant recipients and patients with autoimmune diseases. Nephrotoxicity due to calcineurin inhibitors can be acute, represented by thrombotic microangiopathy and tubular vacuolization, or chronic, represented by interstitial fibrosis, glomerulosclerosis, and tubular atrophy. It is suggested that 20–94% of solid organ transplant patients who are prescribed calcineurin inhibitors will develop nephrotoxicity.[4–6] Clinical risk factors for nephrotoxicity secondary to calcineurin inhibitors have included the exposure to the kidney tubules as mediated through transporters, for example, P-glycoprotein, and through drug metabolism enzymes, for example, CYP3A5. Due to some data linking alterations in exposure to cyclosporine or tacrolimus and presence of certain genetic polymorphisms in the genes encoding P-glycoprotein (*ABCB1*) and CYP3A5 (*CYP3A5*),[7–11] it is reasonable to ascertain that polymorphisms may contribute to the risks of nephrotoxicity secondary to influencing localized drug exposure. In fact, local kidney exposure to cyclosporine has a direct relationship with increased histologic damage as well as decreased kidney function.[12] Additionally, altered kidney expression of P-glycoprotein and CYP3A5 proteins predispose transplant patients to histologically confirmed nephrotoxicity.[13,14]

Human studies have demonstrated susceptibility to calcineurin inhibitor nephrotoxicity based on *CYP3A5* and/or *ABCB1* genotype.[15–20] For tacrolimus, liver donor *CYP3A5*3/*3* genotype (A6986G, rs28383472) was associated with kidney dysfunction.[15] However, the *CYP3A5*1* allele was associated with nephrotoxicity in recipients of kidney allografts.[18] Kidney transplant recipients receiving tacrolimus who exhibited *CYP3A4*1/CYP3A5*1* or *CYP3A4*1B/CYP3A5*1* haplotypes had a higher risk of biopsy-proven nephrotoxicity versus those who exhibited the *CYP3A4*1/CYP3A5*3* haplotype (for *CYP3A4*1*; A-392G, rs2740574).[17] Liver transplant patients with variants in *ABCB1* (G2677T, C3435T, and C1236T) had a higher incidence of kidney dysfunction due to tacrolimus.[20] Hebert et al. supported these findings, reporting an increased frequency of kidney dysfunction in liver transplants patients receiving calcineurin inhibitors who had the *ABCB1* 2677TT genotype.[21] While kidney transplant donor *ABCB1* 3435TT genotype was also found to be a risk factor for cyclosporine nephrotoxicity,[19] *ABCB1* genotype has not been linked with nephrotoxicity in heart transplant patients receiving cyclosporine.[22]

The existing studies also suggest that numerous nongenetic factors (transplant type, donor vs. recipient organ of metabolism vs. toxicity, administered drug, etc.) may account for the variable influences of *CYP3A5* and *ABCB1* genotypes on nephrotoxicity due to calcineurin inhibitors. In addition to DMD genes, polymorphisms in several other genes have been associated with calcineurin inhibitor nephrotoxicity.[23–27]

Cisplatin

Cisplatin is used in the treatment of various cancers of solid organs including head/neck, lung, and cervix. Representative oncology regimens commonly include cisplatin administration every 14–28 days. Nephrotoxicity is common, with damage to the kidney tubules occurring in 30–38% of patients after a single dose of cisplatin.[28–30] Several preclinical studies suggest altered expression of OCT1/2, MRP2, and MATE1/2 transporters.[31–33] *SLC22A2* encodes the OAT2 protein, which is an uptake transporter of cisplatin located on the basolateral membrane of kidney proximal tubule cells. The G808T polymorphism (rs316019) in *SLC22A2* is associated with reduced toxicity to the kidneys.[32] These data suggest the role of genetic polymorphisms in drug transporter genes in modulating cisplatin nephrotoxicity.

Cisplatin is metabolized by several intracellular glutathione *S*-transferases (GSTs) to glutathione derivatives. Variants in *GSTA1* C-69T (rs3957356) and *GSTP1* A313G (rs1695) are associated with survival of cervical cancer patients[34] and *GSTP1* A313G and *ABCC2* C-24T correlate with enhanced efficacy in patients with non-small cell lung cancer[35,36] receiving cisplatin therapy. While these former GST polymorphisms have not been associated directly with cisplatin nephrotoxicity, it is plausible given that cellular toxicity from drugs often occurs in treatments that result in enhanced efficacy.

Genes involved in immunology, inflammation, and apoptosis have also been implicated in cisplatin nephrotoxicity. A genetic study in humans sought to evaluate SNPs that had demonstrated an enhanced susceptibility of cells to cisplatin.[37] These evaluations reported genetic variants in cell recognition and adhesion (*CDH13*), metal-ion binding (*ZNF659*), transcription factor activity (*LRRC3B*, *PITX2*), and RNA binding (*LARP2*) with cisplatin sensitivity.[37] While the available genomic studies suggest a link between polymorphisms in DMD and non-DMD genes and nephrotoxicity, prospective studies conducted in humans receiving cisplatin therapy are needed to more fully evaluate which polymorphisms are risk factors for the occurrence of clinical and subclinical nephrotoxicity.

ALBUMINURIA AND END-STAGE KIDNEY DISEASE

The National Kidney Foundation guidelines (K/DOQI) define the staging of CKD based on the presence of functional and/or structural abnormalities in the kidney.[38] While functional variations are based on clearance represented by calculations employing serum creatinine,[39,40] structural abnormalities are represented by the concentrations or amounts of urinary proteins, especially albumin, that are excreted into the urine.[38] Albumin excretion has also been proposed as a biomarker for AKI.[41] While albumin loss in the urine has classically been viewed as a marker for a problem in the filtration barrier at the level of the glomerulus, modern views also recognize the relevance of the proximal tubule and its protein reabsorptive function in proposing the use of albumin as a marker of tubule function as well. Proteinuria is viewed as a prognostic variable for the progression of kidney disease,[42] a predictor of cardiovascular disease,[43] and a predictor for all-cause mortality.[44] Several studies have linked inflammation to albuminuria.[45-47] Research related to genes that may be involved in the appearance of albuminuria has primarily focused on inflammation pathways, cubilin (*CUBN*), and nonmuscle myosin heavy chain 9 (*MYH9*). Other studies have been conducted to evaluate the role of polymorphisms within the genes of the renin–angiotensin–aldosterone system (RAAS) or in DMD pathways, for prediction of responsiveness to therapies employing ACEIs or ARBs in the reduction of urinary albumin (and protein) excretion.

A recent publication has focused on the contribution of polymorphisms in inflammatory response genes to albuminuria.[48] DNA was collected from 5,321 participants in the Third National Health and Nutrition Examination Survey (NHANES III). The associations between urinary albumin excretion and genetic variants were analyzed. The full models fit to the data incorporated adjustments for age, sex, alcohol consumption, educational attainments, and waist to hip ratio. Genetic variants that were important in predicting urinary albumin excretion were different according to race, defined as non-Hispanic whites, non-Hispanic blacks, and Mexican Americans. In non-Hispanic whites, full models demonstrated that variants in immunoglobulin Fc receptor (*FCGR2A* His166Arg; His167Arg, rs1801274), fibrinogen (*FBG* A-462G, rs1800790), mannose-binding lectin 2 (*MBL2* G-618C; G-550C, rs11003125), nitric oxide synthase (*NOS2A* T-2892C; T-1173C, rs9282799), tumor necrosis factor (*TNF* A-555G, rs1800750 and A-417G; A-238G, rs361525), and glucokinase regulator (*GCKR* Pro446Leu, rs1260326) genes resulted in threshold *P*-values <.05. In non-Hispanic blacks, threshold *P*-values were shown in models for variants in c-reactive protein (*CRP* 3'UTR A/G, rs1205; downstream G/A, rs2808630; promoter T/A, rs3093058), thrombin (*F2* upstream A/G, rs1799963), vitamin D receptor (*VDR*, Ile352Ile, rs731236), and transforming growth factor beta-1 (*TGFB1* A-800G, rs1800468) genes. Lastly, for Mexican Americans, variants in *NOS2A* (promoter C/G, rs1800482), *NOS3* (Asp298Glu, rs1799983; and C-786T, rs2070744), *CRP* (upstream G/A, rs11265260; downstream A/C, rs3093075), interleukin 1-beta (*IL1B* C-2022G, rs1143623), and *TNF* (A-487G; A-308G, rs1800629) genes resulted in models demonstrating *P*-values <.05. Further evaluations are needed to discern the potential mechanistic roles for the identified genes in contributing to an albuminuria phenotype. These results suggest that protein products of targeted genes involved in the inflammation process contribute to albuminuria through various physiological processes.

Cubilin

A missense variant (I2984V, rs1801239) of the *CUBN* gene, representing the protein cubilin, has recently been identified as a gene locus for albuminuria.[49] This finding is interesting given the role of cubulin and megalin in the proximal tubule endocytosis processes of numerous proteins. Mechanistically, deficiency in functional cubulin would reduce the reabsorption of albumin from the urine ultrafiltrate through the usual interactions of cubilin with megalin and albumin.[50] Supportive animal models have shown a 6-fold increase in albuminuria in cubulin genetic deletion models.[51] The missense variant of interest is in a location that is important for the megalin–cubilin interaction.[52] The findings in the recent genetics study demonstrating association between the *CUBN* variant (rs1801239) and urinary albumin excretion were present in both African Americans and patients of European ancestry.[53] Each variant copy was associated with a ~42% increased risk for microalbuminuria at long-term follow-up.[53] However, the *CUBN* variant explains only 0.06–0.15% of the total variance in urinary albumin excretion. A recently published editorial suggests more extensive sequencing of the *CUBN* gene to evaluate for rarer variants that have larger effects.[54] The implications of variants in *CUBN* on urinary elimination of drugs that are highly bound to albumin are currently unknown.

Nonmuscle Myosin Heavy Chain

The nonmuscle myosin protein is expressed in the podocytes of the glomerulus. Other key proteins including nephrin, CD2AP, podocin, and alpha-actinin 4 are also expressed within the podocytes and their genetic variants are being evaluated in various forms of glomerulonephritis (described later in this chapter). Podocytes are outcroppings from the glomerular epithelial membrane that form the so-called foot processes visualized on microscopy. Podocytes help to form the glomerular slit pores that are important for sieving, for example, large molecules are retained in the blood and small molecules are passed into the glomerular filtrate to the proximal tubule. Additionally, podocytes are involved in regulation of the glomerular filtration rate (GFR) through their ability to contract. Several investigators have found associations between polymorphisms in the *MYH9* gene (encoding nonmuscle myosin heavy chain) and kidney disease in African Americans.[55-58] More specifically, associations were found with albuminuria in hypertensives[56] and idiopathic and HIV-associated focal glomerulosclerosis[57] and with end-stage renal disease (ESRD) in hypertensives.[55,58] The investigators found an odds ratio of 4–5 for focal segmental glomerulosclerosis (FSGS) and HIV nephropathy and 1.5–3.4 for hypertensive ESRD in patients with *MYH9* variants.[55,57] Variants in *MYH9* associated with nephropathy include rs4821480 (T36695247G), rs2032487 (T36695428C), rs4821481 (T36695942C), and rs3752462 (C36710183T). The GCCT haplotype, derived from the SNPs consecutively listed in the previous sentence, is recognized as the "at-risk" haplotype for nephropathy.[57] While the association of *MYH9* variants with numerous human kidney diseases is promising research, there is still some concern by scientists given that deletion of the *MYH9* gene in mice has not been found to elevate the risk of CKDs, with the exception of nephropathy induced by Adriamycin.[59]

Renin–Angiotensin–Aldosterone System

Medications aimed at the angiotensin pathway, for example, ACEIs and/or ARBs, have been the cornerstone of treatment for the primary and secondary prevention of CKD, especially in diabetic patients. These therapies have shown positive results in preventing and reducing albumin excretion, slowing kidney disease progression, and reducing the risk for doubling of serum creatinine concentrations and/or requiring dialysis or transplantation. Three decades ago, it was reported that the insertion/deletion (I/D) polymorphism in the angiotensin-converting enzyme (*ACE*) gene explained ~50% of the variability in ACE levels.[60] This variant is located in intron 16 and is defined by a 250 base pair fragment (rs1799782). Since this initial report, numerous studies have sought to evaluate the influence of the I/D polymorphism on the responses to ACE inhibitors, with findings that have been variable from study to study. A meta-analysis published in 2005 reviewed the response data from 11 studies employing ACEIs.[61] While four of the studies evaluated outcomes of one or more kidney-related clinical parameters (proteinuria, serum creatinine, GFR, ESRD), two of them provided the majority of included data.[62,63] The study by Perna et al. included 212 nondiabetic, proteinuric, Caucasians who received ramipril versus placebo and were categorized as ACE D/D, D/I, and I/I.[63] Reductions in proteinuria, GFR, and albumin excretion rate at 30 months were reported. The outcomes favored the D/D genotype, with D/I genotypes demonstrating a response that was between the D/D and I/I genotypes. The overall effect showed a mean ± SD of 0.33 ± 1.2 g per day reduction in proteinuria and 0.08 ± 0.63 mL/min per month increase in GFR. There was also a 0.65 risk reduction in ESRD that favored the D/D genotype.[63] Penno et al. evaluated proteinuria in 530 Caucasian diabetics with normoalbuminuria or microalbuminuria who received lisinopril.[62] The study outcome favored the I/I genotype, with a 7.33 µg/min reduction in albumin excretion rate.[62] A previous genetic study from 1,365 Caucasian patients from the DCCT and EDIC studies showed that patients with the I/I genotype had a lower risk for persistent microalbuminuria and severe nephropathy.[64] More recent studies in Asians reported a benefit of the ACE I/I genotype, lower risk of kidney disease progression from diabetes,[65] more decreases in proteinuria and amelioration of kidney function loss with ARB treatment,[66] and reduced risk of nephropathy from type II diabetes.[67] Two other studies fail to support any association between ACE I/D polymorphism and susceptibility to immunoglobulin A (IgA) nephropathy or autosomal dominant polycystic kidney disease (ADPKD).[68,69] The results from the existing studies suggest race- and disease-related differences in kidney outcomes according to ACE I/D genotypes, suggesting the interplay between genetic and nongenetic factors. There is currently no consensus regarding ACEI therapy or dose selection based on the ACE I/D polymorphism in terms of nephropathy reduction.

There have been investigations into the role of polymorphisms in angiotensinogen (*AGT* M235T, rs699), angiotensin II receptor type I (*AGTR1* A1166C, rs5186), angiotensin II receptor type II (*AGTR2* A1818T, rs5978731), and aldosterone synthase (*CYP11B2* C-344T, rs1799998) and kidney diseases and/or response to treatments employing ARBs. Type I diabetics with the *AGT* T/T genotype (at base position 235) had a 4-fold increased risk for microalbuminuria as compared with M/M and M/T genotypes.[70] A study of nearly 900 Mexican Americans reported an association between the *AGT* T/T genotype and reductions in GFR.[71] In 239 Asian diabetic patients with proteinuria receiving valsartan, the *AGTR1* A1166C homozygous wild-type genotype was associated with a 46% reduction in proteinuria from baseline as opposed to an 11% reduction in patients with the C/C genotype.[72] The *AGTR2* A1818T genetic variant has been associated with the progression of IgA nephropathy in Koreans.[73] A study in Caucasian hypertensive patients reported a possible interaction of the *CYP2B11* C/C genotype with the *AGT* T/T, *AGTR1* A/C, and *ACE* D/D genotypes for the development of kidney insufficiency.[74] These data show that polymorphisms in genes within the RAAS pathway other than *ACE* are being investigated for their potential role in kidney disease, as well as in explaining response to therapies employing ACEIs or ARBs. Evolving data may enable more individualized selection of therapeutic agents in patient with urinary protein excretion.

CYP2C9 Polymorphisms and Losartan Response

Polymorphisms in the cytochrome P450 *2C9* gene have been explored for relationships to blood pressure lowering and influence on proteinuria reduction in patients receiving the ARB, losartan. Losartan is a therapeutically active drug that is further metabolized to E3174, an active metabolite. Reductions in metabolic activity of CYP2C9 would be predicted to reduce the overall pharmacodynamic responses secondary to shunting of metabolism to inactive moieties via other metabolism routes. Thus, while all patients would be exposed to the parent drug, exposure to E3174 would be greatest in patients without alterations resulting in the decreased activity of CYP2C9. *CYP2C9* *2 (Arg144Cys, rs1799853) and *CYP2C9* *3 (Ile359Leu, rs1057910) variants result in a reduced CYP2C9 activity phenotype in patients. However, since the variants are rare in African American patients and more common in Caucasians, their influence would be relevant to blood pressure (systolic and diastolic) and proteinuric responses in the latter group. The influence of *CYP2C9* genotype on losartan pharmacodynamic responses was recently evaluated in Caucasian patients with primary and secondary kidney diseases.[75] Patients with primary kidney diseases who carried variant alleles had less favorable antiproteinuric responses (31% vs. 125% reductions, respectively). Patients with secondary kidney diseases who carried variant alleles had less favorable reductions in diastolic and systolic blood pressures.[75] Lajer et al. evaluated blood pressure responses according to *CYP2C9* genotype in Caucasian type I diabetic nephropathy patients receiving losartan.[76] Diabetic nephropathy would be considered as an etiology for secondary kidney disease. A significant reduction in systolic blood pressure in the non-*3 carriers versus *3 carriers was noted. No differences in diastolic blood pressure or urinary albumin excretion were noted.[76] These two studies suggest reduced pharmacodynamic responses to losartan in Caucasian patients with nephropathy. Since these former studies were of only 4–6 months in duration, the long-term outcomes to losartan therapy based on *CYP2C9* genotype are unknown.

GLOMERULONEPHRITIS

Glomerulonephritis is the third leading cause of CKD in the United States and is ranked as the second leading cause in most Asian populations.[1] Numerous diseases are represented under the category of glomerulonephritis and these include membranous nephropathy, IgA nephropathy, systemic lupus erythematosus (SLE) nephritis, FSGS, and the systemic vasculitides with kidney manifestations. Most experts suggest an immune component and/or a genetic basis for glomerulonephritis. Therapy for these disorders is focused on systemic approaches including glucocorticoids, cytotoxic drugs, antimetabolites, and immunosuppressives. The diseases themselves are associated with chronic relapses and remissions and responses to therapies are often inconsistent between patients and have inadequate outcomes. Due to the progressive nature of these diseases and the lack of consistent therapeutic responses, there is extensive interest within the nephrology community in discerning the role of genes and/or genetic variants that are important as risk factors for glomerulonephritis. Additionally, there is great interest in determining what factors predict initial and subsequent responses to treatments, and what tools may be helpful in determining appropriate therapeutic regimens of prescribed medications.

Phospholipase A$_2$ Receptor

The elusive target antigen in the pathophysiology of human membranous nephropathy has been the focus of numerous research efforts, after the identification of megalin-bound antibodies in the glomerular podocytes of rats.[77,78] A landmark study published in 2009 reported the identification of the M-type phospholipase A$_2$ receptor (PLA$_2$R) in human glomerular extract samples.[79] Additionally, PLA$_2$R was expressed in podocytes and colocalized with IgG in immune deposits. Two genetic variants in the carbohydrate recognition domains (CRD) of *PLA$_2$R* (C1110G, rs35771982; and G3528A, rs3828323) have been evaluated for their role in susceptibility to membranous nephropathy.[80] This CRD is the location where PLA2 binds to PLA$_2$R. The C/C variants in rs35771982 were reported to have a higher susceptibility to idiopathic membranous nephropathy as compared with other genotypes.[80] Variants in *NPHS1* and *TNFα* have also been explored in susceptibility to or progression of membranous nephropathy.[81,82]

Nephrin and Podocin

Nephrin is a transmembrane protein that is localized to the slit diaphragm of the glomerulus, in the area between the podocyte foot processes. In addition to being involved in the slit pore, nephrin is also involved in signaling processes that are integral for podocyte function.[83] Nephrin is encoded by the *NPHS1* gene. Podocin is expressed on the podocyte, involved in signaling and scaffolding, and is encoded by the *NPHS2* gene.[84] Genetic variants in *NPHS1* and *NPHS2* have been associated with congenital nephropathy of the Finnish type, membranous nephropathy, minimal change disease, IgA nephropathy, and FSGS.[81,85–88] The Finnish variant is represented by a frameshift deletion of two base pairs in exon 2 (nt121delCT) of *NPHS1* resulting in a stop codon, for example, the major variant, and a nonsense mutation in exon 26 (R1109X), for example, the minor variant.[85] A study by Franceschini et al. suggested that the Arg229Glu variant of *NPHS2* is associated with a 20–40% risk of FSGS in the European population.[87] A greater frequency of membranous nephropathy was noted in Asian patients with *NPHS2* variant Val763Val (rs437168).[87]

IgG Fc Receptors (FcγR)

Nephritis secondary to SLE is hypothesized to result from deposition of immune complexes in the kidney. The reasons for deposition of these complexes are many, and include a reduction in clearance of the immune complexes. Since complement and IgG Fc receptors (FcγR) are key players in these processes, numerous investigations have explored associations between SLE nephritis susceptibility and polymorphisms in the genes encoding FcγR and complement components. Fcγ receptors are denoted as FcγR1, FcγRII, and FcγRIII, with the first receptor having high affinity for IgG and the latter two having low affinity.[89] Numerous variants in Fcγ receptors have been reported to be associated with various forms of glomerulonephritis, including SLE nephritis and IgA nephropathy.[90–96] A recent meta-analysis reported an elevated likelihood of SLE nephritis in Europeans and Asians with the presence of the *FcγRIIIa* Val158Phe variant (odds ratio of 1.15).[97] Furthermore, patients who were homozygous (F/F) for the variant had an even higher likelihood for nephritis (odds ratio of 1.30). Another recent meta-analysis evaluated the association of *FcγR IIIb* NA1 versus *FcγR IIIb* NA2 on susceptibility to SLE nephritis.[98] Although previous research demonstrated that homozygous NA1 was more efficient for binding certain IgG immune complexes than NA2,[99] genotypes comprising *FcγR IIIb* NA2 were not found to be associated with SLE nephritis.[98] Variants in the *FcγR IIa* and *FcγR IIb* are associated with SLE nephritis. For *FcγR IIa*, homozygosity for the Arg131 versus His131 allele was significantly associated with SLE nephritis in both Caucasians and Asians.[100] Additionally, it appears to be a risk allele in proliferative forms of glomerulonephritis.[101] For *FcγR IIb*, a meta-analysis reported that it only confers susceptibility in Asian patients who have SLE without nephritis.[102] Multiple polymorphisms in the C1q gene (*C1QA*) and associations with SLE nephritis were recently reported in the African American population. These polymorphisms may be related to the reduced serum complement titers commonly encountered in SLE patients in clinical practice.[103]

Rituximab is a monoclonal anti-CD20 antibody that is currently being evaluated as a treatment option in various forms of glomerulonephritis. As CD20 is a B cell marker, rituximab targets the CD20 to enhance contact of B cells with cells such as macrophages in order to reduce the B cell population. The *FcγRIIIa* has a gene dimorphism at amino acid location 158. The receptor's affinity to IgG is higher with valine as opposed to phenylalanine in this amino acid location. One study supports requirements for a 10-fold increase in serum rituximab concentrations in patients with the presence of phenylalanine instead of valine[104] in order to achieve a similar degree of B cell depletion. A genetic variant at location 176 (low-affinity allele) showed greater B cell depletion than the wild-type allele.[105] Further studies will be needed to appropriately understand and model the impact of pharmacogenomics on rituximab pharmacodynamics in patients with glomerulonephritis.

Nuclear Factor-Like 2 (NRF2)

NRF2 is a transcription factor that regulates genes through the antioxidant response element (ARE). It is also known to regulate numerous genes involved in drug metabolism. Given the hypothesis that exposures to environmental chemicals and drugs are risk factors for SLE, polymorphisms in *NRF2* could be important in regulating exposure to drugs and environmental compounds. Promoter variants in genes that are regulated by NRF2 may have their interactions with NRF2 altered, which could have implications for the disposition of compounds that are substrates for the proteins of these pathways, for example, phase II metabolism pathways.[106] Further study of these interactions will be required, especially since an NRF2 activator is currently in phase III clinical trials for the treatment of diabetic nephropathy.[107] *NRF2* has also been suggested as a gene candidate for susceptibility to SLE in European Americans.[108] A recent publication reported the association between a novel *NRF2* variant G-653A and childhood-onset SLE nephritis.[109]

Cytochrome P450S

Cyclophosphamide is a major component in the induction treatment repertoire of patients with glomerulonephritis, especially those with SLE nephritis and systemic vasculitis. It is a prodrug that requires activation to its metabolite 4-hydroxycyclophosphamide via several CYP450 enzymes including CYP2B6, CYP3A4/5, and CYP2C9. Two publications have sought to describe the influence of polymorphisms in CYP450 genes and toxicity and clinical response in patients with SLE nephritis.[110,111] The initial publication genotyped SLE nephritis patients ($n = 62$) from an NIH cohort for common variants in *CYP2B6*, *CYP2C19*, *CYP2C9*, and *CYP3A4/5*. Results showed that patients who carried the *CYP2C19 *2* allele (I331V) had a lower risk of premature ovarian failure, a common complication

of cyclophosphamide therapy.[110] Regarding kidney function, homozygotes for the *CYP2B6 *5* (R487C) or *CYP2C19 *2* (I331V) variants had a higher probability of ESRD, doubling serum creatinine, and a lower probability of achieving a complete renal response.[110] Another study ($n = 237$) of SLE nephritis patients was conducted to explore the kidney-related findings from the original NIH cohort report.[111] However, data on treatment-related kidney outcomes were available for only 36 patients who received cyclophosphamide (in the oral form). It is unclear why only a small number of patients were included in the cohort. The findings from this recent study do not suggest an association between *CYP2B6 *5* or *CYP2C19 *2* variant alleles and cyclophosphamide treatment outcomes in SLE nephritis.[111] The differences in patient races between cohorts could account for at least a portion of the variable findings, with the most recent study including a higher percentage of African American patients (44% vs. 24%). A recently completed study by our own group may provide additional information regarding the link between genetic polymorphisms in CYP2B6, 3A4/5, and CYP2C9 and cyclophosphamide pharmacokinetics and outcomes.

Uridine Diphosphate Glucuronosyltransferases (UGTS)

In addition to its use as a common immunosuppressive agent for kidney transplant recipients, mycophenolate is frequently used in the maintenance regimen of patients with various forms of glomerulonephritis. Mycophenolate is sometimes used as an induction agent in the therapy of glomerulonephritis. It undergoes conversion to mycophenolic acid, the active immunosuppressive moiety. Mycophenolic acid is subsequently metabolized to an inactive glucuronide by numerous UGT isoforms including UGT2B7, UGT1A7, and UGT1A9. There are several publications describing polymorphisms in UGTs on mycophenolic disposition in the transplant population and this is covered in *Chapter 15*. This section focuses on the data from the glomerulonephritis population. One recent manuscript evaluated the effects of genetic polymorphisms in *UGT2B7* and *UGT1A7* on the pharmacokinetics of mycophenolic acid in patients with glomerulonephritis secondary to SLE nephritis and small vessel vasculitis.[112] Increased apparent oral clearance of mycophenolic acid was demonstrated in patients with heterozygosity in the *UGT2B7* C802T and separately in the *UGT1A7* T622C variants. Decreased trough concentrations of mycophenolic acid were also shown in the patients with heterozygosity in *UGT1A7* T622C. Since so few patients exhibited homozygosity for either the *UGT2B7* or *UGT1A7* alleles that were evaluated, a significant difference was notable only between the patients who were heterozygotes and those who were homozygous wild types. Further work is required to discern the effects of other common *UGT* variants in glomerulonephritis patients receiving mycophenolate therapy. Additionally, the role of UGT variants on treatment-related outcomes to mycophenolate requires further study.

DIABETIC NEPHROPATHY

Diabetes mellitus is the leading cause of CKD in the United States and abroad.[1] In fact, approximately 44% of ESRD cases are the result of diabetes mellitus.[1] Much research is focused on understanding the molecular pathways that contribute to kidney complications of diabetes mellitus and on treatments that may prevent or slow kidney disease progression. Numerous investigations have and continue to be conducted to ascertain the role of genes and their variants that contribute to diabetes mellitus and more specifically to diabetic nephropathy. Polymorphisms in genes within the RAAS and their contribution to diabetic nephropathy and efficacy of ACEI and ARB treatments have been previously described in the section "Albuminuria and End-Stage Kidney Disease." Most recently, the glucose transporters GLUT1/2 and SGLT1/2 have attracted considerable attention as potential targets for therapies aimed at managing exposure of the kidney to glucose in diabetes mellitus. Another area of therapeutic research involves determination of genetic variants that alter pharmacokinetics and pharmacodynamics of therapies that are primarily aimed at reducing blood glucose levels and secondarily to minimizing the complications (including nephropathy) of diabetes mellitus.

Glucose Transporters

The glucose transporters in the kidney have attracted considerable attention due to their role in controlling the exposure of the kidney tubules to glucose. The SGLT1 and SGLT2 transporters are located on the apical membrane of proximal tubule cells and, coupled with sodium, are responsible for active reabsorption of 90% and 10%, respectively, of the glucose that is filtered through the glomerulus. The GLUT1 and GLUT2 transporters are located on the basolateral membrane of proximal tubule cells and through facilitated diffusion release glucose from the proximal tubule cell to the interstitium. GLUT1 is also found on other kidney cells including glomerular mesangial cells and podocytes and enables diffusion of glucose into these cell types. Alterations in GLUT1 could have direct relevance to glomerular pathology related to diabetes mellitus, as well as downstream effects at the level of the proximal tubule.

While several variants in the gene encoding SGLT2 (*SLC5A2*) have been reported in patients with renal glucosuria and aminoaciduria, the contributions of these or other variants have not yet been reported in association with diabetic nephropathy.[113–115] The *SLC5A1* gene has been evaluated to an even lesser degree than *SLC5A2*. Since the SGLT2 protein is being explored as a therapeutic target, future research will be required to elucidate the role of genetic polymorphisms on the dosing of these drugs and outcomes to such treatments.

Genetic variants in the *GLUT1* gene have been more extensively evaluated using DNA from the Atherosclerosis Risk in Communities (ARIC) study.[116] It is worthwhile to note that the contribution of a specific variant to a disease process needs to employ consideration of the location of the transporter in relation to the disease process. The GLUT1 protein facilitates *uptake*

into glomerular structures and *efflux from* the proximal tubule. Polymorphisms that increase activity of GLUT1 would actually enhance glucose uptake to the glomerular structure, but reduce exposure of the proximal tubule to glucose. African Americans and European Americans with urinary albumin excretion from the ARIC study were evaluated in reference to six polymorphisms in *GLUT1*.[116] The analyses were stratified by race and type II diabetes status.[116] The *Enh2* polymorphism (C21793T, rs841847) was associated with albuminuria (odds ratio of 2.14) in diabetic European Americans. Additionally, the polymorphism was associated with macroalbuminuria (odds ratio 2.69) in the same population. An interesting finding from this study was the association of the *Enh2* polymorphism with macroalbuminuria in nondiabetic European Americans with high fasting insulin (odds ratio 1.84).[116] While the study by Hsu et al. did not implicate the *XbaI* polymorphism (C23063A, rs841853) in type II diabetes, previous studies have reported both the *XbaI* and *Enh2* polymorphisms with albuminuria.[117–121] Previous research in type I diabetes suggests some association of *XbaI* and *Enh2* with albuminuria.[117]

Other Genes in Diabetic Nephropathy

Several additional genes have been reported to be associated with the diagnosis of diabetic nephropathy. Most interesting are the associations between DMD or drug mechanism of action pathway genes and diabetic nephropathy. One such DMD gene is *SLC22A* that encodes for the organic cation transporters (OCTs). OCT2 is an uptake transporter on the basolateral membrane of proximal tubule cells in the kidney. Variants in *SLC22A1*, *SLC22A2*, and *SLC22A3* are all associated with nephropathy in patients with type I diabetes.[122] A recent publication evaluated several polymorphisms in the *SLC22A1*, *SLC22A2*, and *SLC22A3* genes and their association with diabetic nephropathy in an initial and follow-up cohort, based on the previous published findings.[123] Although there were positive associations with *SLC22A2* and *SLC22A3* polymorphisms from the initial cohort, the authors were not able to replicate the findings in the second cohort of patients.[123] The biguanide antidiabetic agent metformin is a known substrate for renal OCT2 and is now considered first-line therapy for type II diabetes mellitus. Although a variant allele at *SLC22A2* Ala270Ser (rs316019) reduces metformin renal clearance, clinical outcomes related to this polymorphism have not been reported.[124] While this evolving area of research requires much additional study, having polymorphisms in DMD genes could predispose patients to nephropathy, alter efficacy of therapies, and/or alter toxicity to therapies that are prescribed to control diabetes mellitus.

Peroxisome proliferator-activated receptor gamma (PPARγ) is a target for the thiazolidinedione class of antidiabetic compounds, for example, rosiglitazone and pioglitazone. Several publications report on the benefits of PPARγ agonists in the treatment of nephropathy.[125–128] Genetic polymorphisms in *PPARγ* have been reported to result in differential responses to troglitazone and to pioglitazone.[129,130] Interestingly, the *PPARγ*

Pro12Ala polymorphism (rs1801282) has been associated with both response to pioglitazone[130] and new-onset microalbuminuria in type II diabetic patients prescribed ACEI therapy.[131] Alanine carriers were found to have lower albuminuria and better response to pioglitazone than proline homozygotes. It is provocative that selection of patients for therapeutic benefits in terms of diabetic nephropathy may need to consider the *PPARγ* genotype. Since *CYP450* genes are implicated in the metabolism of PPARγ agonists, polymorphisms in these genes may alter disposition as well as benefits to the kidney with these treatments.

Numerous other genes have been suggested to be associated with risk for diabetic nephropathy. For nephropathy due to type I diabetes, the *VDR*, receptor for advanced glycation end products (*RAGE*), matrix metalloproteinase (*MMP*), bone morphogenic protein (*BMP*), and *NOS3* genes and their variants have been reported. For nephropathy due to type II diabetes, the engulfment and cell motility protein 1 (*ELMO1*), adiponectin (*ADIPOQ*), vascular endothelial growth factor (*VEGF*), *VDR*, acetyl-CoA carboxylase beta (*ACACB*), methylenetetrahydrofolate reductase (*MTHFR*), and proteasome (*PSMD9*) genes and their variants have been reported. Several recent genome-wide association studies (GWAS) with or without meta-analysis have also been conducted in patients with diabetic nephropathy.[132–134] The ribosomal protein S12 (*RPS12*), LIM kinase 2 (*LIMK2*), and *SFI1* genes are associated with diabetic nephropathy in African American patients.[132] Genomic regions surrounding the cysteinyl-tRNA synthetase (*CARS*), myosin 16 (*MYO16*), and insulin receptor substrate 2 (*IRS2*) genes are associated with diabetic kidney disease in Caucasians.[134] A random-effects meta-analysis recently reported variants near the *ACE*, aldo-keto reductase family 1, member B1 (*AKR1B1*), apolipoprotein C1 (*APOC1*), apolipoprotein E (*APOE*), erythropoietin (*EPO*), *NOS3*, *heparan sulfate proteoglycan 2* (*HSPG2*), *VEGFA*, FERM domain containing 3 (*FRMD3*), *CARS*, *UNC13B*, carboxypeptidase, vitellogenic-like (*CPVL*), chimerin (chimaerin) 2 (*CHN2*), and gremlin 1 (*GREM1*) genes that were associated with diabetic nephropathy.[133]

OTHER KIDNEY DISEASES WITH GENETIC COMPONENTS

The remainder of this chapter will describe four other kidney diseases that are considered to have a genetic basis. Polycystic kidney disease is characterized by cyst formation in the kidneys and includes ADPKD and autosomal recessive polycystic kidney disease (ARPKD). For ADPKD, cystic lesions can also occur in the liver, pancreas, and lung, and brain aneurysms are common. Autosomal dominant genetic mutations occur in *PKD1* and *PKD2* and these genetic mutations affect the function of the polycystin 1 and polycystin 2 proteins.[135] For ARPKD, the defects are usually present at birth and include oligohydramnios, portal hypertension, and CKD. Autosomal recessive genetic mutations occur in *PKD1*, encoding the protein fibrocystin.[135] The treatments for both disorders include arginine vasopressin V2 receptor antagonists. The implication of polymorphisms in the receptor and response to treatment is an area for investigation.

Bartter syndrome and Gitelman syndrome are autosomal recessive disorders that result from abnormalities in the sodium chloride transporters. Bartter syndrome results in abnormalities in the reabsorption of sodium chloride in the loop of Henle. The transporters that are involved include the Na-2Cl-K cotransporter (NKCC2), renal outer medullary potassium channel (ROMK), and a protein (barttin) in two chloride channels, for example, ClC-Kb and ClC-Ka.[136] The genes implicated include *SLC12A1* (encodes the NKCC2 transporter), *ROMK1*, chloride channel Kb (*CLCNKB*), and *BSDN* (encodes barttin). Gitelman syndrome is an autosomal recessive disorder that results in a reduction in the ability to reabsorb sodium chloride in the distal tubule. Defects in the gene (*SLC12A3*) encoding the sodium chloride cotransporter NCCT are implicated in Gitelman syndrome.[136]

SUMMARY

Patients with kidney diseases are some of the more difficult patients to manage due to abnormalities in numerous clinical laboratories and polypharmacy. In addition to considering many of the laboratory abnormalities in dosing of medications, clinicians will also need to be aware of genetic polymorphisms that may influence how a patient responds to therapies. The application of genomics to the field of nephrology is clearly an emerging area that is ripe for basic and clinical research. Many genetic variants recognized in the susceptibility to kidney diseases are also important in the metabolism and disposition of numerous classes of pharmaceuticals. Clinicians will certainly want to familiarize themselves with the current status of genomics and the kidney, as well as keep abreast of evolving research in this area that may impact patient care.

Case 1

As a clinical pharmacologist who is now responsible for consultation with the renal service, you want to evaluate susceptibility to nephrotoxicity due to calcineurin inhibitors. With an understanding of the pathophysiology of CKD, *what clinical and demographic variables do you plan to assess?*

Based on a literature review of genetic variants in DMD genes and susceptibility to nephrotoxicity secondary to calcineurin inhibitors, *which genetic variants do you plan to evaluate?*

You have a thorough understanding of the mechanism of action of calcineurin inhibitors and their drug metabolism and transport characteristics. *Recommend some other potential genetic targets that you might want to explore for risks of nephrotoxicity.*

Case 2

A Caucasian patient newly evaluated in the kidney clinic has a 12-year history of diabetes mellitus (type II) and a recent diagnosis of FSGS. The patient has a GFR of 70 mL/min and is excreting 4 g per day of proteins in the urine. *You are asked to recommend a treatment strategy to reduce the urinary protein excretion and slow kidney disease progression due to diabetes and FSGS.*

A fellow on the renal service asks you to *review the current state of affairs pertaining to genetic variants that may be risk factors for CKD disease due to diabetes mellitus and FSGS.*

The attending nephrologist later asks you to *comment on genetic polymorphisms relevant to responses to losartan therapy.*

REFERENCES

1. USRDS. Atlas of chronic kidney disease and end-stage renal disease in the United States. In: *Diseases of the Kidney.* Bethesda, MD: NIH, NIDDK; 2010 [report].

2. Schetz M, Dasta J, Goldstein S, Golper T. Drug-induced acute kidney injury. *Curr Opin Crit Care.* 2005;11(6):555–565.

3. Taber SS, Mueller BA. Drug-associated renal dysfunction. *Crit Care Clin.* 2006;22(2):357–374, viii.

4. Nankivell BJ, Borrows RJ, Fung CL, et al. The natural history of chronic allograft nephropathy. *N Engl J Med.* 2003;349(24):2326–2333.

5. Nizze H, Mihatsch MJ, Zollinger HU, et al. Cyclosporine-associated nephropathy in patients with heart and bone marrow transplants. *Clin Nephrol.* 1988;30(5):248–260.

6. Zietse R, Balk AH, vd Dorpel MA, et al. Time course of the decline in renal function in cyclosporine-treated heart transplant recipients. *Am J Nephrol.* 1994;14(1):1–5.

7. Macphee IA, Fredericks S, Tai T, et al. Tacrolimus pharmacogenetics: polymorphisms associated with expression of cytochrome p4503A5 and P-glycoprotein correlate with dose requirement. *Transplantation.* 2002;74(11):1486–1489.

8. Hesselink DA, van Schaik RH, van der Heiden IP, et al. Genetic polymorphisms of the CYP3A4, CYP3A5, and MDR-1 genes and pharmacokinetics of the calcineurin inhibitors cyclosporine and tacrolimus. *Clin Pharmacol Ther.* 2003;74(3):245–254.

9. Tsuchiya N, Satoh S, Tada H, et al. Influence of CYP3A5 and MDR1 (ABCB1) polymorphisms on the pharmacokinetics of tacrolimus in renal transplant recipients. *Transplantation.* 2004;78(8):1182–1187.

10. Haufroid V, Mourad M, Van Kerckhove V, et al. The effect of CYP3A5 and MDR1 (ABCB1) polymorphisms on cyclosporine and tacrolimus dose requirements and trough blood levels in stable renal transplant patients. *Pharmacogenetics.* 2004;14(3):147–154.

11. Anglicheau D, Thervet E, Etienne I, et al. CYP3A5 and MDR1 genetic polymorphisms and cyclosporine pharmacokinetics after renal transplantation. *Clin Pharmacol Ther.* 2004;75(5):422–433.

12. Podder H, Stepkowski SM, Napoli K, Kahan BD. Pharmacokinetic interactions between sirolimus and cyclosporine exacerbate renal dysfunction. *Transplant Proc.* 2001;33(1–2):1086.

13. Joy MS, Hogan SL, Thompson BD, Finn WF, Nickeleit V. Cytochrome P450 3A5 expression in the kidneys of patients with calcineurin inhibitor nephrotoxicity. *Nephrol Dial Transplant.* 2007;22(7):1963–1968.

14. Joy MS, Nickeleit V, Hogan SL, Thompson BD, Finn WF. Calcineurin inhibitor-induced nephrotoxicity and renal expression of P-glycoprotein. *Pharmacotherapy.* 2005;25(6):779–789.

15. Fukudo M, Yano I, Yoshimura A, et al. Impact of MDR1 and CYP3A5 on the oral clearance of tacrolimus and tacrolimus-related renal dysfunction in adult living-donor liver transplant patients. *Pharmacogenet Genomics.* 2008;18(5):413–423.

16. de Denus S, Zakrzewski M, Barhdadi A, et al. Association between renal function and CYP3A5 genotype in heart transplant recipients treated with calcineurin inhibitors. *J Heart Lung Transplant.* 2011;30(3):326–331.

17. Kuypers DR, de Jonge H, Naesens M, et al. CYP3A5 and CYP3A4 but not MDR1 single-nucleotide polymorphisms determine long-term tacrolimus disposition and drug-related nephrotoxicity in renal recipients. *Clin Pharmacol Ther.* 2007;82(6):711–725.

18. Kuypers DR, Naesens M, de Jonge H, et al. Tacrolimus dose requirements and CYP3A5 genotype and the development of calcineurin inhibitor-associated nephrotoxicity in renal allograft recipients. *Ther Drug Monit.* 2010;32(4):394–404.

19. Hauser IA, Schaeffeler E, Gauer S, et al. ABCB1 genotype of the donor but not of the recipient is a major risk factor for cyclosporine-related nephrotoxicity after renal transplantation. *J Am Soc Nephrol.* 2005;16(5):1501–1511.

20. Hawwa AF, McKiernan PJ, Shields M, et al. Influence of ABCB1 polymorphisms and haplotypes on tacrolimus nephrotoxicity and dosage requirements in children with liver transplant. *Br J Clin Pharmacol.* 2009;68(3):413–421.

21. Hebert MF, Dowling AL, Gierwatowski C, et al. Association between ABCB1 (multidrug resistance transporter) genotype and post-liver transplantation renal dysfunction in patients receiving calcineurin inhibitors. *Pharmacogenetics.* 2003;13(11):661–674.

22. Taegtmeyer AB, Breen JB, Smith J, et al. ATP-binding cassette subfamily B member 1 polymorphisms do not determine cyclosporin exposure, acute rejection or nephrotoxicity after heart transplantation. *Transplantation.* 2010;89(1):75–82.

23. Bai JP, Lesko LJ, Burckart GJ. Understanding the genetic basis for adverse drug effects: the calcineurin inhibitors. *Pharmacotherapy.* 2010;30(2):195–209.

24. Cho JH, Huh S, Kwon TG, et al. Association of C-509T and T869C polymorphisms of transforming growth factor-beta1 gene with chronic allograft nephropathy and graft survival in Korean renal transplant recipients. *Transplant Proc.* 2008;40(7):2355–2360.

25. Gallon L, Akalin E, Lynch P, et al. ACE gene D/D genotype as a risk factor for chronic nephrotoxicity from calcineurin inhibitors in liver transplant recipients. *Transplantation.* 2006;81(3):463–468.

26. Grenda R, Prokurat S, Ciechanowicz A, Piatosa B, Kalicinski P. Evaluation of the genetic background of standard-immunosuppressant-related toxicity in a cohort of 200 paediatric renal allograft recipients—a retrospective study. *Ann Transplant.* 2009;14(3):18–24.

27. Klawitter J, Kushner E, Jonscher K, et al. Association of immunosuppressant-induced protein changes in the rat kidney with changes in urine metabolite patterns: a proteo-metabonomic study. *J Proteome Res.* 2010;9(2):865–875.

28. Shord SS, Thompson DM, Krempl GA, Hanigan MH. Effect of concurrent medications on cisplatin-induced nephrotoxicity in patients with head and neck cancer. *Anticancer Drugs.* 2006;17(2):207–215.

29. Arany I, Safirstein RL. Cisplatin nephrotoxicity. *Semin Nephrol.* 2003;23(5):460–464.

30. Daugaard G, Abildgaard U. Cisplatin nephrotoxicity. A review. *Cancer Chemother Pharmacol.* 1989;25(1):1–9.

31. Aleksunes LM, Augustine LM, Scheffer GL, Cherrington NJ, Manautou JE. Renal xenobiotic transporters are differentially expressed in mice following cisplatin treatment. *Toxicology.* 2008;250(2–3):82–88.

32. Filipski KK, Mathijssen RH, Mikkelsen TS, Schinkel AH, Sparreboom A. Contribution of organic cation transporter 2 (OCT2) to cisplatin-induced nephrotoxicity. *Clin Pharmacol Ther.* 2009;86(4):396–402.

33. Nakamura T, Yonezawa A, Hashimoto S, Katsura T, Inui K. Disruption of multidrug and toxin extrusion MATE1 potentiates cisplatin-induced nephrotoxicity. *Biochem Pharmacol.* 2010;80(11):1762–1767.

34. Khrunin AV, Moisseev A, Gorbunova V, Limborska S. Genetic polymorphisms and the efficacy and toxicity of cisplatin-based chemotherapy in ovarian cancer patients. *Pharmacogenomics J.* 2010;10(1):54–61.

35. Booton R, Ward T, Heighway J, et al. Glutathione-S-transferase P1 isoenzyme polymorphisms, platinum-based chemotherapy, and non-small cell lung cancer. *J Thorac Oncol.* 2006;1(7):679–683.

36. Sun N, Sun X, Chen B, et al. MRP2 and GSTP1 polymorphisms and chemotherapy response in advanced non-small cell lung cancer. *Cancer Chemother Pharmacol.* 2010;65(3):437–446.

37. Shukla SJ, Duan S, Badner JA, Wu X, Dolan ME. Susceptibility loci involved in cisplatin-induced cytotoxicity and apoptosis. *Pharmacogenet Genomics.* 2008;18(3):253–262.

38. National Kidney Foundation. K/DOQI clinical practice guidelines for chronic kidney disease: evaluation, classification, and stratification. *Am J Kidney Dis.* 2002;39(2 suppl 2):S1–S246.

39. Cockcroft DW, Gault MH. Prediction of creatinine clearance from serum creatinine. *Nephron.* 1976;16(1):31–41.

40. Levey AS, Coresh J, Greene T, et al. Expressing the Modification of Diet in Renal Disease Study equation for estimating glomerular filtration rate with standardized serum creatinine values. *Clin Chem.* 2007;53(4):766–772.

41. Dieterle F, Marrer E, Suzuki E, et al. Monitoring kidney safety in drug development: emerging technologies and their implications. *Curr Opin Drug Discov Devel.* 2008;11(1):60–71.

42. Bakris GL. Slowing nephropathy progression: focus on proteinuria reduction. *Clin J Am Soc Nephrol.* 2008;3(suppl 1):S3–S10.

43. Sarnak MJ, Levey AS, Schoolwerth AC, et al. Kidney disease as a risk factor for development of cardiovascular disease: a statement from the American Heart Association Councils on Kidney in Cardiovascular Disease, High Blood Pressure Research, Clinical Cardiology, and Epidemiology and Prevention. *Circulation.* 2003;108(17):2154–2169.

44. Go AS, Chertow GM, Fan D, McCulloch CE, Hsu CY. Chronic kidney disease and the risks of death, cardiovascular events, and hospitalization. *N Engl J Med.* 2004;351(13):1296–1305.

45. Jager A, van Hinsbergh VW, Kostense PJ, et al. C-reactive protein and soluble vascular cell adhesion molecule-1 are associated with elevated urinary albumin excretion but do not explain its link with cardiovascular risk. *Arterioscler Thromb Vasc Biol.* 2002;22(4):593–598.

46. Kshirsagar AV, Bomback AS, Bang H, et al. Association of C-reactive protein and microalbuminuria (from the National Health and Nutrition Examination Surveys, 1999 to 2004). *Am J Cardiol.* 2008;101(3):401–406.

47. Stehouwer CD, Gall MA, Twisk JW, et al. Increased urinary albumin excretion, endothelial dysfunction, and chronic low-grade inflammation in type 2 diabetes: progressive, interrelated, and independently associated with risk of death. *Diabetes.* 2002;51(4):1157–1165.

48. Ned RM, Yesupriya A, Imperatore G, et al. Inflammation gene variants and susceptibility to albuminuria in the U.S. population: analysis in the Third National Health and Nutrition Examination Survey (NHANES III), 1991–1994. *BMC Med Genet.* 2010;11:155.

49. Boger CA, Chen MH, Tin A, et al. CUBN is a gene locus for albuminuria. *J Am Soc Nephrol.* 2011;22(3):555–570.

50. Christensen EI, Verroust PJ, Nielsen R. Receptor-mediated endocytosis in renal proximal tubule. *Pflugers Arch.* 2009;458(6):1039–1048.

51. Amsellem S, Gburek J, Hamard G, et al. Cubilin is essential for albumin reabsorption in the renal proximal tubule. *J Am Soc Nephrol.* 2010;21(11):1859–1867.

52. Birn H, Christensen EI. Renal albumin absorption in physiology and pathology. *Kidney Int.* 2006;69(3):440–449.

53. Boger CA, Heid IM. Chronic kidney disease: novel insights from genome-wide association studies. *Kidney Blood Press Res.* 2011;34(4):225–234.

54. O'Toole JF, Sedor JR. Are cubilin (CUBN) variants at the heart of urinary albumin excretion? *J Am Soc Nephrol.* 2011;22(3):404–406.

55. Freedman BI, Hicks PJ, Bostrom MA, et al. Polymorphisms in the non-muscle myosin heavy chain 9 gene (MYH9) are strongly associated with end-stage renal disease historically attributed to hypertension in African Americans. *Kidney Int.* 2009;75(7):736–745.

56. Freedman BI, Kopp JB, Winkler CA, et al. Polymorphisms in the nonmuscle myosin heavy chain 9 gene (MYH9) are associated with albuminuria in hypertensive African Americans: the HyperGEN study. *Am J Nephrol.* 2009;29(6):626–632.

57. Kopp JB, Smith MW, Nelson GW, et al. MYH9 is a major-effect risk gene for focal segmental glomerulosclerosis. *Nat Genet.* 2008;40(10):1175–1184.

58. Kao WH, Klag MJ, Meoni LA, et al. MYH9 is associated with non-diabetic end-stage renal disease in African Americans. *Nat Genet.* 2008;40(10):1185–1192.

59. Johnstone DB, Zhang J, George B, et al. Podocyte-specific deletion of Myh9 encoding nonmuscle myosin heavy chain 2A predisposes mice to glomerulopathy. *Mol Cell Biol.* 2011;31(10):2162–2170.

60. Rigat B, Hubert C, Alhenc-Gelas F, et al. An insertion/deletion polymorphism in the angiotensin I-converting enzyme gene accounting for half the variance of serum enzyme levels. *J Clin Invest.* 1990;86(4):1343–1346.

61. Scharplatz M, Puhan MA, Steurer J, Perna A, Bachmann LM. Does the angiotensin-converting enzyme (ACE) gene insertion/deletion polymorphism modify the response to ACE inhibitor therapy?—A systematic review. *Curr Control Trials Cardiovasc Med.* 2005;6:16.

62. Penno G, Chaturvedi N, Talmud PJ, et al. Effect of angiotensin-converting enzyme (ACE) gene polymorphism on progression of renal disease and the influence of ACE inhibition in IDDM patients: findings from the EUCLID Randomized Controlled Trial. EURODIAB Controlled Trial of Lisinopril in IDDM. *Diabetes.* 1998;47(9):1507–1511.

63. Perna A, Ruggenenti P, Testa A, et al. ACE genotype and ACE inhibitors induced renoprotection in chronic proteinuric nephropathies1. *Kidney Int.* 2000;57(1):274–281.

64. Boright AP, Paterson AD, Mirea L, et al. Genetic variation at the ACE gene is associated with persistent microalbuminuria and severe nephropathy in type 1 diabetes: the DCCT/EDIC Genetics Study. *Diabetes.* 2005;54(4):1238–1244.

65. Tien KJ, Hsiao JY, Hsu SC, et al. Gender-dependent effect of ACE I/D and AGT M235T polymorphisms on the progression of urinary albumin excretion in Taiwanese with type 2 diabetes. *Am J Nephrol.* 2009;29(4):299–308.

66. Nonoguchi H, Nakayama Y, Shiigai T, et al. Low-responders to angiotensin II receptor blockers and genetic polymorphism in angiotensin-converting enzyme. *Clin Nephrol.* 2007;68(4):209–215.

67. Ng DP, Tai BC, Koh D, Tan KW, Chia KS. Angiotensin-I converting enzyme insertion/deletion polymorphism and its association with diabetic nephropathy: a meta-analysis of studies reported between 1994 and 2004 and comprising 14,727 subjects. *Diabetologia.* 2005;48(5):1008–1016.

68. Schena FP, D'Altri C, Cerullo G, Manno C, Gesualdo L. ACE gene polymorphism and IgA nephropathy: an ethnically homogeneous study and a meta-analysis. *Kidney Int.* 2001;60(2):732–740.

69. Pereira TV, Nunes AC, Rudnicki M, et al. Influence of ACE I/D gene polymorphism in the progression of renal failure in autosomal dominant polycystic kidney disease: a meta-analysis. *Nephrol Dial Transplant.* 2006;21(11):3155–3163.

70. Gallego PH, Shephard N, Bulsara MK, et al. Angiotensinogen gene T235 variant: a marker for the development of persistent microalbuminuria in children and adolescents with type 1 diabetes mellitus. *J Diabetes Complications.* 2008;22(3):191–198.

71. Thameem F, Voruganti VS, He X, et al. Genetic variants in the renin–angiotensin system genes are associated with cardiovascular-renal-related risk factors in Mexican Americans. *Hum Genet.* 2008;124(5):557–559.

72. Lee YJ, Jang HR, Kim SG, et al. Renoprotective efficacy of valsartan in chronic non-diabetic proteinuric nephropathies with renin–angiotensin system gene polymorphisms. *Nephrology (Carlton).* 2011;16(5):502–510.

73. Yoon HJ, Chin HJ, Na KY, et al. Association of angiotensin II type 2 receptor gene A1818T polymorphism with progression of immunoglobulin A nephropathy in Korean patients. *J Korean Med Sci.* 2009;24(suppl):S38–S43.

74. Fabris B, Bortoletto M, Candido R, et al. Genetic polymorphisms of the renin–angiotensin–aldosterone system and renal insufficiency in essential hypertension. *J Hypertens.* 2005;23(2):309–316.

75. Joy MS, Dornbrook-Lavender K, Blaisdell J, et al. CYP2C9 genotype and pharmacodynamic responses to losartan in patients with primary and secondary kidney diseases. *Eur J Clin Pharmacol.* 2009;65(9):947–953.

76. Lajer M, Tarnow L, Andersen S, Parving HH. CYP2C9 variant modifies blood pressure-lowering response to losartan in type 1 diabetic patients with nephropathy. *Diabet Med.* 2007;24(3):323–325.

77. Couser WG, Salant DJ. In situ immune complex formation and glomerular injury. *Kidney Int.* 1980;17(1):1–13.

78. Couser WG, Steinmuller DR, Stilmant MM, Salant DJ, Lowenstein LM. Experimental glomerulonephritis in the isolated perfused rat kidney. *J Clin Invest.* 1978;62(6):1275–1287.

79. Beck LH Jr, Bonegio RG, Lambeau G, et al. M-type phospholipase A_2 receptor as target antigen in idiopathic membranous nephropathy. *N Engl J Med.* 2009;361(1):11–21.

80. Kim S, Chin HJ, Na KY, et al. Single nucleotide polymorphisms in the phospholipase A_2 receptor gene are associated with genetic susceptibility to idiopathic membranous nephropathy. *Nephron Clin Pract.* 2011;117(3):c253–c258.

81. Lo WY, Chen SY, Wang HJ, et al. Association between genetic polymorphisms of the NPHS1 gene and membranous glomerulonephritis in the Taiwanese population. *Clin Chim Acta.* 2010;411(9–10):714–718.

82. Bantis C, Heering PJ, Aker S, et al. Tumor necrosis factor-alpha gene G-308A polymorphism is a risk factor for the development of membranous glomerulonephritis. *Am J Nephrol.* 2006;26(1):12–15.

83. Patrakka J, Kestila M, Wartiovaara J, et al. Congenital nephrotic syndrome (NPHS1): features resulting from different mutations in Finnish patients. *Kidney Int.* 2000;58(3):972–980.

84. Saleem MA, Ni L, Witherden I, et al. Co-localization of nephrin, podocin, and the actin cytoskeleton: evidence for a role in podocyte foot process formation. *Am J Pathol.* 2002;161(4):1459–1466.

85. Beltcheva O, Martin P, Lenkkeri U, Tryggvason K. Mutation spectrum in the nephrin gene (NPHS1) in congenital nephrotic syndrome. *Hum Mutat.* 2001;17(5):368–373.

86. Koziell A, Grech V, Hussain S, et al. Genotype/phenotype correlations of NPHS1 and NPHS2 mutations in nephrotic syndrome advocate a functional inter-relationship in glomerular filtration. *Hum Mol Genet.* 2002;11(4):379–388.

87. Franceschini N, North KE, Kopp JB, McKenzie L, Winkler C. NPHS2 gene, nephrotic syndrome and focal segmental glomerulosclerosis: a HuGE review. *Genet Med.* 2006;8(2):63–75.

88. Zhu L, Yu L, Wang CD, et al. Genetic effect of the NPHS2 gene variants on proteinuria in minimal change disease and immunoglobulin A nephropathy. *Nephrology (Carlton).* 2009;14(8):728–734.

89. Bournazos S, Woof JM, Hart SP, Dransfield I. Functional and clinical consequences of Fc receptor polymorphic and copy number variants. *Clin Exp Immunol.* 2009;157(2):244–254.

90. Wu J, Ji C, Xie F, et al. FcalphaRI (CD89) alleles determine the proinflammatory potential of serum IgA. *J Immunol.* 2007;178(6):3973–3982.

91. Norsworthy P, Theodoridis E, Botto M, et al. Overrepresentation of the Fcgamma receptor type IIA R131/R131 genotype in caucasoid systemic lupus erythematosus patients with autoantibodies to C1q and glomerulonephritis. *Arthritis Rheum.* 1999;42(9):1828–1832.

92. Jonsen A, Gunnarsson I, Gullstrand B, et al. Association between SLE nephritis and polymorphic variants of the CRP and FcgammaRIIIa genes. *Rheumatology (Oxford).* 2007;46(9):1417–1421.

93. Tanaka Y, Suzuki Y, Tsuge T, et al. FcgammaRIIa-131R allele and FcgammaRIIIa-176V/V genotype are risk factors for progression of IgA nephropathy. *Nephrol Dial Transplant.* 2005;20(11):2439–2445.

94. Bazilio AP, Viana VS, Toledo R, et al. Fc gamma RIIa polymorphism: a susceptibility factor for immune complex-mediated lupus nephritis in Brazilian patients. *Nephrol Dial Transplant.* 2004;19(6):1427–1431.

95. Salmon JE, Millard S, Schachter LA, et al. Fc gamma RIIA alleles are heritable risk factors for lupus nephritis in African Americans. *J Clin Invest.* 1996;97(5):1348–1354.

96. Duits AJ, Bootsma H, Derksen RH, et al. Skewed distribution of IgG Fc receptor IIa (CD32) polymorphism is associated with renal disease in systemic lupus erythematosus patients. *Arthritis Rheum.* 1995;38(12):1832–1836.

97. Li LH, Yuan H, Pan HF, et al. Role of the Fcgamma receptor IIIA-V/F158 polymorphism in susceptibility to systemic lupus erythematosus and lupus nephritis: a meta-analysis. *Scand J Rheumatol.* 2010;39(2):148–154.

98. Yuan H, Ni JD, Pan HF, et al. Lack of association of FcgammaRIIIb polymorphisms with systemic lupus erythematosus: a meta-analysis. *Rheumatol Int.* 2011;31(8):1017–1021.

99. Salmon JE, Edberg JC, Kimberly RP. Fc gamma receptor III on human neutrophils. Allelic variants have functionally distinct capacities. *J Clin Invest.* 1990;85(4):1287–1295.

100. Yuan H, Pan HF, Li LH, et al. Meta analysis on the association between FcgammaRIIa-R/H131 polymorphisms and systemic lupus erythematosus. *Mol Biol Rep.* 2009;36(5):1053–1058.

101. Gelmetti AP, Freitas AC, Woronik V, et al. Polymorphism of the FcgammaRIIalpha IgG receptor in patients with lupus nephritis and glomerulopathy. *J Rheumatol.* 2006;33(3):523–530.

102. Lee YH, Ji JD, Song GG. Fcgamma receptor IIB and IIIB polymorphisms and susceptibility to systemic lupus erythematosus and lupus nephritis: a meta-analysis. *Lupus.* 2009;18(8):727–734.

103. Namjou B, Gray-McGuire C, Sestak AL, et al. Evaluation of C1q genomic region in minority racial groups of lupus. *Genes Immun.* 2009;10(5):517–524.

104. Anolik JH, Campbell D, Felgar RE, et al. The relationship of FcgammaRIIIa genotype to degree of B cell depletion by rituximab in the treatment of systemic lupus erythematosus. *Arthritis Rheum.* 2003;48(2):455–459.

105. Albert D, Dunham J, Khan S, et al. Variability in the biological response to anti-CD20 B cell depletion in systemic lupus erythaematosus. *Ann Rheum Dis.* 2008;67(12):1724–1731.

106. Nakamura A, Nakajima M, Higashi E, Yamanaka H, Yokoi T. Genetic polymorphisms in the 5′-flanking region of human UDP-glucuronosyltransferase 2B7 affect the Nrf2-dependent transcriptional regulation. *Pharmacogenet Genomics.* 2008;18(8):709–720.

107. Pergola PE, Raskin P, Toto RD, et al. Bardoxolone methyl and kidney function in CKD with type 2 diabetes. *N Engl J Med.* 2011;365(4):327–336.

108. Xing C, Sestak AL, Kelly JA, et al. Localization and replication of the systemic lupus erythematosus linkage signal at 4p16: interaction with 2p11, 12q24 and 19q13 in European Americans. *Hum Genet.* 2007;120(5):623–631.

109. Cordova EJ, Velazquez-Cruz R, Centeno F, Baca V, Orozco L. The NRF2 gene variant, −653G/A, is associated with nephritis in childhood-onset systemic lupus erythematosus. *Lupus.* 2010;19(10):1237–1242.

110. Takada K, Arefayene M, Desta Z, et al. Cytochrome P450 pharmacogenetics as a predictor of toxicity and clinical response to pulse cyclophosphamide in lupus nephritis. *Arthritis Rheum.* 2004;50(7):2202–2210.

111. Winoto J, Song H, Hines C, Nagaraja H, Rovin BH. Cytochrome P450 polymorphisms and the response of lupus nephritis to cyclophosphamide therapy. *Clin Nephrol.* 2011;75(5):451–457.

112. Joy MS, Boyette T, Hu Y, et al. Effects of uridine diphosphate glucuronosyltransferase 2B7 and 1A7 pharmacogenomics and patient clinical parameters on steady-state mycophenolic acid pharmacokinetics in glomerulonephritis. *Eur J Clin Pharmacol.* 2010;66(11):1119–1130.

113. Santer R, Kinner M, Lassen CL, et al. Molecular analysis of the SGLT2 gene in patients with renal glucosuria. *J Am Soc Nephrol.* 2003;14(11):2873–2882.

114. Magen D, Sprecher E, Zelikovic I, Skorecki K. A novel missense mutation in SLC5A2 encoding SGLT2 underlies autosomal-recessive renal glucosuria and aminoaciduria. *Kidney Int.* 2005;67(1):34–41.

115. Yu L, Lv JC, Zhou XJ, et al. Abnormal expression and dysfunction of novel SGLT2 mutations identified in familial renal glucosuria patients. *Hum Genet.* 2011;129(3):335–344.

116. Hsu CC, Kao WL, Steffes MW, et al. Genetic variation of glucose transporter-1 (GLUT1) and albuminuria in 10,278 European Americans and African Americans: a case–control study in the Atherosclerosis Risk in Communities (ARIC) study. *BMC Med Genet.* 2011;12:16.

117. Ng DP, Canani L, Araki S, et al. Minor effect of GLUT1 polymorphisms on susceptibility to diabetic nephropathy in type 1 diabetes. *Diabetes.* 2002;51(7):2264–2269.

118. Hodgkinson AD, Millward BA, Demaine AG. Polymorphisms of the glucose transporter (GLUT1) gene are associated with diabetic nephropathy. *Kidney Int.* 2001;59(3):985–989.

119. Grzeszczak W, Moczulski DK, Zychma M, et al. Role of GLUT1 gene in susceptibility to diabetic nephropathy in type 2 diabetes. *Kidney Int.* 2001;59(2):631–636.

120. Makni K, Jarraya F, Rebai M, et al. Risk genotypes and haplotypes of the GLUT1 gene for type 2 diabetic nephropathy in the Tunisian population. *Ann Hum Biol.* 2008;35(5):490–498.

121. Hodgkinson AD, Page T, Millward BA, Demaine AG. A novel polymorphism in the 5′ flanking region of the glucose transporter (GLUT1) gene is strongly associated with diabetic nephropathy in patients with type 1 diabetes mellitus. *J Diabetes Complications.* 2005;19(2):65–69.

122. McKnight AJ, Maxwell AP, Sawcer S, et al. A genome-wide DNA microsatellite association screen to identify chromosomal regions harboring candidate genes in diabetic nephropathy. *J Am Soc Nephrol.* 2006;17(3):831–836.

123. Sallinen R, Kaunisto MA, Forsblom C, et al. Association of the SLC22A1, SLC22A2, and SLC22A3 genes encoding organic cation transporters with diabetic nephropathy and hypertension. *Ann Med.* 2010;42(4):296–304.

124. Wang ZJ, Yin OQ, Tomlinson B, Chow MS. OCT2 polymorphisms and in-vivo renal functional consequence: studies with metformin and cimetidine. *Pharmacogenet Genomics.* 2008;18(7):637–645.

125. Joy MS, Gipson DS, Dike M, et al. Phase I trial of rosiglitazone in FSGS: I. Report of the FONT Study Group. *Clin J Am Soc Nephrol.* 2009;4(1):39–47.

126. Cabezas F, Lagos J, Cespedes C, et al. Megalin/LRP2 expression is induced by peroxisome proliferator-activated receptor -alpha and

-gamma: implications for PPARs' roles in renal function. *PLoS One.* 2011;6(2):e16794.

127. Setti G, Hayward A, Dessapt C, et al. Peroxisome proliferator-activated receptor-gamma agonist rosiglitazone prevents albuminuria but not glomerulosclerosis in experimental diabetes. *Am J Nephrol.* 2010;32(5):393–402.

128. Zuo Y, Yang HC, Potthoff SA, et al. Protective effects of PPARγ agonist in acute nephrotic syndrome. *Nephrol Dial Transplant.* 2012;27(1): 174–181.

129. Wolford JK, Yeatts KA, Dhanjal SK, et al. Sequence variation in PPARγ may underlie differential response to troglitazone. *Diabetes.* 2005;54(11): 3319–3325.

130. Hsieh MC, Lin KD, Tien KJ, et al. Common polymorphisms of the peroxisome proliferator-activated receptor-gamma (Pro12Ala) and peroxisome proliferator-activated receptor-gamma coactivator-1 (Gly482Ser) and the response to pioglitazone in Chinese patients with type 2 diabetes mellitus. *Metabolism.* 2010;59(8):1139–1144.

131. De Cosmo S, Motterlini N, Prudente S, et al. Impact of the PPAR-gamma2 Pro12Ala polymorphism and ACE inhibitor therapy on new-onset microalbuminuria in type 2 diabetes: evidence from BENEDICT. *Diabetes.* 2009;58(12):2920–2929.

132. McDonough CW, Palmer ND, Hicks PJ, et al. A genome-wide association study for diabetic nephropathy genes in African Americans. *Kidney Int.* 2011;79(5):563–572.

133. Mooyaart AL, Valk EJ, van Es LA, et al. Genetic associations in diabetic nephropathy: a meta-analysis. *Diabetologia.* 2011;54(3):544–553.

134. Pezzolesi MG, Poznik GD, Skupien J, et al. An intergenic region on chromosome 13q33.3 is associated with the susceptibility to kidney disease in type 1 and 2 diabetes. *Kidney Int.* 2011;80(1):105–111.

135. Igarashi P, Somlo S. Genetics and pathogenesis of polycystic kidney disease. *J Am Soc Nephrol.* 2002;13(9):2384–2398.

136. Naesens M, Steels P, Verberckmoes R, Vanrenterghem Y, Kuypers D. Bartter's and Gitelman's syndromes: from gene to clinic. *Nephron Physiol.* 2004;96(3):p65–p78.

Index

Page numbers followed by *f* or *t* indicate figures or tables, respectively.

CPSIA information can be obtained
at www.ICGtesting.com
Printed in the USA
BVHW011504040819

554824BV00020B/24/P